Spinal Imaging

AF902972

Heung Sik Kang • Joon Woo Lee
Editors

Spinal Imaging

Springer

PANMUN

Editors
Heung Sik Kang
Department of Radiology
Seoul National University College of Medicine, Seoul National University Bundang Hospital
Seongnam, Korea (Republic of)

Joon Woo Lee
Department of Radiology
Seoul National University College of Medicine, Seoul National University Bundang Hospital
Seongnam, Korea (Republic of)

Jointly published with Panmun Education Co., Ltd.

ISBN 978-981-95-1385-7 ISBN 978-981-95-1386-4 (eBook)
https://doi.org/10.1007/978-981-95-1386-4

The print edition is not for sale in the Republic of Korea. Customers from the Republic of Korea please order the print book from: Panmun Education Co., Ltd.

The original submitted manuscript has been translated into English. The translation was done using artificial intelligence. A subsequent revision was performed by the author(s) to further refine the work and to ensure that the translation is appropriate concerning content and scientific correctness. It may, however, read stylistically different from a conventional translation.

Translation from the Korean language edition: "Spinal Imaging" by Heung Sik Kang and Joon Woo Lee, © Panmun Education Co., Ltd. 2020. Published by Panmun Education Co., Ltd.. All Rights Reserved.

© Panmun Education Co., Ltd. 2025

This work is subject to copyright. All rights are solely and exclusively licensed by the Publisher, whether the whole or part of the material is concerned, specifically the rights of reprinting, reuse of illustrations, recitation, broadcasting, reproduction on microfilms or in any other physical way, and transmission or information storage and retrieval, electronic adaptation, computer software, or by similar or dissimilar methodology now known or hereafter developed.
The use of general descriptive names, registered names, trademarks, service marks, etc. in this publication does not imply, even in the absence of a specific statement, that such names are exempt from the relevant protective laws and regulations and therefore free for general use.
The publishers, the authors, and the editors are safe to assume that the advice and information in this book are believed to be true and accurate at the date of publication. Neither the publishers nor the authors or the editors give a warranty, express or implied, with respect to the material contained herein or for any errors or omissions that may have been made. The publishers remain neutral with regard to jurisdictional claims in published maps and institutional affiliations.

This Springer imprint is published by the registered company Springer Nature Singapore Pte Ltd.
The registered company address is: 152 Beach Road, #21-01/04 Gateway East, Singapore 189721, Singapore

If disposing of this product, please recycle the paper.

Preface

It has been 7 years since the publication of *Spinal Imaging*. At that time, spinal imaging was in a situation where there were no textbooks specifically dealing with the Korean language, *Spinal Imaging* has established itself as a basic textbook for understanding spinal imaging for residents and full-time teachers. As medicine has advanced at a terrifying speed, and there have been many changes in spine-related medicine, we have published a revised edition that includes the latest opinions. In this revised edition, we have added eight chapters including congenital spinal diseases, clinical diagnostic methods for patients with spinal pain, osteoporosis, bone marrow diseases, spinal alignment disorders, non-tumor spinal diseases, spinal motion therapy, brachial plexus diseases, and imaging diagnostic tips for major spinal diseases, which were not deeply covered before. Clinical diagnostic methods for patients with spinal pain, spinal alignment disorders, and spinal motion therapy were written by professors from neurosurgery, orthopedics, and rehabilitation medicine, and a wide range of clinical perspectives from various fields, not limited to the perspective of radiologists, were added. Congenital spinal diseases are described in terms of content that can be helpful in actual clinical practice, focusing on diseases that can commonly be observed in adults. Also, osteoporosis, bone marrow diseases, non-tumor spinal diseases, and brachial plexus diseases, which were not deeply covered before, are deeply covered as separate chapters, reflecting the trend that their importance is increasing day by day. The last chapter is a newly established chapter called "Imaging Diagnosis Tips for Major Spinal Diseases", where the author has described in an easy-to-understand manner with cases, things to consider when interpreting spinal images, the order of interpretation, and lesions that are easy to miss, which the author has been orally telling residents and full-time teachers for years. Also, the previous ten chapters have been extensively revised to include the latest opinions, and they have been organized so that there is no shortage as a completely revised edition. This book, as a textbook in Korean, tried to mark medical terms in Korean as much as possible and mark English as needed, and used the original words as they are to reduce confusion for terms that are commonly used in actual clinical practice, just like the previous book. I would like to express my deep gratitude to the 19 authors who participated in the writing. Also, I would like to express my deep gratitude to the employees, including the representative of Panmun Education, who participated in the publication of this revised edition and made a good book. I sincerely hope that the revised edition of *Spinal Imaging* will be helpful for all doctors dealing with spinal diseases to understand spinal imaging.

Seongnam, Korea (Republic of)

Heung Sik Kang
Joon Woo Lee

Contents

Contributors

Jee Won Chai Department of Radiology, Seoul National University College of Medicine, Seoul, Republic of Korea

Suk-joo Hong Department of Radiology, Korea University College of Medicine, Seoul, Republic of Korea

Joon-Yong Jung Department of Radiology, Seoul St. Mary's Hospital, College of Medicine, The Catholic University of Korea, Seoul, Republic of Korea

Heung Sik Kang Department of Radiology, Seoul National University College of Medicine, Seoul National University Bundang Hospital, Seongnam, Korea (Republic of)

Ho-Joong Kim Department of Orthopedic Surgery, Seoul National University College of Medicine, Seoul, Republic of Korea

Ji Young Kim Department of Radiology, Seoul National University Bundang Hospital, Seongnam-si, Republic of Korea

Sungjun Kim Department of Radiology, Yonsei University College of Medicine, Seoul, Republic of Korea

Wan Tae Kim Department of Radiology, Veterans Health Service Medical Center, Seoul, Republic of Korea

Jong Won Kwon Department of Radiology, Dongcheon Donggang Hospital, Ulsan, Republic of Korea

Guen Young Lee Department of Radiology, Chung-Ang University College of Medicine, Seoul, Republic of Korea

In Sook Lee Department of Radiology, Pusan National University College of Medicine, Yangsan-si, Republic of Korea

Jun Ho Lee Department of Neurosurgery, Kyung Hee University College of Medicine, Seoul, Republic of Korea

Joon Woo Lee Department of Radiology, Seoul National University College of Medicine, Seoul National University Bundang Hospital, Seongnam, Korea (Republic of)

Seunghun Lee Department of Radiology, Hanyang University College of Medicine, Seoul, Republic of Korea

Eugene Lee Department of Radiology, Seoul National University Bundang Hospital, Seongnam-si, Republic of Korea

Jung Mee Park Department of Radiology, College of Medicine, The Catholic University of Korea, Seoul, Republic of Korea

Ju Seok Ryu Department of Rehabilitation Medicine, Seoul National University College of Medicine, Seoul, Republic of Korea

Kyung Nam Ryu Department of Radiology, Kyung Hee University Hospital, Seoul, Republic of Korea

Hyejin Yoo Department of Radiology, Seoul National University Hospital, Seoul, Republic of Korea

Spinal Anatomy

1

Joon-Yong Jung

Each osseous vertebra is connected at the front by the intervertebral disc and at the back by the facet joint, forming the central axis of our body, the spinal column. It consists of a total of 32–33 vertebral segments, typically 7 cervical spine, 12 thoracic spine, 5 lumbar spine, 5 sacrum, and 3–4 coccyx. These vertebral segments are arranged along the characteristic dorsolateral curvature across the entire spinal column, with the cervical and lumbar showing a convex lordotic curvature forward, and the thoracic and sacrum showing a convex kyphotic curvature backward. Inside the spinal column, a central canal is formed, through which the spinal cord surrounded by the dura mater and cerebrospinal fluid passes, and the spinal nerves and vessels connected to the spinal cord pass through the neural foramen formed between each vertebral segment.

1.1 Osseous Anatomy

Each vertebra consists largely of the anterior vertebral body and the posterior vertebral arch and bone appendage. Like other bones, the vertebra is surrounded by cortical bone and the interior is composed of trabecular bone and marrow. The vertebral arch consists of the pedicle, which connects to the vertebral body, and the posterior arch formed by the lamina. A neural foramen is formed between the pedicles of adjacent vertebral segments. The transverse process, superior articular process, and inferior articular process are each directed outward, upward, and downward at the transition point of the pedicle and lamina (Fig. 1.1). The pars interarticularis refers to the narrow part located at the transition point of the superior articular process and the inferior articular process, meaning between the upper and lower posterior joints ('pars' 5 part, 'inter' 5 between, 'articularis' 5 joint). The spinous process is formed where the two laminae meet.

1.1.1 Cervical Spine

The first cervical spine (C1), also known as the atlas, is a structure where the bony mass supporting the occipital bone on both sides is connected by the anterior and posterior vertebral arches without a vertebral body. There is a posterior facet that articulates with the odontoid process of the second cervical spine in the center of the inner side of the anterior arch. On the upper surface of the posterior arch, there is a groove formed on both sides for the vertebral artery to pass (Fig. 1.2).

The second cervical spine (C2), also known as the axis, has an odontoid process that articulates with the posterior facet of the C1 anterior arch protruding upward in the center of the vertebral body, and on both sides, there is a large facet that articulates with the lateral bony mass of C1 (Fig. 1.2).

J.-Y. Jung (✉)
Department of Radiology, Seoul St. Mary's Hospital, College of Medicine, The Catholic University of Korea, Seoul, Republic of Korea

© The Author(s), under exclusive license to Springer Nature Singapore Pte Ltd. 2025

H. S. Kang, J. W. Lee (eds.), *Spinal Imaging*, https://doi.org/10.1007/978-981-95-1386-4_1

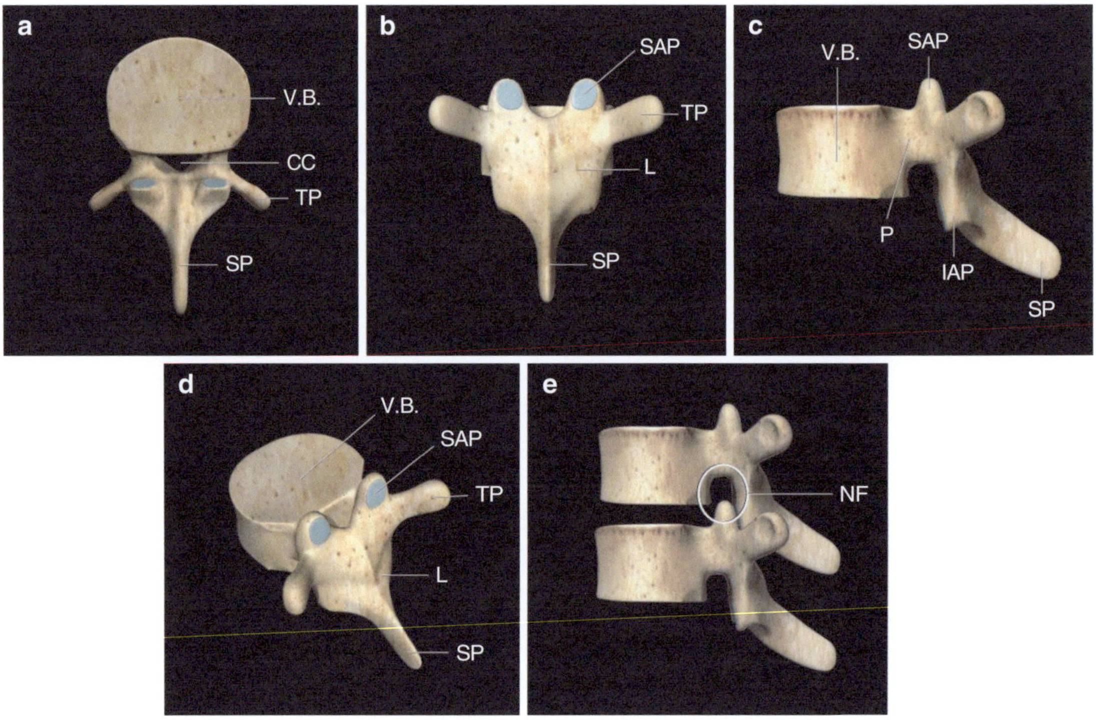

Fig. 1.1 Schematic diagram of the spine
Vertebral body (VB), Vertebral arch: pedicle (P) and lamina (L), Bone appendage: transverse process (TP), superior articular process (SAP), inferior articular process (IAP), spinous process (SP); central canal (CC), neural foramen (NF)

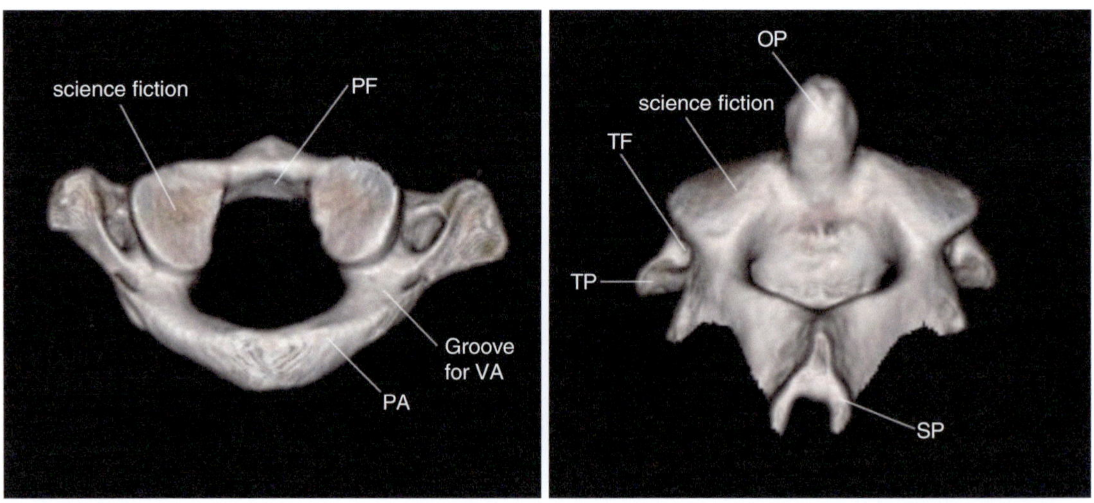

Fig. 1.2 Schematic of atlas and axis
Schematic of C1 (Atlas): posterior facet (PF), posterior arch (PA), Groove for vertebral artery (VA), superior facet (SF), Schematic of C2 (axis): odontoid process (OP), superior facet (SF), Spinous process (SP), Transverse process (TP), Transverse foramen (TF)

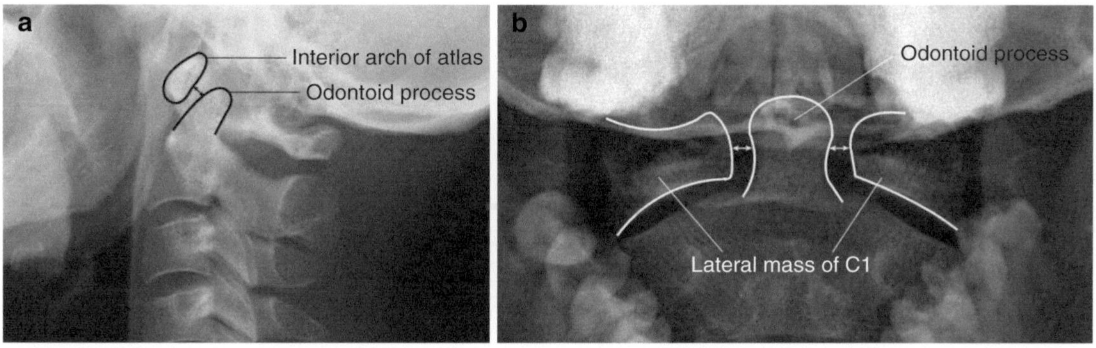

Fig. 1.3 Simple radiograph of C1–2. (**a**) Lateral view: The distance (atlantodental interval, both arrows) between the posterior facet of the C1 anterior arch and the C2 odontoid process is normally 3 mm in adults and 5 mm in children on the lateral view, (**b**) open mouth AP view: the difference in the distance (both arrows, left and right) between the bilateral lateral mass and the odontoid process is within 2 mm

The distance between the posterior facet of the C1 anterior arch and the C2 odontoid process should normally be <3 mm in adults and <5 mm in children in the lateral view, and the difference in the distance between the lateral mass and the odontoid process in the open mouth AP view should be <2 mm (Fig. 1.3).

The third and lower cervical spine increases in size as it goes down, and the left-right length becomes larger than the front-back. The upper surface of the vertebral body is concave, and the lower surface is convex. Unlike the thoracolumbar spine, the cervical spine has an uncinated processes on the posterolateral aspect of the upper surface of the vertebral body. This forms a joint by contacting the demifacet of the lower surface of the adjacent segmented vertebral body, so it is called the uncovertebral joint or joint of Luschka. This is a common site of degenerative changes in the cervical spine and forms the anterior boundary of the neural foramen, so if there is osteophyte formation, foraminal stenosis and nerve root compression symptoms can occur (Fig. 1.4).

In the cervical spine, a bone appendage is formed outside of the vertebral body, forming a relatively large bone mass compared to the vertebral body, which is called the lateral mass. In contrast, the articular pillar refers to the outer pillar formed by the superior articular process and the inferior articular process, excluding the transverse process. In the cervical spine, it is normal for the spinous process to appear bifid. In the lateral plain radiograph of the cervical spine, imaginary lines can be drawn to determine whether the alignment is abnormal, including the anterior vertebral line that follows the front boundary of the vertebral body, the posterior vertebral line that follows the back boundary of the vertebral body, the spinolaminar line that follows the transition part of the lamina and spinous process, and the posterior spinous line that follows the back boundary of the spinous process. In normal cervical spine, these lines should be smoothly connected without angles or breaks (Fig. 1.5a).

The neural foramen of the cervical spine is open to the anterolateral direction, and the neural foramen of the opposite side of the detector with the back is observed under the pedicle in the oblique view. The uncovertebral joint is observed in front of the neural foramen, and the facet joint is observed in the back. The pedicle on the side with the back appears overlapped with the vertebral body (Fig. 1.6b, c).

1.1.2 Thoracolumbar Spine

The thoracic spine looks similar to the closer side of the cervical spine and lumbar spine. Most thoracic vertebral bodies are concave in front, but the first and second are flat in front, and the third thoracic spine is slightly convex in front. The

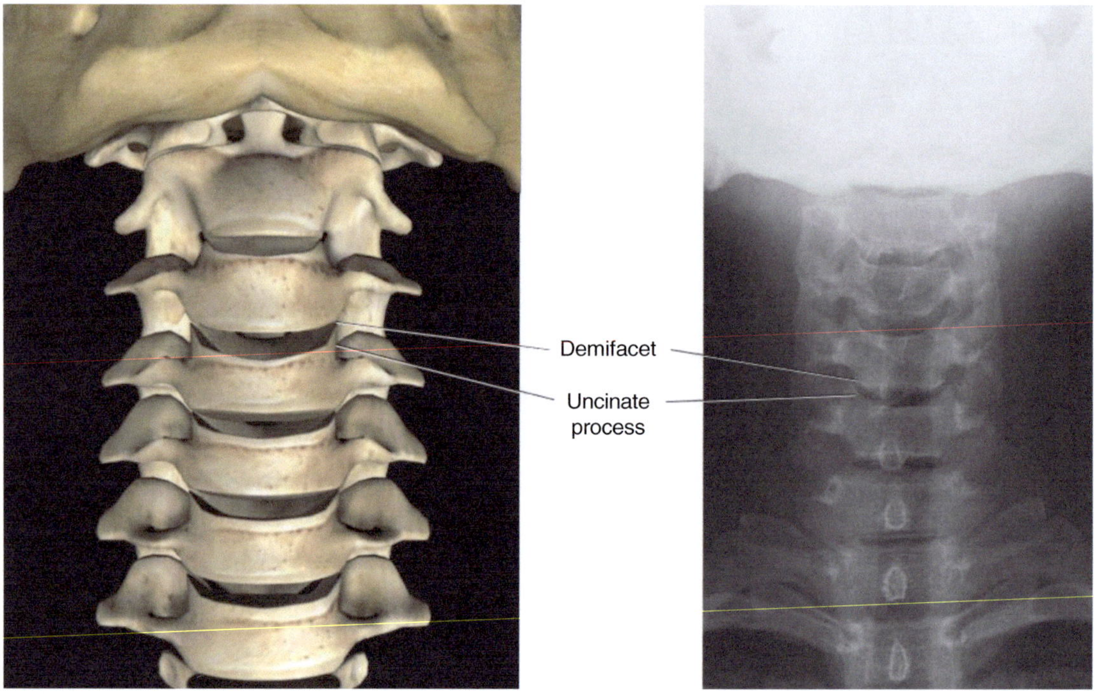

Fig. 1.4 Uncovertebral joint (Joint of Luschka) in cervical spine

vertebral body of the third thoracic vertebra is the smallest, and it gets bigger as it goes down. The pedicles of the thoracic spine, unlike the cervical or lumbar spine, run parallel to each other front and back. The pedicle also gets bigger as it goes down. The upper surface of the pedicle is convex or flat, but the lower surface is very concave and has a deep groove.

The thoracic spine forms joints with about 12 pairs of ribs and the sides of the vertebral body. The first costovertebral joint is located on the side of the first vertebral body, while the second to tenth costovertebral joints are located across two adjacent vertebral bodies. However, the 11th and 12th costovertebral joints are located on the lateral side of the corresponding vertebral body.

The lumbar spine has the largest vertebral body, and the pedicle runs slightly obliquely from the vertebral body in the posterior lateral direction. The lumbar spine also has larger superior articular processes, inferior articular processes, and spinous processes compared to the thoracic spine. The normal lumbar spine shows a convex lordotic curve anteriorly when viewed from the lateral. The neural foramen, like the thoracic spine, faces laterally. Therefore, it can be confirmed under the pedicle in a lateral plain radiograph (Fig. 1.6). The articular surface of the facet joint faces anteromedially, so in the oblique view, the facet joint on the side facing the detector appears open, and the surrounding superior, inferior articular processes and pars interarticularis can be identified. In particular, these structures show a scotty dog appearance in the oblique view (Fig. 1.7).

1.1.3 Bone Marrow

The spine is an important hematopoietic organ, with bone marrow filling between the trabecular

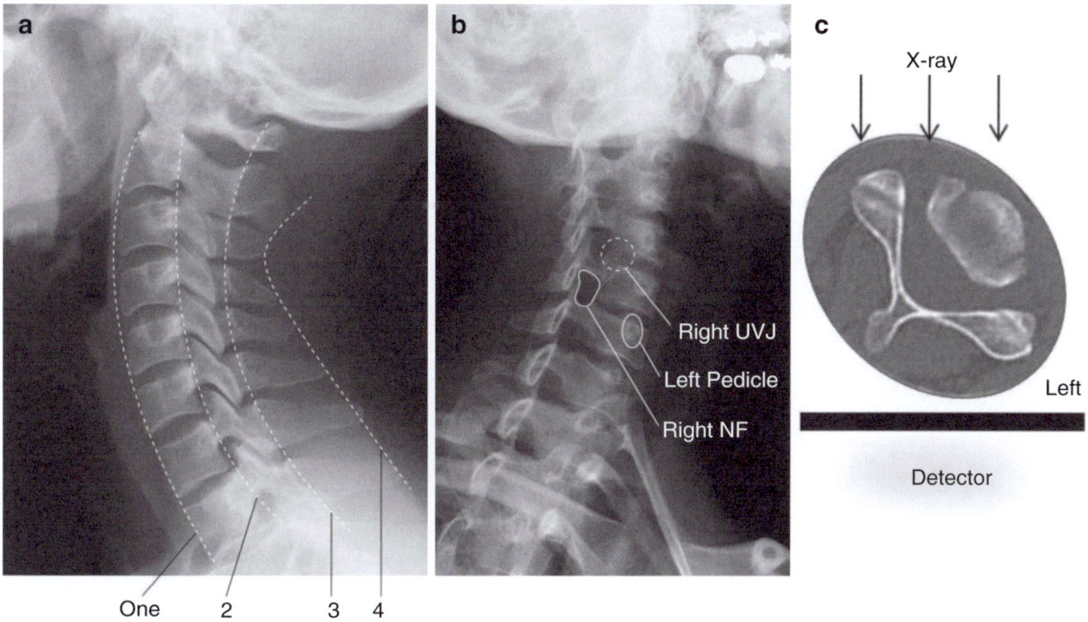

Fig. 1.5 Uncovertebral joint, neural foramen. (**a**) C-spine Lateral, 1: anterior vertebral line, 2: posterior vertebral line, 3: spinolaminar line, 4: posterior spinous line, (**b**) C-spine Left posterior oblique, UVJ (uncovertebral joint), NF (neural foramen), (**c**) direction of X-ray projection in left posterior oblique

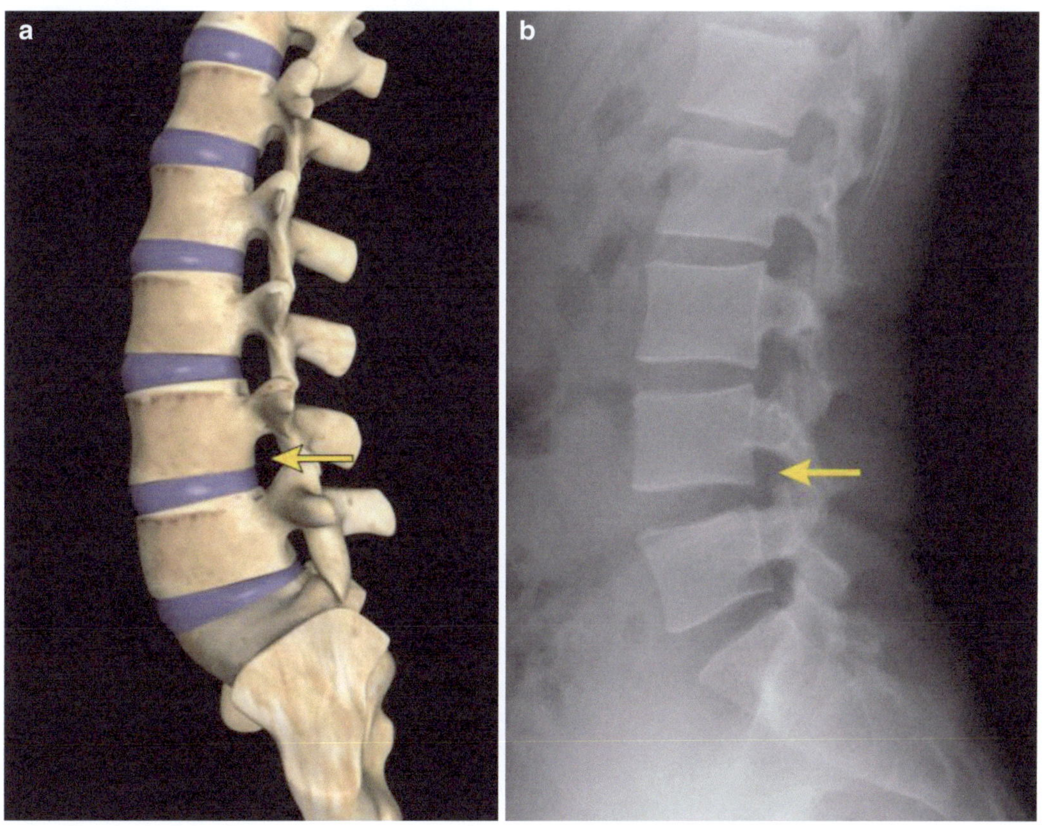

Fig. 1.6 L-spine lateral
In the L-spine, the neural foramen is oriented laterally, so it can be seen below the pedicle on the L-spine lateral view (arrow)

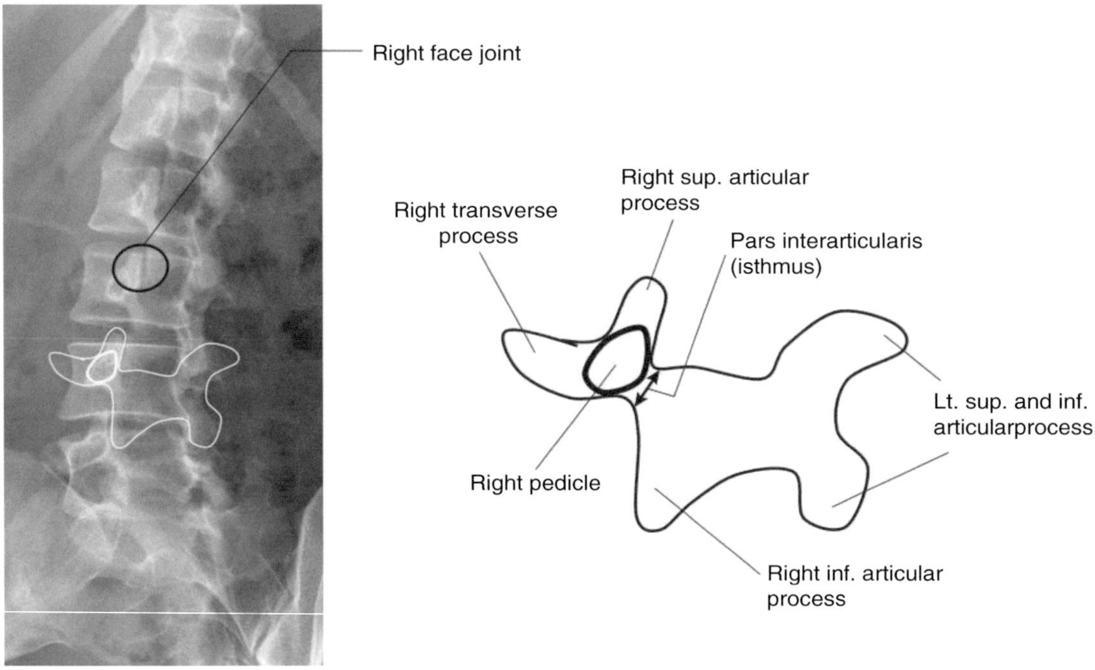

Fig. 1.7 Scotty dog appearance seen in L-spine right posterior oblique
The articular surface of the facet joint is oriented antero-medially, so in the oblique view, the facet joint on the side facing the detector appears open, and the surrounding superior, inferior articular process and pars interarticularis of the same side can be confirmed. In particular, these structures appear as a scotty dog appearance in the oblique view

bone inside the vertebral body. Bone marrow can be divided into red marrow, which is rich in hematopoietic cells, and fatty marrow, which is rich in fat cells, each showing different signals on MRI. Red marrow shows moderate signal intensity in both T1- and T2-weighted images, while fatty marrow shows high signal intensity in both T1- and T2-weighted images. Generally, it is mostly composed of red marrow in infancy, but gradually replaced with fatty marrow after adolescence (Fig. 1.8) [1].

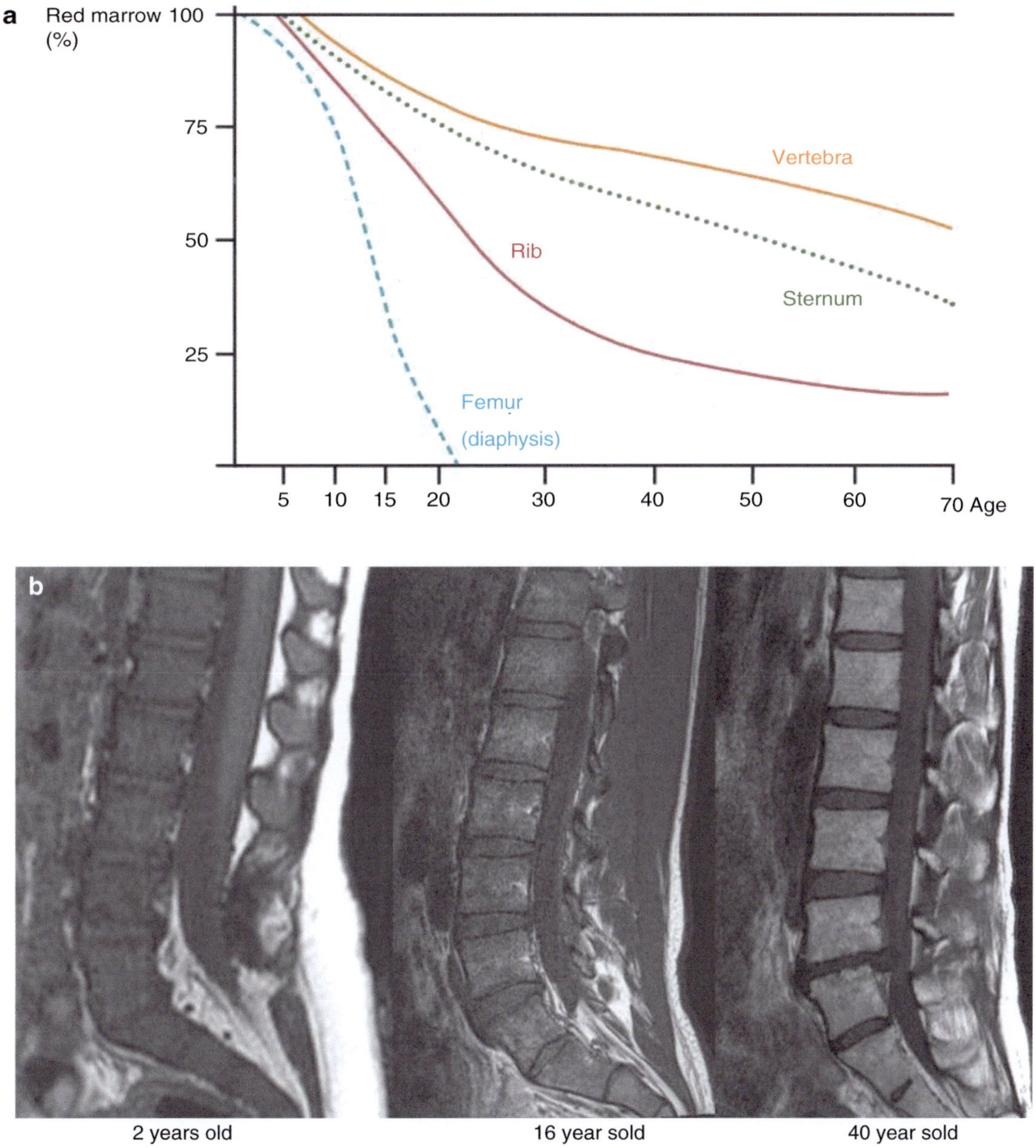

Fig. 1.8 Bone marrow graph, MR (red marrow, fatty marrow)
(**a**) The process of normal hematopoietic marrow changing to fat marrow. (**b**) Changes in bone marrow signal intensity in T1-enhanced images with age: as the proportion of fat marrow gradually increases, the signal intensity in the bone marrow gradually increases

1.2 Joints and Soft Tissues

The joints between spinal segments are divided into the discovertebral joint between the vertebral bodies in the front and the facet joint between the articular processes in the back [2]. Also, there are various muscles around the spine that are involved in the movement of the spine through these joints and the stability of the spine.

1.2.1 Discovertebral Joint and Surrounding Ligaments

1.2.1.1 Intervertebral Disk

The intervertebral disk has a gelatinous nucleus pulposus in the center, surrounded by a layered structure of annulus fibrosus (Fig. 1.9a) [3]. The nucleus pulposus, composed of water, proteoglycans, and loose collagen fibers, serves as a shock absorber. The water content decreases with age, reaching 90% after birth and dropping to 70% in the 40 s. Excluding water, 65% of the dry weight of the nucleus pulposus is proteoglycans, and 15–20% is collagen [2]. When pressure is applied, the nucleus pulposus flattens, transmitting shock to the periphery, and the annulus fibrosus blocks it. The annulus fibrosus is a structure surrounded by several layers of fibrocartilage, connected to the vertebral body by Sharpey's fibers on the outside. In the cervical spine, the annulus fibrosus at the back of the intervertebral disk is very thin.

The nucleus pulposus, which has a high water content, shows low signal intensity on MRI T1-weighted images and high signal intensity on T2-weighted images. However, as the water content decreases due to degenerative changes, it gradually changes to low signal intensity on T2-weighted images. The annulus fibrosus, due to its fibrocartilage component, shows low signal on both T1- and T2-weighted images (Fig. 1.9b) [4, 5].

1.2.1.2 Cartilaginous Endplate

The cartilaginous endplate (CEP) is a thin hyaline cartilage layer between the intervertebral disk and vertebral body, serving as a mechanical barrier and a route for nutritional transport [6]. In a normal intervertebral disk, most of the interior lacks blood vessels, so nutrients are supplied by diffusion through the CEP from the adjacent vertebral body. However, the peripheral part of the annulus fibrosus has blood vessels, so nutrients are directly supplied.

On MRI, the CEP shows low signal intensity in both T1- and T2-weighted images, indistinguishable from the adjacent cortical bone. However, by capturing ultrashort echo time MR images that receive signals from tissues with such short T2 values, the CEP and cortical bone can be distinguished [7].

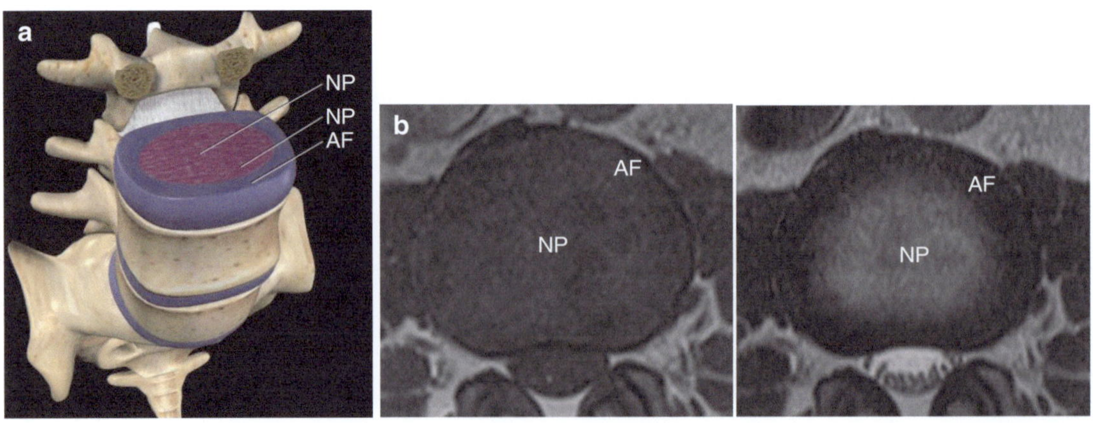

Fig. 1.9 Intervertebral disk
(**a**) NP (nucleus pulposus), AF (annulus fibrosus). (**b**) Axial T1- and T2-enhanced images of the intervertebral disk. The annulus fibrosus shows low signal in both T1- and T2-enhanced images due to its fibrocartilage component. The nucleus pulposus, which has a high water content, shows low signal intensity in MRI T1-enhanced images and high signal intensity in T2-enhanced images

1.2.1.3 Anterior and Posterior Longitudinal Ligament

The anterior longitudinal ligament (ALL) is a ligament that connects the front of the vertebral body vertically. It connects from the occipital bone to the first segment of the sacrum. The ALL is strongly attached to the front of the vertebral body and intervertebral disk. The posterior longitudinal ligament (PLL) is a ligament that connects the back of the vertebral body vertically, extending from the tectorial membrane to connect from C2 to S1. The PLL is strongly attached to the intervertebral disk, but loosely attached in the middle of the back of the vertebral body. As a result, venous plexus and epidural fat are located between the middle of the vertebral body and the PLL. The ALL and PLL appear as low signal intensity lines running anterior and posterior to the vertebral body on MRI and are not distinguishable from the cortex of the vertebral body or the periphery of the annulus fibrosus (Fig. 1.10).

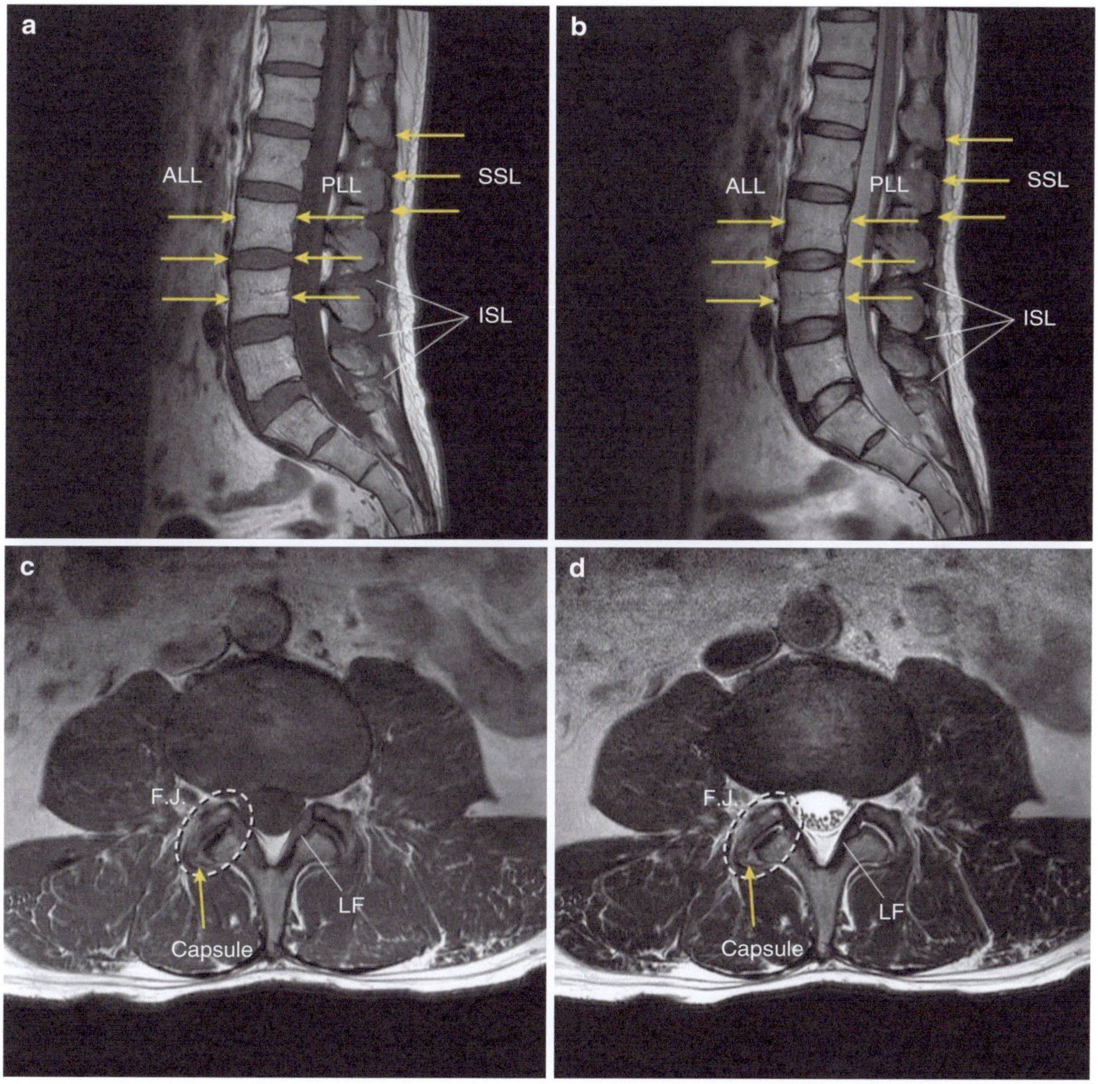

Fig. 1.10 MRI of L-spine. (**a**) Sagittal T1-enhanced image. (**b**) Sagittal T2-enhanced image. (**c**) Axial T1-enhanced image. (**d**) Axial T2-enhanced image Anterior longitudinal ligament (ALL), Posterior longitudinal ligament (PLL), Facet joint (FA), Ligament flavum (LF), Supraspinous ligament (SSL), Interspinous ligament (ISL)

1.2.2 Facet Joint and Ligaments of Posterior Element

The facet joint is a joint located on both sides of the back of the spine, formed by the superior articular process of the lower vertebra and the inferior articular process of the upper vertebra [8]. Like other joints, the facet joint is covered with hyaline cartilage and synovium, and a synovial joint is surrounded by a joint capsule, with a slight range of motion. The hyaline cartilage inside the facet joint shows high signal intensity on MRI T2-weighted images, which can be mistaken for synovial fluid, and the facet joint capsule shows low signal intensity (Fig. 1.10).

The articular surface of the facet joint shows various orientations depending on the location. The facet joint of the cervical spine forms a slightly horizontal plane forward and backward, while in the thoracic spine, it is parallel to the coronal plane, and in the lumbar spine, it is slightly oblique in the sagittal plane (Fig. 1.11). Due to this orientation of the articular surface, spondylolisthesis of the spinal segment due to degenerative arthritis of the facet joint is common in the lumbar spine. The synovial cavity of the facet joint is often not limited to the area where the articular surface is located, but extends around it, especially in cases with degenerative changes. This expansion of the synovial cavity can extend to the inside of the ligament flavum on the front side and can even connect to the synovial cavity of the opposite facet joint in severe cases.

The ligamentum flavum, also known as the yellow ligament, is located in front of the lamina, filling the interlaminar space between the lamina and connecting to the lamina of the lower segment. Laterally, it connects to the anterior capsule of the facet joint. The interspinous

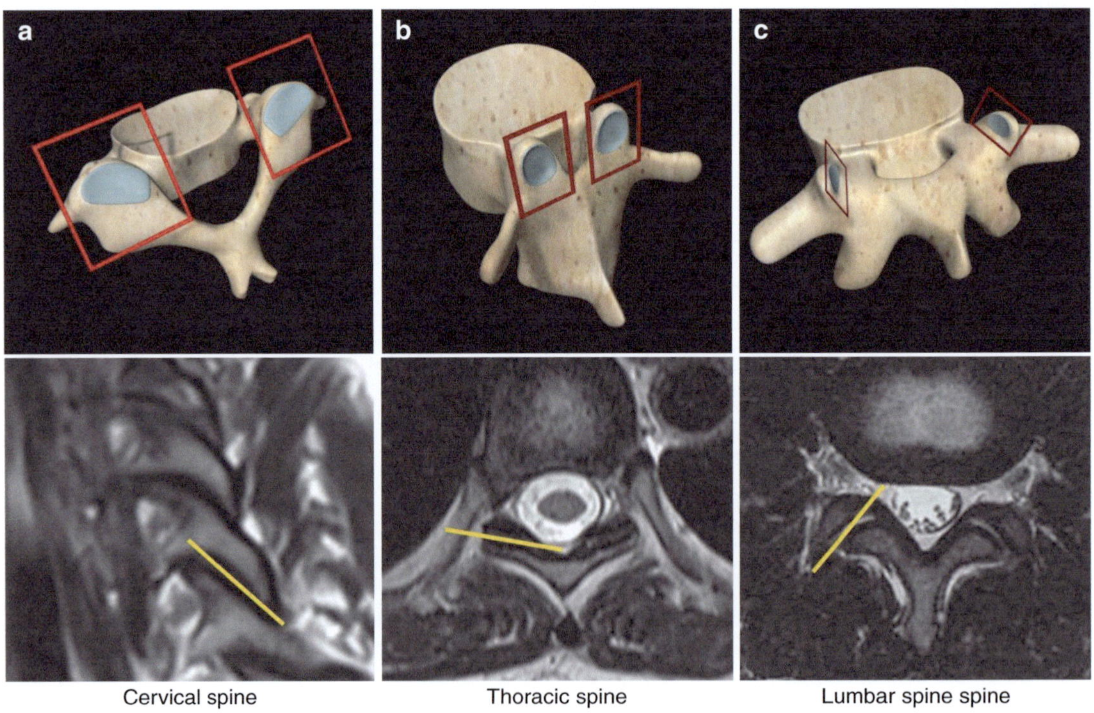

Fig. 1.11 Facet joint orientation
Facet joint orientation by area

ligament connects between the spinous processes, and the supraspinous ligament connects the tips of the spinous processes (Fig. 1.12). The ligament in the cervical spine is transformed into the nuchal ligament. The ligamentum flavum and supraspinous ligament both show low signal intensity in T1- and T2-enhanced images, but the interspinous ligament shows various signal intensities due to internal fat degeneration (Fig. 1.10).

1.2.3 Paraspinal Muscles

The muscles around the spine can be divided into the superficial group involved in shoulder movement and the deep group involved in spine extension and rotation. The superficial group includes the levator scapulae, trapezius, latissimus dorsi, etc. The deep group mainly occupies most of the soft tissue located posterolaterally to the spinal column, and when viewed in axial MRI images of the thoracic and lumbar spine, it is composed of the multifidus, longissimus, and iliocostalis muscles from the inside to the outside (Fig. 1.13). The psoas muscle and quadratus lumborum muscle are located anterolaterally to the spinal column. The cervical spine involves various muscles in the movement of the neck and head compared to the thoracolumbar spine.

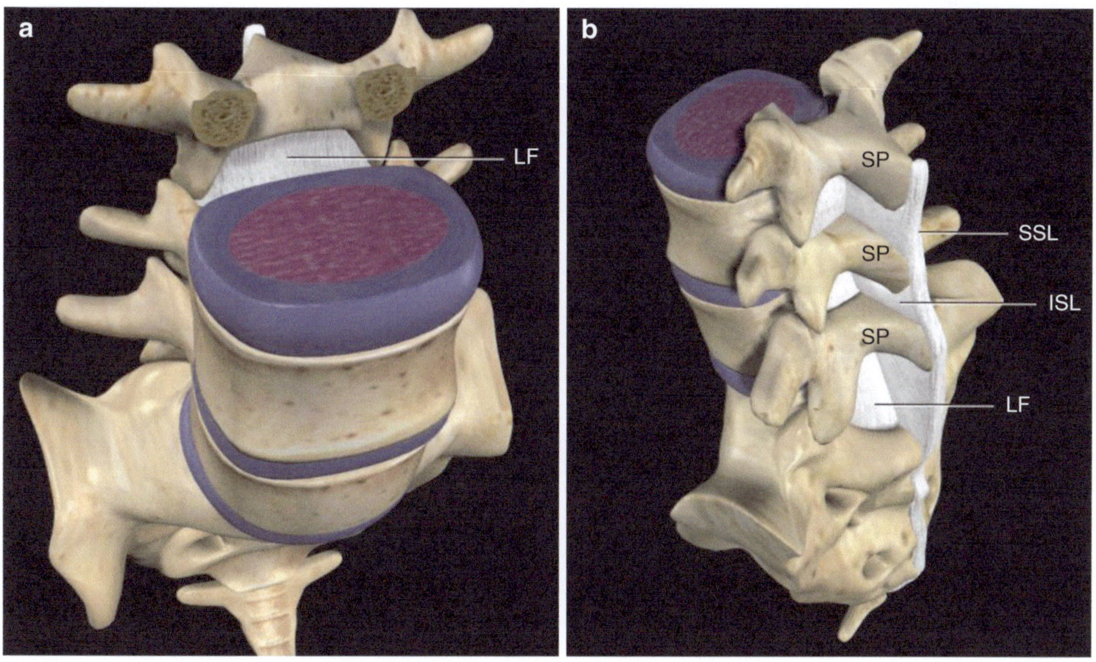

Fig. 1.12 Ligament, MRI
Ligamentum flavum (LF), Interspinous ligament (ISL), Supraspinous ligament (SSL), SP (spinous process)

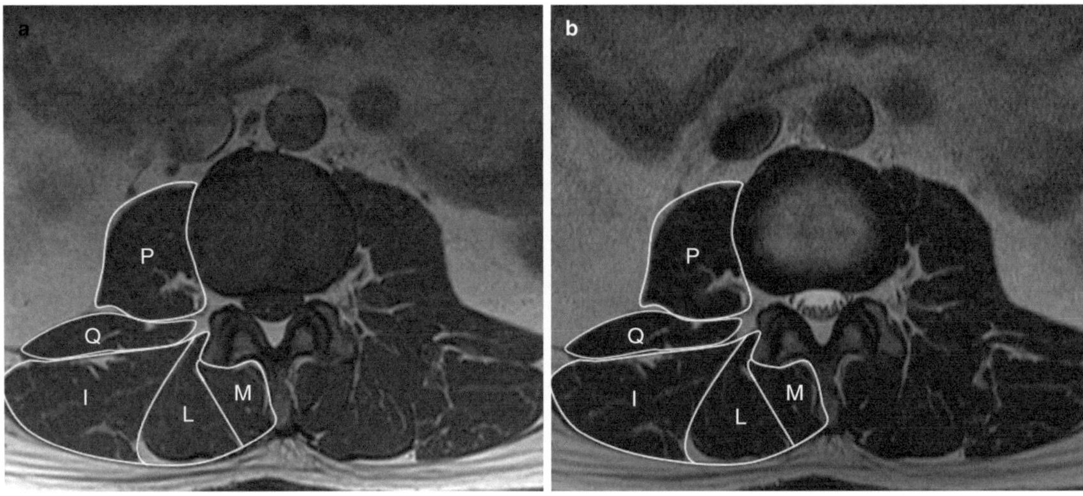

Fig. 1.13 Paraspinal muscles. A. Axial T1-enhanced image. B. Axial T2-enhanced image M (multifidus), L (Longissimus dorsalis), I (Iliocostalis lumborum), Q (quadratus lumborum), P (psoas)

1.3 Spinal Cord and Spinal Nerves

1.3.1 Spinal Cord

The spinal cord is a central nervous system located within the dura, connected downwards from the medulla oblongata. The spinal cord starts from the foramen magnum and ends at the first or second lumbar spine level [9]. The spinal cord is normally thickened at the lower cervical spine and thoracolumbar junction, these parts are called the cervical enlargement and lumbar enlargement, respectively, and are connected to the brachial plexus and lumbosacral plexus, respectively. The upper part of the spinal cord appears funnel-shaped, and this part is called the conus medullaris. Below the conus medullaris, nerve roots are observed, which are called the "cauda equina (horse's tail)" because they look like a horse's tail (Fig. 1.14). The connective tissue filament connected downwards from the tip of the conus medullaris is called the filum terminale, which pierces the dura at the S2 level and attaches to the first segment of the coccyx.

In MR images, the cerebrospinal fluid shows low signal intensity in T1-enhanced images and high signal intensity in T2-enhanced images due to its water content, and the spinal cord shows moderate signal intensity in both T1- and T2-enhanced images (Fig. 1.15). Outside the dural sac, there is epidural fat tissue, which shows high signal intensity in both T1- and T2-enhanced images, and the nerve roots that pass through this and exit through the neural foramen show the same moderate signal intensity as the spinal cord (Fig. 1.16).

1.3.2 Nerve Roots

The nerve root is a peripheral nerve system that comes out of the spinal cord and exits the spine to the left and right through the neural foramen. The ventral root, which carries motor nerves, passes in front of the neural foramen, and the dorsal root, which is responsible for sensory nerves, passes behind it, and the swollen area where the sensory nerve cells are located is called the dorsal root ganglion (Fig. 1.16) [10]. Outside the neural

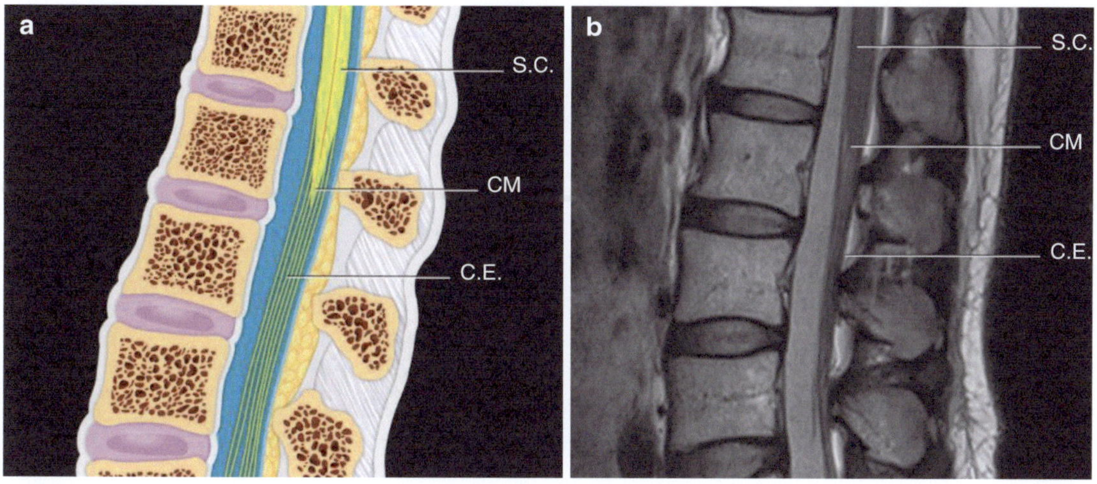

Fig. 1.14 Upper part of the spinal cord
Spinal cord (SC), Conus medullaris (CM), Cauda equina (CE)

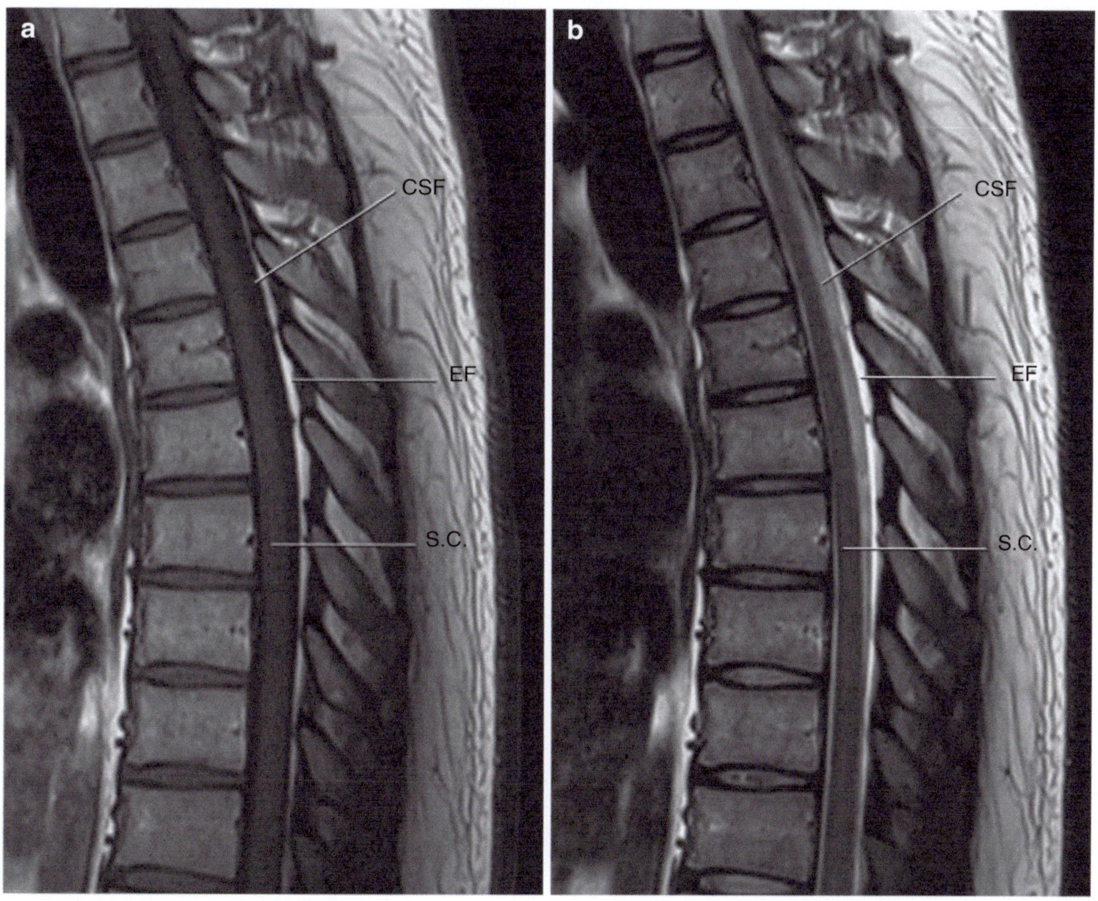

Fig. 1.15 Cerebrospinal fluid, spinal cord, and epidural fat in MRI

T1(left) and T2(right) enhanced images, Spinal cord (SC), Cerebrospinal fluid (CSF), Epidural fat (EF)

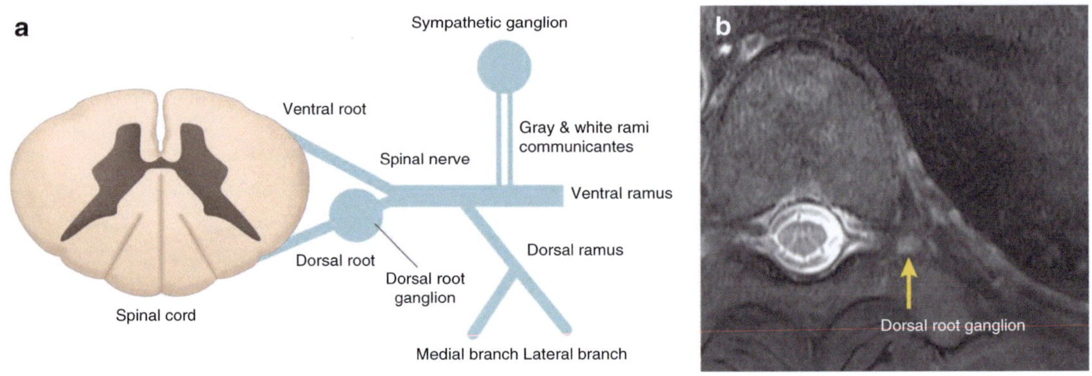

Fig. 1.16 Spinal cord and nerve root

foramen, the dorsal root and ventral root combine to form the spinal nerve, which then branches into the ventral ramus and dorsal ramus.

Knowing the level of the nerve root that exits from each neural foramen is fundamental in determining the consistency between imaging findings and symptoms such as radiculopathy. In the cervical spine, the C1 nerve root to the C7 nerve root exits through the pedicle with the same number. For example, the C6 nerve root exits through the C6. The pedicle above the C5–6 neural foramen exits. However, in the cervical spine, there is a C8 nerve root, but there are only up to C7 vertebrae, so the C8 nerve root exits through the C7–T1 neural foramen. Therefore, below the thoracic spine, the nerve root exits under the pedicle of the same number. That is, the T1 nerve root exits through the T1–2 neural foramen, and the L4 nerve root exits through the L4–5 neural foramen (Fig. 1.17). In the cervical spine or thoracic spine, the nerve root runs almost horizontally, but in the lumbar spine, the nerve root exits from the dural sac higher and runs obliquely downward in the epidural space to exit the neural foramen. For example, the L5 nerve root exits the dural sac at the L4–5 intervertebral disk level, passes through the narrow epidural space in front of the superior articular process, the lateral recess, and runs downward to exit through the L5–S1 neural foramen. Therefore, when the L4–5 intervertebral disk is escaped from the central zone or subarticular zone, it compresses the L5 nerve root that exits through the neural foramen below, the L5–S1.

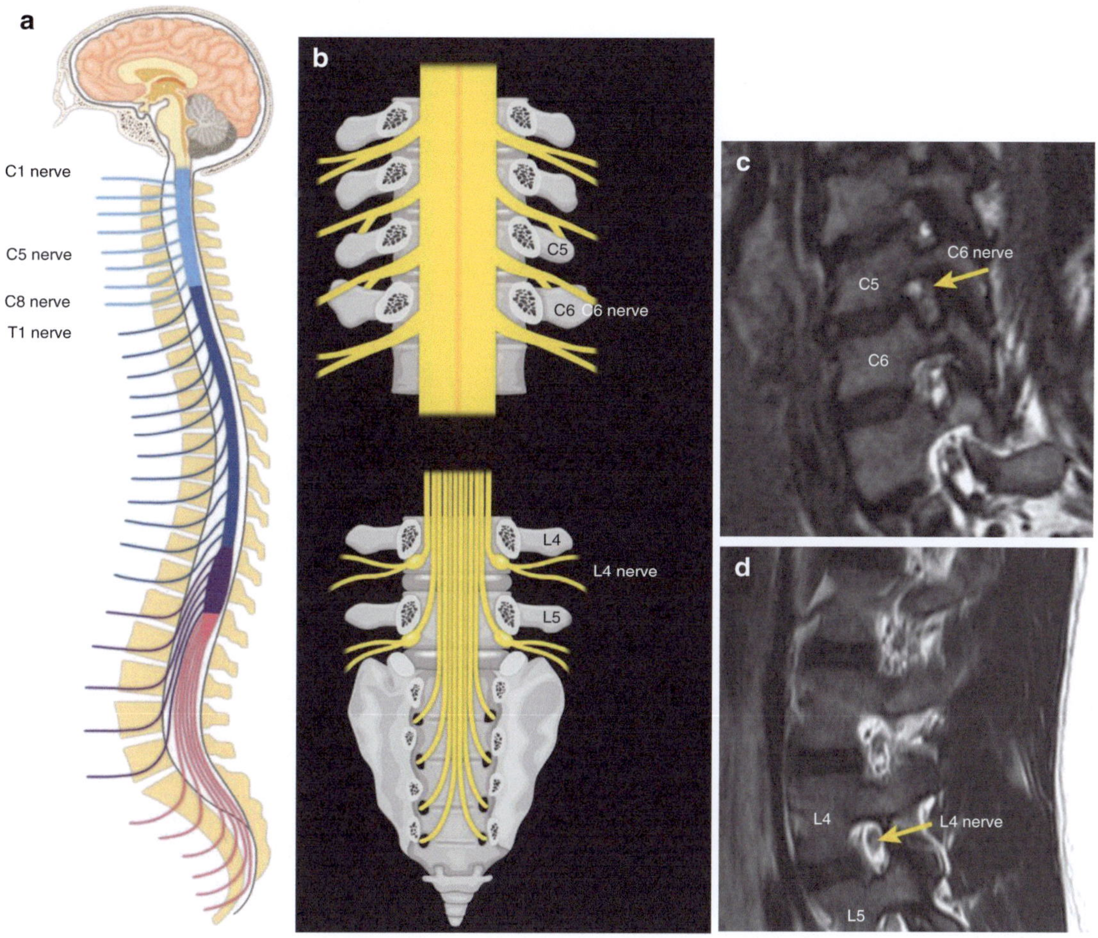

Fig. 1.17 Nerve root count

Bibliography

1. Ricci C, Cova M, Kang YS, Yang A, Rahmouni A, Scott WW Jr, et al. Normal age-related patterns of cellular and fatty bone marrow distribution in the axial skeleton: MR imaging study. Radiology. 1990;177(1):83–8.
2. Del Grande F, Maus TP, Carrino JA. Imaging the intervertebral disk: age-related changes, herniations, and radicular pain. Radiol Clin North Am. 2012;50(4):629–49.
3. Rumboldt Z. Degenerative disorders of the spine. Semin Roentgenol. 2006;41(4):327–62.
4. Castillo M, Malko JA, Hoffman JC Jr. The bright intervertebral disk: an indirect sign of abnormal spinal bone marrow on T1-weighted MR images. AJNR Am J Neuroradiol. 1990;11(1):23–6.
5. Aguila LA, Piraino DW, Modic MT, Dudley AW, Duchesneau PM, Weinstein MA. The intranuclear cleft of the intervertebral disk: magnetic resonance imaging. Radiology. 1985;155(1):155–8.
6. Moon SM, Yoder JH, Wright AC, Smith LJ, Vresilovic EJ, Elliott DM. Evaluation of intervertebral disc cartilaginous endplate structure using magnetic resonance imaging. Eur Spine J. 2013;22(8):1820–8.

7. Bae WC, Statum S, Zhang Z, Yamaguchi T, Wolfson T, Gamst AC, et al. Morphology of the cartilaginous endplates in human intervertebral disks with ultrashort echo time MR imaging. Radiology. 2013;266(2):564–74.
8. Xu GL, Haughton VM, Carrera GF. Lumbar facet joint capsule: appearance at MR imaging and CT. Radiology. 1990;177(2):415–20.
9. Macdonald A, Chatrath P, Spector T, Ellis H. Level of termination of the spinal cord and the dural sac: a magnetic resonance study. Clin Anat. 1999;12(3):149–52.
10. Hasegawa T, Mikawa Y, Watanabe R, An HS. Morphometric analysis of the lumbosacral nerve roots and dorsal root ganglia by magnetic resonance imaging. Spine (Phila Pa 1976). 1996;21(9):1005–9.

Clinical Diagnosis in Patients with Spinal Pain

2

Jun Ho Lee

2.1 Introduction

Spinal pain, especially back pain, is the second most common reason for visiting medical institutions after respiratory diseases and is a symptom that almost everyone experiences at least once in their lifetime. It can be said that it is the most frequently encountered symptom in actual clinical practice. More than 90% of all patients with back pain are believed to be caused by mechanical lesions (degenerative changes, disc herniation, spinal stenosis, spondylolisthesis, etc.), but it is rare that the exact pathological anatomical lesion is revealed [1]. Therefore, to evaluate back pain early, general medical history and physical examination alone can find clues to the answer, but in a minority, other special tests may be needed for accurate diagnosis.

Neurological examination begins the moment the patient enters the clinic, and a general physical examination must be performed before starting a neurological examination. This is because physical findings can help differentiate diagnosis from other diseases that show similar symptoms, even if the patient's main symptom suggests a neurological abnormality. The most important thing in conducting a neurological examination is to exclude other diseases that can show symptoms similar to spinal diseases. In patients suspected of spinal and spinal cord diseases, the approximate location of the lesion is identified through a neurological examination, and based on this, radiological examination is performed for confirmation. Neurological examination should be conducted without omission, and it is important to have a certain process and format to facilitate subsequent analysis [2].

J. H. Lee (✉)
Department of Neurosurgery, Kyung Hee University College of Medicine, Seoul, Republic of Korea
e-mail: moo9924@khu.ac.kr

2.2 Terminological Clarification and Classification of Musculoskeletal and Spinal Pain

Pain can be divided into dermatomal pain, sclerotomal pain, and myotomal pain. Dermatomal pain refers to pain in the distribution area of a single nerve root that controls a specific part of the skin. Sclerotomal pain refers to pain caused by stimulation of structures originating from the mesoderm of the spine (muscles, ligaments, periosteum, joint capsules, fibrous rings), which is vague and felt deep in our body.

It refers to a referred pain. Myotomal pain refers to pain in the distribution area of the muscle group controlled by a single nerve root. Also, it is necessary to know the difference between radicular pain and referred pain. The former refers to pain in the distribution area of a single

© The Author(s), under exclusive license to Springer Nature Singapore Pte Ltd. 2025
H. S. Kang, J. W. Lee (eds.), *Spinal Imaging*, https://doi.org/10.1007/978-981-95-1386-4_2

nerve root, meaning that the anterior primary ramus of the nerve root has been compromised. The latter refers to feeling pain far from the site of the lesion, which is thought to occur due to an error in the brain's cognitive function, complaining of unclear pain in the back and somewhere in the leg, meaning that the structure controlled by the posterior primary ramus of the nerve root has been compromised.

This classification approach helps to classify spinal pain into (1) nonspecific spinal pain [referring to spinal pain without signs corresponding to specific spinal diseases such as serious underlying diseases (e.g., cancer, infection, and cauda equina syndrome), spinal stenosis/radiculopathy or ankylosing spondylitis or spinal compression fractures], (2) spinal pain associated with radiculopathy, and (3) spinal pain caused by other specific spinal diseases [3]. The third category, pain caused by specific spinal diseases, includes (1) serious or progressive neurological deficits, (2) diseases requiring immediate additional tests such as tumors, infections, cauda equina syndrome, and (3) diseases responding to special treatments such as spinal compression fractures, ankylosing spondylitis. Cases corresponding to the third category, pain caused by specific spinal diseases, are relatively few in primary care settings, appearing at frequencies of compression fractures (4%), cancer (0.7%), and spinal infections (0.01%) [4]. To distinguish spinal pain caused by these specific spinal diseases, the presence or absence of so-called red flags (Table 2.1) should be confirmed by questioning [5].

This classification of the three types of spinal pain helps determine the next steps in diagnosis and treatment. It is particularly important to distinguish between back pain associated with radiculopathy and back pain caused by specific spinal causes at the initial stage.

Table 2.1 Potentially serious pathologies and specific causes of low back pain that warrant additional investigation

Cancer
• History of cancer
• Unexplained weight loss
• Night pain or pain at rest
• Age 50 years or 20 years
Spinal infection
• Persistent fever
• History of intravenous drug abuse
• Recent bacterial infection
• Immunocompromised states
• Pain at rest
Cauda equina syndrome
• Urinary incontinence or retention
• Saddle anesthesia
• Decrease in anal sphincter tone
• Bilateral lower extremity weakness
• Progressive neurological deficit
Major nerve root compression
• Radicular pain
• Major muscle weakness
• Foot drop
Vertebral fracture
• Prolonged use of corticosteroids
• Mild trauma at age 50 years
• Age 70 years
• History of osteoporosis
• Recent substantial trauma at any age
Abdominal aortic artery aneurysm
• Abdominal pulsating mass
• Atherosclerotic vascular disease
• Pain at rest or nocturnal pain
• Age 60 years

Red flags, courtesy from Verhagen AP et al. Red flags presented in current low back pain guidelines: a review. Eur Spine J. 2016

2.3 Physical Evaluation of Spinal Pain Prior to History Taking

As spinal pain can be caused by various reasons, taking a medical history and physical examination are very important processes for accurate diagnosis. Since the exact cause of spinal pain is often not revealed even through advanced equipment, classifying and treating patients based on information obtained through history taking and physical examination can yield good results. However, it is not easy for patients to always accurately point out this pain area during the initial questioning in the clinic. It is not. Anderson and others have investigated the sensitivity and specificity of history taking and physical examination in patients with disc herniation. They stated that there is no information obtained from individual patients that has sufficient diagnostic value [6]. For example, the sensitivity of sciatica is relatively high at 0.98, which can be useful in diagnosing disc herniation, but the specificity is not clear at about 0.88, and if the prevalence of disc herniation itself is low, the positive predictive value is also low [7, 8]. There are not many studies on the usefulness of history and physical examination in the diagnosis of spinal stenosis, and the positive likelihood ratios of radiculopathy and pseudoclaudication are 2.2 and 1.2, respectively [9]. Therefore, during the history taking of patients with low back pain, it is always necessary to check for the presence or absence of leg pain. For example, if the patient complains of pain below the knee, a nerve root lesion can be suspected. You should ask when and why it occurred, and what factors exacerbate the pain. If the patient complains of pain when bending the waist, disc herniation can be suspected, and if it hurts when bending the waist backwards, spinal stenosis or spondylolisthesis can be suspected. If there is unusual weight loss in patients with spinal pain or if the symptoms do not improve even with bed rest, it is necessary to check for the presence of systemic diseases instead of the spine. Also, in patients with chronic low back pain, there may be an imbalance in the muscles of the lumbar pelvic area, so this should be checked in advance during history taking.

2.4 Physical Examination

The physical examination for evaluating musculoskeletal pain is recommended to be performed in order(see Table 2.2), always checking for the presence or absence of nerve root disease and the relevance of the problematic local area and spinal segment, and determining the affected segment based on a comprehensive evaluation [10, 11].

Table 2.2 Suggested sequence of physical examination for musculoskeletal pain

(1) His taking including event, duration, worsening factor, relieving factor
(2) Check posture, gait
(3) Palpation on painful soft tissue and joint
(4) Palpation on spine, interspinous process, transverse process
(5) Range of motion of spine
(6) Neurologic examination
(7) Segmental diagnosis (peripheral change on palpation whichinnervated by same spinal nervel spine changes on palpation of the same segment)

Courtesy from Ahn K. Segmental palpation for radiculopathy. Anesth Pain Med 2011

2.4.1 Inspection

The most important process in physical examination is inspection, where the patient's posture and gait are observed to determine whether they are out of the normal range or unnatural. It is also necessary to check the range of motion of the spine. In the measurement of lumbar flexion, the distance between the ground and the fingers when the upper body is flexed forward is commonly measured, but this alone cannot represent the flexibility of the spine, so it is important to observe the overall curvature of the spine. Evaluation of muscle spasm and tenderness through palpation of the spine and surrounding areas is also necessary, and palpation should be performed in various states such as standing, sitting, bending, or stretching the spine.

2.4.2 Palpation

Maigne [12] expressed the examination of the nerve innervation segment, called cellulalgia, by palpating the skin and fascia, which has considerable diagnostic value. The examination relies on the pinch roll test, which involves pinching and rubbing the skin. Generally, this

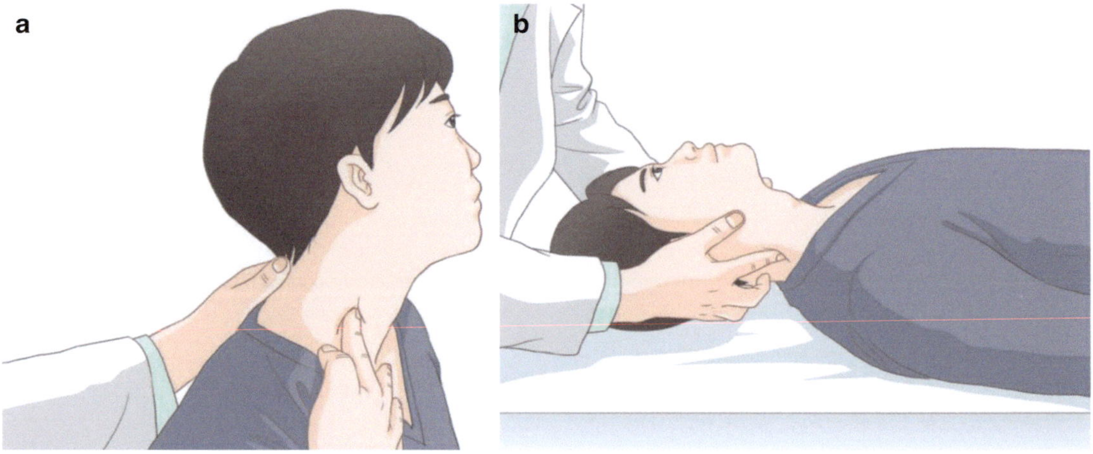

Fig. 2.1 Palpation of the posterior tubercle with the patient's neck side flexed at 15° to the opposite side. Notice the SCM muscle in front of it. To facilitate the palpation, draw an imaginary line along the transverse processes and trace the locations of the posterior tubercles. (**a**) Palpation of the cervical zygopophyseal joints with an examiner's index finger at the sides of the semispinal muscles while the patient is lying on the back maintaining the natural C-curve of the neck. (**b**) (Courtesy from Ahn K. Segmental palpation for radiculopathy. Anesth Pain Med 2011)

examination should be conducted with the muscles, but if there is abnormally hypersensitive pain in the posterior joint or transverse process and cellulalgia is present, the treatment target is not the skin but the corresponding spinal area [10, 13]. Cellulalgia involves examining the skin and fascia together, so it should be remembered that it is different from a simple skin segment.

2.4.2.1 Stimulation of the Cervical Joint

Stimulation of the cervical joint involves fixing the thumb or index finger on the cervical joint and diagnosing by checking for tenderness or resistance to movement while flexing the cervical spine forward and sideways or by rubbing the thumb or index finger fixed on the joint back and forth. Although this is a more accurate method, it is generally easier to touch the interspinous space or stimulate the facet joint while the patient is lying flat [12, 13]. First, stimulate the transverse process or facet joint from the outside, then use a method to stimulate the facet joint from the back of the neck. It is easier to touch when stimulated from the outside and pressure must be applied when stimulated from the back. After applying pressure, the muscles may tense up, making stimulation difficult (Fig. 2.1).

Stimulation of the transverse process or facet joint involves lightly pressing the finger on the transverse process or facet joint and rubbing it back and forth to the extent that the transverse process or joint surface can be felt. The degree of tenderness at this time is divided into four stages.

Stage 1 is the degree of tenderness felt during stimulation, Stage 2 is severe tenderness during stimulation causing the body to avoid or grimace, Stage 3 is severe pain causing the body to avoid, and Stage 4 is pain as soon as the transverse process or joint surface touches, causing the body to avoid. Usually, Stages 1–2 are not definitive, so the same level of stimulation should be applied to the opposite joint for comparison. However, if Stages 3 and 4 occur, this indicates the presence of tenderness in the transverse process or joint surface and the possibility of segmental hypersensitivity. From the outside of the neck, stimulation is possible from the C2.3 facet joint to the C3–4, C4–5, C5–6, C6–7, C7–T1 joint. Also, according to Maigne's interspinous touch method, stimulation is possible from the C2.3 spinous process to the T1–2 spinous process. In thin people, the facet joint surface can also be stimulated from the back of the neck, 1 cm lateral to the interspinous gap [11].

2.4.2.2 Stimulation of the Thoracic and Lumbar Joints

First, a spinal examination is conducted for the segmental examination of the lower extremities. In the spinal examination, tests are performed by lying down with a pillow and touching the spinous process of the spine with the abdomen touching the floor, or by bending the waist 45° forward and touching the spinous process. It is important to identify pain or instability in the spine [14, 15]. Palpation between the spinous processes is a useful method for diagnosing spinal diseases, and if the space between the spinous processes is loose, pain can easily be induced by pressing. If a gap is felt between the spinous processes and spondylolisthesis is suspected, it is essential to perform a flexion-extension view to check for any minor displacements. Even if displacement has occurred, if there is no tenderness between the spinous processes, it is likely that this is not the cause of the pain.

(1) Thoracolumbar Junction

Pain in the thoracolumbar junction appears in two forms: one is pain in the thoracolumbar junction or lower back, and the other is pain in the lower abdomen and lateral thigh, which appears through the anterior primary ramus, and pain in the hip joint area and lateral thigh, which exists along the branches of the posterior primary ramus [16]. This is often confused with lesions of the lower lumbar spine and can be difficult to identify without careful observation. The distinction between pain in the thoracolumbar junction and pain in the lumbosacral junction is based on the following three points. First, pain in the thoracolumbar junction does not result in segmental abnormalities below the knee. Second, pain in the thoracolumbar junction, except for L2, does not accompany segmental abnormalities of the medial part of the facet joint. Third, it is rare to cause tenderness at the attachment of the great trochanter. Pain from the subcutaneous segment of the thoracolumbar junction appears in the buttocks, lateral thigh, and lateral thigh, and these can appear alone or together. Pain in the thoracolumbar junction is often confirmed by pressing between the spinous processes or if the space between the spinous processes is significantly stretched compared to other spinous processes, and it shows a form of cellulagia as shown in the figure, it has a clear significance (Fig. 2.2).

(2) Segmental abnormalities of the lumbar and sacral nerves

A method of evaluating by examining a few common muscles and abnormalities in or around the spine is followed. If there is pain between the L4–5 spinous processes or if there is a gap when bent compared to other spinous processes, this can mean not only a problem with spinal segmentation but also instability that does not appear on spinal imaging. Therefore, to confirm the presence or absence of abnormalities in the picture, a flexion and extension view of the waist should be taken to find the possibility of minor instability. If tenderness between the spinous processes or instability of the spine appears, first check if there is pain in the unstable joint, and confirms the abnormality of the nerve that controls that joint and the nerve that exists on the outermost side of the dural tube passing through that joint. For example, if an abnormality appears between the L2 and L3 spinous processes, the L2, especially, the possibility of abnormalities in the L4 nerve, which is located on the outermost side of the dura mater from the L3 nerve and its joint, is high, and similarly, between the L3 and L4 spinous processes, there is a high possibility of abnormalities in the L3, especially the L4 or L5 nerves. Between the L4 and L5 spinous processes, there is a high possibility of abnormalities in the L4, especially the L5 or S1 nerves. If there is a problem between the L5 and S1 spinous processes, there are many problems with the L5, especially the S1 and S2 nerves.

Characteristically, the tender point of the gluteus medius often harbors problems with

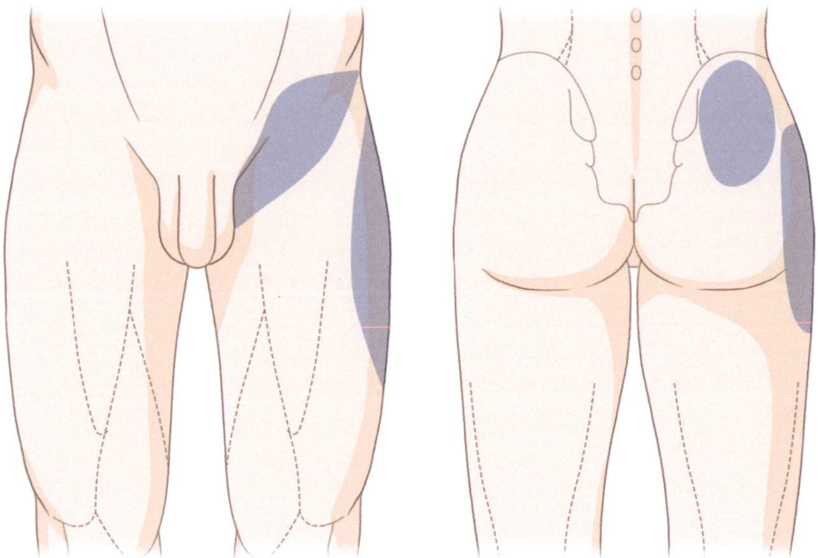

Fig. 2.2 Cellulalgia at T12 and L1 innervation
The dysfunction in the thoracolumbar junction is associated with the pain in the dermatome of the posterior primary ramus and that of the anterior primary ramus as well as the back pain. This is confirmed by the pinch and roll test with the affected skin and the existence of tenderness at the interspinous space in the thoracolumbar junction. (Courtesy from Ahn K. Segmental palpation for radiculopathy. Anesth Pain Med 2011)

the L5 nerve. The weakening of the gluteus medius expresses a more powerful weakening of the L5 nerve-controlled muscles, often unable to stand on one foot, or walking with legs spread and bending the body. This is a very common symptom in the elderly. Also, abnormalities in the S1 nerve often accompany neuropathic pain, radiculopathy, and physical examination of cellulalgia in the L5 or S2 nerve-controlled segments (Fig. 2.3).

Especially, there are cases where clear problems such as L4/5 disc herniation, spinal stenosis, and spondylolisthesis are found, but symptoms often appear without these problems. However, clear abnormalities are found in the physical examination. Although there are cases where abnormalities in the L5 and S1 nerves exist alone in the spinal examination, it is not common compared to between the L4 and L5 vertebrae. It is usually accompanied by tenderness between the L4 and L5 spinous processes. However, if it hurts more than between the L4–5 vertebrae, it can be assumed that the problem is mainly in the lumbosacral junction. When there are problems not only in the calf but also in the back of the knee, the heel, and the sole of the foot, it is often accompanied by abnormalities in the S1 and S2 nerves in the physical examination.

2.4.3 Percussion, Deep Tendon Reflex (DTR), Muscle Stretch Reflex

It can be said to be a useful test method to find lesions in patients who do not cooperate well or cannot express or appeal appropriately. In order to maintain consistency in the grading classification, it is a principle that the same examiner performs as much as possible. The basic test method is to perform on both sides in a relaxed state of the patient and to test other areas for comparison between the two sides to find differences. Deep tendon reflexes are classified from 0 to 4 grades in the order of loss, decrease, normal, hyperactive, and very hyperactive depending on the strength, speed, and range of muscle contraction.

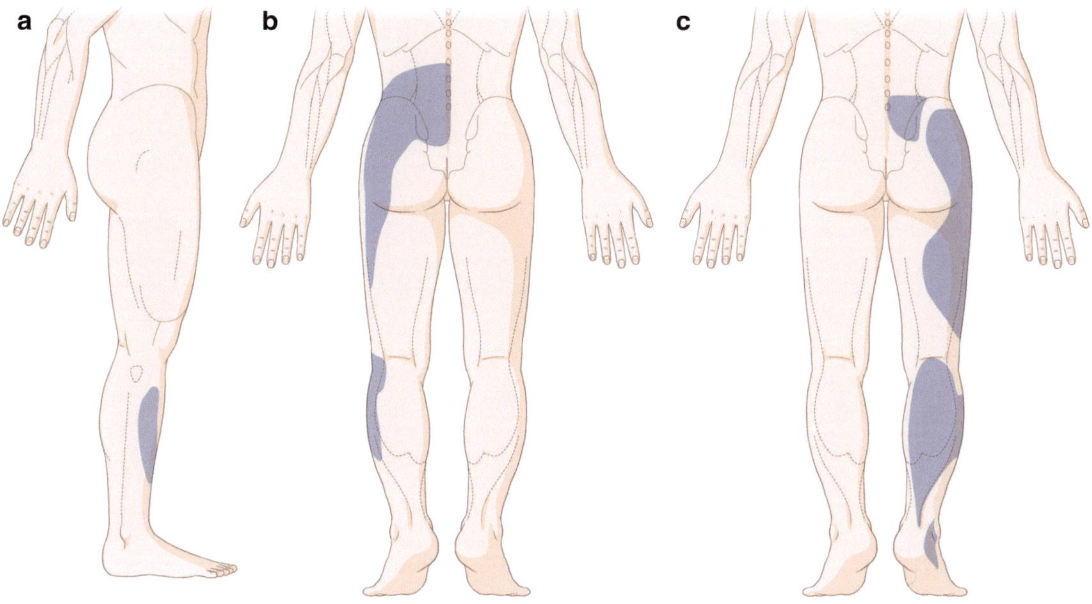

Fig. 2.3 Cellulalgia and pain from the dorsal ramus of L5 (**a** and **b**) vs S1 (**c**) (Courtesy from Ahn K. Segmental palpation for radiculopathy. Anesth Pain Med 2011)

Generally, the reflexes of the biceps, brachioradialis, triceps, patellar, and Achilles tendons are tested, and in 3–10% of normal people, tendon reflexes may disappear. If the reflex action is symmetrical when the deep tendon reflex is performed on both sides, it can be seen as normal unless there is a lesion on both sides. The reflex arc consists of a receptor, afferent nerve, intercalated neuron, and motor unit. If there are lesions in the efferent nerve fiber, deep tendon reflexes may be lost or reduced. This can occur not only in common degenerative spinal pain diseases such as spinal stenosis, but also in neuritis, radiculoneuritis, syringomyelia, diabetic neuropathy, etc. On the other hand, lesions in the cerebral premotor area or pyramidal tract, spinal cord injuries, etc., excite the neural pathway that facilitates the spinal cord from the brainstem or induce the excitation of spinal nerves, causing deep tendon reflexes to be hyperactive.

(1) Biceps reflex (Biceps reflex, C5, 6: musculocuatenous nerve)
The patient stands or sits with the elbow bent close to a right angle and rests it on the examiner's left forearm. With the patient's elbow held in the examiner's left hand, the examiner places his left thumb on the biceps tendon and strikes it with a hammer. Normally, the contraction of the biceps causes the forearm to flex and supinate (Fig. 2.4).

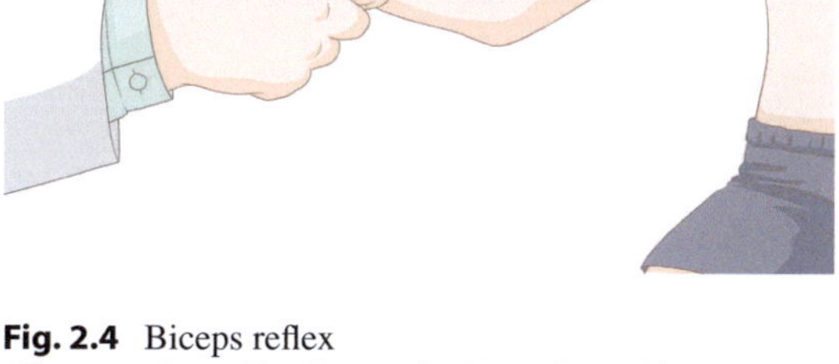

Fig. 2.4 Biceps reflex (Courtesy from Cho Sung-min, Hong Soon-ki, Koo Yeonmoo. Chapter 5 Neurological Examination. Spine Study 3rd Edition, 2018)

(2) Brachioradialis reflex (Brachioradialis reflex, C5, 6: radial nerve)

When the forearm is in a semi-flexed and semi-pronated state, striking the tendon above the styloid process of the radius causes the forearm to supinate and flex.

(3) Triceps reflex (Triceps reflex, C7, 8: radial nerve)

Striking above the triceps insertion on the ulna, the olecranon causes the triceps to contract and the forearm to extend. However, if the forearm flexes when struck, it is called a paradoxical triceps reflex, which occurs when the triceps reflex arc is damaged.

(4) Patellar reflex or knee jerk (Patellar reflex or knee jerk, L3, 4: femoral nerve)

The examinee is seated on the examination table with their legs hanging down below the table or lying down. After the examiner supports the examinee's knee with their hand, when the patellar tendon just below the patella is struck, the contraction of the quadriceps femoris can be observed as the knee extends (Fig. 2.5).

(5) Achilles tendon reflex or ankle jerk (Achilles tendon reflex or ankle jerk, S1: Tibial nerve)

After making the examinee lie comfortably, bend and externally rotate the knee, and dorsiflex the foot with the examiner's hand, or make them lie prone, bend the knee, and lightly dorsiflex the foot, when the Achilles tendon is struck, the ankle joint can be seen to extend (Fig. 2.6).

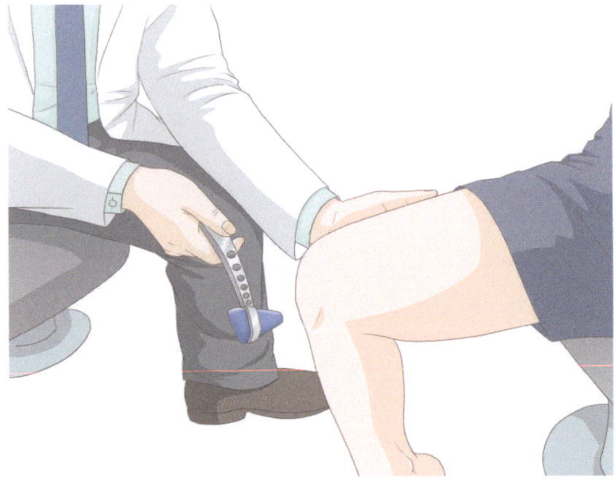

Fig. 2.5 Patellar reflex
(Courtesy from Cho Sung-min, Hong Soon-ki, Koo Yeonmoo. Chapter 5 Neurological Examination. Spine Study 3rd Edition, 2018)

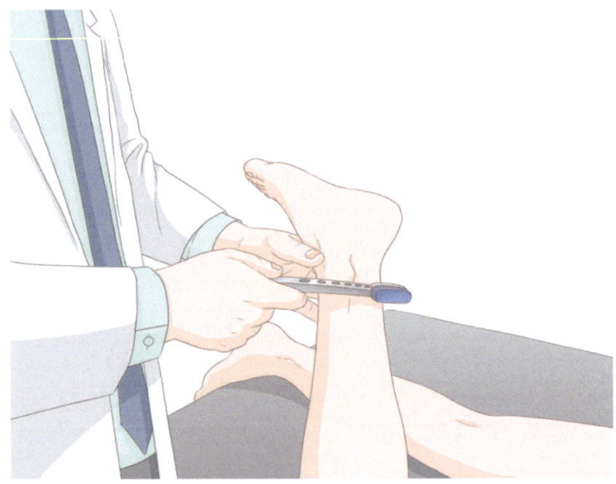

Fig. 2.6 Achilles tendon reflex
(Courtesy from Cho Sung-min, Hong Soon-ki, Koo Yeonmoo. Chapter 5 Neurological Examination. Spine Study 3rd Edition, 2018)

2.4.4 Neurological Examination and Evoked Tests

2.4.4.1 Neurological Examination for Spinal Cord Disease

(1) Hoffman's sign

Once relieving the tensed arm and hand, the examiner might scratch the patient's thumbnail to inflict the pain. If the patient's thumb or other fingers are triggered and responded with flickering, it is considered positive and has the pathway of the 6th cervical vertebra, and it is a pathological reaction that can be expected to have abnormalities in the pyramidal tract. However, in cases where the patient's muscle tension is severe, it can appear positive in generalized reflex hyperactivity and even in healthy people (Fig. 2.7).

(2) Ankle clonus reflex

When the patient's ankle joint is quickly flexed, if the calf muscle's intermittent contraction and relaxation occur more than 4–5 times, it is considered positive. It can normally appear in infants (Fig. 2.8).

(3) Lhermitte's sign

When the patient is sitting and flexes the head as much as possible, if there are symptoms like electricity flowing down the back or

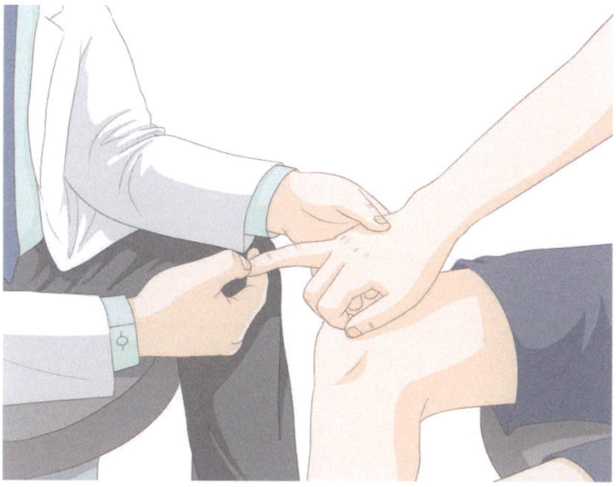

Fig. 2.7 Hoffman's sign
(Courtesy from Cho Sung-min, Hong Soon-ki, Koo Yeon-moo. Chapter 5 Neurological Examination. Spine Study 3rd Edition, 2018)

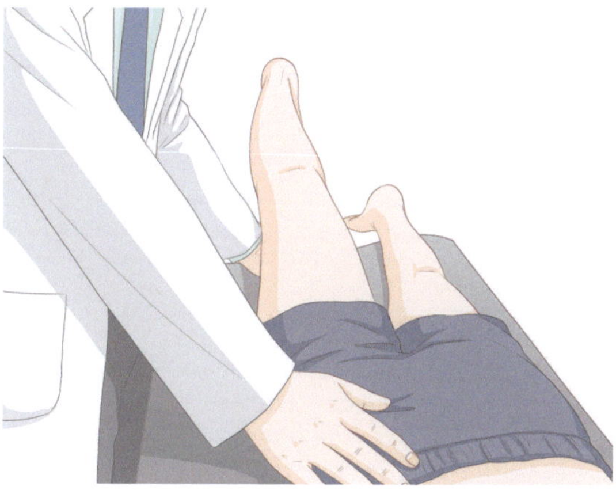

Fig. 2.8 Ankle clonus reflex
(Courtesy from Cho Sung-min, Hong Soon-ki, Koo Yeon-moo. Chapter 5 Neurological Examination. Spine Study 3rd Edition, 2018)

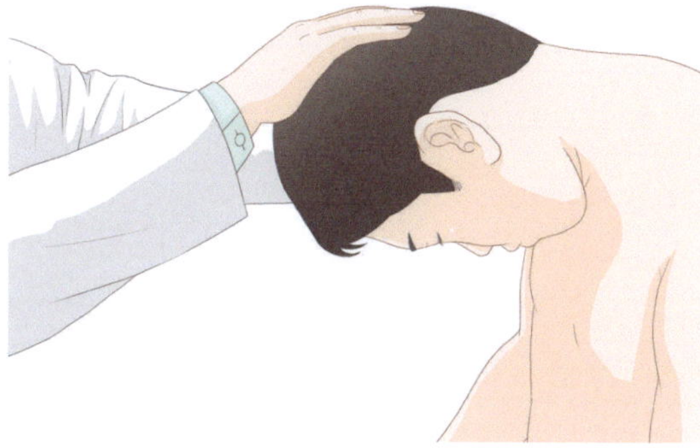

Fig. 2.9 Lhemitte sign
(Courtesy from Cho Sung-min, Hong Soon-ki, Koo Yeon-moo. Chapter 5 Neurological Examination. Spine Study 3rd Edition, 2018)

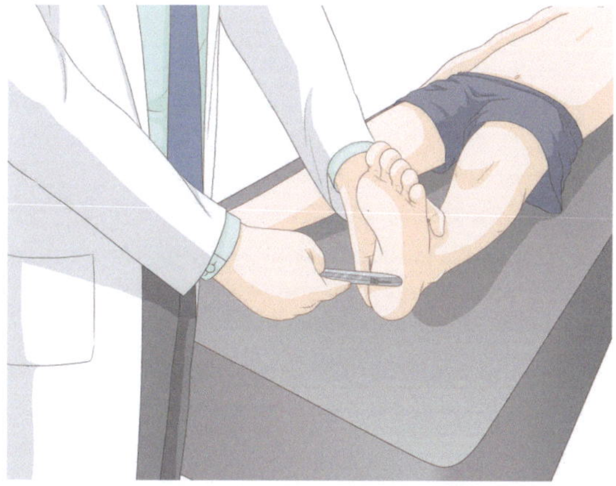

Fig. 2.10 Babinski's sign (Plantar reflex)
(Courtesy from Sungmin Jo, Soonki Hong, Yeonmu Koo. Chapter 5 Neurological Examination. Spine Study 3rd Edition, 2018)

limbs, it is considered positive and can suspect pathological conditions of the cervical spine, multiple sclerosis, spinal tumors, cervical spondylosis, ossification of the posterior longitudinal ligament (OPLL), etc. (Fig. 2.9).

(4) Babinski's sign (plantar reflex)
When the outside of the sole is stimulated in the longitudinal direction, if the thumb extends and all toes spread, it is called a Fan sign, and it can be seen as a normal reaction from 6 months to 12 months after birth. It is a pathological reaction that can be expected to have abnormalities in the pyramidal tract (Fig. 2.10).

2.4.4.2 Cervical Muscle Strength, Sensation, and Reflex Test

In the case of major cervical disc herniation, the working muscles, sensory change areas, and decreased reflexes that are transferred according to the compressed nerve root are different in distinguishing the escape site clinically (Table 2.3).

2.4.4.3 Lumbar Muscle Strength Test and Sensory Test

During the lumbar muscle strength test, the corresponding muscle must be isometrically contracted for at least 5 s [17]. Except for acute

Table 2.3 Differentiation of cervical disc herniation sites

	Cervical 4/5	Cervical 5/6	Cervical 6/7	Cervical 7/ Thoracic 1
Compressed nerve root	5th nerve root	6th nerve root	7th nerve root	8th nerve root
Working muscles	Deltoid	Forearm flexion	Forearm extension (wrist drop)	Hand intrinsics
Sensory changes	Shoulder	Upper arm, thumb, radial forearm	2nd, 3rd fingers All finger tips	4th, 5th fingers
Reflex decrease	Deltoid and pectoralis	Biceps and brachioradialis	Triceps	Finger reflex

Courtesy from Sungmin Jo, Soonki Hong, Yeonmu Koo. Chapter 5 Neurological Examination. Spine Study 3nd Edition, 2018

injuries, it is rare for more than one nerve root to be invaded at the same time. Deyo emphasized that the strength and sensory tests of the ankle joint and big toe extensor and the deep tendon reflex of the ankle joint should be tested at the same time [3]. The muscle strength test includes the hip flexor (L1–L3), quadriceps (L2–L4), tibialis anterior (L4), big toe dorsiflexor (L5), gastrocnemius/soleus (S1), etc. Especially in the case of gastrocnemius/soleus, the examiner holds the subject's hands, lifts the opposite leg, and lifts the heel 10 times for the test.

In the sensory test, both sides should be compared. The corresponding parts are proximal thigh (L3), medial leg (L4), lateral leg (L5), calf (S1), medial malleolus (L4), the sacral promontory (L5), and and the lateral malleolus (S1).

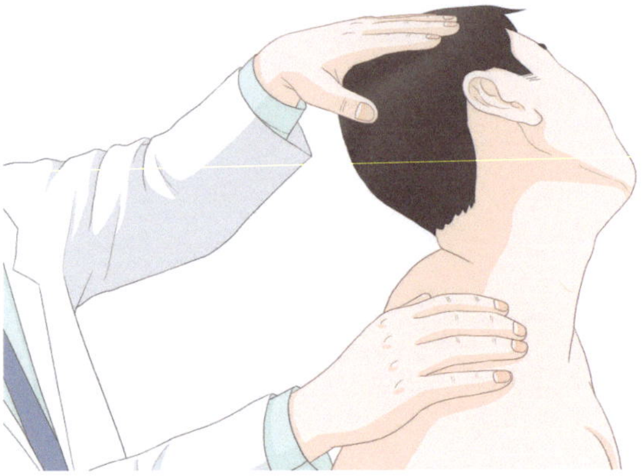

Fig. 2.11 Spurling's sign (Courtesy from Sungmin Jo, Soonki Hong, Yeonmu Koo. Chapter 5 Neurological Examination. Spine Study 3rd Edition, 2018)

2.4.4.4 Provocation Test

(1) Cervical nerve root disease test

- Foraminal compression test (modified Spurling's maneuver); a test to confirm the presence or absence of nerve root compression due to lack of space in the intervertebral foramen. The examiner stands behind the seated patient, placing one hand on the patient's head above the ear and the other hand on the opposite shoulder joint to prevent the patient's upper body posture from collapsing during the test. The patient's head is laterally flexed, and the neck is extended in the direction of upper limb pain. Once the posture is fixed, the head is pressed down axially, causing the intervertebral foramen of the lesion site to narrow further and compress the nerve root. If radicular pain is provoked, it is considered a positive Spurling's sign, suggesting cervical disc herniation and foraminal stenosis. If the head is tilted to the opposite side of the lesion, the radicular pain disappears (Fig. 2.11).
- Shoulder abduction relief test; when the symptomatic arm is abducted and the hand is raised above the head, the patient's radicular pain and numbness disappear or decrease, which is considered positive (Bakody's sign). If the symptoms are relieved due to decreased tension in the cervical nerve root, it implies secondary radicular pain caused by cervical disc lesions, but it does not necessarily mean cervical spondylosis.

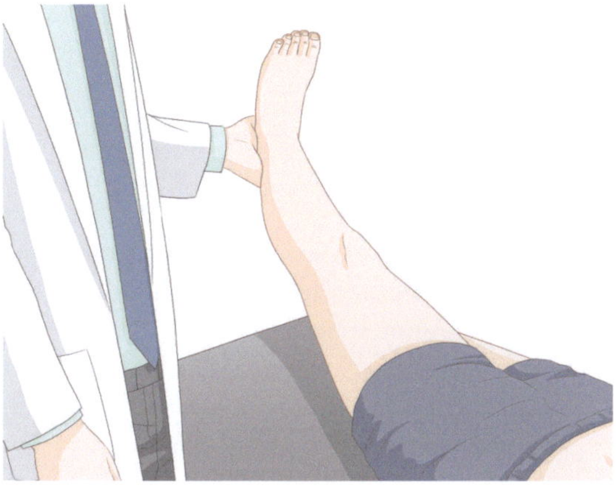

Fig. 2.12 Straight leg raising test (Courtesy from Sungmin Jo, Soonki Hong, Yeonmu Koo. Chapter 5 Neurological Examination. Spine Study 3rd Edition, 2018)

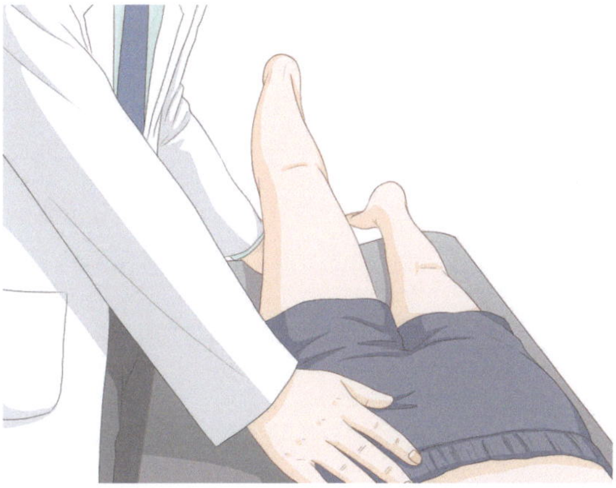

Fig. 2.13 Femoral nerve stretching test (Courtesy from Jo Sung-min, Hong Soon-ki, Koo Yeon-moo. Chapter 5 Neurological Examination. Spine Study 3rd Edition, 2018)

(2) Lumbar dural tension testing
- Straight leg raise (SLR) test: after fully extending the knee joint, the lower limb is lifted. If symptoms are provoked between 30 and 70 degrees, it implies that the L5, S1, and S2 spinal nerves are compromised. Also, symptoms may increase if the ankle joint is extended, the lower limb is internally rotated, or the neck is flexed (Fig. 2.12).
- Crossed straight leg raising test: if the nucleus pulposus has severely herniated into the central part of the nerve canal or herniated as an axillary type, and radicular pain on the symptomatic side is weakened or provoked when the asymptomatic lower limb is raised, it is considered positive. This is because the nerve root on the lesion side is compressed by the herniated nucleus pulposus due to traction of the nerve root on the asymptomatic side. It is also called the "Peyton sign."
- Slump test: in a sitting position on the bed, the patient's hands are directed behind the back and clasped together, then the waist is flexed and the neck is extended. Next, the examiner flexes the neck and extends the lower limb to provoke nerve root symptoms, which is considered positive [18].
- Femoral stretch test, also known as reverse straight leg raise (reverse SLR) also known as the test. In the abdomen and stomach, the examiner flexes the knee joint almost until the heel of the foot touches the buttock. Then, while pressing the left hip bone with one hand to prevent the pelvis from rotating forward, the other hand extends the hip joint. If pain is induced in the anterior thigh or anterior thigh, it is positive and means that the L1–L3 or sometimes L4 spinal nerve root is compromised (Fig. 2.13).

(3) Sacroiliac joint test: There is no single test that can confirm the function of the sacroiliac joint, and it is meaningful to show a positive response to various tests [18, 19].
- Anterior flexion test (standing or sitting): The examiner places both thumbs on the PSIS and extends the knee and bends it forward as much as possible. The thumb on the side where the movement of the sacroiliac joint is limited goes up a bit more, which is also called the "jump sign" and means positive.
- Gillet or Stork test (standing): The examiner places both thumbs on the PSIS and the examinee bend the knee of the other leg, grab it with both hands, and stand in a

posture where it is pulled up to the chest. If the thumb on the side of the leg with the bent knee moves up, it is positive, and if it moves down, it is normal.

- Fabere test (Patrick test): Bend the knee and place it on the knee of the other leg, place one hand on the iliac crest, and place the other hand on the inside of the bent leg's knee and push it down. If you feel pain in the ipsilateral anterior thigh, it means degenerative joint disease of the hip joint, and if you feel pain on the opposite side, it means dysfunction of the sacroiliac joint.
- Gaenslen test: Lie on the edge of the bed in a supine position, flex the knee and hip joint of one leg, and apply pressure to the thigh of the other leg to overextend the hip joint. If you feel pain in the anterior thigh on the overextended side, it may mean dysfunction of the sacroiliac joint (Fig. 2.14).
- Yeoman test: In the abdomen and stomach, the examiner applies pressure downward from the iliac crest with one hand while placing the other hand on the anterior thigh above the knee and extending the hip joint. If you feel pain in the anterior thigh, it is positive.

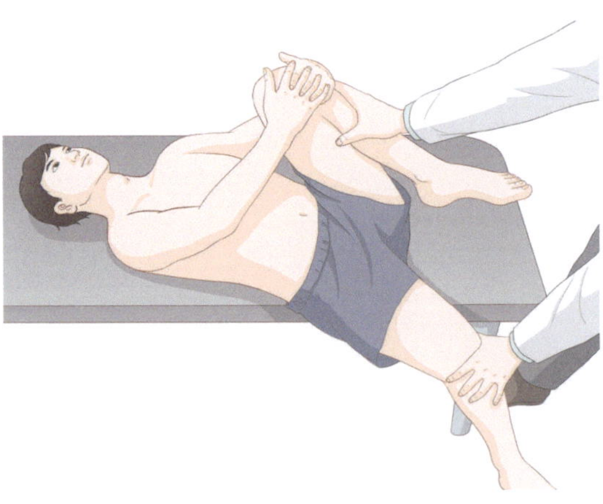

Fig. 2.14 Gaenslen test
(Courtesy from Jo Sung-min, Hong Soon-ki, Koo Yeon-moo. Chapter 5 Neurological Examination. Spine Study 3rd Edition, 2018)

(4) Posterior facet syndrome
Symptoms include complaints of pain in the buttocks, thighs, and lower back, mainly spasmodic leg pain occurring above the knee joint, lower back stiffness that occurs when lying down or sitting in the morning and is relieved by light movement, no paresthesia, and when bending and twisting the waist, or when straightening the waist. Sharp pain occurs, and there may be tenderness around the lumbar region (mainly confined to 1–2 in. from the spinous process), and pain in the waist, buttocks, and thigh during straight leg raising. Diagnosis is possible when pain is induced and then disappears by injecting physiological saline into the spinal facet joint [20–22]

(5) Piriformis syndrome
The piriformis originates from the anterior of the second to fourth sacral vertebrae, passes through the sciatic notch, and terminates at the upper part of the greater trochanter. Its function is involved in the position of the hip joint, rotation of the hip joint during extension, abduction during flexion, and it is the only connecting muscle of the sacroiliac joint. The sciatic nerve is formed from the lumbosacral plexus, which consists of the fourth and fifth lumbar and first sacral nerve roots, passes through the sciatic notch, and divides into the tibial nerve and perineal nerve. Most of the time, it passes as a single sciatic nerve under the piriformis, but in some cases, it passes through the piriformis.

Symptoms of piriformis syndrome occur when the sciatic nerve is compressed by the piriformis, that is, during the stance phase of the gait cycle, during internal rotation of the hip joint due to piriformis stretch. It can occur due to excessive use of the buttocks and hip joints, repetitive trauma leading to the formation of microhematoma in the piriformis, abnormal gait due to leg length discrepancy, and hypertrophy of the piriformis. Examination methods are diverse, including the Piriformis stretch (Fig. 2.15), and it is

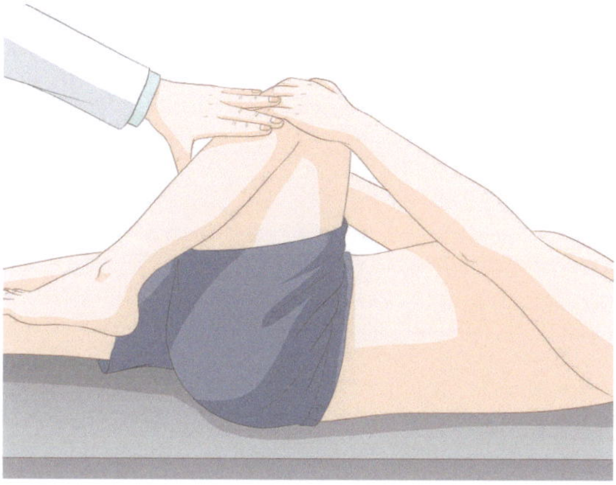

Fig. 2.15 Piriformis stretch
In the supine position, the patient is asked to hold their own knee and pull it to flex the hip joint to 90°, and when pain occurs during adduction and internal rotation, it is considered positive. (Courtesy from Jo Sung-min, Hong Soon-ki, Koo Yeon-moo. Chapter 5 Neurological Examination. Spine Study 3rd Edition, 2018)

necessary to compare with the opposite side and concurrently test for lumbar radiculopathy.

(6) Clinical Diagnosis of Spinal Stenosis
According to Katz et al. [23, 24], in the elderly over 65 years old, if there is no pain when sitting, they walk with a wide-based gait, and thigh pain is induced by continuous lumbar extension for 30 s, it can be diagnosed as spinal stenosis. Fritz et al. [25] used a two-stage treadmill test. This test is performed on a treadmill at level (the spine is in extension) and inclined (the spine is flexed) walking, with three variables. That is, the time until symptoms appear or worsen, the total walking time, and the time it takes to recover to baseline. Therefore, if symptoms appear early during level walking, the walking time increases during inclined walking, and the recovery time after level walking is long, it has value in diagnosing lateral type spinal stenosis.

2.5 Summary

The important goal of initial history taking and physical examination in patients with spinal pain is to make an accurate diagnosis for proper treatment. Such history taking and physical examination will be the first step in solving the inherent problem, and although the accuracy of each test or history may be low, it will be comprehensive and repetition will increase the reliability of the evaluation. Therefore, it is important to ensure that nothing is omitted in the neurological examination, and to have a consistent process and format to facilitate subsequent analysis.

Bibliography

1. White AA 3rd, Gordon SL. Synopsis: workshop on idiopathic low back pain. Spine. 1982;7:141–9.
2. Sung-min C, Soon-ki H, Yeon-moo K. Chapter 5: Neurological examination. In: Korean spine neurosurgery society: spine study. 3rd ed. Seoul: Gunja Publishing Company; 2018. p. 163–78.
3. Deyo RA, Rainville J, Kent DL. What can the history and physical examination tell us about low back pain? JAMA. 1992;268:760–5.
4. Jarvik JG, Deyo RA. Diagnostic evaluation of low back pain with emphasis on imaging. Ann Intern Med. 2002;137:586–97.
5. Verhagen AP, Downie A, Popal N, Maher C, Koes BW. Red flags presented in current low back pain guidelines: a review. Eur Spine J. 2016;25:2788–802.
6. Andersson GB, Deyo RA. History and physical examination in patients with herniated lumbar disc. Spine. 1996;21:10s–8s.
7. van den Hoogen HM, Koes BW, van Eijk JT, Bouter LM. On the accuracy of history, physical examination, and erythrocyte sedimentation rate in diagnosing low back pain in general practice. A criteria-based review of the literature. Spine. 1995;20:318–27.
8. Vroomen PC, de Krom MC, Knottnerus JA. Diagnostic value of history and physical examination in patients suspected of sciatica due to disc herniation: a systematic review. J Neurol. 1999;246:899–906.
9. de Graaf I, Prak A, Bierma-Zeinstra S, Thomas S, Peul W, Koes B. Diagnosis of lumbar spinal stenosis: a systematic review of the accuracy of diagnostic tests. Spine. 2006;31:1168–76.

10. Ahn K, Lee SC. Segmental radiculopathic model and chronic musculoskeletal pain. Korean J Anesthesiol. 2002;43:535–41.
11. Ahn K. Segmental palpation for radiculopathy. Anesth Pain Med. 2011;6:101–8.
12. Maigne R. Diagnosis and treatment of pain of vertebral origin. 2nd ed. CRC Press; 2006. p. 133–61.
13. Fligg B. Lower cervical spine motion palpation (C2–7). J Can Chiropr Assoc. 1984;28:219–21.
14. Johnston WL, Allan BR, Hendra JL, Neff DR, Rosen ME, Sills LD, et al. Interexaminer study of palpation in detecting location of spinal segmental dysfunction. J Am Osteopath Assoc. 1983;82:839–45.
15. Schneider M, Erhard R, Brach J, Tellin W, Imbarlina F, Delitto A. Spinal palpation for lumbar segmental mobility and pain provocation: an interexaminer reliability study. J Manipulative Physiol Ther. 2008;31:465–73.
16. Maigne R. Diagnosis and treatment of pain of vertebral origin. 2nd ed. CRC Press; 2006. p. 103–32.
17. Magee DJ. Orthopaedic physical assessment. 3rd ed. W.B. Saunders; 1997.
18. Geraci MC, Alleva JT. Physical examination of the spine and its functional kinetic chain. In: Cole A, Herring S, editors. The low back pain handbook. A practical guide for the primary care clinician. Philadelphia: Hanley and Belfus; 1997. p. 49–70.
19. DonTigny RL. Mechanics and treatment of the sacroiliac joint. In: 2nd Interdisciplinary world congress on low back pain. p. 515–28.
20. Destouet JM, Murphy WA. Indications and technique for lumbar facet block. Orthop Rev. 1985;14:57–65.
21. Helbig T, Lee CK. The lumbar facet syndrome. Spine. 1988;13:61–4.
22. Lippitt AB. The facet joint and its role in spine pain. Spine. 1984;9:746–50.
23. Katz JN, Dalgas M, Stucki G, et al. Degenerative lumbar spinal stenosis. Diagnostic value of the history and physical examination. Arthritis Rheumatism. 1995;38:1236–41.
24. Katz JN, Dalgas M, Stucki G, et al. Diagnosis of lumbar spinal stenosis. Rheum Dis Clin North Am. 1994;20:471–83.
25. Fritz JM, Erhard RE, Delitto A, et al. Preliminary results of the use of a two stage treadmill test as a clinical diagnostic tool in the differential diagnosis of lumbar spinal stenosis. J Spinal Dis. 1997;10:410–6.

3 Imaging Techniques for Spinal Magnetic Resonance Imaging

Kyung Nam Ryu and Hyejin Yoo

Various imaging techniques are used in spinal magnetic resonance imaging, so it is important to understand the types and pros and cons of each imaging technique. It is also important to understand the various ways and principles to optimize each imaging technique, in order to apply the optimized imaging technique for each spinal disease. It is also important to understand the ways to reduce the metallic artifact caused by the increasing spinal surgery metal, and the pros and cons of the widely used 3T device, for the optimization and diagnosis of the image.

3.1 Imaging Techniques Used in Spinal Magnetic Resonance Imaging

3.1.1 Fast Spin Echo (Fast Spin Echo)

The general spin echo pulse sequence uses 90-degree and 180-degree radio frequency (RF) pulses. However, in fast spin echo, multiple rephasing 180° are given between TR (repetition time) to generate echoes and fill the k-space. The number of echoes generated by the repeated 180-degree radio frequency is called the echo train length (ETL).

The shooting time in spin echo is [TR 3 NEX (number of excitation) 3 Number of phase encoding], but in fast spin echo, it is [TR 3 NEX 3 Number of phase encoding/echo train length], so the time is shortened. For example, if the ETL is 8, the time is reduced to 1/8 compared to the spin echo pulse technique (Fig. 3.1). Thus, the fast spin echo technique has a shorter shooting time than spin echo, and the reduced time can be used to improve the quality of the image, and artifacts due to movement or magnetization are relatively less, so better images can be obtained than spin echo images. However, the disadvantage is that the number of image sections decreases by increasing the ETL, which is to compensate, the TR may be increased and the section divided to repeat the video twice (2 packages, doubling the shooting time in this case). Also, the signal from the adipose tissue may be high, which may result in a low detection rate of lesions, so fat suppression imaging may be needed as necessary. Also, the sensitivity to hemorrhage or calcification may decrease, so gradient echo imaging may be needed. Despite these drawbacks, the image quality is excellent, so most use the fast spin echo technique [1, 2].

3.1.2 Fat Suppression Imaging

Fat suppression techniques are commonly used in magnetic resonance imaging to suppress or

K. N. Ryu (✉)
Department of Radiology, Kyung Hee University Hospital, Seoul, Republic of Korea

H. Yoo
Department of Radiology, Seoul National University Hospital, Seoul, Republic of Korea

© The Author(s), under exclusive license to Springer Nature Singapore Pte Ltd. 2025
H. S. Kang, J. W. Lee (eds.), *Spinal Imaging*, https://doi.org/10.1007/978-981-95-1386-4_3

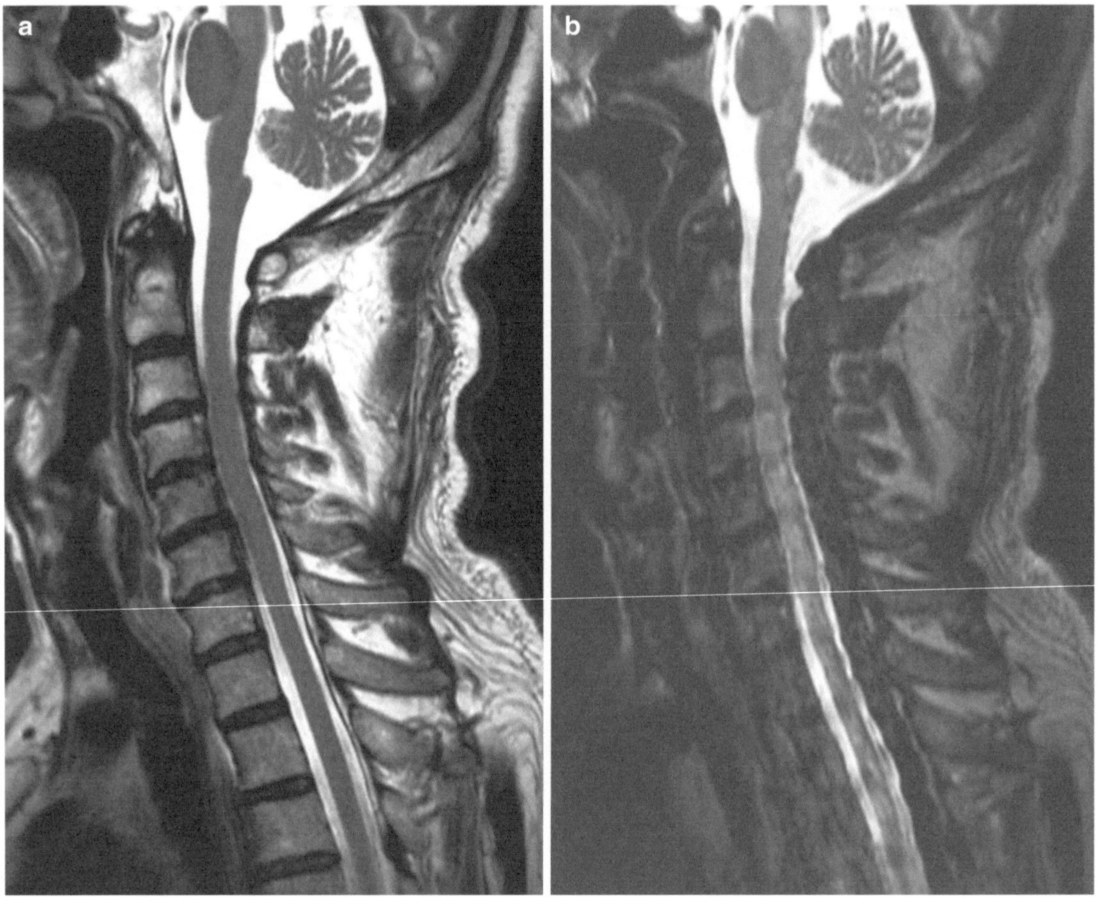

Fig. 3.1 A 76-year-old male patient. Fast spin echo and spin echo images of the cervical spine. (**a**) Fast spin echo images. Shooting time; 3 min 2 s [TR(2276 ms) 3 NEX(4) 3 Number of phase encoding(256)/echo train length(27)] 3 2 packages. (**b**) Spin echo images. Shooting time; 12 min 35 s [TR(2098 ms) 3 NEX(2) 3 Number of phase encoding(179)]

find signals from adipose tissue and can be obtained in three ways: fat saturation, inversion recovery, and in-phase/opposed-phase. Depending on the purpose of fat suppression and the amount of fat in the area being examined, a method can be selected. Fat suppression techniques have two main indications. One is to suppress signals from normal adipose tissue to reduce chemical shift artifacts or maximize contrast effects, and the other is to distinguish tissue characteristics in adrenal gland tumors, bone marrow infiltration, fatty tumors, etc.

Fat suppression imaging utilizes two different characteristics of water (H_2O) and fat (CH_3). One is the difference in frequency (chemical shift effects) and the other is the difference in T1 relaxation time. Hydrogen, the main component of water and fat, can feel different magnetic field strengths even within the same magnetic field depending on its bonding state with other elements. In the case of hydrogen belonging to adipose tissue, it feels a weaker magnetic field due to these shielding effects compared to water tissue. This difference in magnetic fields results in a difference in precessional frequency, which shows a frequency difference of about 450 Hz at 3T. Due to this difference, when obtaining an image, the image can move in the direction of frequency encoding even at the same location, which is called a chemical shift. In addition, hydrogen in water and fat shows different T1 relaxation times, with water hydrogen having a long T1 and fat hydrogen having a short T1.

The fat saturation technique is a method that utilizes the difference in frequency between water and fat. It is a method of giving an invert pulse that only corresponds to the area representing fat. Other tissues are not affected, so the signal-to-noise ratio (SNR) is good compared to the short tau inversion recovery (STIR), and almost no additional time is needed. It also has the advantage of being able to be used with contrast agents because it is not greatly affected by T1 relaxation time. However, because it uses a frequency that only selects fat tissue, it is greatly affected by the inhomogeneity of the magnetic field or RF filter, and it has a disadvantage that it is difficult to obtain uniform fat suppression images.

The inversion recovery technique is a method that utilizes the fact that the T1 relaxation time of hydrogen atoms in fat is shorter than that of hydrogen atoms in water. This method is sensitive to T1 relaxation time, so it cannot be used with contrast agents, and it has the disadvantage of a decreased signal-to-noise ratio. However, it has the advantage of being able to obtain uniform fat-suppressed images regardless of the homogeneity of the magnetic field in images with a wide imaging area (Fig. 3.2).

The opposed-phase technique is a quick and easy-to-apply technique that helps distinguish lesions with a small amount of fatty tissue. The problem is that it has low reliability in distinguishing small tumors buried in fatty tissue [3, 4].

3.1.3 Three-Dimensional MR T2 High-Resolution

This is an isotropic high-resolution 3D image, also called a three-dimensional (3D) CISS (constructive interference in steady state), 3D True-FISP (fast imaging with steady-state procession), or FIESTA (fast imaging employing steady-state acquisition) sequence. This image has the advantage of being able to reconstruct to other planes without image distortion because it is a high-resolution image that clearly shows small structures and is an isotropic image. Another 3D T2 high-resolution image is the SPACE (sampling perfection with application optimized contrasts using different flip angle evolution), CUBE, or VISTA (volume isotropic turbo spin echo acquisition) sequence of the fast spin echo series. This has the advantage of being less sensitive to flow and susceptibility artifacts and clearly showing the nerve root [5, 6].

These images can be used as MR myelography, which can non-invasively obtain anatomical information about the subarachnoid space because of the excellent contrast between the high signal intensity of the cerebrospinal fluid and the low signal intensity of the nerves. It is used to evaluate spinal nerves, thin walls of syringes, internal structures of cystic tumors, pseudomeningoceles after trauma, cerebrospinal fluid leaks, Tarlov cysts, etc.

It can also be used as MR neurography, which visualizes small peripheral nerves using the advantages of high resolution and signal-to-noise ratio. It is mainly used to evaluate the brachial plexus, lumbosacral plexus, thoracic outlet, etc. in diseases such as nerve damage, nerve tumors, inflammation, nerve compression associated with disc herniation, nerve compression syndrome, etc. (Fig. 3.3) [7].

3.1.4 Diffusion-Weighted Imaging (DWI)

Diffusion-weighted imaging (DWI) can show the random motion of water molecules in the body. Water molecules are constantly undergoing random Brownian motion when contained in a vessel outside the body. This unrestricted motion of water molecules is called free diffusion. In contrast, the movement of water molecules within tissues is restricted and altered by cell membranes and macromolecules. In tissues, the signal in DWI comes from the movement of water molecules in the extracellular space, intracellular space, and intravascular space. Water molecules in the blood vessels show greater diffusion than those in the extracellular or intracellular space

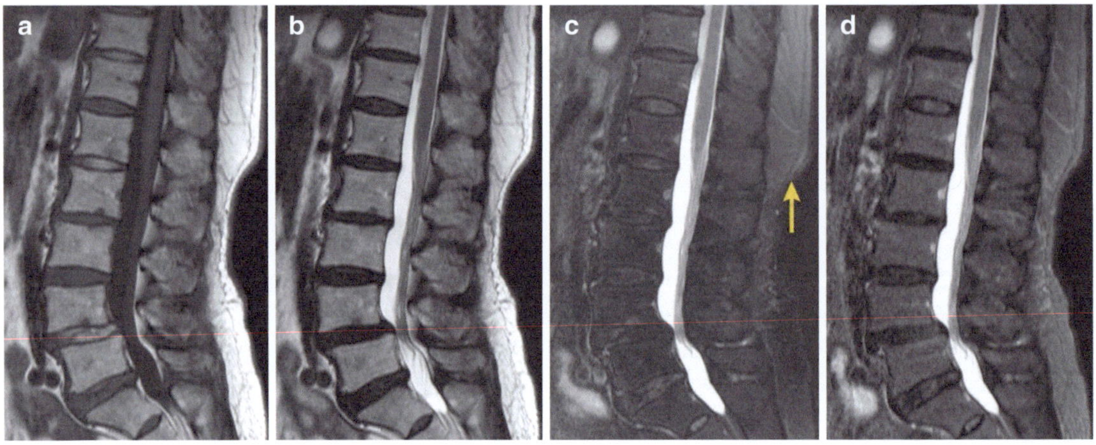

Fig. 3.2 A 58-year-old female patient. Degenerative spondylolisthesis of the fourth lumbar vertebra accompanied by spinal stenosis at the fourth-fifth lumbar region. (**a**) Fast spin echo T1-enhanced sagittal image. (**b**) Fast spin echo T2-enhanced sagittal image. (**c**) Fat-suppressed T2-enhanced sagittal image. Incomplete fat suppression is observed in the upper lumbar posterior fat tissue (arrow). (**d**) Short tau inversion recovery image. In this image, all areas of fat tissue show homogeneous fat suppression

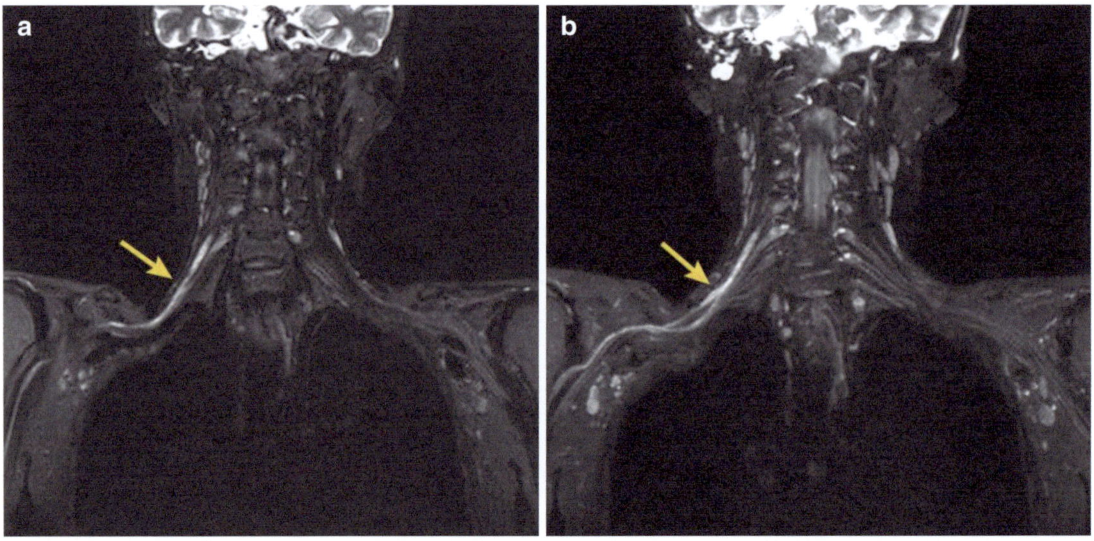

Fig. 3.3 A 55-year-old female patient. Right brachial plexopathy. (**a**) Three-dimensional high-resolution T2-enhanced coronal image. (**b**) 3D high-resolution T2-enhanced coronal image with maximum intensity projection reconstruction. The lesion site of the right brachial plexus shows a high T2 signal intensity

due to blood flow. In tumors showing an increase in blood flow, the diffusion of water in the blood vessels occupies a large part. The diffusion of water within the tissue is proportional to tissue cellularity and the integrity of the cell membrane. Therefore, the movement of water molecules is more restricted in tissues composed of numerous cells with normal cell membranes. In contrast, it is less restricted where the cell membrane is broken or there are fewer cells. The diffusion within the tissue is represented as apparent diffusion. Tissues can be defined by comparing the differences in apparent diffusion within the tissue. For example, tumors show restricted apparent diffusion compared to cysts because the free movement of water molecules is restricted due to the maintenance of the cell membrane [8, 9].

One simple method to obtain DWI images is to apply paired gradients (opposing and balanced magnetic field gradients) around the T2 emphasized spin echo refocusing pulse. Stationary water molecules are not affected by the paired gradients and maintain the original signal. However, moving water molecules lose the overall signal by not being rephased in the second gradient after receiving phase information from the first gradient. In DWI images, the decrease in signal is proportional to the amount of water molecule diffusion that occurs during the examination. As a result, tumors show less signal attenuation compared to normal tissue because the diffusion of water molecules is restricted, and they show signal intensity. The degree of applied diffusion emphasis is indicated by the b-value, which represents the time between the paired gradients and the duration and size of the applied gradient. By applying a variety of b-values, the sensitivity to the degree of diffusion movement changes. Using a large b-value is more sensitive to slow movement of water molecules and small diffusion distances. In the case of investigating malignant tumors, different b-values are used, through which the apparent diffusion coefficient (ADC; unit mm^2/s) can be calculated [10, 11].

In spinal imaging, these characteristics can be used to distinguish between benign and malignant fractures of the vertebral body. In DWI, benign fractures show similar or lower signal intensity to the surrounding vertebral bodies (Fig. 3.4), while malignant fractures show high signal intensity due to restricted diffusion of water molecules (Fig. 3.5).

3.1.5 Diffusion Tensor Imaging (DTI)

Diffusion tensor imaging (DTI) is an imaging test that can show the diffusion of water molecules within the tissue. Under conditions where water molecules can freely diffuse, they can spread equally in all directions [isotropic diffusion], but under conditions with physical restrictions (myelin sheath, neurofilaments, axonal membranes, etc.), diffusion can only be restricted in a specific direction [anisotropic [anisotropic diffusion]. Therefore, by observing how much or how little water molecules have diffused, we can verify the physical environment of the tissue. Diffusion tensor imaging, unlike diffusion-weighted imaging, measures diffusion in multiple directions to detect not only the magnitude of diffusion but also its direction. By applying a diffusion gradient in at least six directions, diffusion tensor images can be obtained. In white matter of the spinal cord, water molecules show anisotropic diffusion, which occurs most significantly in the same direction as the tract, whereas in gray matter, the degree of anisotropic diffusion is small. The most important variables in diffusion tensor imaging are mean diffusivity (MD) and fractional anisotropy (FA). MD refers to the total diffusion distance that occurred within a given voxel, and FA refers to the ratio of diffusions that occurred in different directions. A color-coded average FA map is typically used to indicate the direction of anisotropic diffusion. Generally, right/left diffusion directions are marked in red, up/down diffusion directions in blue, and front/back diffusion directions in green [12–14].

Echo planar imaging, which can sensitively reflect the uneven magnetic field strength, is used to obtain diffusion tensor images. However, in cases like the spinal cord where the magnetic field cannot be uniformly formed due to the relationship with various surrounding tissues, the quality of echo planar imaging has been problematic due to its decrease. Recently, with technological advancements, the quality of diffusion tensor imaging has improved, and its clinical usefulness has been confirmed. In the case of spinal cord tumors, it can be used to identify the boundary between the tumor and surrounding nerve fibers before surgery (Fig. 3.6). In the case of spinal cord injuries, there is research suggesting that a decrease in FA values can help assess the extent of actual nerve fiber damage. However, due to difficulties in image acquisition and image quality issues, it is not yet widely used clinically [13, 14].

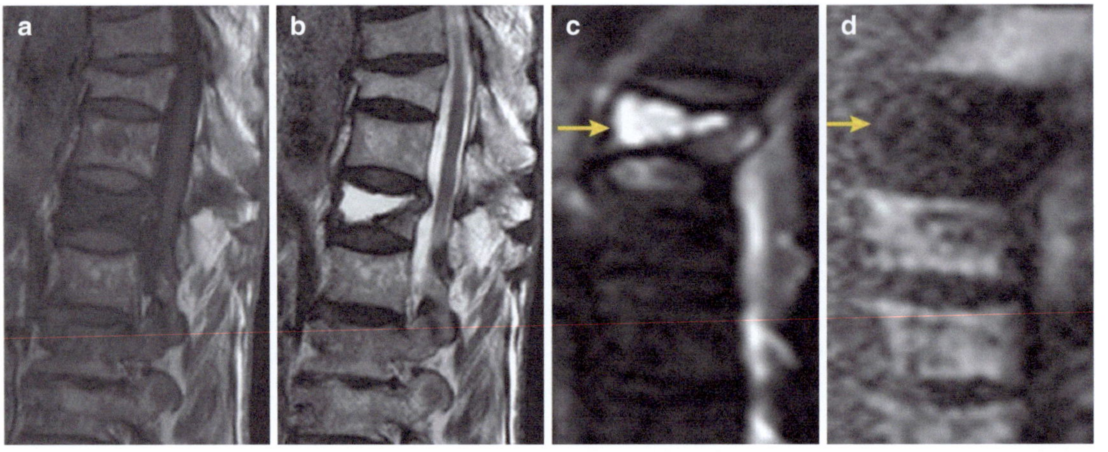

Fig. 3.4 A 79-year-old male patient. Benign compression fracture of the twelfth thoracic vertebra. (**a**) Fast spin echo T1-enhanced sagittal image. (**b**) Fast spin echo T2-enhanced sagittal image. (**c**) Diffusion-enhanced image (*b*-value, 0). The twelfth thoracic vertebra shows a high signal intensity (arrow). (**d**) Diffusion-enhanced image (*b*-value, 1400). The twelfth thoracic vertebra shows a low signal intensity (arrow)

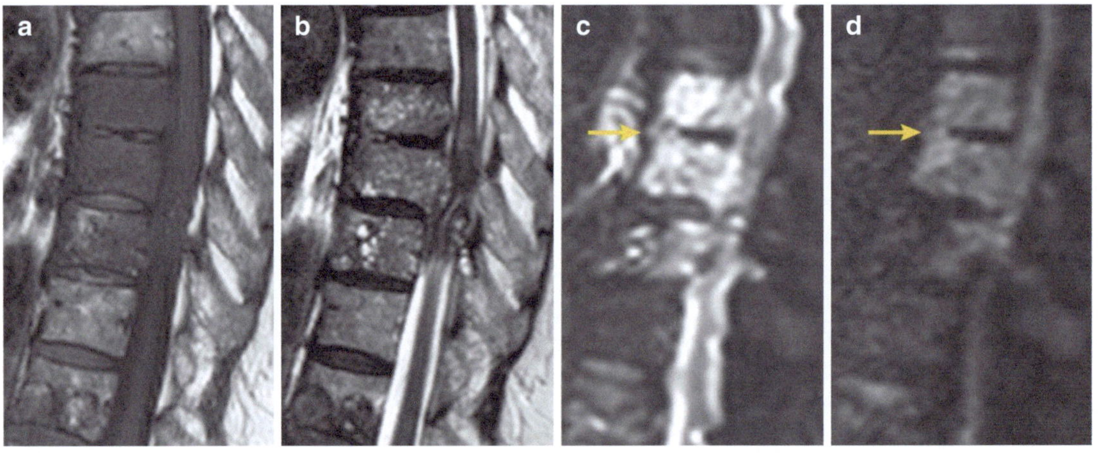

Fig. 3.5 A 77-year-old male patient. Metastatic carcinoma of the eighth-tenth and twelfth thoracic vertebrae. (**a**) Fast spin echo T1-enhanced sagittal image. (**b**) Fast spin echo T2-enhanced sagittal image. (**c**) Diffusion-enhanced image (*b*-value, 0) (arrow). (**d**) In the diffusion-enhanced image (*b*-value, 1400), the lesion site shows a high signal intensity (arrow)

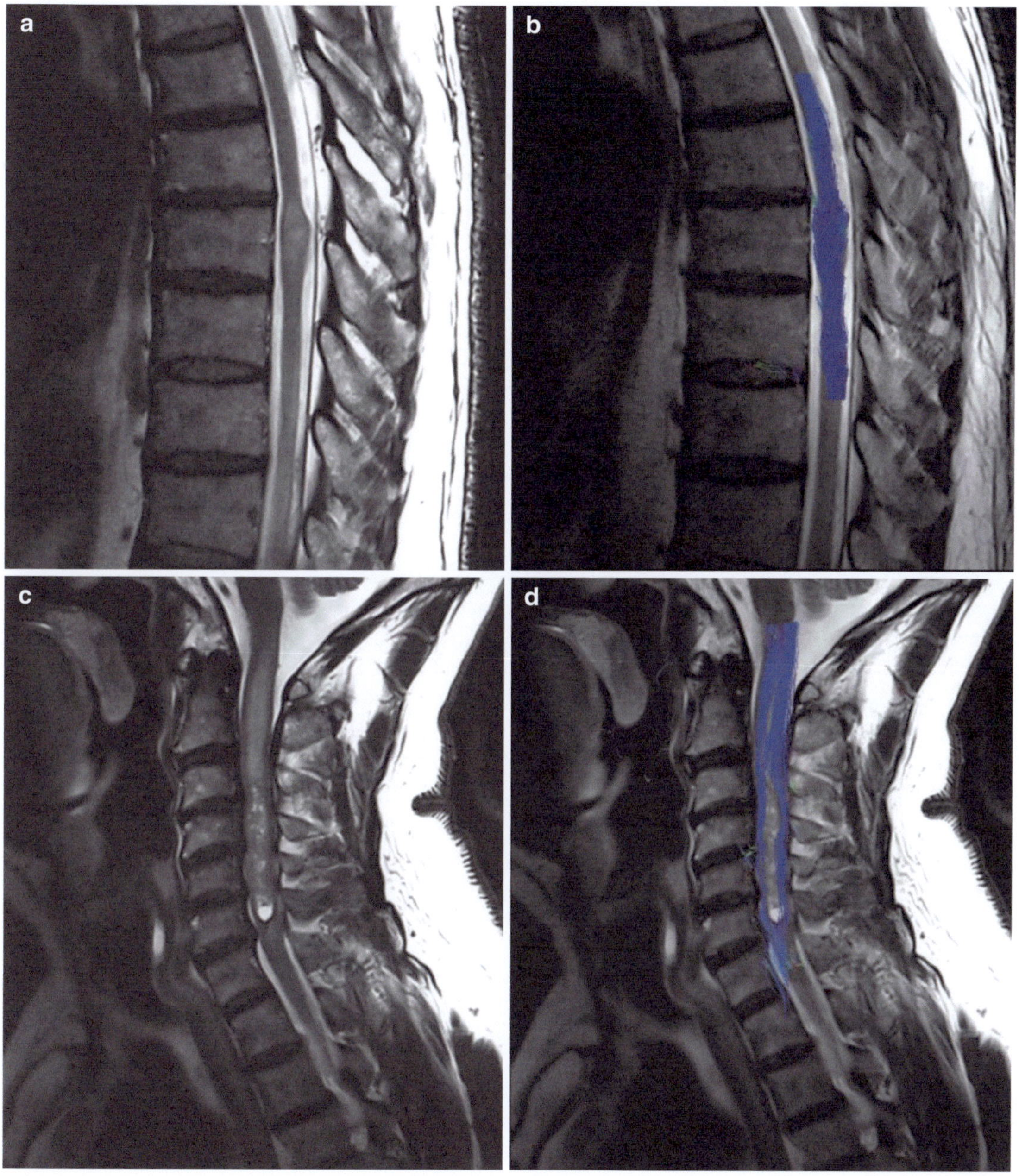

Fig. 3.6 Diffusion tensor imaging. (**a**) T2-enhanced image of astrocytoma. (**b**) Diffusion tensor image of astrocytoma. (**c**) T2-enhanced image of ependymoma. (**d**) Diffusion tensor image of ependymoma. In the diffusion tensor image, astrocytoma suggests a poor tumor boundary mixed with surrounding nerve fibers. However, ependymoma shows a good tumor boundary clearly distinguished from surrounding nerve fibers

3.2 Optimal Imaging Techniques for Spinal Magnetic Resonance Imaging

There can be many combinations depending on imaging techniques, shooting planes, shooting thickness/direction, etc. for spinal magnetic resonance imaging, but the following methods are mainly used.

Basic imaging techniques include

- T1-weighted sagittal images
- T2-weighted sagittal images
- T1-weighted axial images
- T2-weighted axial images

Other images used when there are symptoms but no findings in the basic imaging techniques, or to distinguish between benign and malignant compression fractures, and to identify the characteristics of infections or tumors, are as follows.

- Fat-suppressed images
- Diffusion-enhanced imaging
- Contrast-enhanced imaging
- Magnetic resonance myelography

3.2.1 T1-Weighted Imaging

T1-weighted imaging shows a high signal-to-noise ratio and helps distinguish anatomical structures. It is important to check for any abnormalities in the signal intensity of the bone marrow. Also, the height of the disc and the area of bone hardening are well observed.

3.2.2 T2-Weighted Imaging

It is good for distinguishing intervertebral disc lesions and can determine whether there is an abnormal signal intensity in the spinal cord. Normal intervertebral discs, cerebrospinal fluid, epidural fat, and most pathological findings show high signal intensity in T2-weighted images.

3.3 Utilization of Contrast-Enhanced Imaging

In magnetic resonance imaging of spinal lesions, most common diseases (such as disc herniation and spinal metastasis) can be diagnosed without the use of contrast agents, and the diversity of other components of the spine (spinal cord and nerve roots and nerves, intervertebral discs, vertebral bodies and joints, epidural tissues and vascular structures, etc.) can make it more complex when contrast-enhanced.

Anatomical structures of the spine can be divided into bone parts, epidural parts, extradural spinal parts, and intraspinal parts. Each of these has a unique anatomical structure and shows different diseases and pathological phenomena, so individual imaging strategies are needed.

Most lesions in the spine show low signal intensity in T1-weighted images, so the vertebral body, soft tissues around the spine, and fat tissues in the epidural space show high contrast in non-contrast T1-weighted images. To highlight abnormal findings against a background of many fat tissues, fat suppression images can be applied to T2-weighted images or contrast-enhanced T1-weighted images [15, 16].

3.3.1 Intraspinal Part

The spinal cord, part of the central nervous system, has a blood–spinal cord barrier that prevents contrast enhancement of the spinal cord and leptomeninges when normal. Like in the brain, the normal background contrasting with the lesion is the cerebrospinal fluid. The spinal cord has a similar anatomical structure to the brain and similar diseases occur, so similar images to brain images are used. Also, in certain diseases, increasing the amount of contrast agent or obtaining delayed images can help find the contrast-enhanced area.

In patients with multiple sclerosis or other demyelinating diseases, the time interval between contrast injection and image acquisition can be lengthened to find an abnormal blood–spinal cord barrier. In demyelinating diseases, contrast enhancement within the lesion can be seen as inflammation, and changes due to treatment can be confirmed. In the case of tumorous lesions, the extent of the tumor can be distinguished by the contrast-enhanced area, and it helps to determine the scope of surgical resection by distinguishing it from the T2 signal abnormality area due to accompanying edema.

In the spinal cord, contrast enhancement along the wall of the cystic lesion helps to distinguish between the non-contrast-enhanced syrinx cavity and the cystic tumor. In addition, contrast enhancement is important in diagnosing vascular lesions invading the spinal cord, and in the case of spinal vascular malformations, performing contrast-enhanced magnetic resonance angiography (MR angiography) helps in diagnosis.

3.3.2 Intrathecal Extramedullary Part

This corresponds to the subarachnoid space, and important anatomical structures include nerve roots, meninges (dura mater and arachnoid), pachymeninges, and spinal vessels.

Normally, the meninges and nerve roots do not show prominent contrast enhancement. In contrast-enhanced T1-weighted images, spinal arteries are small and not easily visible due to flow void phenomena, but normal veins show contrast enhancement findings due to slow flow. The normal veins that are contrast-enhanced from the back of the conus medullaris should not be confused with vascular malformations or meningeal diseases. Diseases that can be distinguished by contrast enhancement include infections, inflammations, and tumor diseases of the meninges, as well as meningiomas, neurofibromas, lymphomas, and metastases.

The basic imaging techniques for this area are T1-weighted images, T2-weighted images (fat-suppressed or non-fat-suppressed), and fat-suppressed contrast-enhanced T1-weighted images. In the case of tumors, multiplanar fat-suppressed T1-weighted images help to understand the contrast enhancement pattern and the relationship with surrounding structures. The most common tumors in this area are Schwannomas and Meningiomas.

3.3.3 Epidural Part

The epidural part is the space between the spinal canal and the dura mater, containing adipose tissue and vessels. An important point in the contrast-enhanced images of epidural diseases is to include fat suppression techniques. Because the epidural space, spinal marrow, and perispinal area are rich in fat, fat-suppressed images are used to reduce background signals. After contrast injection, normal contrast enhancement findings of the dorsal root ganglion and epidural plexus can be seen.

Common lesions in the epidural area are abscesses, hematomas, and tumors. Especially, abscesses and hematomas require caution as they can lead to severe neurological sequelae. Epidural hematomas are observed with various signal intensities depending on the degradation products of hemoglobin. Initially, hematomas do not show contrast enhancement. These findings should be distinguished from abscesses or tumors. It is an important opinion for discernment. The fat-suppressed T1-enhanced image obtained after contrast enhancement helps diagnose epidural abscesses that do not enhance in the center and show enhancement along the border, or confirm the site of infection (Fig. 3.7). Inflammatory reactions and swelling areas are also enhanced, so this should be considered when interpreting. Tumors in the epidural space are common when tumors around the adjacent vertebrae or spine invade the epidural space.

3.3.4 Spinal Bone Disease

The contrast-enhanced fat-suppressed T1-enhanced image is very useful for diagnosing tumors. The imaging techniques mainly used are T1-enhanced images, fat-suppressed T2-enhanced images or STIR images, contrast-enhanced fat-suppressed T1-enhanced images,

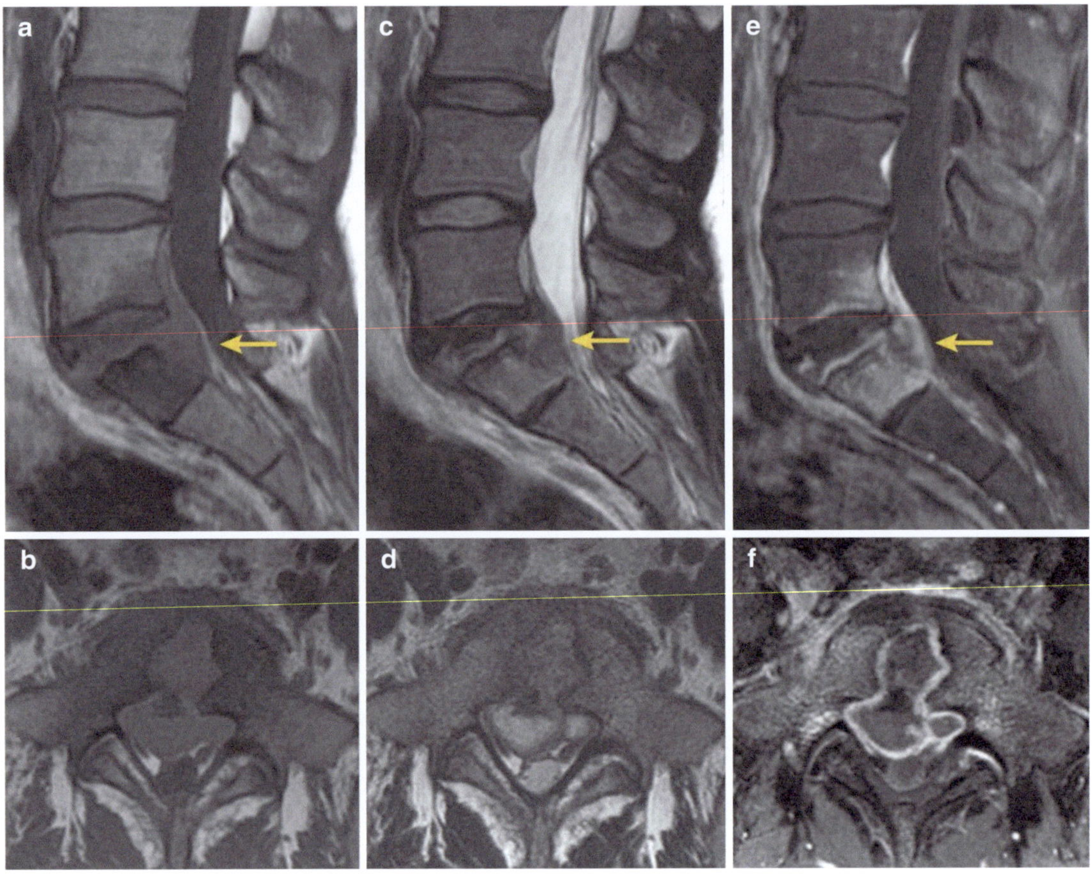

Fig. 3.7 A 26-year-old male patient. Tuberculous spondylitis of the fifth lumbar-first sacral region. (**a**) Fast spin echo T1-enhanced sagittal image (arrow). (**b**) Fast spin echo T2-enhanced sagittal image (arrow). (**c**) Fat-suppressed T1-enhanced sagittal image (arrow). (**d**) Fast spin echo T1-enhanced axial image. E. Fast spin echo T2-enhanced axial image. F. Fat-suppressed T1-enhanced contrast-enhanced axial image

etc. The marrow seen in the spine shows various signal intensities depending on the degree of fat marrow and hematopoietic marrow, but it shows relatively high signal intensity in non-contrast T1-enhanced images due to fat marrow. These findings help confirm local or widespread marrow abnormalities. Contrast-enhanced images are necessary to confirm the degree of vascularization of bone tumors or to distinguish vascular tumors like aggressive hemangiomas.

3.4 Magnetic Resonance Imaging Artifacts

An artifact refers to a signal that occurs regardless of the patient's anatomical structure, and it is a complex result of imaging equipment, gradient coils, high-frequency transceivers, and image reconstruction systems. Since artifacts can sometimes be mistaken for pathological findings, it is very important to know the findings and causes of these artifacts. The types of artifacts are very diverse and can be largely divided into equipment-related artifacts and patient-related artifacts. The artifacts that are mainly observed in the magnetic resonance imaging of the spine are as follows [17].

3.4.1 Equipment-Related Artifacts

(1) Susceptibility artifact

When the susceptibility of adjacent tissues in the body is different, local distortion of the magnetic field or signal reduction occurs, which is called a susceptibility artifact. Air and bone show lower susceptibility than soft tissue, so they are mainly observed at the boundary between air and soft tissue or bone and soft tissue. Artifacts caused by metallic implants are the same because they have higher susceptibility than body tissues, showing more severe distortion (Fig. 3.8). Recently, as there are many cases of performing magnetic resonance imaging in patients who have undergone surgery, the number of cases observing artifacts caused by metal is increasing. To reduce artifacts caused by metal, surgical devices should be positioned as much as possible in the direction of the main magnetic field. In terms of material, titanium alloy has less artifact than stainless steel. It is less. Among the imaging techniques, the fast spin echo technique is more advantageous than the gradient echo technique in reducing artifacts. In cases where fat-suppressed images are needed while minimizing artifacts, the short tau inversion recovery technique is better than the frequency-selective fat saturation technique. If you are using a high-field device, adjusting image variables (reduction of the shooting area, increase of the image grid, shooting of thin thickness, increase of ETL, increase of gradient intensity) can help. Recently, the SEMAC (Slice Encoding for Metal Artifact Correction) technique, which reduces metallic artifacts, has been introduced (Fig. 3.8) [18–20].

(2) Aliasing or wraparound artifact

This is a common artifact observed in magnetic resonance imaging, where if the imaging area is smaller than the examination area, the image of one peripheral part overlaps on the opposite side. It can occur in both frequency encoding and phase encoding directions, but usually occurs in the phase encoding direction (Fig. 3.9).

(3) Truncation, gibbs, or ringing artifact

In magnetic resonance imaging, it is observed as a bright or dark line parallel to the boundary where a sudden change in signal intensity is shown. This occurs because the number of samples measuring the signal is limited, and

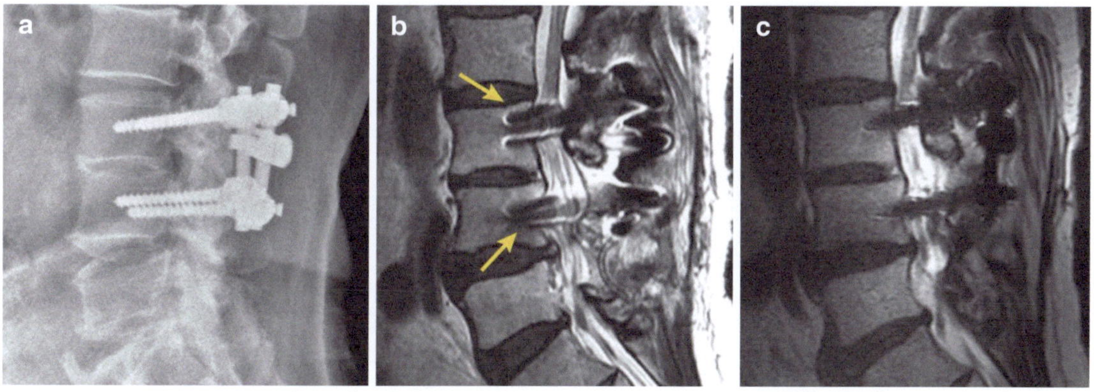

Fig. 3.8 A 69-year-old male patient. Ferromagnetic artifact at the site of posterior fixation of the third and fourth lumbar vertebrae. (**a**) The posterior fixation device at the third and fourth lumbar vertebrae is visible in the plain image. (**b**) The ferromagnetic artifact is observed in the fast spin echo T2-enhanced sagittal image (arrow). (**c**) The artifact is reduced in the SEMAC image that minimizes metallic artifacts

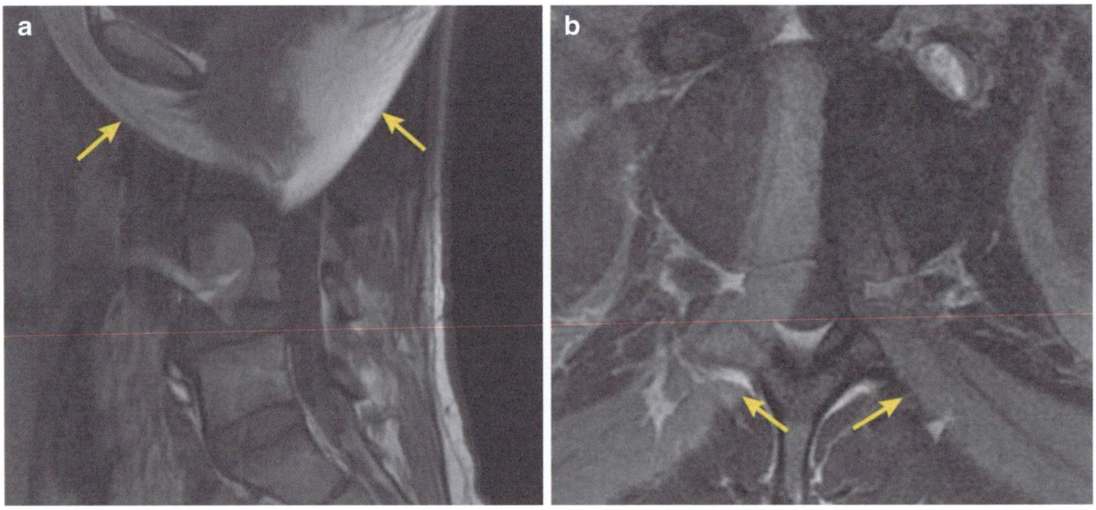

Fig. 3.9 A 40-year-old female patient. Image overlap artifact due to small imaging area. (**a**) In the fast spin echo T1-enhanced sagittal image, the image of the pelvic area overlaps with the lumbar area (arrow). (**b**) In the fast spin echo T1-enhanced axial image, the lateral side of the lumbar and body overlaps (arrow)

although there are degrees of difference, it is an artifact that exists in all images (Fig. 3.10).

(4) Chemical shift artifact
The hydrogen atoms of water and fat have different resonance frequencies, and this difference is called a chemical shift. The chemical shift between water and fat occurs in the frequency encoding direction, and the signal intensity of the fat tissue in the image is slightly shifted to the side. As a result, it shows a bright signal in the direction of low frequency and a low signal in the direction of high frequency. It is mainly observed in places surrounded by fat (Fig. 3.11).

3.4.2 Patient-Related Artifacts

(1) Motion artifact
The patient's movement during shooting creates artifacts, which makes the boundaries of the image unclear. Breathing or heartbeat creates artifacts in the phase encoding direction. Generally, periodic movements create artifacts of a certain shape, and non-periodic movements blur the boundaries of tissues. In spinal imaging, the movement of cerebrospinal fluid is mainly observed in the thoracic spine images, and care should be taken as it

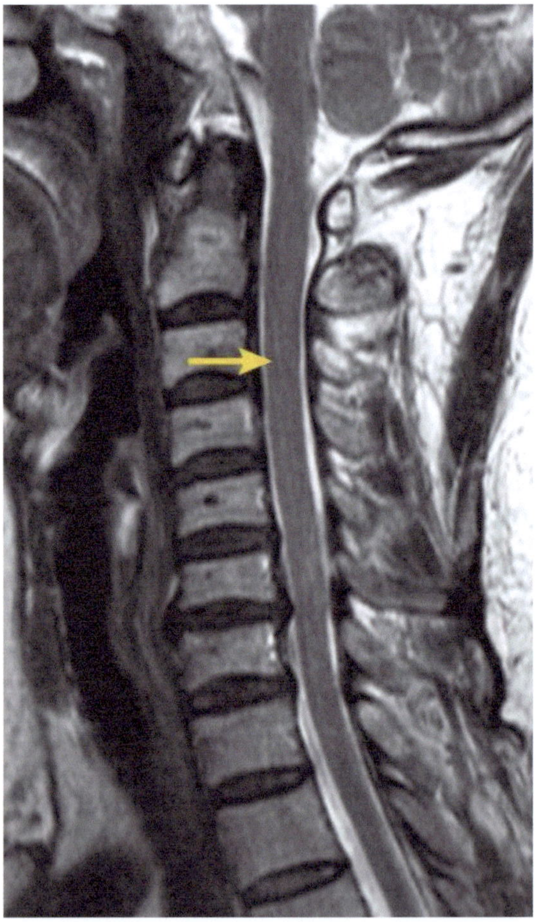

Fig. 3.10 A 63-year-old female patient. Truncation artifact A high signal intensity band is seen in the spinal cord in the fast spin echo T2-enhanced sagittal image (arrow)

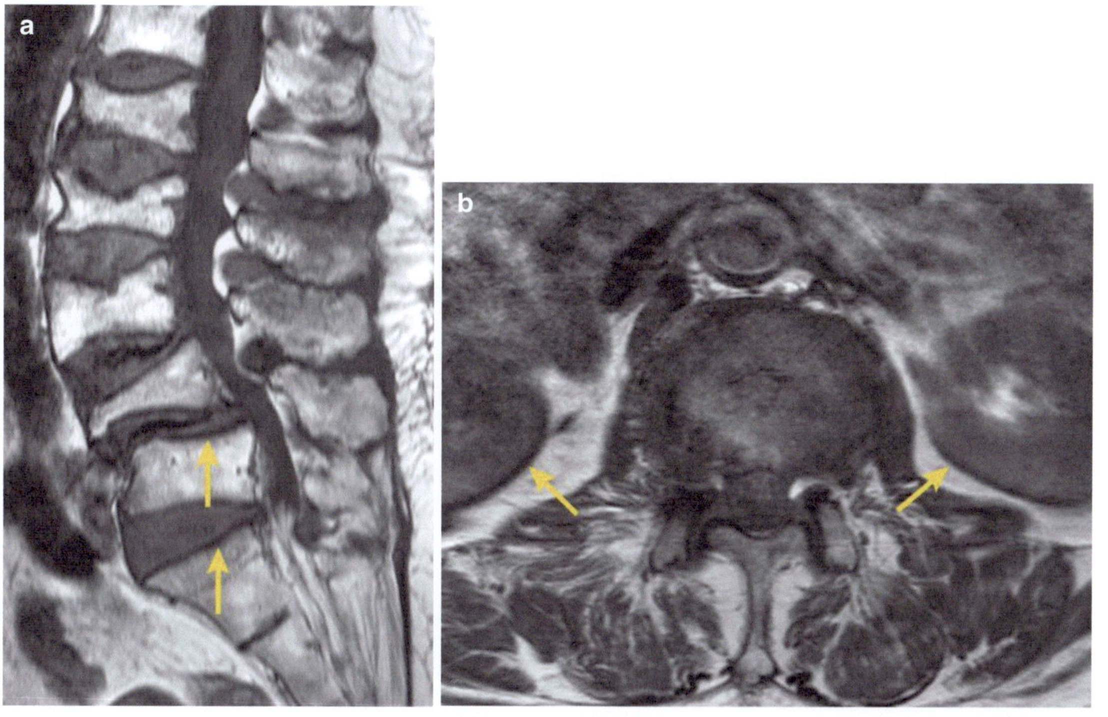

Fig. 3.11 A 69-year-old female patient. Chemical shift artifact. (**a**) In the fast spin echo T1-enhanced sagittal image, the superior endplate of the fifth lumbar and first sacral vertebrae shows a thick band of low signal intensity (arrow). (**b**) In the fast spin echo T1-enhanced axial image, a band of low signal intensity is seen along the posterior border of the right kidney (arrow)

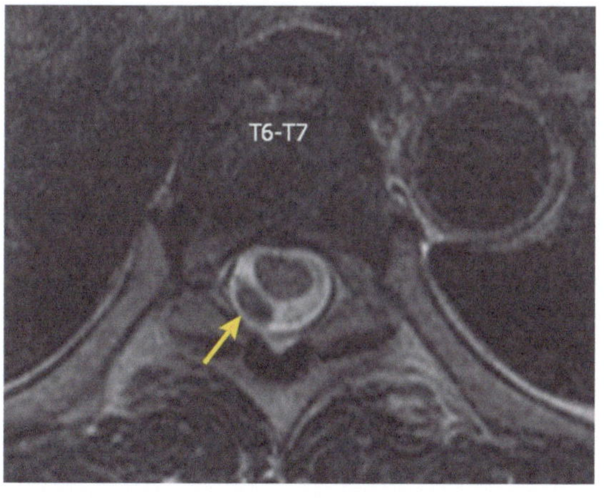

Fig. 3.12 A 60-year-old female patient. Motion artifact due to cerebrospinal fluid in the thoracic vertebrae
A low signal intensity artifact is seen in the cerebrospinal fluid in the fast spin echo T2-enhanced axial image (arrow)

can be mistaken for intradural tumors or vascular malformations (Fig. 3.12).

(2) Flow artifact

Blood flow is a form of motion artifact that causes signal loss in the phase encoding direction. In the spin echo technique, the blood flow leaves the imaging area before the 180-degree refocusing pulse after being exposed to the 90-degree excitation pulse, resulting in black (Fig. 3.13). It also creates phenomena that appear bright in gradient echo images.

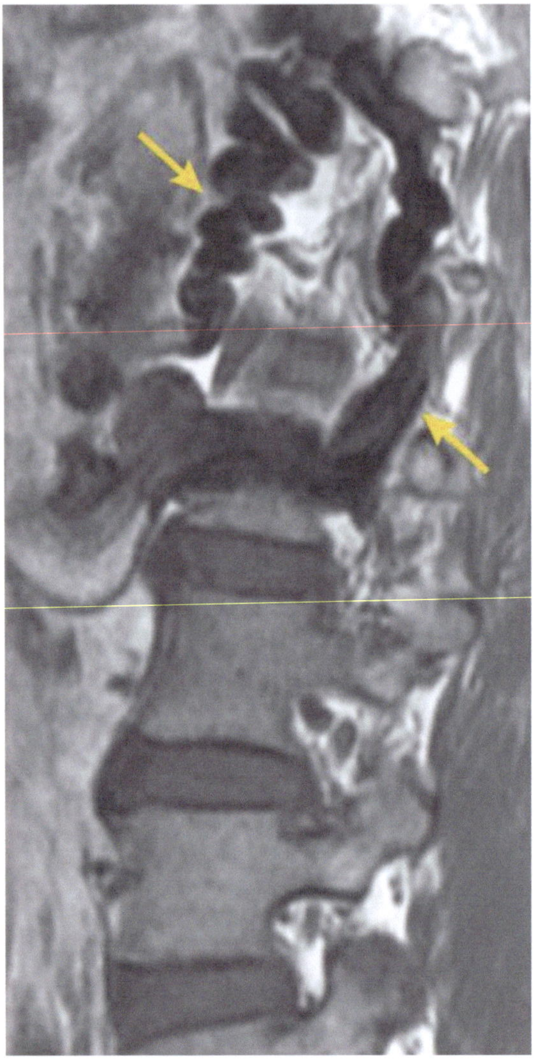

Fig. 3.13 A 60-year-old male patient. Flow artifact seen in a patient with Budd–Chiari syndrome
The lateral circulation vessels show low signal intensity due to signal loss in the fast spin T1-enhanced sagittal image (arrow)

3.5 3T Imaging

High-field imaging has many advantages, but new challenges must be overcome to optimize image quality. The resonance frequency given by the Larmor equation is proportional to the magnetic field strength. When the magnetic field strength increases from 1.5T to 3T, the difference in resonance frequency between fat and water hydrogen atoms doubles. This phenomenon causes data errors in k-space and leads to chemical shift artifacts in the image. Chemical shifts can be reduced by increasing the receiver bandwidth. A similar effect can be seen by reducing the imaging area. These changes reduce the signal-to-noise ratio, but this is more than compensated for by the improvement in image quality at 3T.

As the strength of the magnetic field increases, the sensitivity to magnetic field inhomogeneity also increases. Also, at 3T, signal loss or geometric distortion increases due to shortening of T2 and T2*. To maintain good image quality at 3T in patients with iron-containing implants after spinal surgery, sensitivity must be mitigated. This can be achieved by increasing the receiver bandwidth, maximizing ETL, reducing slice thickness and echo time, and positioning frequency encoding parallel to the long axis of the metal, which can reduce artifacts.

As the strength of the magnetic field increases, artifacts due to flow and pulsation also increase. This can make it difficult to find lesions in T1-weighted images, especially in T1-fast spin echo techniques.

Regardless of the magnetic field, the quality of spinal MRI is improved by placing saturation bands between pulsating vessels and these vessels and important anatomical structures. Along with this, avoiding the use of anterior-posterior direction for phase encoding also helps prevent these artifacts.

Theoretically, the signal-to-noise ratio of 3T imaging is twice that of 1.5T imaging. The increase in signal can be used to optimize the image. At 3T, a thin anatomical slice can maintain the same or higher signal-to-noise ratio as 1.5T. Especially at 3T, the slice thickness can be halved when using the same grid as 1.5T. This helps in 3D imaging techniques using thin slices. If the same slice is maintained as 1.5T, the grid size can be doubled to increase spatial resolution. Other conditions at 3T can maintain the same spatial resolution and signal-to-noise ratio as 1.5T, but can shorten the examination time (21).

Bibliography

1. Gillams AR, Soto JA, Carter AP. Fast spin echo vs conventional spin echo in cervical spine imaging. Eur Radiol. 1997;7:1211–4.
2. à Nijeholt GL, Castelijns JA, Weerts J, Ader H, van Waesberghe JH, Polman C, Barkhof F. Sagittal MR of multiple sclerosis in the spinal cord: fast versus conventional spin-echo imaging. AJNR Am J Neuroradiol. 1998;19:355–60.
3. Delfaut EM, Beltran J, Johnson G, Rousseau J, Marchandise X, Cotton A. Fat suppression in MR imaging: techniques and pitfalls. Radiographics. 1999;19:373–82.
4. Dennis R. Optimal magnetic resonance imaging of the spine. Vet Radiol Ultrasound. 2011;52:S72–80.
5. Chhabra A, Andreisek G, Soldatos T, et al. MR neurography: past, present, and future. AJR Am J Roentgenol. 2011;197:583–91.
6. Chhabra A, Zhao L, Carrino JA, et al. MR Neurogr: Adv Radiol Res Pract. 2013;2013:809568.
7. Carpenter EL, Bencardino JT. Focus on advanced magnetic resonance techniques in clinical practice: magnetic resonance neurography. Radiol Clin North Am. 2015;53:513–29.
8. Bammer R. Basic principles of diffusion-weighted imaging. Eur J Radiol. 2003;45:168–84.
9. Koh DM, Padhani AR. Diffusion-weighted MRI: a new functional clinical technique for tumour imaging. Br J Radiol. 2006;79:633–5.
10. Baur A, Dietrich O, Reiser M. Diffusion-weighted imaging of bone marrow: current status. Eur Radiol. 2003;13:1699–708.
11. Parker GJM. Analysis of MR diffusion weighted images. Br J Radiol. 2004;77:S176–85.
12. Nagayama M, Wadanave Y, Okumura A, Amoh Y, Nakashita S, Dodo Y. High -resolution single-slice MR myelography. AJR Am J Roentgenol. 2002;179:515–21.
13. O'Connell MJ, Ryan M, Powell T, Eustace S. The value of routine MR myelography at MRI of the lumbar spine. Acta Radiol. 2003;44:665–72.
14. Mahnken AH, Wildverger JE, Adam G, et al. Is there a need for contrast-enhanced T1-weighted MRI of the spine after inconspicuous short T inversion recovery imaging? Eur Radiol. 2005;15:1387–92.
15. Colosimo C, Cianfoni A, Lella GMI, Gaudino S. Contrast-enhanced MR imaging of the spine: when, why and how? How to optimize contrast protocols in MR imaging of the spine. Neuroradiology. 2006;48:18–33.
16. Zhuo J, Gullapalli RP. MR artifacts, safety, and quality control. Radiographics. 2006;26:275–97.
17. Lu W, Pauly KB, Gold GE, Pauly JM, Hargreaves BA. SEMAC: slice encoding for metal artifact correction in MRI. Magn Reson Med. 2009;62(1):66–76.
18. Lee MJ, Kim SJ, Lee SA, et al. Overcoming artifacts from metallic orthopedic implants at high field strength MR imaging and multidetector CT. Radiographics. 2007;27:791–803.
19. Rutherford EE, Tarplett LJ, Davies EM, Harley JM, King LJ. Lumbar spine fusion and stabilization: hardware, techniques, and imaging appearances. Radiographics. 2007;27:1737–49.
20. Shapiro MD. MR imaging of the spine at 3T. Magn Reson Imaging Clin N Am. 2006;14:97–108.

Development of Normal Pediatric Spine and Congenital Spinal and Spinal Cord Disorders

4

Ji Young Kim

The immature spine of a child, which has not undergone sufficient ossification, not only differs in basic shape from an adult spine, but can also be mistaken for abnormal findings such as fractures due to various secondary ossification centers that are not visible in adults. Also, the ligaments supporting the spine are looser than in adults, leading to hypermobility, which can result in changes in spinal alignment. This chapter aims to understand the normal shape of the pediatric spine, anatomical structures appearing during spinal ossification, and normal variations of the spine, and to facilitate the distinction between normal variations and pathological conditions of the spine. Also, it aims to focus on congenital spinal and spinal cord disorders that can commonly be seen in adult age.

4.1 Development of the Normal Spine

4.1.1 Normal Morphology of the Pediatric Spine

In young children, including newborns (up to about 2 years old), the vertebral body appears oval. As age increases, it changes to a rectangular shape with rounded corners, and in adolescence, it becomes similar to the shape of an adult vertebral body (Fig. 4.1). The curvature of the newborn spine is gentler than that of an adult. After the first year of life, as the head support structure develops to hold the head, cervical lordosis is enhanced. Then, as upright walking becomes possible, lumbar lordosis begins to become distinct at about 2 years of age. The spinal curvature then becomes more pronounced, and after puberty, it settles into a shape similar to that of an adult (Fig. 4.2).

4.1.2 Ossification of the Normal Spine

During development, the spine forms one ossification center in the center of the vertebral body and one ossification center in each neural arch, resulting in a total of three primary ossification centers at birth (Fig. 4.3). The ossification centers of the vertebral body and the neural arch are connected by a cartilaginous part called the neurocentral synchondrosis. The neurocentral synchondrosis is a site of endochondral ossification, similar to the growth plate of a long bone. The ossification centers of the vertebral body and the neural arch fuse around the ages of 3–6, and the ossification centers of the bilateral neural arches fuse around the ages of 2–3. In a newborn's simple spinal radiograph where fusion between the neural arches has not occurred, the unfused cartilaginous part between the neural

J. Y. Kim (✉)
Department of Radiology, Seoul National University Bundang Hospital, Seongnam-si, Republic of Korea

© The Author(s), under exclusive license to Springer Nature Singapore Pte Ltd. 2025

H. S. Kang, J. W. Lee (eds.), *Spinal Imaging*, https://doi.org/10.1007/978-981-95-1386-4_4

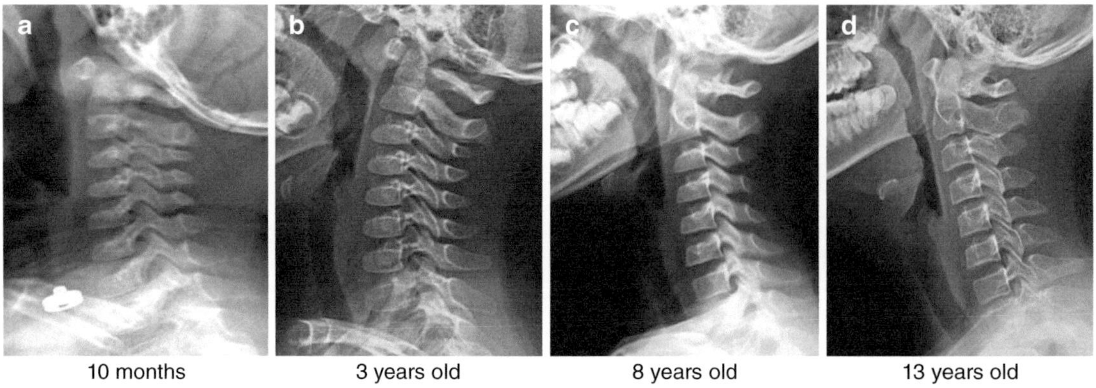

Fig. 4.1 The shape of a normal spine
When looking at the lateral plain radiographs of children by age, a 10-month-old infant shows a round vertebral body shape, which changes to a rectangular shape with rounded corners as age increases, and shows a rectangular shape similar to an adult vertebral body when reaching adolescence

arches appears as a gap, which can look like spina bifida (Fig. 4.3d, e). During puberty, a total of five secondary ossification centers develop in the spine, one at the end of each transverse process, one in the spinous process, and one at the top and bottom corners of the vertebral body, located on the epiphyseal plate of the vertebral body. The vertebral body epiphyseal plate is a "C"-shaped cartilage plate located at the top and bottom corners of the vertebral body, and the secondary ossification center that occurs on this growth plate is called the ring apophysis. The ring apophysis appears between the ages of 6 and 12 and fuses with the vertebral body around the age of 18. The ring apophysis appears as a small sclerotic linear shadow (step-like recess) at the top and bottom front corners of the vertebral body in a lateral simple radiograph of the spine (Fig. 4.4). This can be mistaken for a fracture if one is not familiar with the stages of spinal ossification. In a lateral photograph of a newborn's spine where the ossification of the vertebral body is not sufficiently progressed, anterior and posterior clefts of the vertebral body are commonly seen, which are thought to be due to vascular passages (Fig. 4.5). The posterior cleft can persistently be seen even in adults. The axis (C2) differs from other vertebrae in that it has a total of four primary ossification centers [vertebral body, bilateral neural arches, odontoid process] and undergoes a somewhat complex ossification process. At birth, the top of the odontoid process appears divided, and the odontoid process and the axis body fuse around the age of 6. The secondary ossification center of the odontoid process, the Os terminale, appears around the age of 3 and fuses with the odontoid process around the age of 12 (Fig. 4.6).

4.1.3 Magnetic Resonance Imaging of the Pediatric Spine

Magnetic resonance imaging of the pediatric spine in newborns, the bone marrow is composed of hematopoietic marrow with little fat content, which appears as low signal intensity on T1-weighted images, similar to or slightly lower than the signal intensity of the intervertebral disc. After the age of 1, the degree of low signal intensity of the bone marrow on T1-weighted images gradually decreases, and after the age of 5, it mostly shows higher signal intensity than the intervertebral disc (Fig. 4.2).

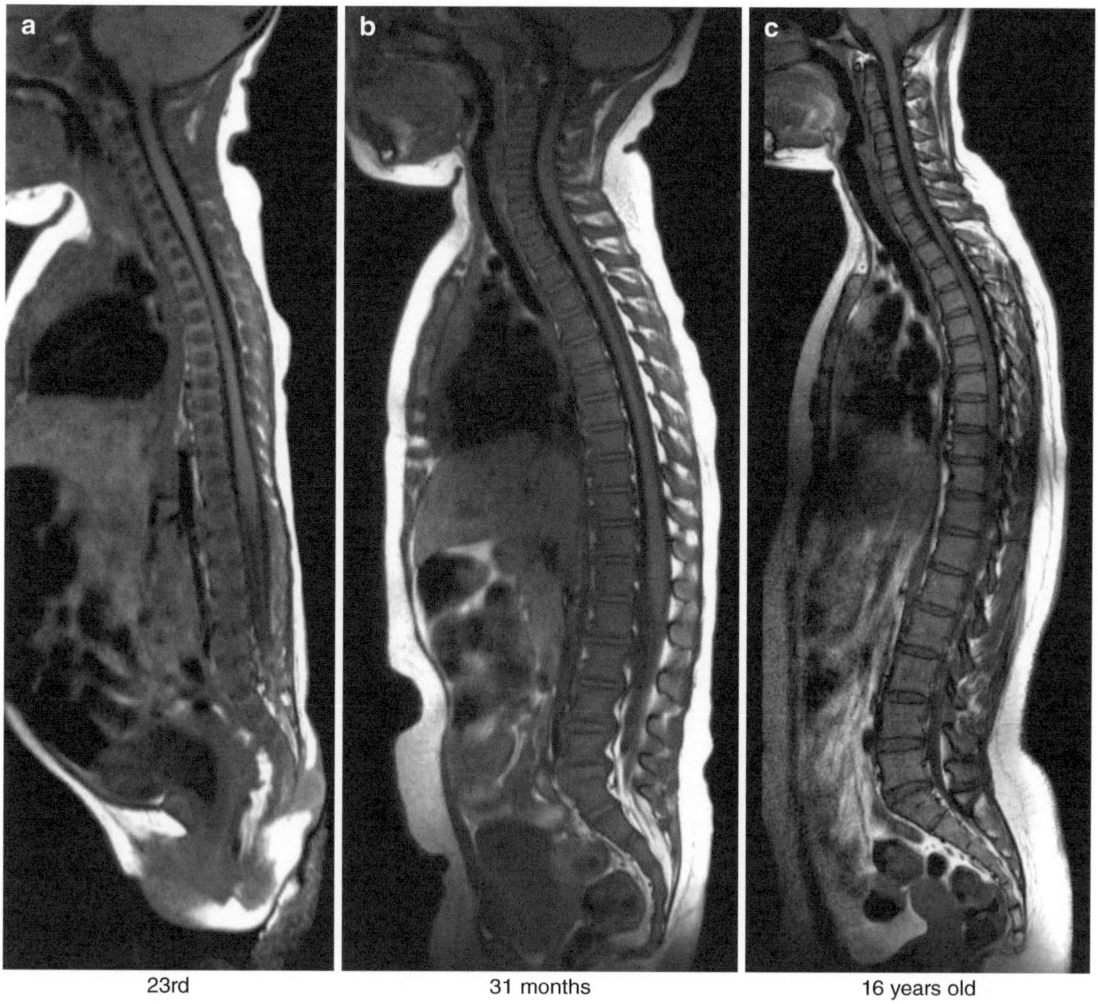

Fig. 4.2 The curvature and MRI of a normal spine
The gentle spinal curvature in newborns becomes similar to adults as the cervical lordosis and lumbar lordosis are enhanced with growth. In the sagittal view of T1-weighted MRI, the spinal marrow of a 23-day-old newborn shows a lower signal intensity than the intervertebral disc, but the signal intensity gradually increases, and the 16-year-old spinal marrow shows a higher signal intensity than the intervertebral disc

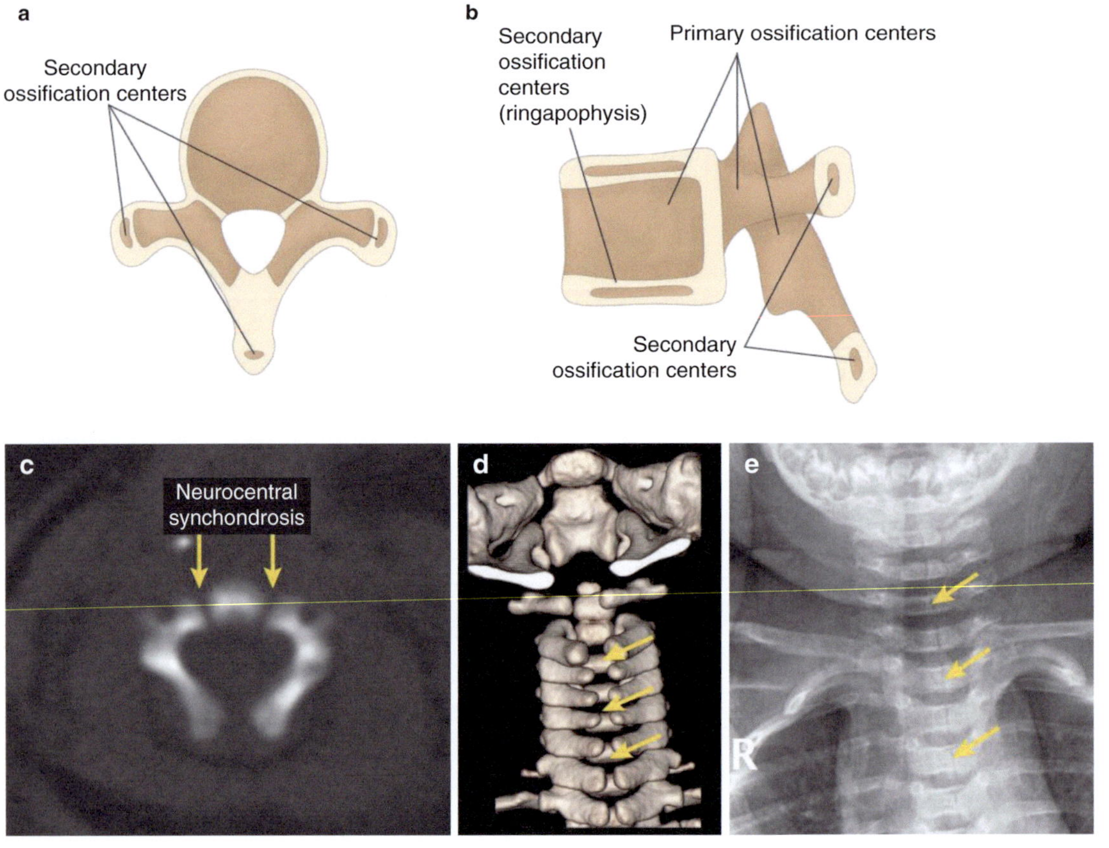

Fig. 4.3 Ossification of the spine. (**a**–**c**) The spine is born with three primary ossification centers (one in the center of the vertebral body, one on each side of the vertebral arch) and a total of five secondary ossification centers appear as it grows. (**d**, **e**) The ununited cartilage part between the infantile vertebral arches is shown on CT. The gap between the spinal arches (arrow) can be seen in simple spinal imaging or video, which can look like spina bifida

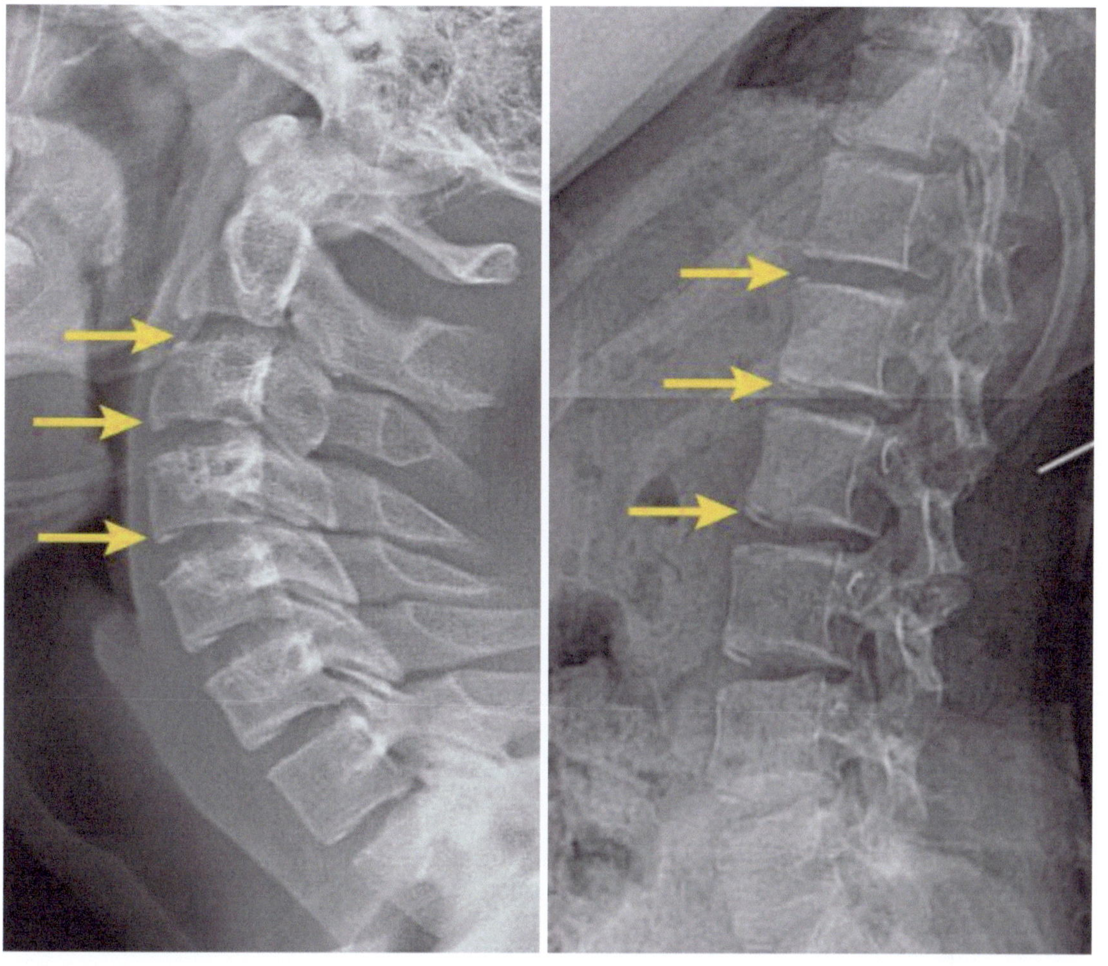

Fig. 4.4 Ring apophysis
As a secondary ossification center that occurs in the vertebral body growth plate, it can be mistaken for a fracture as it appears as a sclerotic linear shadow on the upper and lower edges of the anterior corner of the cervical and lumbar vertebrae in simple lateral imaging (arrow)

Fig. 4.5 Anterior and posterior cleft of the vertebral body
In the lateral photo of a newborn's spine taken one day after birth, the anterior and posterior clefts of the vertebral body, known to be caused by vascular pathways, are visible

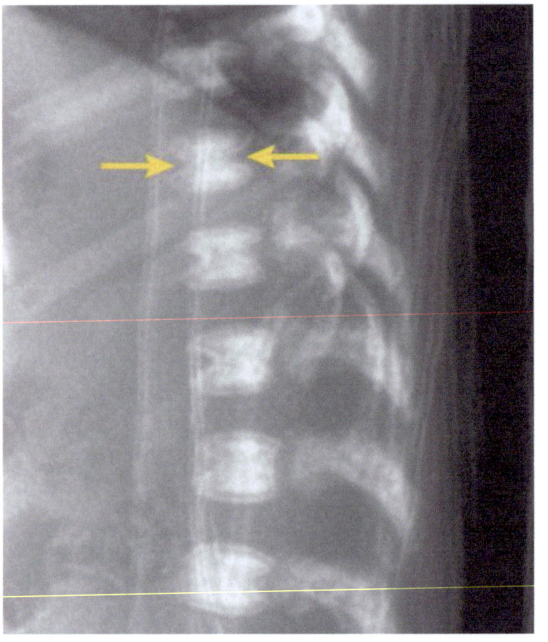

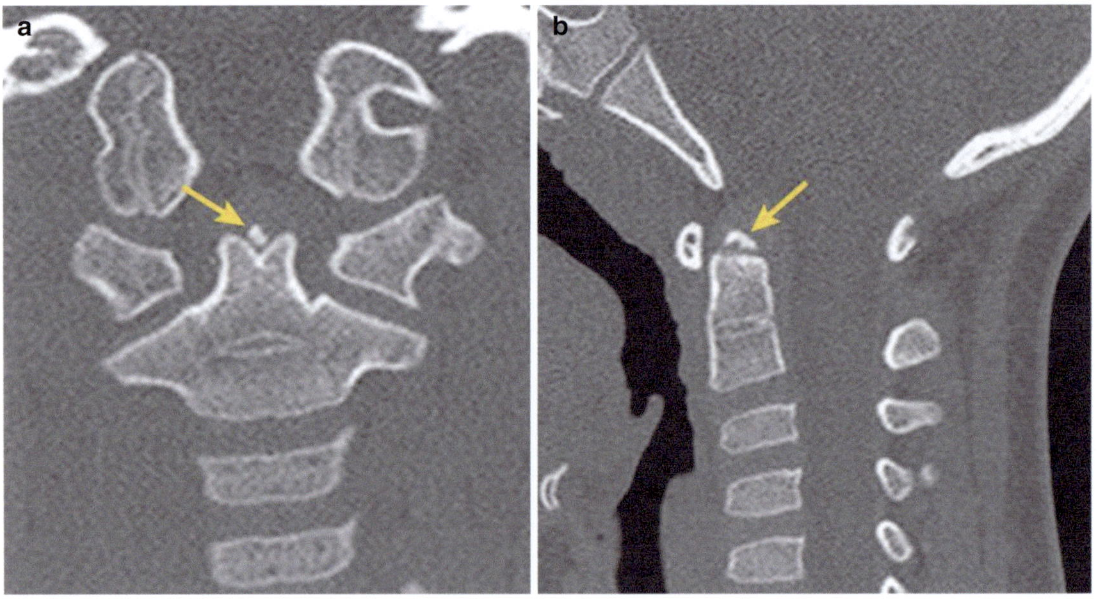

Fig. 4.6 Os terminale
In the cervical CT image of a 5-year-old boy, the divided upper part of the odontoid process and the small secondary ossification center at the end of the odontoid process, the os terminale (arrow), are visible

4.2 Normal Anatomical Variations of the Pediatric Spine

In infants or young children, the arrangement of the spine shows normal hypermobility due to the flexibility of the ligaments that help stabilize the spine. The changes in the shape and arrangement of the spine caused by this hypermobility can be mistaken for pathological conditions. These changes due to spinal hypermobility commonly occur in the upper cervical spine, as the apex of the cervical curve is located at the upper cervical spine level of C2–3 during cervical flexion in children. In contrast, the apex of the adult cervical curve is located at the mid cervical level of C4–6, and degenerative changes often start at the level of C4–5.

4.2.1 Pseudo-Jefferson Fracture

This is a pseudospread finding where the atlas appears to be spread out compared to the axis in the open mouth view of the cervical spine plain radiograph (Fig. 4.7). This is a false finding that appears because the cartilage part of the spine, which is not fully ossified, is not visible in the plain radiograph. Up to the age of 4, the atlas can appear to be displaced laterally up to 6 mm, and sometimes it can be seen up to the age of 7.

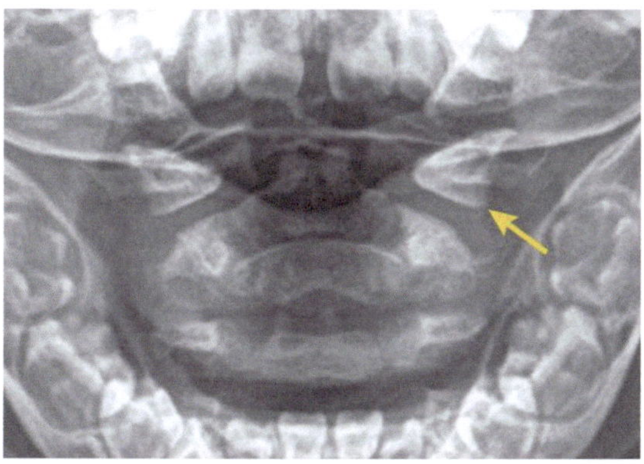

Fig. 4.7 Pseudo-Jefferson fracture
In the open mouth view simple imaging, the atlas appears to be spread out compared to the axis, a phenomenon known as pseudospread

4.2.2 High Anterior Arch of C1

This is when the anterior arch of the atlas is located so high that it appears to be displaced, a finding is commonly seen in young infants when the cervical spine is hyperextended (Fig. 4.8). This is due to the hypermobility of C1 during hyperextension.

4.2.3 Exaggerated C1–2 Interspinous Distance

This is a finding that the distance between the spinous processes of C1 and C2 increases, which appears due to the hypermobility of C1 when the cervical spine is flexed (Fig. 4.9). This finding can be seen not only in infants but also in relatively older children. The interspinous distance of C1–2 can normally increase up to 10 mm, even up to 12 mm, but in this case, it can be differentiated from pathological conditions by confirming that the predental distance (C1-dens distance) is maintained normally.

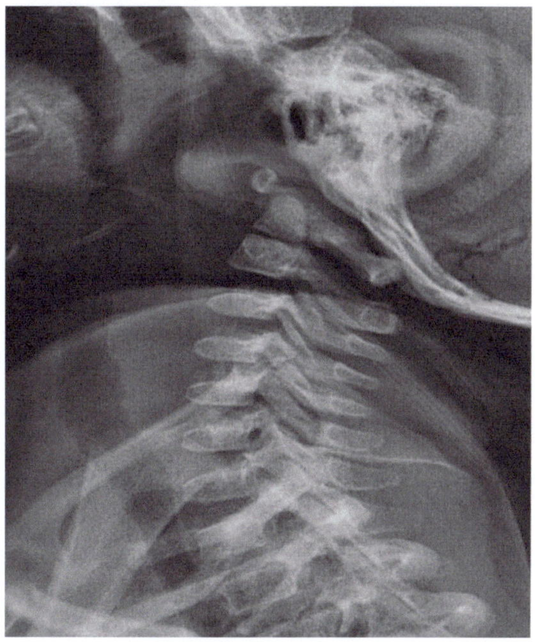

Fig. 4.8 High anterior arch of C1
The anterior arch of the atlas is positioned higher than the odontoid process, making it look as if it has moved forward, but this is a normal variant seen in infants

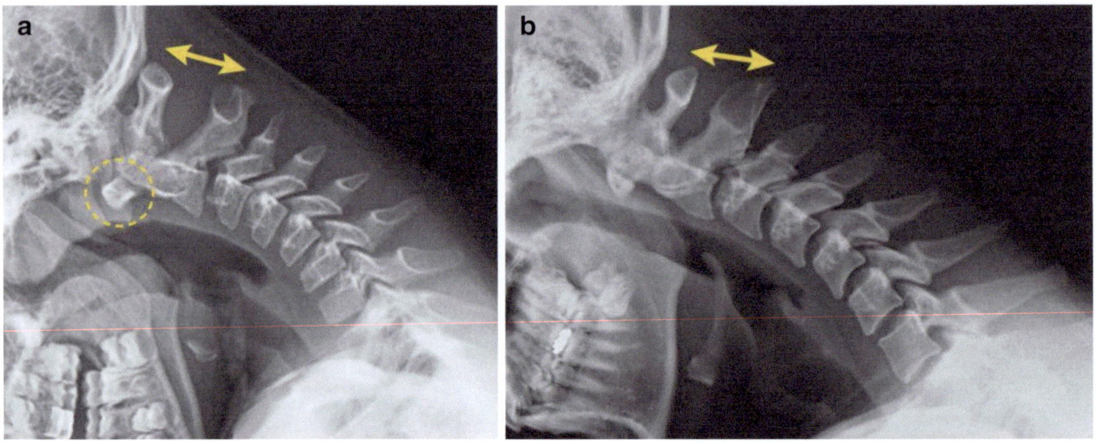

10 years old 19 years old

Fig. 4.9 Exaggerated C1–2 interspinous distance
In the image of a 10-year-old patient's flexed cervical spine, the C1–2 interspinous distance is increased, but the predental distance (C1-dens distance) is maintained normally. At the age of 19, closer to adulthood, the C1–2 interspinous distance does not increase even when flexed

4.2.4 Cervical Pseudosubluxation

In the lateral view of the cervical spine plain radiograph, anterolisthesis of the vertebral body can be seen between C2–3 or C3–4, which is a normal variation due to ligament flexibility (Fig. 4.10). In this case, it can be differentiated from pathological conditions by confirming that the posterior cervical line connecting the spinous processes is normal.

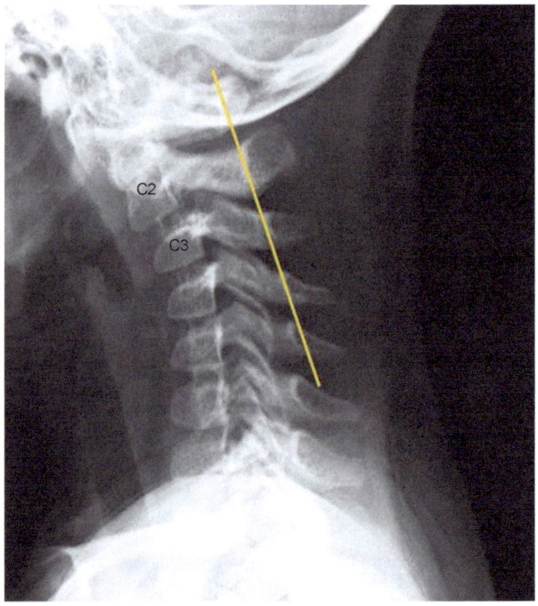

Fig. 4.10 Pseudosubluxation of C2 on C3
Although C2 is anteriorly displaced compared to C3, the posterior cervical line (yellow straight line) is well maintained, indicating that it is a pseudosubluxation, a normal variant of the cervical spine

4.2.5 Anterior Vertebral Wedging

This is a finding where the height of the anterior part of the vertebral body appears slightly reduced, a finding that appears in infancy (Fig. 4.11). It is accepted that this appears due to a growth disorder occurring in the upper front of the lower vertebral body as the angulation between the vertebral bodies deepens due to the hypermobility of the spine when the spine is flexed. Therefore, this finding is prominently seen in the upper cervical spine, especially in C3, C4. Therefore, in infancy, anterior vertebral wedging of about 3 mm should not be mistaken for pathological conditions such as compression fractures. Anterior vertebral wedging improves and disappears as it grows.

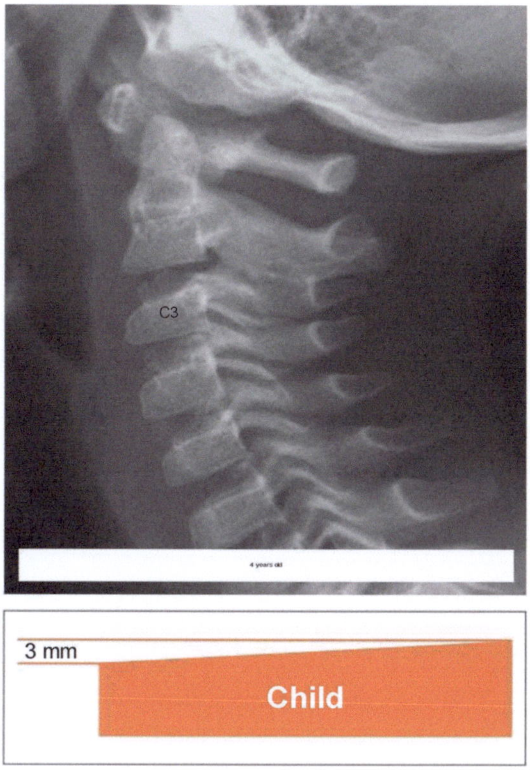

Fig. 4.11 Anterior vertebral wedging

4.3 Congenital Spinal and Spinal Cord Diseases Commonly Encountered in Adults

4.3.1 Segmentation Abnormality

4.3.1.1 Block Vertebra

(1) Mechanism of occurrence and dynamics
It is a congenital anomaly that appears due to a failure in segmentation during the development of the fetal spine. Two or more adjacent vertebrae partially or completely fuse into a single bone block. It most commonly appears in the lumbar region.

(2) Clinical features
Developmental abnormalities such as hemivertebra or vertebral aplasia may be accompanied at the levels above and below the fused spine. Segmentation abnormalities can also be accompanied on the posterior arch of the fused spine, and if the posterior arch is also fused, spinal curvature abnormalities such as scoliosis or kyphosis can occur.

(3) Imaging findings
The fused spine takes on a concave shape due to growth failure at the fusion site, and the anteroposterior diameter decreases (Fig. 4.12). It can also appear in two or more vertebral bones, and a rudimentary intervertebral disc that has not developed properly may be seen between the fused vertebral bodies.

4.3.1.2 Klippel–Feil Syndrome

(1) Mechanism of occurrence and dynamics
It is a disease caused by a failure of segmentation of the cervical vertebrae, characterized by partial or complete fusion of two or more cervical vertebrae, and it occurs more frequently in girls. Most of the affected patients show characteristic triad (short neck, low posterior hairline, severe cervical motion restriction).

(2) Clinical findings
Not only cervical malformations such as Sprengel deformity, atlanto-occipital assimilation, basilar invagination, and hemivertebra, but also kidney abnormalities, congenital heart disease, deafness, and rib fusion can be accompanied. Pain due to degenerative changes of the adjacent non-fused cervical vertebrae or neurological symptoms caused by basilar invagination or atlantoaxial instability can also be induced.

(3) Imaging findings
It is common for the posterior lateral part of the C2–3 level cervical vertebrae to be fused. Although most of the time, one level of the cervical vertebrae is fused, in about 1/3 of the cases, two or more levels of the cervical vertebrae are fused (Fig. 4.13). Degenerative changes and spinal canal stenosis can occur in the cervical vertebrae proximal or superior to the fusion level. Instability of the occipitocervical junction, atlanto-occipital assimilation, malformation of the odontoid process, and basilar invagination may be associated. It can be accompanied by deformities, such as brain flattening.

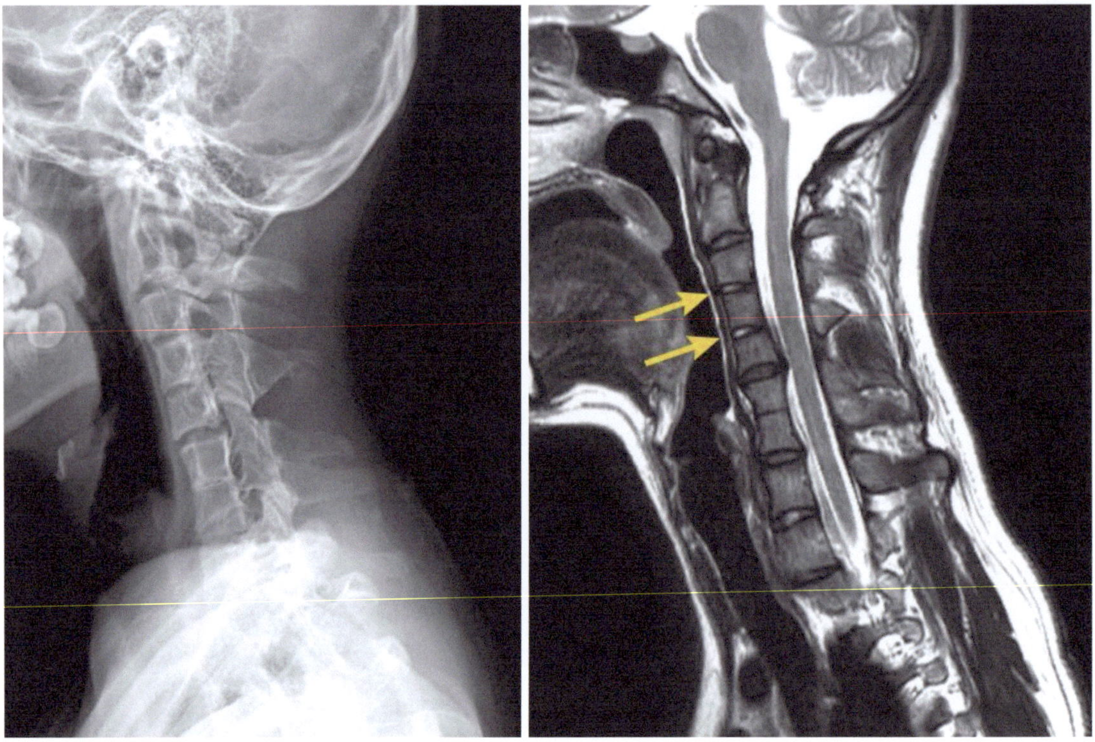

Fig. 4.12 Block vertebra
Three vertebrae from C3 to C5 and two vertebrae from C6–7 are fused into a single bone block. A small intervertebral disc (arrow) that has not developed properly is visible between the bodies of the fused C3–5 vertebrae. The anterior and posterior diameters of the fused vertebrae are reduced, and both the front and back appear concave

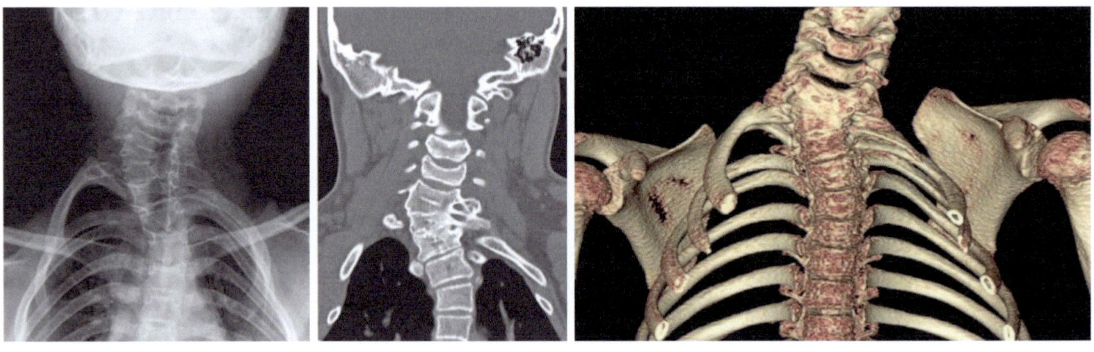

Fig. 4.13 Klippel-Feil syndrome
The patient has multiple levels of fusion mainly on the left lateral part from C6 to the T2 level. The hump is prominent and is accompanied by scoliosis. This patient also has a Sprengel deformity where the left scapula is raised

4.3.2 Chiari Malformation

It is known to occur due to a congenital defect of caudal displacement of the cerebellum and brainstem and was described in three types by Chiari in 1891. Type II and type III appear to be related, and type I is accepted as a different category.

4.3.2.1 Chiari I Malformation

The most common type, the cerebellar tonsils descend into the upper cervical spinal canal through the foramen magnum, showing a "peg-like configuration" (Fig. 4.14). Usually, it is considered an abnormal position when the cerebellar tonsils are more than 5 mm below the foramen magnum. Most patients are asymptomatic, but symptoms can include headaches, neck pain, sleep apnea, and balance disorders. Syringomyelia can occur in the cervical spine, or spinal cord swelling can occur due to cerebrospinal fluid flow disorders.

4.3.2.2 Chiari II Malformation

It is a complex malformation involving the hind brain, spine, skull base, and spinal column. In fact, almost all patients with Chiari II malformation have myelomeningocele. The medulla oblongata, fourth ventricle, and cerebellar vermis are seen to be displaced downward through the foramen magnum (Fig. 4.15). About 2/3 show a "kink" in the upper cervical spine toward the back, and symptoms are common in these cases.

4.3.2.3 Chiari III Malformation

This refers to cases where encephalocele is accompanied in the occipital or upper cervical region, showing similar findings to Chiari II.

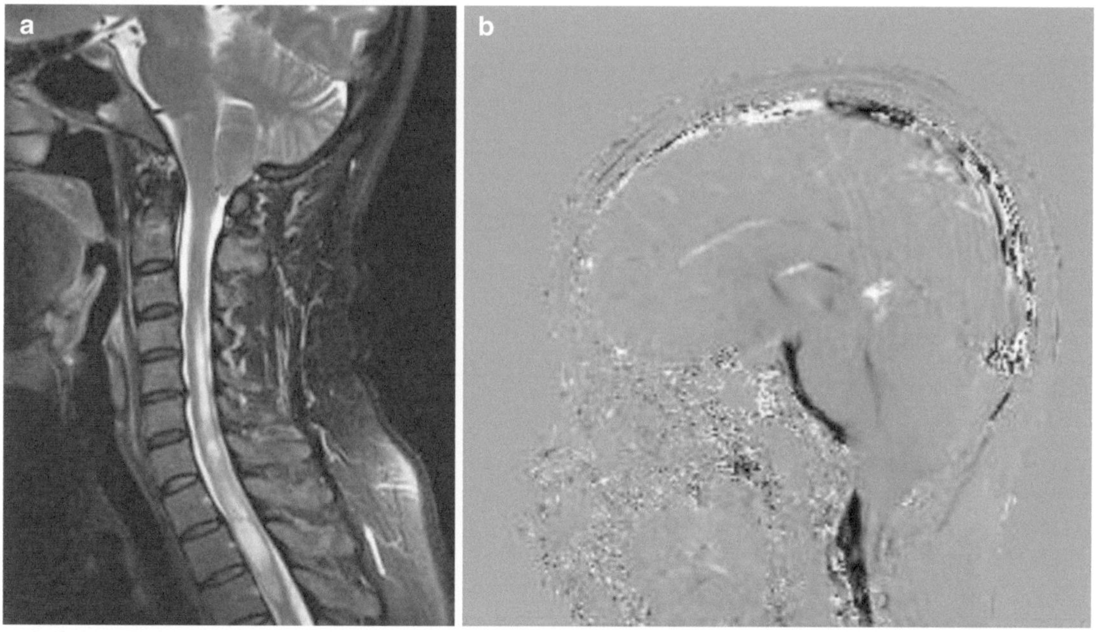

Fig. 4.14 Chiari I malformation. (**a**) In the sagittal T2-weighted magnetic resonance image, the cerebellar tonsils are descended below the foramen magnum, and syringomyelia is accompanied in the cervical and upper thoracic spine. (**b**) In the brain cine magnetic resonance image, it can be confirmed that the flow of cerebrospinal fluid in the foramen magnum is significantly reduced

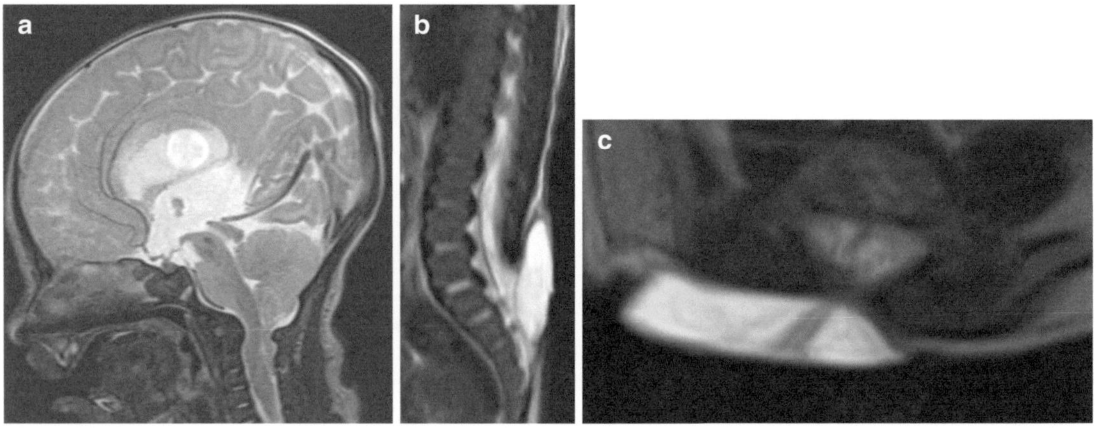

Fig. 4.15 Chiari II malformation. (**a**) In the sagittal T2-weighted magnetic resonance image, the cerebellar vermis and medulla are descended through the foramen magnum, and a cervicomedullary kinking where the upper cervical spine is bent is seen. (**b**, **c**) In the spinal magnetic resonance image, a concurrent myelomeningocele is seen in the lumbar spine

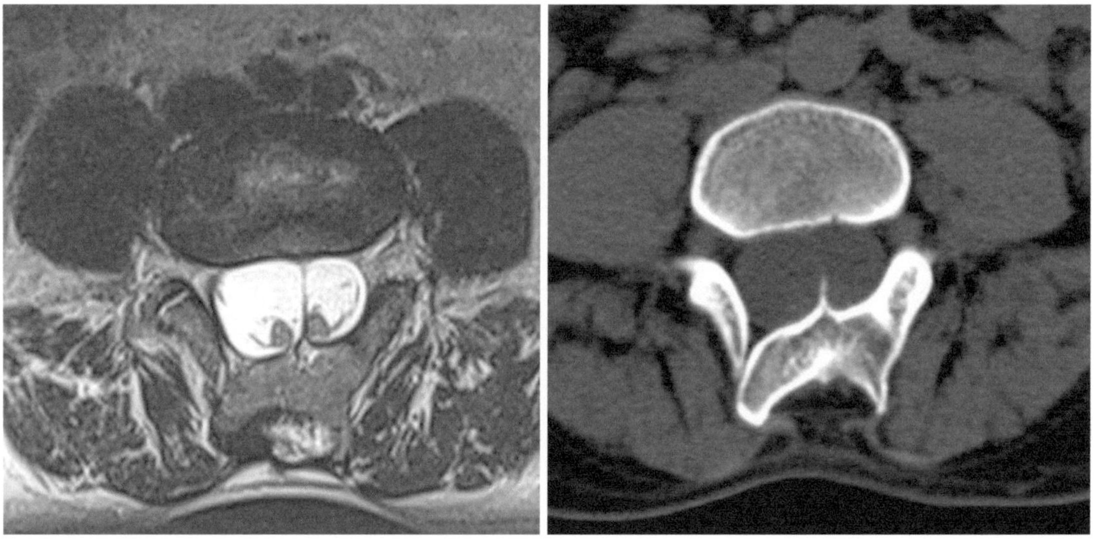

Fig. 4.16 Type I diastematomyelia
Two symmetrical hemispines are seen divided by a bony spur centered on the sagittal plane

4.3.3 Diastematomyelia

4.3.3.1 Mechanism of Occurrence and Dynamics

Diastematomyelia refers to the division of the spinal cord into two symmetrical or asymmetrical hemicords by bone, cartilage, or fibrous spurs centered on the sagittal plane (Fig. 4.16). Each of the two hemicords has one central canal, one dorsal horn, and one ventral horn, each giving off one posterior and one anterior nerve root. Diastematomyelia is divided into two types: Type I, where there are fibrous, cartilaginous, or bony spurs dividing the two hemicords, each surrounded by separate dural sacs and subarachnoid spaces, and Type II, where the two hemicords are located within one dural sac and subarachnoid space, with no spurs crossing the spinal cord. Diastematomyelia is more common in girls and frequently occurs in the thoracic and lumbar regions, and can appear in 1–5% of cases of scoliosis.

4.3.3.2 Clinical Findings

Visible hypertrichosis, nevus, lipoma, hemangioma, etc. Signs of skin abnormalities appear in more than half. Gastric atrophy, loss of deep organ reflexes, foot deformities, and urinary system deformities are commonly accompanied.

4.3.3.3 Imaging findings

The typical protrusion or duplication that appears in Type I spinal dysraphism is located in the tail of the spinal dysraphism, which is because the spinal cord moves relatively toward the head during development. Syringohydromyelia is commonly accompanied in spinal dysraphism, and the position of the spinal cone (conus medullaris) is low and the terminal cord (filum terminale) often thickens. Therefore, during surgery, it is important not only to remove the divided protrusion but also to cut the terminal cord to eliminate traction. Segmental malformations such as fused spine or butterfly-shaped spine appear at a very high frequency in conjunction with spinal dysraphism, and this leads to spinal kyphosis or spinal scoliosis.

4.3.4 Caudal Regression Syndrome

4.3.4.1 Mechanism of Occurrence and Dynamics

It is a congenital disease that shows dysplasia of the lower lumbar and sacral spine, and other tissues derived from the caudal cell mass in embryology can also show abnormal development. The caudal cell mass is a tissue where totipotent cells cluster during development, forming the terminal cord, ventriculus terminalis, spinal cone, upper lumbar and sacral spine, and urorectal septum. Therefore, it can be accompanied by anal atresia, genital malformations, kidney malformations, lung hypoplasia, and limb malformations.

4.3.4.2 Clinical Findings

About 20% of patients with caudal regression syndrome are born to mothers with diabetes (excluding gestational diabetes). In particular, sacral agenesis syndrome, characterized by aplasia of the lumbar-sacral-coccyx and hypoplasia of the lower limbs, is a well-known congenital malformation associated with maternal diabetes. The degree of dysplasia of the lumbar and sacral spine varies, and appropriate treatment is needed depending on the accompanying abnormal disease. Caudal regression syndrome can be accompanied by OEIS (omphalocele, cloacal extrophy, imperforate anus, and spinal deformities), VACTERAL (vertebral abnormality, anal malformation, cardiac anomalies, tracheoesophageal fistula, renal abnormality, limb deformity), or Currarino triad (partial sacral agenesis, anorectal malformation, presacral mass).

4.3.4.3 Imaging Findings

The lower lumbar and sacral spine do not develop normally, and the end of the spinal cord is positioned higher than normal, taking on a "wedge-shaped" shape (Fig. 4.17). In caudal regression syndrome, if the end of the spinal cord is located below the L1 level, spinal traction, spinal dysraphism, lipoma of the terminal cord, and hydromyelia can be accompanied. Abnormalities of the urinary and digestive systems are commonly accompanied.

4.3.5 Tight Filum Terminale Syndrome

The tight filum terminale syndrome occurs due to abnormalities in the retrogressive differentiation process of the caudal cell mass during embryonic development. This results in the development of an abnormally short and thick terminal thread, which may be accompanied by a lipoma or cyst within the terminal thread. The tight filum terminale syndrome causes spinal traction, causing the spinal cone to be abnormally low. Clinical symptoms may include neurological abnormalities or musculoskeletal abnormalities caused by spinal traction. Symptoms such as lower back pain, gait

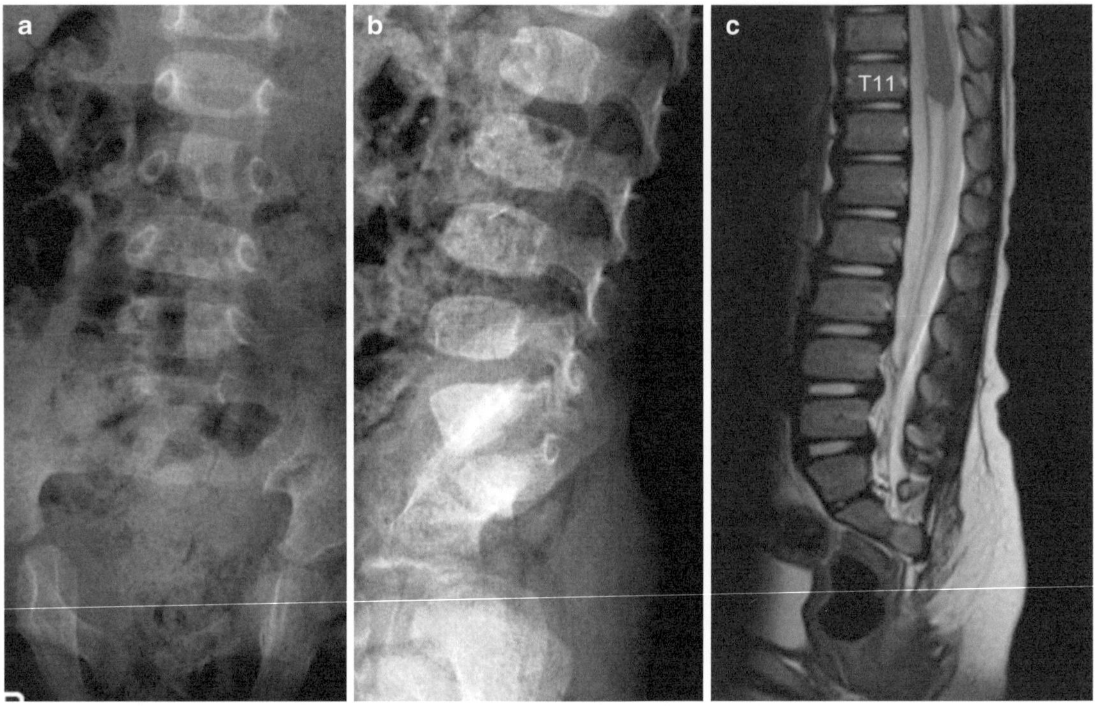

Fig. 4.17 Caudal regression syndrome
In the plain radiograph, the sacrum below S2 is not properly formed (**a**, **b**), and in the sagittal T2-weighted magnetic resonance image, the spinal cone is relatively high at the T11 level and has a "wedge-shaped" form (**c**)

disorders, and abnormalities in the digestive and urinary systems may appear.

4.3.6 Fibrolipoma of the Filum Terminale

4.3.6.1 Mechanism of Occurrence and Dynamics

The terminal thread is a thin, long fibrous filament that starts from the spinal cone, passes through the subarachnoid space and dura mater, and attaches to the ventral side of the first coccyx. The fibrolipoma of the terminal thread is thought to be a minor malformation induced during the communication and retrogressive differentiation process during the development of the central nervous system. In MRI scans of adults without symptoms of spinal traction, fat within the terminal thread can be found at a frequency of 1.5–5%, and it is sometimes considered a normal variant.

4.3.6.2 Clinical Findings

Once the fatty change of the terminal thread is confirmed, a detailed medical history and physical examination are necessary, and follow-up examinations should be conducted with the possibility of spinal traction in mind.

4.3.6.3 Imaging Findings

On MRI, the fibrolipoma of the terminal thread appears as a high signal intensity lesion within the thickened terminal thread on the sagittal T1-weighted image. It can be helpful to also perform axial images as the lipoma may be small or off-center (Fig. 4.18).

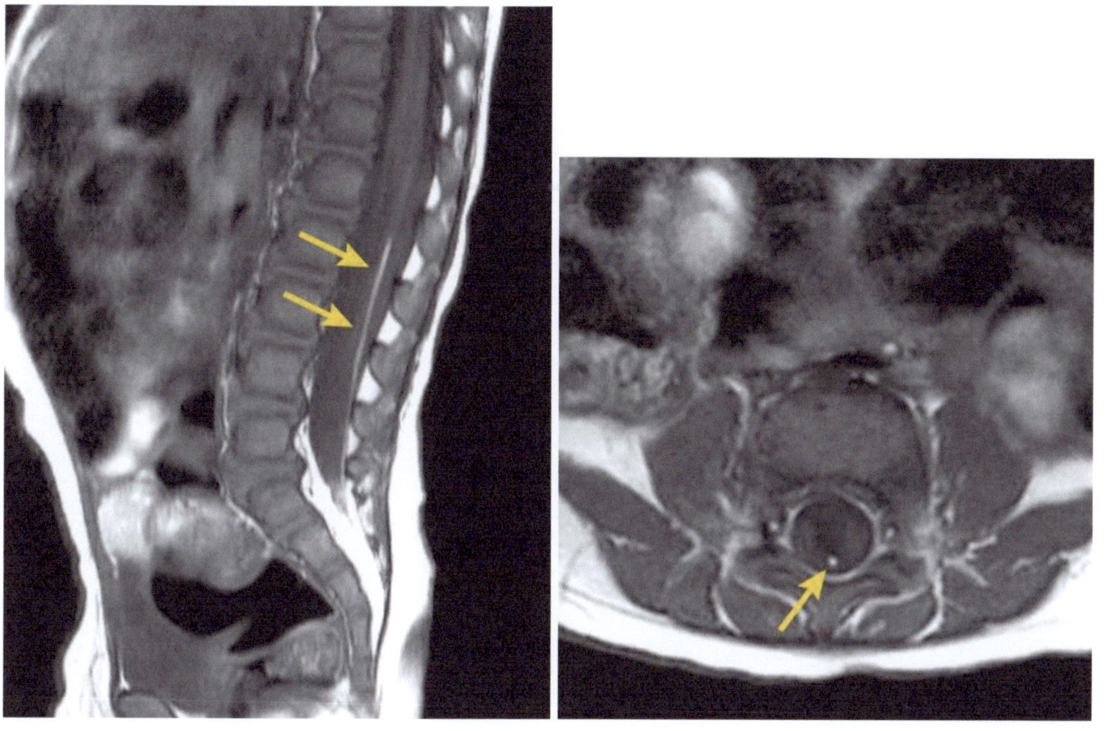

Fig. 4.18 Filum terminale lipoma
In the T1-weighted image, there is a high signal intensity lesion in the filum terminale, indicating a filum terminale lipoma. The height of the spinal cone is normal and there is no evidence of spinal traction in the magnetic resonance image

Bibliography

1. Barkovich AJ. Pediatric neuroimaging. Lippincott Williams & Wilkins; 2005.
2. Lustrin ES, et al. Pediatric cervical spine: normal anatomy, variants, and trauma. Radiographics. 2003;23(3):539–60.
3. Jaremko JL, et al. Common normal variants of pediatric vertebral development that mimic fractures: a pictorial review from a national longitudinal bone health study. Pediatr Radiol. 2015;45(4):593–605.
4. Rossi A, et al. Diagnostic Approach to pediatric spine disorders. Magn Reson Imaging Clin N Am. 2016;24(3):621–44.
5. Chaturvedi A, et al. Malformed vertebrae: a clinical and imaging review. Insights Imaging. 2018;9(3):343–55.
6. Herman MJ, Pizzutillo PD. Cervical spine disorders in children. Orthop Clin N Am. 1999;30(3):457–66.
7. Lee E. Pediatric radiology: practical imaging evaluation of infants and children. Lippincott Williams & Wilkins; 2017.
8. Guille JT, Sherk HH. Congenital osseous anomalies of the upper and lower cervical spine in children. JBJS. 2002;84(2):277–88.
9. Hensinger RN, Lang JE, MacEwen GD. Klippel-Feil syndrome; a constellation of associated anomalies. J Bone Joint Surg Am Vol. 1974;56(6):1246–53.
10. Grimme JD, Castillo M. Congenital anomalies of the spine. Neuroimaging Clin N Am. 2007;17(1):1–16.
11. McLone DG, Knepper PA. The cause of Chiari II malformation: a unified theory. Pediatr Neurosurg. 1989;15(1):1–12.
12. Wolpert SM, et al. Chiari II malformation: MR imaging evaluation. Am J Roentgenol. 1987;149(5):1033–42.
13. Coley BD. Caffey's pediatric diagnostic imaging E-book. Elsevier Health Sciences; 2018.
14. Korean Society of Spine Radiology, Spine radiology. vol. 1. Korea Medicine.
15. Choi In-ho, et al. Pediatric orthopedics. 4th ed. Gunja Publishing Company.

Degenerative Spinal Disease

5

Joon Woo Lee

5.1 Lumbosacral Spine

5.1.1 Anatomy

The lumbar spine and sacral spine are each composed of five vertebrae. The lumbar spine is connected by fibrocartilage called the intervertebral disc between the vertebral bodies, and the rear part is connected by the articular process as a synovial joint (Fig. 5.1). The sacral spine is fused with the vertebral body, and the sacral ala on both sides forms a joint with the ilium.

The intervertebral disc consists of a gelatinous component called the nucleus pulposus, which acts as a cushion in the center, and the annulus fibrosus that surrounds it. The nucleus pulposus is soft, elastic, shock absorber and composed of water, proteoglycans, and loose collagen fibers. The water content decreases with age, reaching 90% after birth and dropping to 70% in the 40s. When pressure is applied, the nucleus pulposus flattens and disperses the shock around it, and the annulus fibrosus surrounding the nucleus pulposus blocks the transmitted shock. The annulus fibrosus is composed of several concentric layers of fibrocartilage. The outermost layer is called Sharpey's fiber and is connected to the posterior longitudinal ligament and vertebral body [1–3].

Most of the normal intervertebral disc interior does not have blood vessels, so nutrients are supplied by diffusion from the adjacent vertebral body, but the peripheral part of the annulus fibrosus has blood vessels, so nutrients are directly supplied. If there is a rupture in the intervertebral disc, the central part does not heal because it does not have blood vessels, but the peripheral part can fill the ruptured part with a granulation plug, etc., because it has blood vessels. This can cause a High-Intensity Zone (HIZ) that appears as a high signal intensity at the site of annulus fibrosus rupture on MR T2-weighted images [4].

The intervertebral disc is innervated by nerves only up to the outer 1/3 of the annulus fibrosus. The anterior and lateral parts of the annulus fibrosus are innervated by the "ventral ramus" or "gray ramus communicans," and the posterior part is innervated by the "sinuvertebral nerve." The "sinuvertebral nerve" has both somatic and sympathetic fibers and receives nerve supply from the "dorsal root." The "ganglion" and "gray ramus communicans" are both connected. The "gray ramus communicans" is a nerve that connects the "dorsal root ganglion" and the "sympathetic trunk." The "sinuvertebral nerve" contains nociceptive C-fibers that transmit pain, making it a pathway for pain transmission (Fig. 5.2) [2, 5].

In the lumbar spine, the synovial joints located at the back between the articular processes are called "zygapophyseal joints," commonly referred to as "facet joints" in clinical terms. In the lumbar spine, the facet joint faces the anteromedial direction (Fig. 5.3), and due to this characteristic, spon-

J. W. Lee (✉)
Department of Radiology, Seoul National University College of Medicine, Seoul National University Bundang Hospital, Seongnam, Korea (Republic of)

© The Author(s), under exclusive license to Springer Nature Singapore Pte Ltd. 2025

H. S. Kang, J. W. Lee (eds.), *Spinal Imaging*, https://doi.org/10.1007/978-981-95-1386-4_5

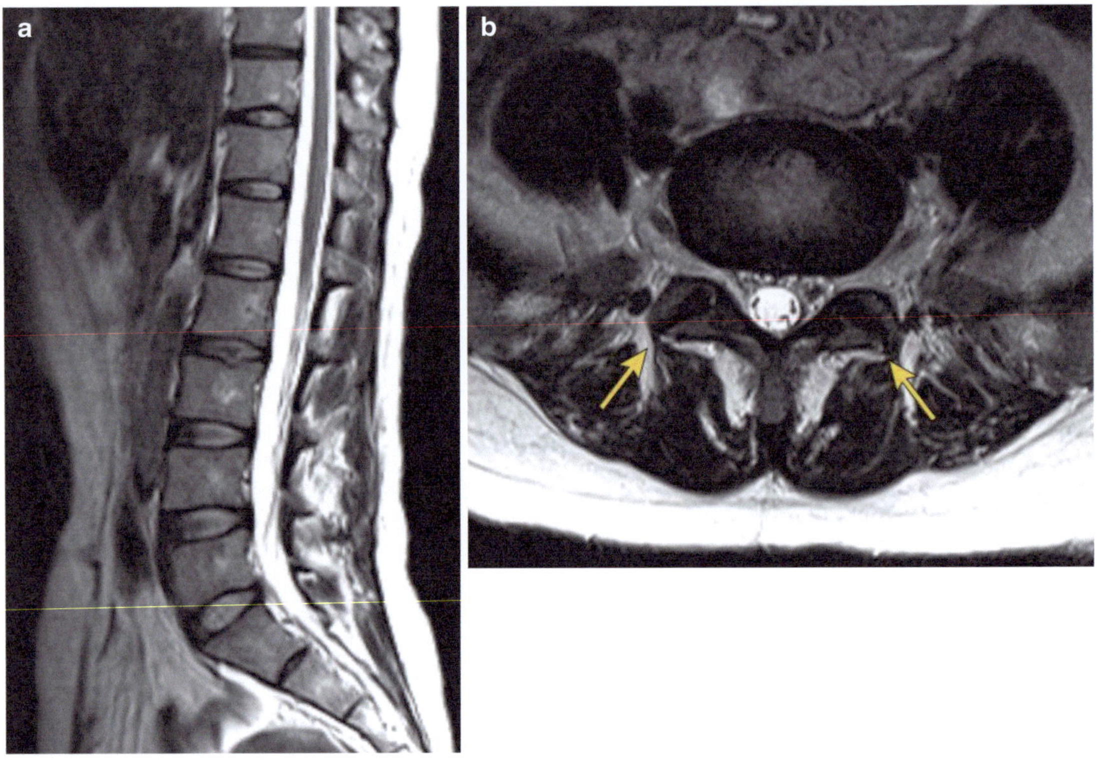

Fig. 5.1 Lumbar spine MR images
The lumbar spine is connected by a fibrocartilage called the intervertebral disc between the vertebral bodies, and the posterior part is connected by a synovial joint between the articular processes (arrow)

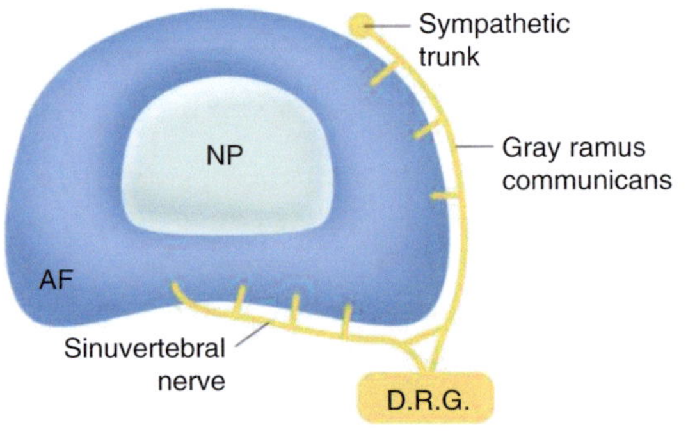

Fig. 5.2 Nerve supply of the intervertebral disc
The intervertebral disc is innervated only up to the outer 1/3 of the annulus fibrosus. The anterior and lateral parts of the annulus fibrosus are innervated by the "ventral ramus" or "gray ramus communicans," and the posterior part is innervated by the "sinuvertebral nerve." The "sinuvertebral nerve" has both somatic and sympathetic fibers and is connected to the "dorsal root ganglion" and "gray ramus communicans" of the segment. The "gray ramus communicans" is a nerve that connects the "dorsal root ganglion" and the "sympathetic trunk." NP: nucleus pulposus, AF: annulus fibrosus, DRG: dorsal root ganglion

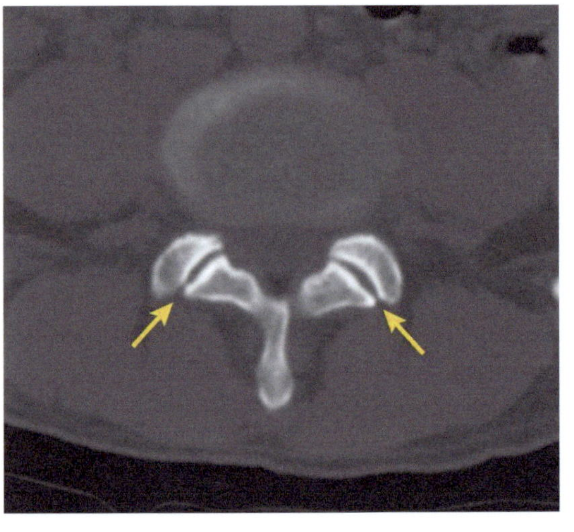

Fig. 5.3 Cross-sectional CT image of the lumbar spine
In the lumbar spine, the facet joint faces the anteromedial direction (arrow). Due to this characteristic, unlike the cervical spine or thoracic spine, spondylolisthesis or retrolisthesis can easily occur due to degenerative changes

dylolisthesis or retrolisthesis caused by degenerative changes can easily occur, unlike in the cervical spine or thoracic spine [6].

A vertebral body that has the characteristics of both the lumbar spine and sacral spine can be seen, and this is called a "lumbosacral transitional vertebra." Although it's not an exact term, in actual clinical practice, when the L5 vertebral body looks like the sacral spine, it's called "sacralization of L5," and when S1 looks like the lumbar spine, it's called "lumbarization of S1." Castellvi et al. [7] divided the lumbosacral transitional vertebra according to its shape as shown in Table 5.1 (Figs. 5.4, and 5.5).

Regarding the shape of the S1/2 intervertebral disc, O'Driscoll et al. [8] divided it into four types as shown in Table 5.2.

To accurately determine whether the lumbosacral transitional vertebra is L5 or S1, the level should be counted from the entire spinal image, but in actual clinical practice, there are many cases where the level must be determined with only the lumbar spine image. In this case, the last vertebral body attached to the rib can be considered as thoracic spine 12, but since there are differences in the number and shape of the ribs, other parameters are also referred to. There are studies that the right renal artery can be seen as the L1/2 disc level, and the transverse process where the iliolumbar ligament attaches can be seen as the L5 level, but these findings do not match in all cases [9].

Table 5.1 Classification of lumbosacral transitional vertebra

Type I	Dysplastic transverse process (unilateral: 1a, bilateral: 1b)
Type II	Incomplete lumbarization/sacralization showing enlarged transverse processes with unilateral (IIa) or bilateral (IIb) pseudoarthrosis with the adjacent sacral ala
Type III	Complete lumbarization/sacralization showing enlarged transverse processes, with unilateral (IIIa) or bilateral (IIIb) fusion with the adjacent sacral ala
Type IV	Mixed (e.g., type IIa on one side and type IIIa on the other)

5.1.2 Intervertebral Disc Degeneration

Degeneration of the intervertebral disc is a process that occurs in almost all patients with age.

The most important finding that appears as the intervertebral disc degenerates is the loss of water content, which appears as a low signal intensity shadow on MR T2-weighted images. Pfirrmann et al. [10] described disc degeneration in five stages, which is the most commonly used stage for disc degeneration to date (Table 5.3, Figs. 5.6, 5.7, and 5.8).

Spondylosis deformans and intervertebral osteochondrosis are representative terms describing changes in adjacent bones due to intervertebral disc degeneration [3, 11–13].

Spondylosis deformans is a change associated with degenerative changes in the annulus fibrosus, with marginal osteophytes being a characteristic feature (Fig. 5.9). In spondylosis deformans, there is no or minimal disc space narrowing. The mechanism of marginal osteophytes is that stress is applied to the ring apophysis attached to the intervertebral disc and adjacent vertebral body due to intervertebral disc degeneration, and by this force, the ring apophyses are slightly separated from the discovertebral joint in the direction of Sharpey's fiber, forming a hook shape. Osteophytes grow. In Spondylosis deformans, osteophytes initially grow in a triangular shape, a little away from the discovertebral junction, and grow toward the disc like a hook. Other differential diagnoses that can show such bony overgrowth include DISH (diffuse idiopathic skeletal hyperostosis), ankylosing spondylitis, and psoriatic spondyloarthropathy. In DISH, characteristic ossification flows along the front and side of the vertebral body across multiple levels. Syndesmophytes seen in ankylosing spondylitis initially ossify along the outer layer of the annulus fibrosus, so unlike spondylosis deformans, they are attached to the periphery of the vertebral body and are thin. In psoriatic spondyloarthropathy, irregular and thick spinal periphery ossification is seen away from the vertebral body [3].

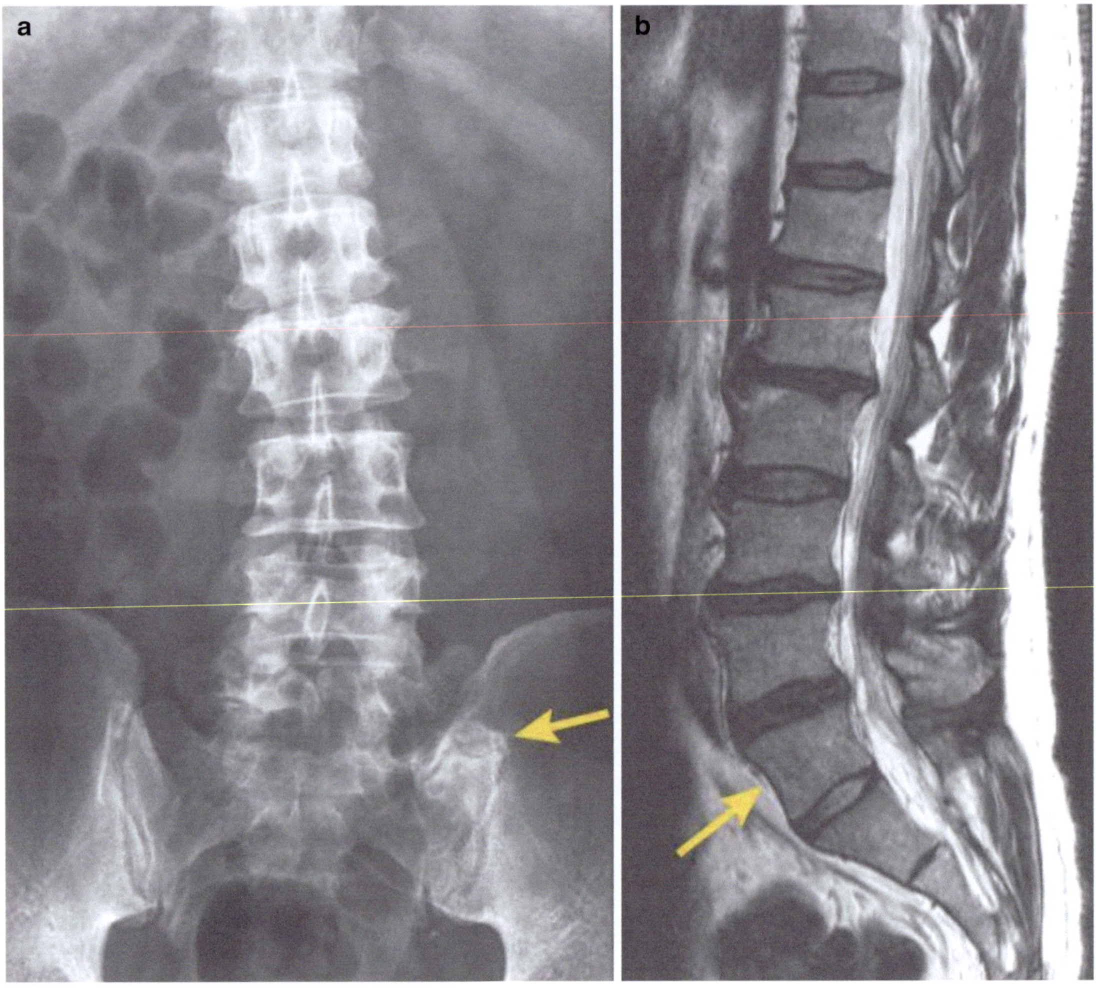

Fig. 5.4 Lumbosacral transitional vertebra type IIa
In the anterior and posterior simple radiographs (**a**), the left transverse process of the first lumbar vertebra forms a pseudoarthrosis with the sacral spine below (arrow), so it is type IIa. In the MR image (**b**) of the same patient, the vertebral body of the first lumbar vertebra (arrow) is separated from the sacral spines below by a complete intervertebral disc, and the first lumbar vertebra shows a rectangular shape, so the shape of the S1/2 intervertebral disc is type 4 in O'Driscoll classification

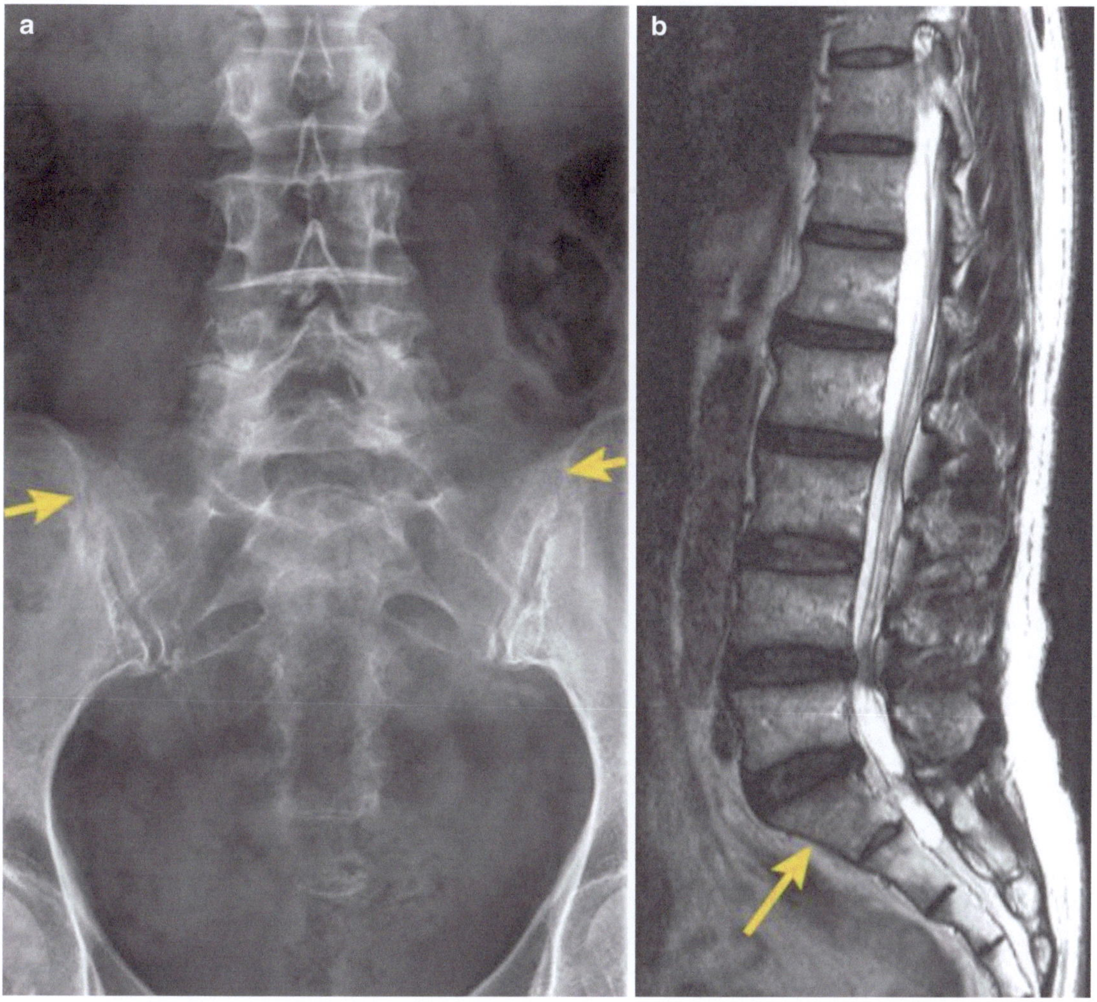

Fig. 5.5 Lumbosacral transitional vertebra type IIIb
In the anterior and posterior simple radiographs, the transverse process of the first lumbar vertebra is fused with the lumbar spine below on both sides (arrow), so it is type IIIb. In the MR image, the vertebral body of the first lumbar vertebra (arrow) is separated from the lumbar spines below by an intervertebral disc, but the shape of the first lumbar vertebra is not deformed and appears trapezoidal, so the shape of the S1/2 intervertebral disc is type 3 in O'Driscoll classification

Table 5.2 Classification of first acral intervertebral disk morphology

Type 1	No disk material between S1 and the sacrum
Type 2	A small residual disk between S1 and the sacrum
Type 3	A well-formed residual disk between S1 and the sacrum
Type 4	A well-formed disk between S1 and the remainder of the sacrum, in addition to an abnormal sagittal outline to the sacrum("squaring" of the first sacral element)

Table 5.3 Stages of intervertebral disc degeneration (Pfirrmann classification)

Grade 1	Discs exhibiting a homogeneous structure with bright hyperintense white signal intensity and a normal height
Grade 2	Discs exhibiting an inhomogeneous structure (with or without horizontal bands)
Grade 3	Discs showing gray, inhomogeneous structure with unclear distinction of nucleus and annulus
Grade 4	Discs exhibiting inhomogeneous, gray to black structure with a loss of distinction of nucleus and annulus
Grade 5	Discs showing black structure with collapsed disc space

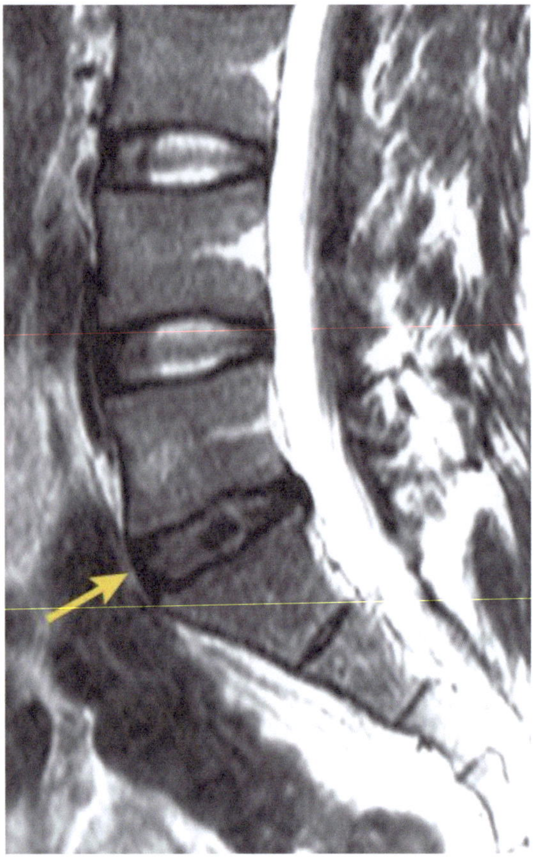

Fig. 5.6 Pfirrmann grade 2 and 3
In the T2-enhanced image of a 30-year-old male, the intervertebral disc of Lumbar spine 3/4, 4/5 maintains a high signal shadow in the center, and a low signal shadow band is observed in the middle, indicating Pfirrmann grade 2 intervertebral disc degeneration. The intervertebral disc between lumbar spine 5 and sacrum 1 shows a loss of high signal shadow and is observed as a gray shadow (arrow), indicating Pfirrmann grade 3 intervertebral disc degeneration

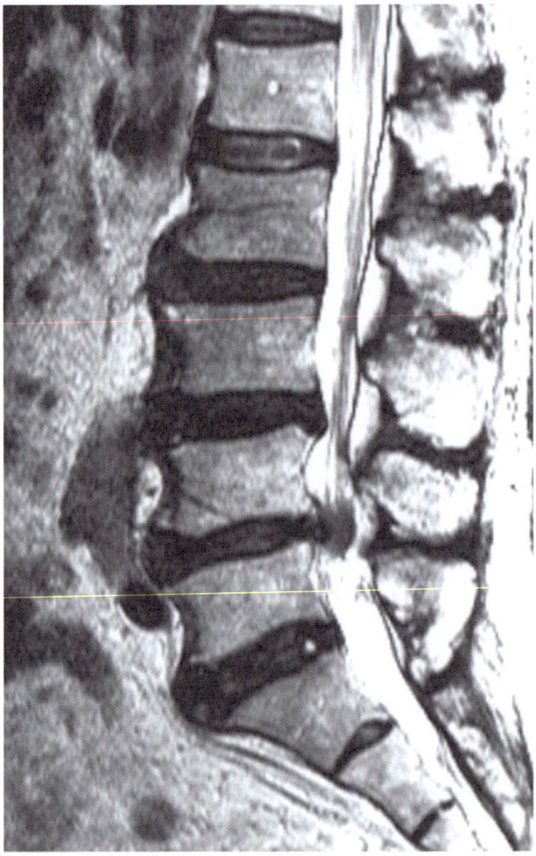

Fig. 5.7 Pfirrmann grade 4
In the T2-enhanced image of a 75-year-old male, the intervertebral disc of lumbar spine 2/3, 3/4, 4/5, L5/S1 shows a low signal shadow overall, and the distinction between the nucleus pulposus and annulus fibrosus is lost, indicating Pfirrmann grade 4 intervertebral disc degeneration

Intervertebral osteochondrosis is a finding associated with the degeneration of the nucleus pulposus. This results in disc height loss, the "vacuum phenomenon," and changes in the adjacent vertebral body. When space is created by intervertebral disc degeneration, air fills this space, which is called the "vacuum phenomenon," a finding that suggests intervertebral osteochondrosis (Fig. 5.10) [3, 12–15].

Modic et al. [16] divided the MR signal changes of the vertebral body due to intervertebral disc degeneration into three types, which are currently most widely applied (Table 5.4, Figs. 5.11, 5.12, and 5.13).

5.1.3 Internal Disc Disruption

The term internal disc disruption (IDD) was first described by Crock in 1970 and emphasized again by Crock at the International Society for the Study of the Lumbar Spine (ISSLS) in 1986 [17]. Crock defined IDD as follows: "A 'disruption' of the internal architecture of the disc without signs of disc protrusions or without positive signs for nerve root compression."

In 1995, Schwarzer et al. [18] performed discography on 92 patients with chronic back pain and reported that 39% of the patients met the diagnostic criteria for IDD. They announced through their research that IDD is a common cause of chronic back pain.

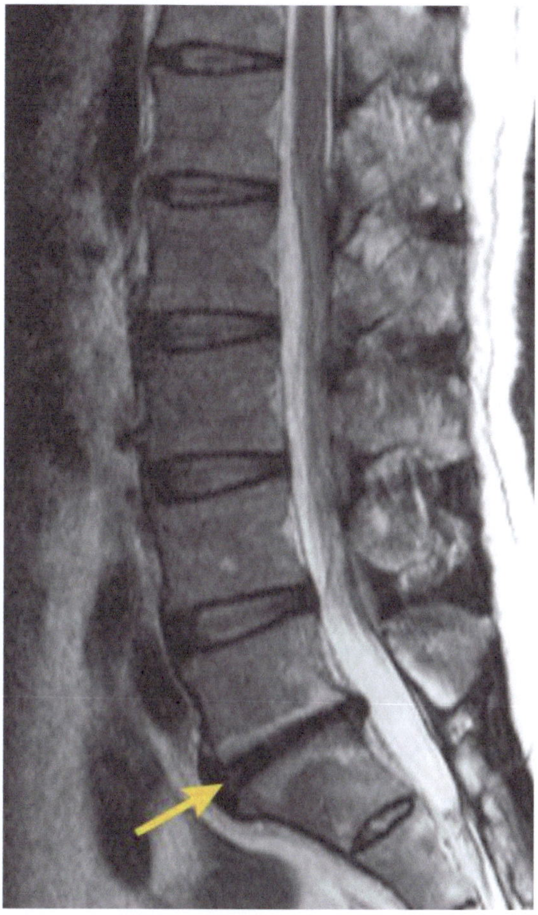

Fig. 5.8 Pfirrmann grade 5
In the T2-enhanced image, the L5/S1 intervertebral disc shows a low signal shadow overall, and the intervertebral disc height is significantly reduced, indicating Pfirrmann grade 5 intervertebral disc degeneration (arrow)

There is still controversy over whether IDD is an actual disease. Therefore, it is recommended by various societies that before performing invasive procedures such as surgery for IDD, strict diagnostic criteria must be applied to the patient's treatment. The "North American Spine Society (NASS)," "International Association for the Study of Pain (IASP)," "International Spine Intervention Society (ISIS)," and other societies have proposed strict diagnostic criteria for diagnosing IDD, and it is said that a diagnosis of IDD can be made through these diagnostic criteria [19, 20].

5.1.3.1 Pathophysiology

IDD is primarily caused by annular fissures occurring due to acute shock or chronic repetitive shock. Annular fissures are divided into transverse (rim lesion, peripheral), concentric (circumferential), and radial fissures (Fig. 5.14). Transverse annular fissures occur when the connection between the annulus fibrosus (AF) and the ring apophysis (RA) separates, usually occurring at the front. Concentric annular fissures are ruptures between the fibrocartilage concentric lamellae of the annulus fibrosus. Radial annular fissures are fissures that cross the layers from the nucleus pulposus to the outer annulus fibrosus, and it is usually triggered at the back. Among the three types of annulus fissures, radial annular fissure is known to be the main cause of IDD. When a full-thickness radial annular fissure occurs, the nucleus pulposus material meets the sinuvertebral nerve ending, and this nucleus pulposus material chemically stimulates the sinuvertebral nerve ending, causing an inflammatory response. This inflammatory response generates a pain signal. Also, through the rupture of the annulus fibrosus, the nerve grows inward, allowing contact with the nucleus pulposus material to occur even in the inner part close to the nucleus pulposus. The pain mechanism of IDD can be due to mechanical pressure as well as chemical stimulation of the sinuvertebral nerve ending. If the annular fissure is extensive, the interior of the disc can no longer support the body weight, and the load is transferred to the posterior annulus fibrosus. This added load mechanically stimulates the sinuvertebral nerve, causing pain [21, 22].

5.1.3.2 Clinical Symptoms

IDD's main symptom is back pain, described as "burning or aching." Sometimes, it can be so severe that the patient has difficulty moving. In young adults, there may be a history of trauma. This back pain tends to worsen during activities that increase pressure on the spine. Patients experience worsening pain when sitting forward, showing "sitting intolerance" where it is difficult to sit for more than 30 minutes (Table 5.5). Even when IDD is in the lower lumbar spine, patients often complain of inguinal pain. This is inter-

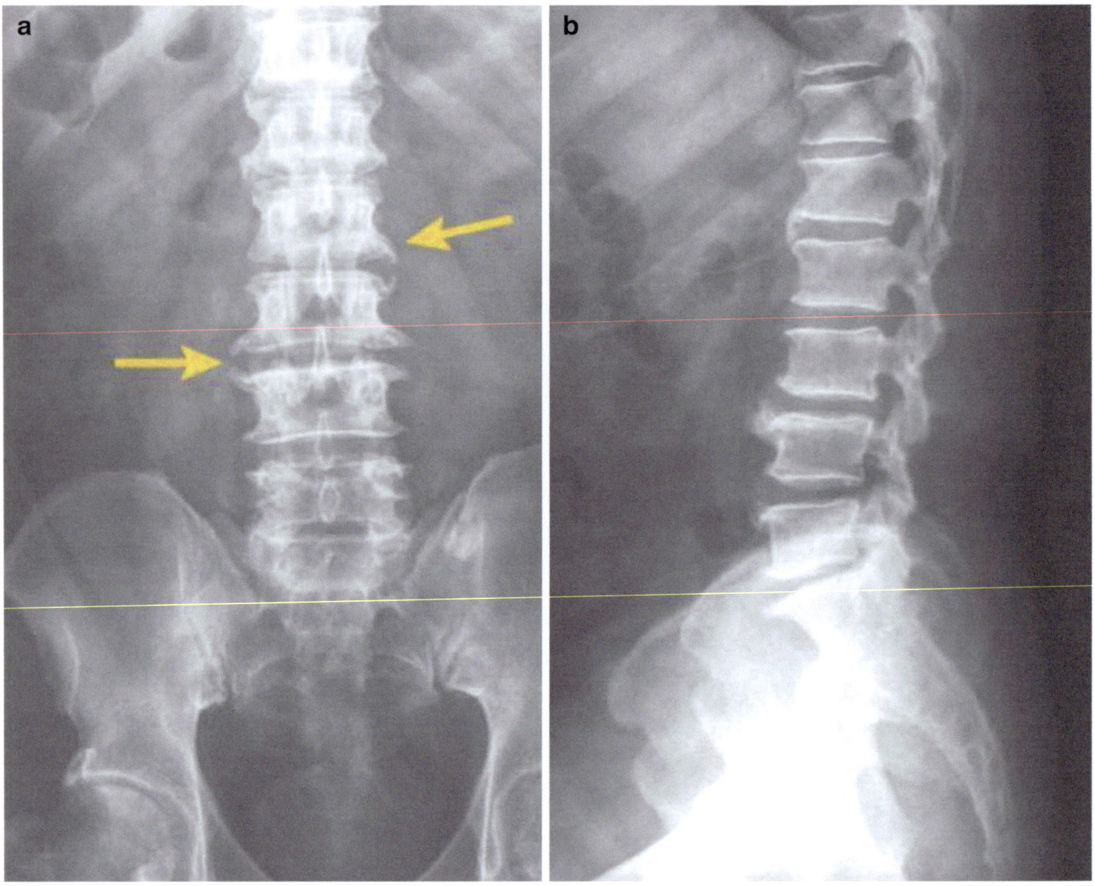

Fig. 5.9 Spondylosis deformans
Spondylosis deformans is a change associated with degenerative changes in the annulus fibrosus, with marginal osteophytes being a characteristic feature. Osteophytes growing toward the intervertebral disc from the vertebral body of the Lumbar spine are observed in the plain radiograph (arrow). The height of the intervertebral disc is relatively maintained

preted as the pain signal from the lower lumbar spine being transmitted to the L2 dorsal root ganglion via the gray ramus communicans from the sinuvertebral nerve, and again through the sympathetic trunk. Regarding the association between the location of the annulus fissure and the pain site, Slipman et al. [23] retrospectively analyzed 40 patients and reported that there was no correlation between the annular fissure and the pain site. Prospective analysis will be needed in the future. In diagnosing IDD, MR is less sensitive than provocation discography. IDD has been reported even in cases that appear normal on MR, confirmed by abnormal discography or surgery. In 1992, April and Bogduk et al. [4] first described the term HIZ (high-intensity zone). HIZ refers to the part that shows high signal shadow separated from the nucleus pulposus in the annulus fibrosus on MR T2-enhanced images (Fig. 5.15). They compared provocation discography and MR and described that the positive predictive rate for seeing a painful disc on provocation discography when HIZ is visible is 86%. In 2000, Carragee et al. [24] published opposing research results. They conducted a prospective study on 109 discs from 42 patients. In their study, the prevalence of HIZ was 59% in the syndrome group and 24% in the asymptomatic group. Although HIZ was common in the syndrome group, it was also seen in a significant number in the asymptomatic group, so they concluded that HIZ does not suggest symptomatic IDD. Smith et al. described

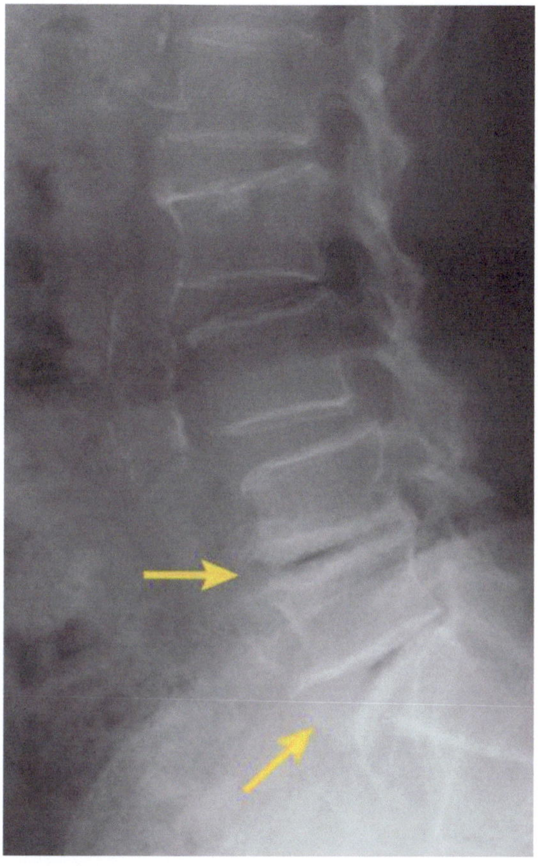

Fig. 5.10 Intervertebral osteochondrosis
Intervertebral osteochondrosis is thought to be a finding due to degeneration of the nucleus pulposus. This shows a decrease in intervertebral disc height, a "vacuum phenomenon," and changes in the adjacent vertebral body. In the lateral view of the Lumbar spine plain radiograph, a decrease in the height of the L4/5 and L5/S1 intervertebral disc and a "vacuum phenomenon" are observed (arrow), and sclerotic changes are observed in the adjacent vertebral body

Table 5.4 Degenerative endplate changes (by Modic)

Modic type	MR signal characteristics	Histopathology
Type 1	Low signal intensity on T1-weighted image, high signal intensity on T2-weighted image	Fibrovascular marrow
Type 2	High signal intensity on T1-weighted and T2-weighted image	Fatty marrow
Type 3	Low signal intensity on T1-weighted and T2-weighted image	Sclerosis

IDD as the specificity of HIZ in diagnosis is reported to be high at 90%, but the sensitivity is low at 31%.

The exact cause of HIZ is not clear, but it is thought to be a secondary inflammatory area associated with annular fissure. If an MR is taken after injecting a contrast agent, the granulation tissue formed in the annular fissure is contrasted.

5.1.3.3 CT Discography

After provocation discography, if a CT is taken (CT discography), the shape of the annular fissure can be more accurately known. On CT discography, radial annular fissure is divided into 5 stages according to the modified Dallas discogram scale (Table 5.6, Fig. 5.16) [25].

5.1.4 Disc Herniation

It is called disc herniation when the intervertebral disc locally exceeds the normal boundaries of the disc space [11–13, 26]. However, the terms used for disc herniation are diverse, and there are many parts that are not completely agreed upon among doctors. In the United States, since 1995, the NASS (North American Spine Society), ASSR (American Society of Spine Radiology), ASNR (American Society of Neuroradiology) combined task force team has organized terms describing the state of the intervertebral disc and announced the results in 2001 [12]. This terminology arrangement is a groundbreaking one that can prevent a lot of confusion related to disc herniation, and it has been accepted and used in various societies since then, and the nomenclature version 2.0 was announced in 2013 [26].

5.1.4.1 Definition of Disc Herniation Terms

When NASS, ASSR, ASNR defined the terms of disc herniation (recommendation by NASS, ASSR, ASNR), the premise was to describe only morphologically without directly implying causes, symptoms, prognosis, treatment, etc.

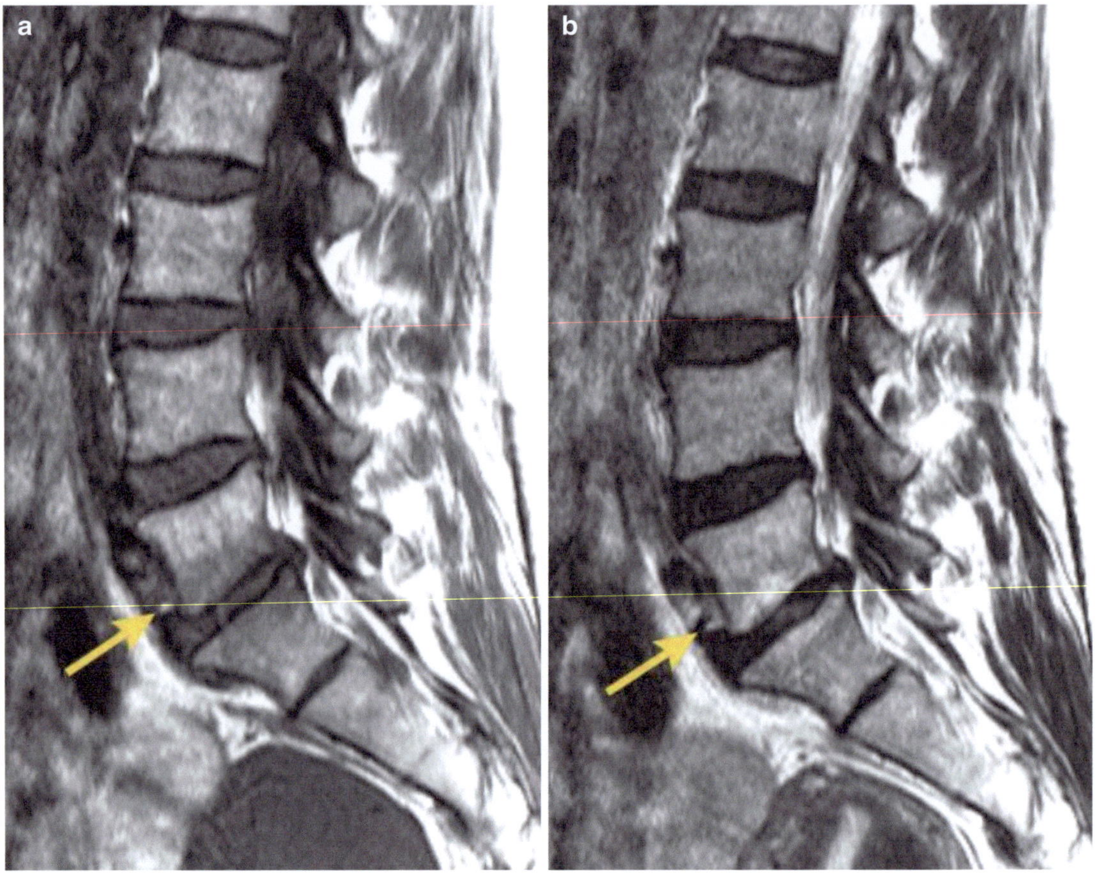

Fig. 5.11 Modic type 1 endplate change
In the lumbar spine MR image, Modic type 1 change is observed in the vertebral body around the L5/S1 disc. Modic type 1 change is due to fibrovascular marrow. It is thought to be a finding due to, low signal intensity on T1-weighted images (**a**), and high signal intensity on T2-weighted images (**b**) (arrow)

Disc herniation is defined as a localized displacement of the intervertebral disc from the boundary of the disc space. Here, the displaced intervertebral disc material can be nucleus pulposus, endplate, annulus fibrosus, bone, etc. The definition of disc space is the vertebral body endplate above and below, and the outer side is the outer edge of the vertebral body ring apophysis, excluding osteophytes. In the past, the definition of "localized" in the definition of locally displaced was defined as displacement within 50% of the disc periphery, and if it was <25%, it was defined as "focal," and if the displacement was between 25% and 50%, it was defined as "broad-based." However, in the revised version 2.0, the definition of localized was changed to <25%, so broad-based herniation disappeared, and only the previous focal herniation was defined as herniation (Fig. 5.17). If the disc displacement is 25% or more, it is not called disc herniation, but is expressed as bulging. This bulging is divided into symmetric bulging and asymmetric bulging. When the intervertebral disc collapses toward the vertebral body, it is defined as intravertebral herniation (Schmorl's node).

In the past, the term herniated nucleus pulposus (HNP) was also used to emphasize that the nucleus pulposus was displaced, but in fact, the

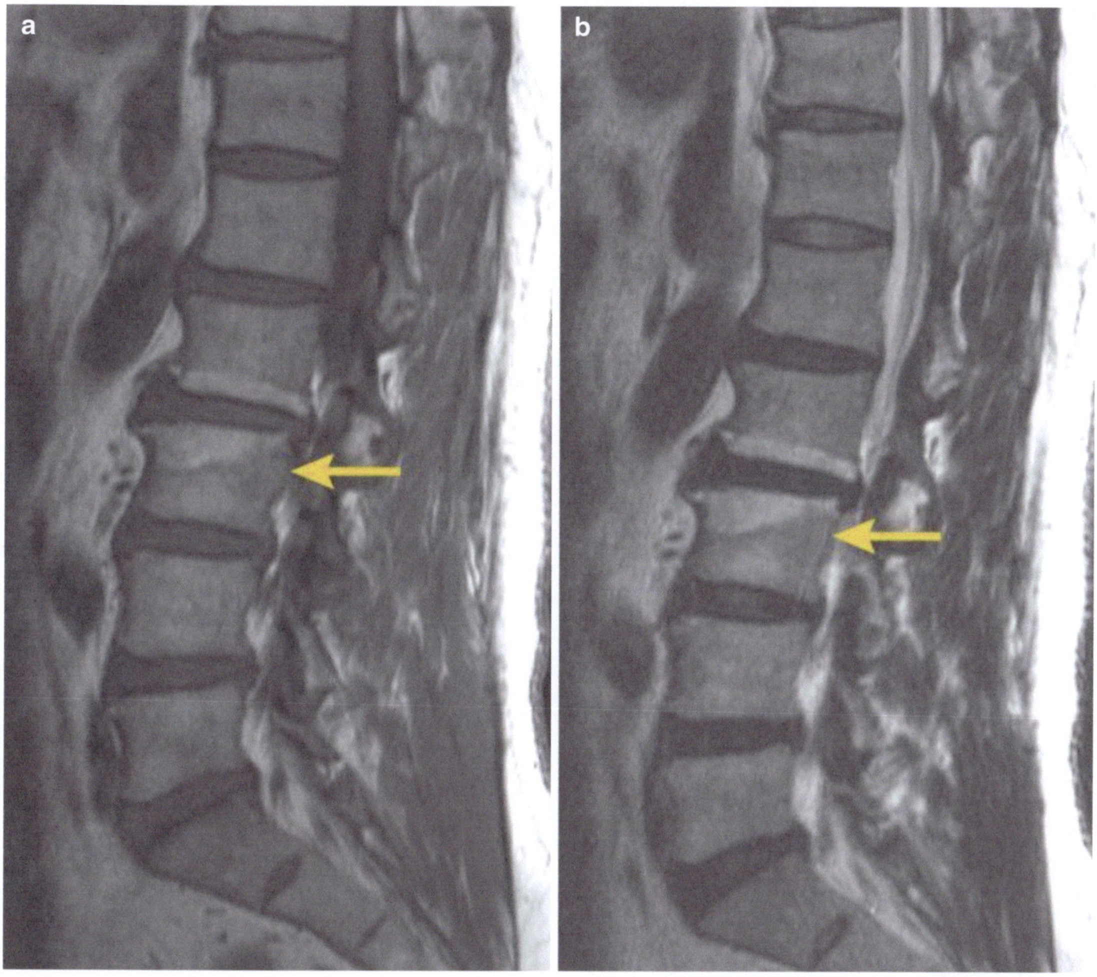

Fig. 5.12 Modic type 2 endplate change
On lumbar spine MR, Modic type 2 change is observed around the L2/3 disc vertebral body. Modic type 2 change is thought to be a finding due to fatty marrow, showing high signal intensity on T1-weighted images and high signal intensity on T2-weighted images (arrow)

displaced components can be as diverse as mentioned earlier, so the term HNP is not appropriate, and it is recommended to name it herniated disc or disc herniation. Among the terms used in the past, the term prolapse is used when the disc herniation moves downward and is located at the suprapedicle level. The term was commonly used, but it was recommended not to use it for disc herniation because the definition of the term is ambiguous and it is a term used when the workplace or uterus comes down. The term rupture gives the impression of rupture due to trauma, so it was recommended not to use it. In conclusion, it was recommended that "disc herniation" (herniated disc) is the most appropriate term. Various shapes of herniated discs can appear from one intervertebral disc and can be accompanied by bulging.

According to the announced term definition, protrusion and extrusion are divided not only by anatomical criteria, but also by morphological criteria. Protrusion is when the distance between the displaced discs in the axial image or coronal image is less than the distance between the base on the same surface. If there is a part where the distance between the displaced discs in the axial image or coronal image is longer than the distance between the base on the same surface, or if

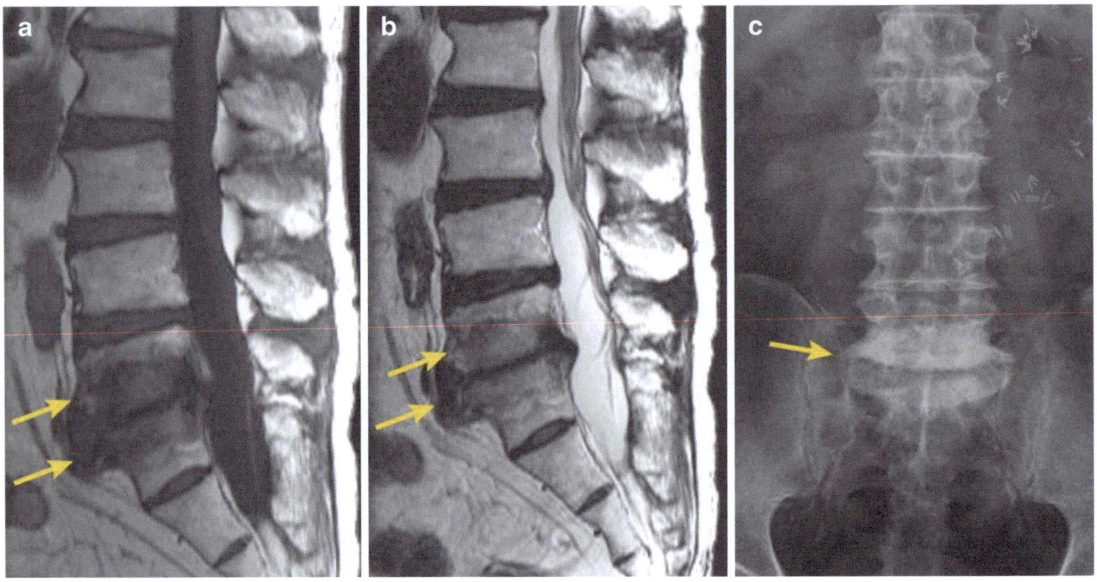

Fig. 5.13 Modic type 3 endplate change
On lumbar MR, Modic type 3 change is observed around the L5/S1 disc vertebral body. Modic type 3 change is thought to be a finding due to sclerosis, showing low signal intensity on T1-weighted images and low signal intensity on T2-weighted images, and observed as a hardened shadow on general X-ray images (arrow)

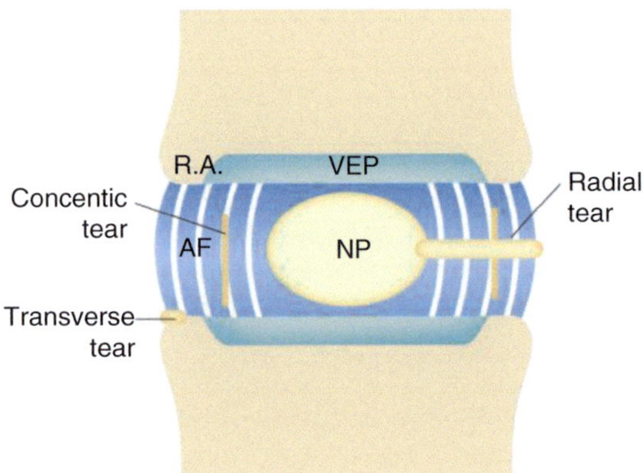

Fig. 5.14 Annular fissure
A transverse fissure is when the part connected to the annulus fibrosus (AF) and ring apophysis (RA) falls off, mainly occurring in the front. A concentric fissure is a fissure between the fibrocartilage concentric lamellae of the annulus fibrosus. A radial fissure is a fissure that crosses the layer from the nucleus pulposus to the outer annulus fibrosus, mainly occurring in the back. *VEP* vertebral endplate, *NP* nucleus pulposus

Table 5.5 Findings suggesting discogenic low back pain

Low back pain
Cumulative loading intolerance (can stand for only a short period of time)
Sitting intolerance (can sit for only a short period of time)
Normal neurologic exam (sensory change, weakness, reflex)

it is separated from the parent disc, it is called extrusion (Fig. 5.18). Therefore, if there is migration up and down, it also belongs to extrusion (Fig. 5.19). Sequestration separated from the parent disc also belongs to extrusion.

The location of disc herniation in the horizontal plane is divided into several zones, which are described as four: central, subarticular, foraminal, and extraforaminal zone (Fig. 5.20). The subarticular zone corresponds to the lateral recess, from the inner boundary of the facet joint

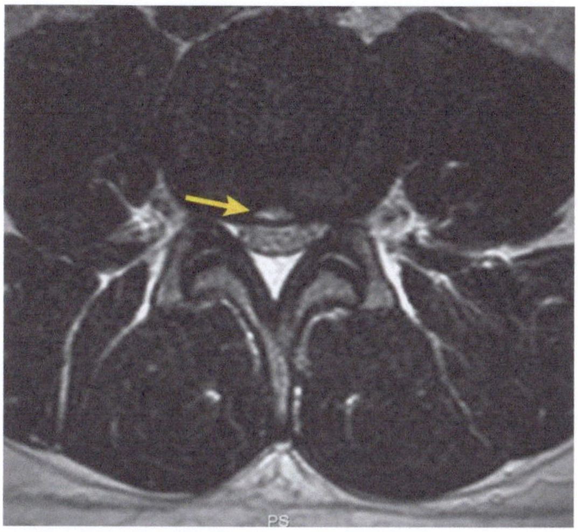

Fig. 5.15 High-intensity zone (HIZ)
HIZ refers to the part that shows high signal intensity separated from the nucleus pulposus within the annulus fibrosus on MR T2-weighted images (arrow), and it is a finding that appears as a secondary change due to an annular fissure

Table 5.6 Modified Dallas discogram scale

Grade 0	Contrast medium confined to a normal nucleus pulposus
Grade 1	Radial tear confined to the inner third of the annulus fibrosus
Grade 2	Radial tear extending to the middle third of the annulus fibrosus
Grade 3	Radial tear extending to the outer third of the annulus fibrosus
Grade 4	Grade 3 tear with dissection into the outer third of the annulus to involve more than 30 degrees of the disc circumference
Grade 5	Any full-thickness tear with extra-annular leakage of contrast

Fig. 5.16 Modified Dallas Discogram scale Radial annular fissure in CT discography is divided into 5 stages according to the Modified Dallas Discogram scale

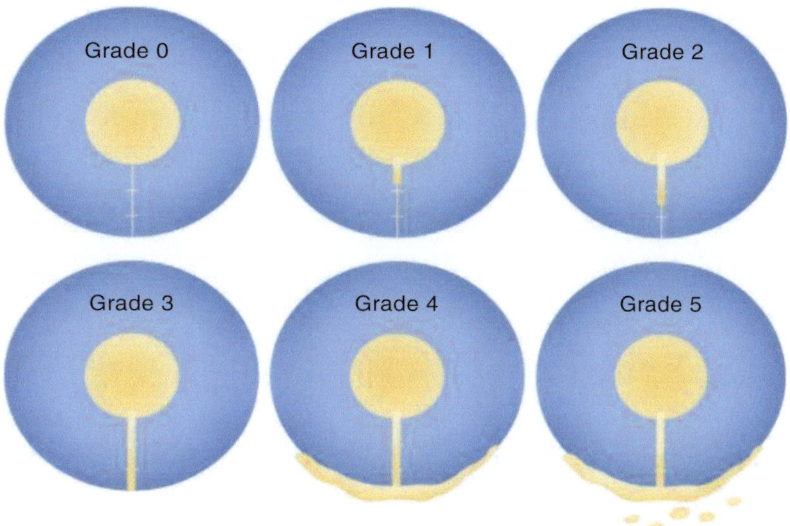

to the inner side of the pedicle (Fig. 5.21). The foraminal zone is the area where the neural foramen is located, from the inner boundary of the pedicle to the outer boundary (Fig. 5.22). Therefore, the boundary between the central zone and the subarticular zone is the inner boundary of the facet joint, the boundary between the subarticular zone and the foraminal zone is the inner boundary of the pedicle, and the boundary between the foraminal zone and the extraforaminal zone is the outer boundary of the pedicle. In the central zone, when there is a slightly biased shape to the left or right, it is described as right central, left central. It was recommended not to use terms used in the past such as central to right or central to left. Also, the term paracentral is not

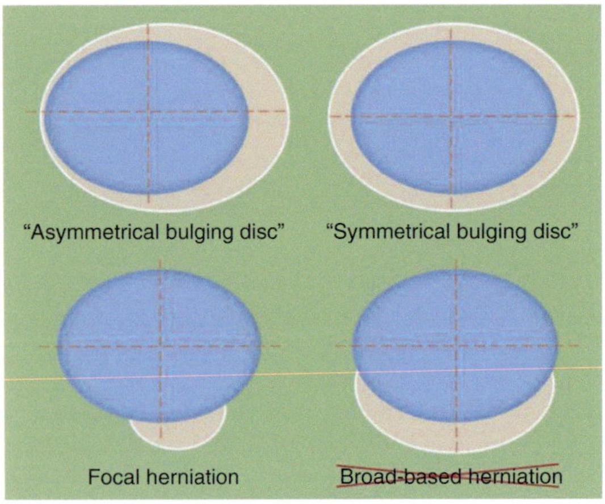

Fig. 5.17 Definition of herniated disc
Disc herniation is defined as the localized displacement of the intervertebral disc from the boundary of the disc space. Previously, the term "localized" in the definition of localized displacement was defined as displacement within 50% of the periphery of the intervertebral disc, with <25% defined as "focal," and displacement between 25% and 50% defined as "broad-based." However, in the revised version 2.0, the definition of localized has been changed to <25%, eliminating broad-based herniation, and only the previous focal herniation is defined as herniation. If the displacement of the intervertebral disc is more than 25%, it is not called disc herniation, but bulging

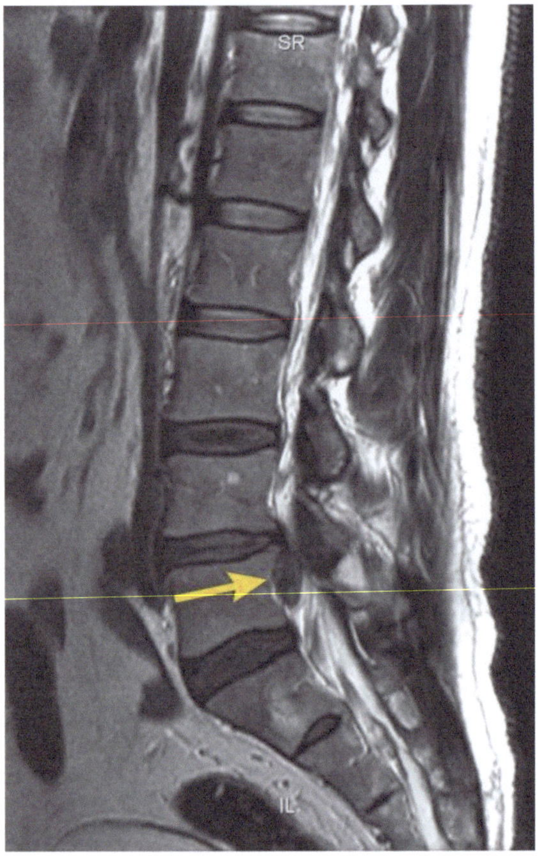

Fig. 5.19 HIVD with inferior migration
In the lumbar spine MR T2-enhanced image, the intervertebral disc between the 4th and 5th lumbar vertebrae is herniated and migrated downwards (arrow), corresponding to extrusion

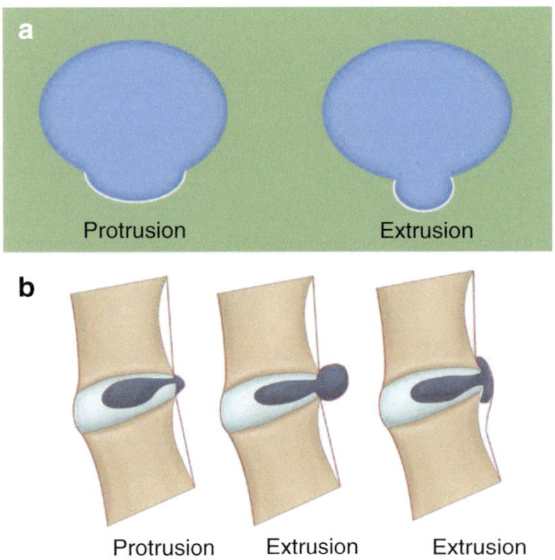

Fig. 5.18 Protrusion and extrusion
Protrusion is when the distance between the displaced intervertebral discs in both the axial and sagittal images is less than the distance between the base on the same plane. If there is a part where the distance between the displaced intervertebral discs in the axial or sagittal image is longer than the distance between the base on the same plane, or if it is separated from the parent intervertebral disc, it is called extrusion

accurate, so it was decided to use the terms right central or left central. When the intervertebral disc displacement spans multiple zones, it is expressed as central-right central-right subarticular-right foraminal zone.

The location of disc herniation in the coronal plane is called level, and it is distinguished based on the intervertebral disc and pedicle. The area where the intervertebral disc is located is called the disc level, the area where the pedicle is located is called the pedicle level, and the area above the pedicle is divided into the suprapedicle level, and the area below the pedicle is the infrapedicle level (Fig. 5.23).

The volume of disc herniation is described as mild if it is <1/3 of the dural sac in the cross-section where the compression of the dural sac is most severe, moderate if it is between 1/3 and

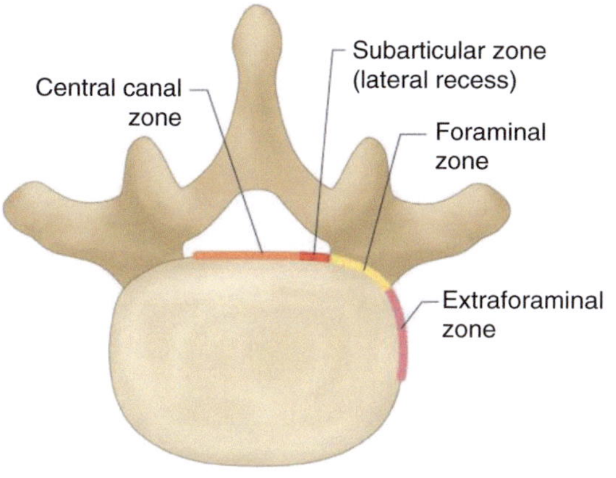

Fig. 5.20 The direction of disc herniation in the horizontal plane is central, subarticular, It is described in four terms: foraminal, extraforaminal zone
The boundary between the central zone and the subarticular zone is the inner surface of the facet joint, the boundary between the subarticular zone and the foraminal zone is the inner surface of the pedicle, and the boundary between the foraminal zone and the extraforaminal zone is the outer surface of the pedicle

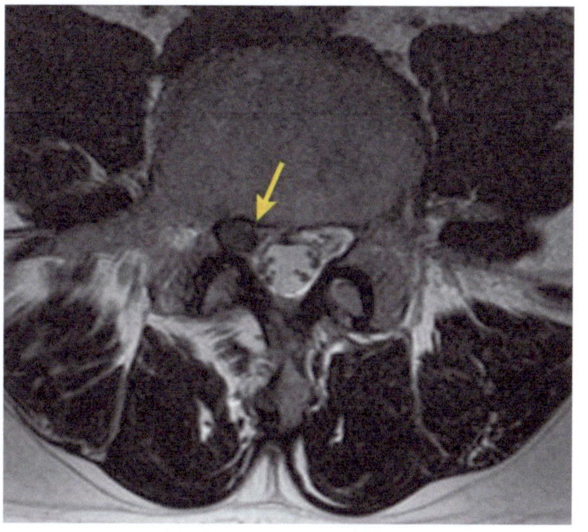

Fig. 5.21 Herniated disc at right subarticular zone
Disc herniation into the subarticular zone is observed in the axial T2-weighted image (arrow). The subarticular zone is the area corresponding to the lateral recess, from the inner surface of the facet joint to the inner surface of the pedicle

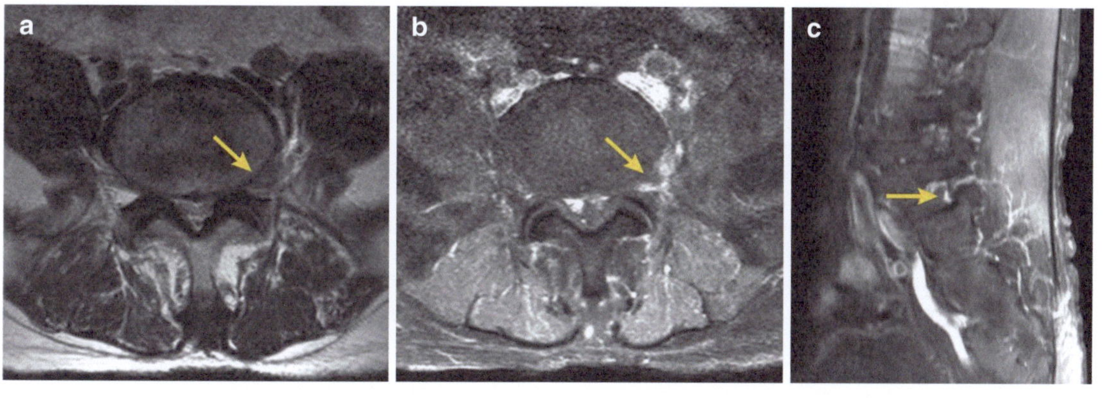

Fig. 5.22 Herniated disc at left foraminal zone
In the T2-enhanced axial image (**a**) and fat-suppressed post-contrast axial (**b**) and sagittal (**c**) images, L5/S1 disc herniation is observed in the left foraminal zone. The foraminal zone is the area where the neural foramen is located, from the inner boundary of the pedicle to the outer boundary

2/3, and severe if it is more than 2/3. These criteria also divide the foramen into three stages based on the foramen in the foraminal zone.

Chronic disc herniation is a term used when calcification, ossification, and air are observed in the herniated disc, and such cases can be said to be not recently occurring disc herniation. However, the term chronic disc herniation is not used in disc herniation where calcification, ossification, and air components are not observed. A similar concept is the term hard disc, which refers to a herniated disc with calcification or ossification and adjacent vertebral. The term is used when observed with osteophytes of the body, mainly used in contrast to disc herniation caused by displacement of the nucleus pulposus itself in the cervical spine.

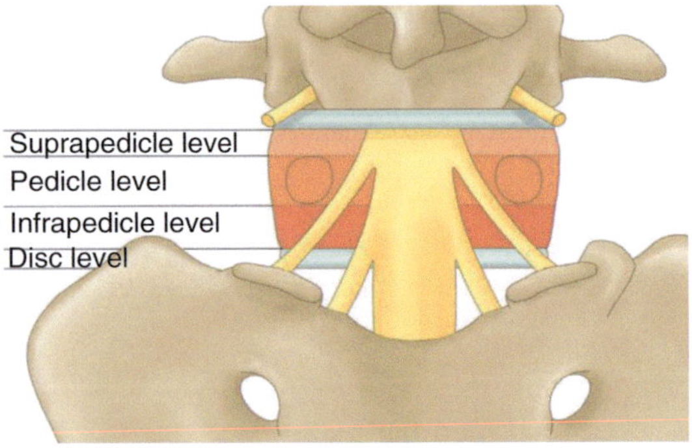

Fig. 5.23 The location of disc herniation in the sagittal plane is distinguished based on the intervertebral disc and pedicle
The area where the intervertebral disc is located is called the disc level, the area where the pedicle is located is called the pedicle level, the area above the pedicle is called the suprapedicle level, and the area below the pedicle is called the infrapedicle level

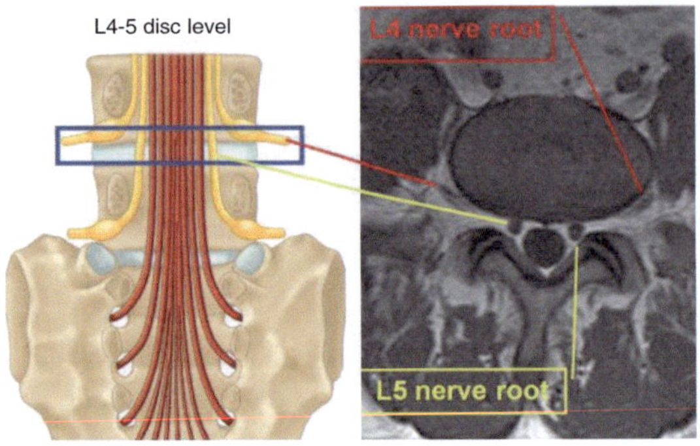

Fig. 5.24 In the lumbar spine, the nerve root exits early from the dura mater and exists in the epidural space, so at the lumbar 4/5 intervertebral disc level, the lumbar 5 nerve is already out of the dural sac and located in the epidural space, and the lumbar 4 nerve is located in the lumbar 4/5 neural foramen

The revised nomenclature version 2.0 presents findings that can suggest acute disc herniation, which are (1) high signal shadows on T2-enhanced images and (2) contrast enhancement around the herniated disc [26].

Describing the relationship between disc herniation and the posterior longitudinal ligament, it is described as transligamentous when it has passed through the posterior longitudinal ligament, and subligamentous when it has not.

5.1.4.2 Relationship Between Disc Herniation and Nerve Root

The number of nerve roots differs between the cervical spine and the thoracolumbar spine because there are 8 cervical spinal nerves compared to 7 cervical spines. Since the C1 nerve comes out above the first cervical spine bone, in the cervical spine, the nerve of the same number comes out above the cervical spine bone of the same number. For example, the C6 nerve comes out of the C5/6 neural foramen. However, since the C8 nerve comes out of the C7/T1 neural foramen, the nerve of the same number comes out below the spine bone of the same number below this. But in the lumbar spine, the nerve root exits early from the dural sac and exists in the epidural space. For example, the L4 nerve comes out of the L4/5 neural foramen. However, at the L4/5 intervertebral disc level, the L5 nerve is already out of the dural sac and located in the epidural space (Fig. 5.24). The L5 nerve, while located on the inner side of the L5 pedicle of the same number, goes down and rides on the lower side of the L5 pedicle and exits to the L5/S1 neural foramen. Due to these anatomical features, if the L4/5 intervertebral disc herniates to the central zone or subarticular zone, the L5 nerve root is compressed. If the L4/5 intervertebral disc escapes to the foraminal zone or extraforaminal zone, the L4 nerve root is compressed.

The relationship between disc herniation and nerve root can be described as contact, deviation (or displacement), compression. Contact is when the herniated disc touches the nerve root when the nerve root is in its normal position, deviation is when the nerve root is pushed back from its normal position but maintains its round shape, and compression is when the nerve root is flattened and its round shape is lost due to the herniated disc.

5.1.5 Segmental Instability and Alignment Disorder

The stability of the spine means to withstand physiological shocks without mechanical deformation or progressive neurological symptoms. The loss of such stability is called instability, and if this instability continues, the arrangement of the vertebral body is damaged.

5.1.5.1 Structures for Spinal Stability

According to the theory of Panjabi et al. [27] spinal stability is composed of three subsystems: passive subsystem, active subsystem, and neural control subsystem. The passive subsystem consists of the vertebral body, facet joint, spinal ligaments, etc. Among them, the main stabilizing structures in the flexion position are the posterior ligaments (interspinous and supraspinous ligaments), facet joint, intervertebral disc, etc. In the extension position, they are the anterior longitudinal ligament, the anterior part of the annulus fibrosus, facet joint, etc. Rotational movements are mainly regulated by the intervertebral disc or facet joint, and side-bending movements are important for the inter-transverse ligament. The active subsystem consists of muscles and tendons. Muscles and tendons play a role in providing information to the neural control subsystem by detecting changes in posture. Unisegmental muscles and plurisegmental muscles play different roles. Unisegmental muscles, such as intertransversarii and interspinalis, are muscles adjacent to the center of the spine, mainly providing information to the nerve control subsystem for movement or posture control. Plurisegmental muscles, such as abdominal muscles and erector spinae, play a role in creating the movement of the lumbar spine. The nerve control subsystem consists of transducers and a neural control center. Panjabi defined clinical instability as follows: "A significant decrease in the capacity of the stabilizing system of the spine to maintain the intervertebral neutral zones within the physiologic limits, so that there is no neurologic dysfunction, no major deformity, and no pain."

5.1.5.2 Diagnostic Criteria

To date, the diagnostic criteria for segmental instability have not been established. Findings suggesting segmental instability in simple X-ray imaging taken in a neutral position include mild intervertebral disc space narrowing, vertebral body sclerosis, "traction osteophyte" growing horizontally 2–3 mm away from the vertebral endplate, and "vacuum phenomenon" [6] Simple X-ray imaging in flexion/extension position, which can observe changes due to spinal movement, is the most commonly used test for diagnosing segmental instability. Spinal instability is suspected when changes in the angle or displacement between spinal segments are observed in simple X-ray images in flexion/extension position (Fig. 5.25). However, since the angle or displacement of flexion/extension can also be observed in actual asymptomatic groups and the range varies depending on the study, it is unreasonable to diagnose instability based on a certain value. It is understood that alignment disorder appears as a result of segmental instability. Such alignment disorders include spondylolisthesis, retrolisthesis, laterolisthesis, kyphosis, scoliosis, etc.

Spondylolisthesis refers to the condition where the vertebral body is anterior to the adjacent lower vertebral body [3, 6, 28, 29]. The main causes are spondylolysis and degeneration. Spondylolysis is a case with a defect in the pars interarticularis, and spondylolisthesis caused by spondylolysis is called spondylolytic spondylolisthesis. If spondylolysis is ambiguous in lateral simple X-ray imaging, oblique imaging can more clearly observe the presence or absence of spondylolysis. In the oblique view, the lumbar spine shows a "scotty dog appearance," where the part corresponding to the dog's eye is the pedicle, the part corresponding to the dog's ear is the superior articular process, the part corresponding to the dog's front leg is the inferior articular process, and the part corresponding to the dog's neck is the pars interarticularis. Therefore, the presence or absence of a defect in the pars interarticularis, which corresponds to the dog's neck, can be directly confirmed in the oblique view (Fig. 5.26).

Spondylolisthesis caused by degeneration without spondylolysis is called degenerative spondylolisthesis. In the lumbar spine, the articular surface of the posterior facet joint is oriented anteromedially, making it vulnerable to spondylolisthesis due to degeneration.

In degenerative spondylolisthesis, both the central canal and neural foramen often narrow (Fig. 5.27), while in spondylolytic spondylolis-

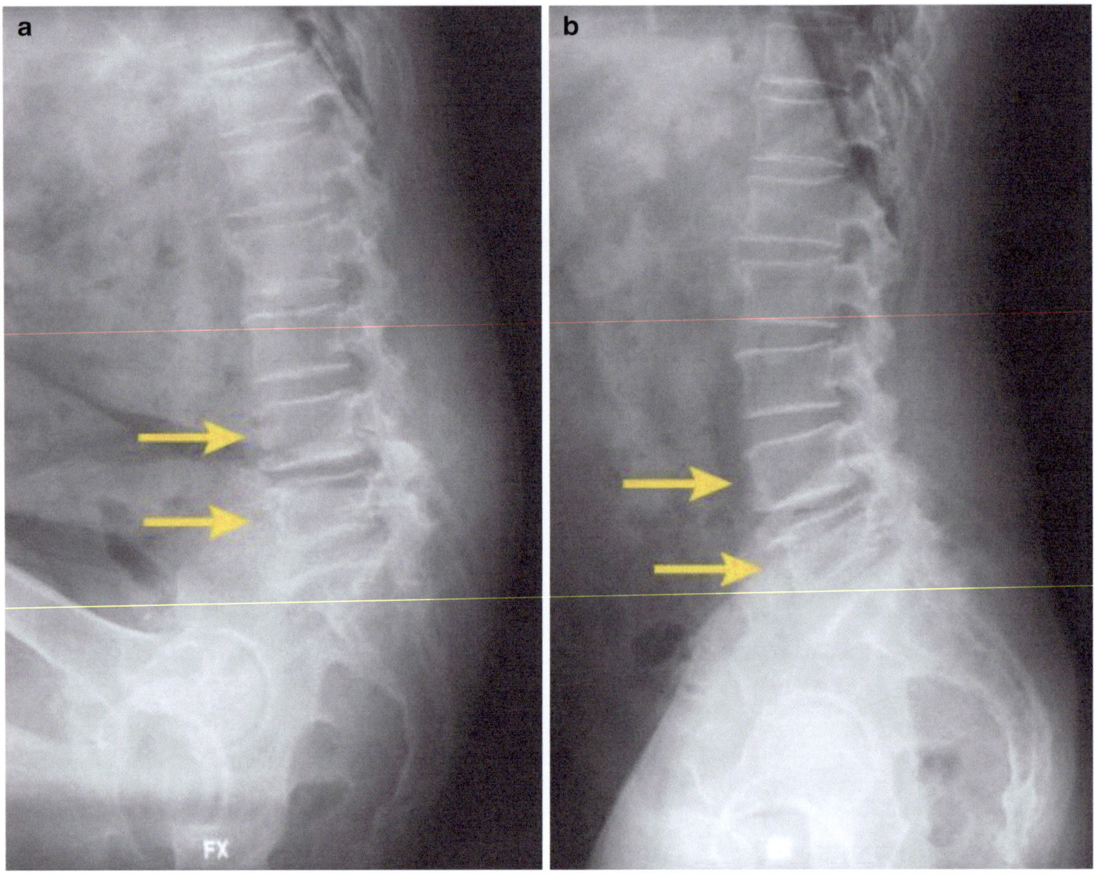

Fig. 5.25 Segmental instability
Changes in the angle and displacement between the lumbar 4/5 vertebrae are observed in the simple X-ray image of the flexed posture, so segmental instability is suspected. Also, there is a finding of spondylolisthesis where the lumbar 4 is displaced forward relative to the lumbar 5

thesis, the central canal does not narrow but rather appears widened, and the neural foramen often narrows (Fig. 5.28). In lateral simple X-ray imaging, the spinous process also remains in place in spondylolytic spondylolisthesis, even though it is anteriorly displaced.

Spondylolisthesis is classified into grade 1 when the displacement is <1/4 of the upper endplate of the lower vertebral body, grade 2 when it is 1/4–2/4, grade 3 when it is 2/4–3/4, and grade 4 when it is 3/4.

Retrolisthesis is when the vertebral body is displaced backward compared to the lower vertebral body, which occurs due to degeneration. This retrolisthesis can cause central canal stenosis and symptoms. The vertebral body can also be displaced sideways due to degeneration, which is called lateral displacement.

Degeneration can cause kyphosis, which is called lumbar degenerative kyphosis (LDK). Characteristically, the forward bending is emphasized in erect X-ray images, and patients show clinical symptoms of leaning forward when walking. It is common in patients who have done a lot of work like farming. If the alignment disorder caused by degeneration spans multiple segments, it can become degenerative scoliosis.

5.1.6 Spinal Stenosis

Spinal stenosis refers to the compression of the nerve due to narrowing in the spinal canal where

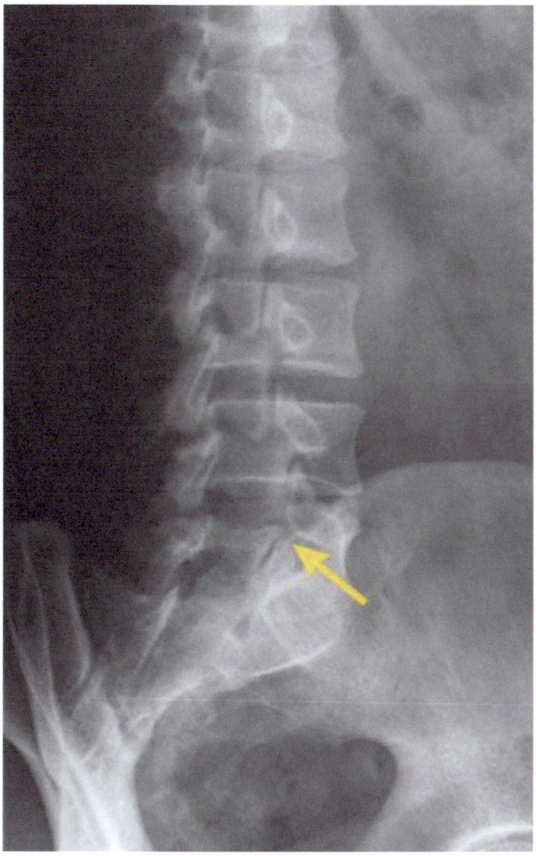

Fig. 5.26 Spondylolysis
When the lumbar spine is photographed in the oblique view, the lumbar spine shows a "scotty dog appearance," where the part corresponding to the dog's eye is the pedicle, the part corresponding to the dog's ear is the superior articular process, the part corresponding to the dog's front leg is the inferior articular process, and the part corresponding to the dog's neck is the pars interarticularis. A defect in the pars interarticularis, which corresponds to the dog's neck, is observed in the lumbar spine 5 (arrow), so it is lumbar 5 spondylosis

the nerve runs. Broadly, spinal stenosis includes all cases where the spinal canal narrows due to various causes, with congenital causes including chondrodysplasia, Morquio syndrome, short pedicle syndrome, and acquired causes including degeneration, disc herniation, spondylolisthesis, ossification of the posterior longitudinal ligament, Paget's disease, and acromegaly. Narrow spinal stenosis refers to narrowing due to structural changes caused by long-term degeneration, and clinically, it is often used in the narrow sense. In the lumbar spine, spinal stenosis is divided into central canal stenosis, lateral recess stenosis, and foraminal stenosis depending on its location.

5.1.6.1 Central Canal Stenosis

Central canal stenosis is mainly caused by intervertebral disc degeneration and height reduction due to disc bulging and ligamentum flavum hypertrophy, and posterior osteophytes from the vertebral body or degenerative arthritis of the facet joint can also be a concurrent cause. As mentioned earlier, degenerative spondylolisthesis and retrolisthesis are also important causes of central canal stenosis (Fig. 5.29) [3, 11, 30, 31].

In the lumbar spine, if the cross-sectional area of the dural sac in the central canal is <100 mm^2, it is diagnosed as central canal stenosis, and if it is <75 mm^2, it is diagnosed as severe central canal stenosis (Fig. 5.29) [32]. However, there is a problem that these figures do not consider individual differences or segmental differences.

Another definition diagnoses lumbar spine central canal stenosis based on the presence or absence of cerebrospinal fluid loss in front of the cauda equina and between the nerve roots of the cauda equina on MR, and can divide the severity [33]. If the intradural cerebrospinal fluid part in front of the cauda equina is not visible due to loss on T2-weighted images, it is diagnosed as central canal stenosis, and if each nerve root of the intradural cauda equina is completely separated, it is mild, and if some are clustered together, it is moderate. If all nerve roots appear as a single bundle, it is described as severe (Table 5.7, Fig. 5.30).

In the lumbar spine, due to central canal stenosis, the nerve roots of the cauda equina are continuously compressed, and the flow of cerebrospinal fluid causes the nerve roots to roll upwards, causing the nerve roots of the compressed proximal parts to stretch. Depending on the case, the nerve roots of the compressed proximal parts can also stretch. These stretched nerve roots can sometimes be mistaken for intradural tumors, so careful observation is required. It can be distinguished from tumors by findings such as the stretched appearance of the nerve root bundles, central canal stenosis in the lower lum-

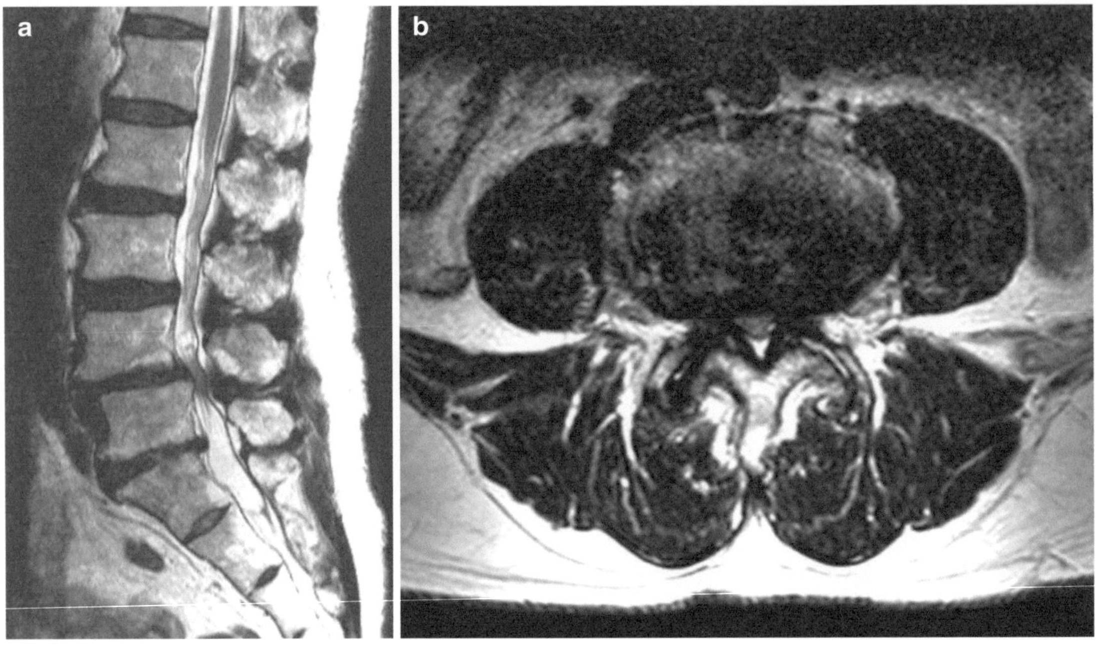

Fig. 5.27 Degenerative spondylolisthesis
Degenerative spondylolisthesis is observed between lumbar 4/5 in the MR T2-weighted sagittal image (**a**). Severe central canal stenosis is observed at L4/5 in the MR T2-weighted sagittal image (**a**) and axial image (**b**)

bar spine, and elongation of the proximal nerve roots (Fig. 5.31).

5.1.6.2 Foraminal Stenosis

In the lumbar spine, foraminal stenosis is caused by a decrease in intervertebral disc height, intervertebral disc bulging, alignment disorder due to facet joint arthrosis, and osteophytes. Spondylolytic spondylolisthesis can cause neural foraminal stenosis even in relatively young adults.

The method of diagnosing and grading lumbar foraminal stenosis is the degree of fat tissue loss around the nerve root in the coronal plane and the presence or absence of nerve root compression. If fat tissue loss is observed in both directions (up-down or front-back), it is diagnosed as foraminal stenosis. If there is fat tissue loss in only one direction (up-down or front-back), it is considered mild (grade 1), and if there is fat tissue loss in two or more directions, it is considered moderate (grade 2). Even if the fat tissue is not completely lost, if the nerve root is compressed and flattened, it is divided into severe (grade 3) (Table 5.8, Figs. 5.32, 5.33, and 5.34).

5.1.6.3 Lateral Recess Stenosis

The lateral recess is a passage where the nerve root descends before exiting the neural foramen in the lumbar spine, and it is the space between the medial side of the pedicle, the superior articular process, and the posterior surface of the vertebral body. Lateral recess stenosis is less common than central canal stenosis or foraminal stenosis and is diagnosed when the distance between the posterior surface of the vertebral body and the superior articular process is <3 mm. Lateral recess stenosis mainly occurs due to osteophytes originating from the posterior surface of the vertebral body, osteophytes growing forward from the facet joint, and degenerative scoliosis.

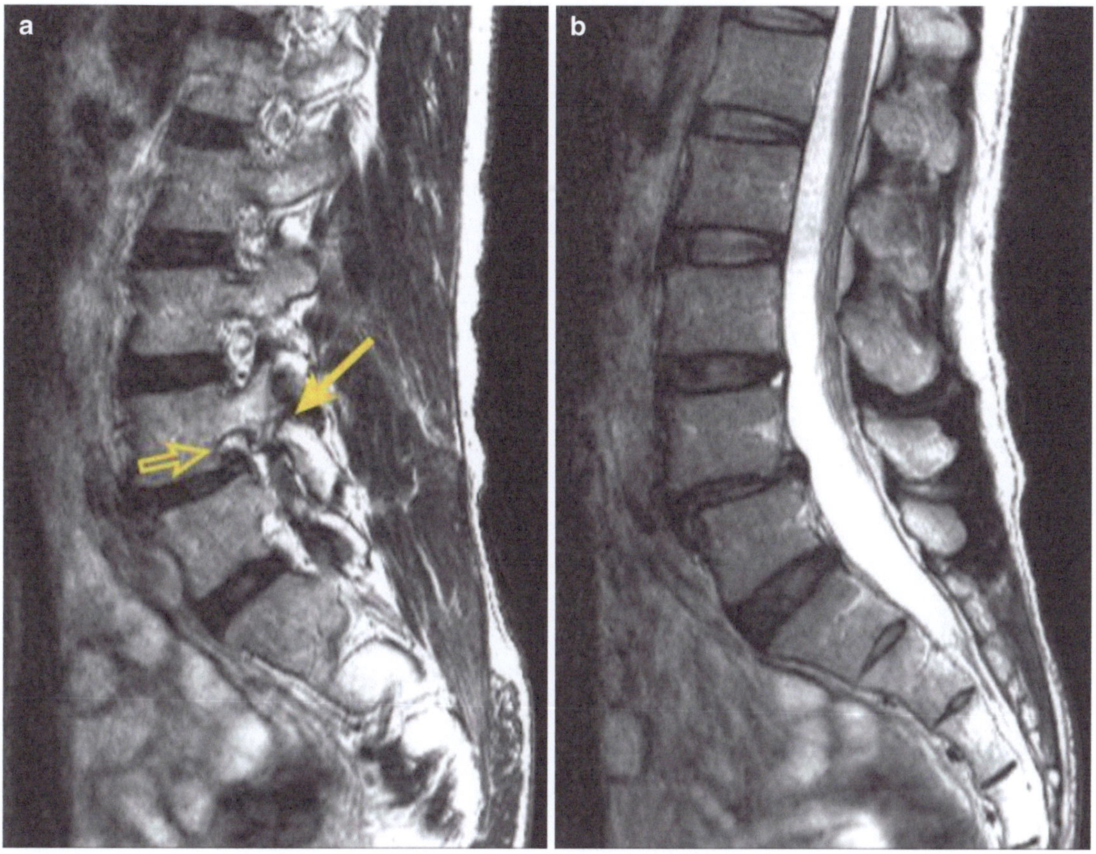

Fig. 5.28 Spondylolytic spondylolisthesis
In the MR T2-weighted image, spondylolisthesis due to spondylolysis is observed at L4/5 (arrow), and foraminal stenosis is accompanied (empty arrow). In spondylolisthesis due to spondylolysis, the central canal appears to be widened

5.1.7 Degeneration of posterior tissues

Normally, the intervertebral disc supports about 2/3 of the load and absorbs shock. However, as this intervertebral disc degenerates, it can only support about half of the load, and the remaining shock is absorbed by the posterior tissues, accelerating degenerative changes. These degenerative changes in the posterior tissues appear in the ligamentum flavum, facet joint, interspinous ligament, spinous process, etc.

The ligamentum flavum thickens due to degenerative changes, and this hypertrophied ligamentum flavum is a cause of the previously mentioned spinal stenosis.

The facet joint is a synovial joint, so it shows similar degenerative changes to other joints. That is, joint space narrowing, subchondral sclerosis, subchondral erosion and cyst, osteophytes formation, etc. Such facet joints are a major cause of the previously mentioned spinal instability or alignment disorder. Due to the degenerative changes of the facet joint, joint effusion can sometimes occur. When this joint effusion leaks into the surrounding space and shows a mass shape, it is called a synovial cyst of facet joint origin (Fig. 5.35). Such a synovial cyst can cause clinical symptoms by compressing the nerve root when it occurs in front of the facet joint, but it does not show any clinical symptoms when it occurs behind the facet joint.

Due to the degenerative changes of the spinous process and interspinous ligament, the spi-

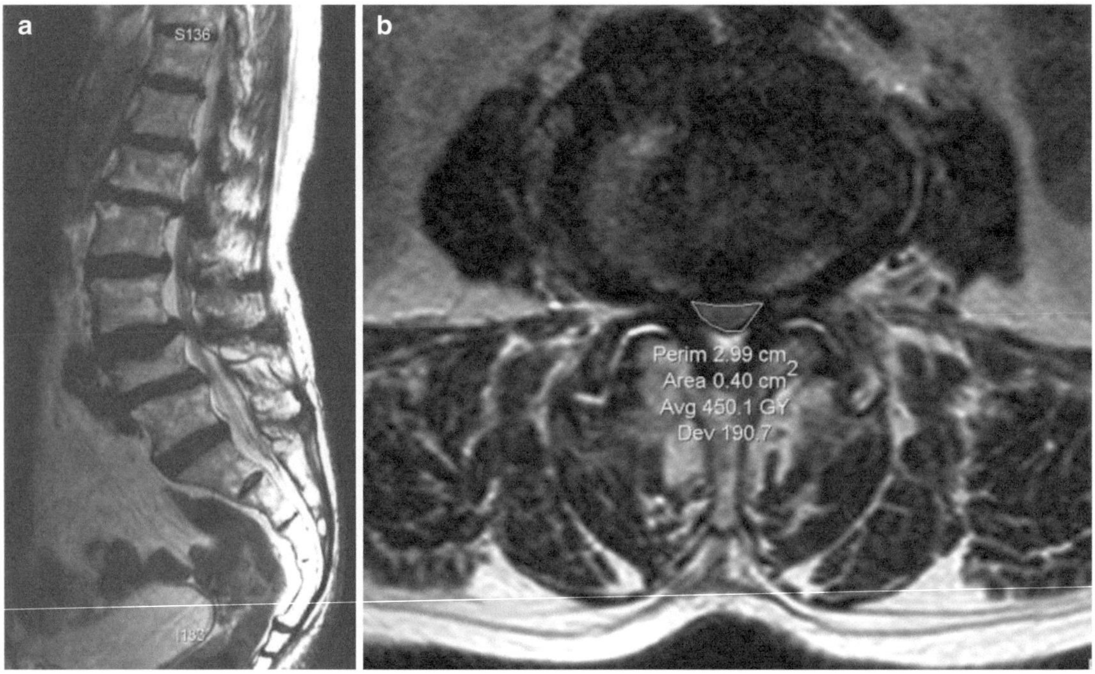

Fig. 5.29 Lumbar central canal stenosis
Degenerative spondylolisthesis is observed between lumbar 3/4 in the MR T2-weighted sagittal image (**a**), and central canal stenosis is observed in the axial image (**b**). The cross-sectional area of the dural sac was measured as 40 mm^2

Table 5.7 Diagnostic criteria and grades of lumbar spine central canal stenosis

Mild central canal stenosis	Obliterated CSF space in front of cauda equina on T2W axial image, but clear separation of all cauda equina
Moderate central canal stenosis	With aggregation of some cauda equina
Severe central canal stenosis	With none of cauda equina separated, showing one bundle-like appearance

nous process can enlarge, and pseudoarthrosis and bursitis can form in the interspinous ligament. Such degenerative changes of the spinous process and interspinous ligament are called Baastrup's phenomenon (Fig. 5.36) [11].

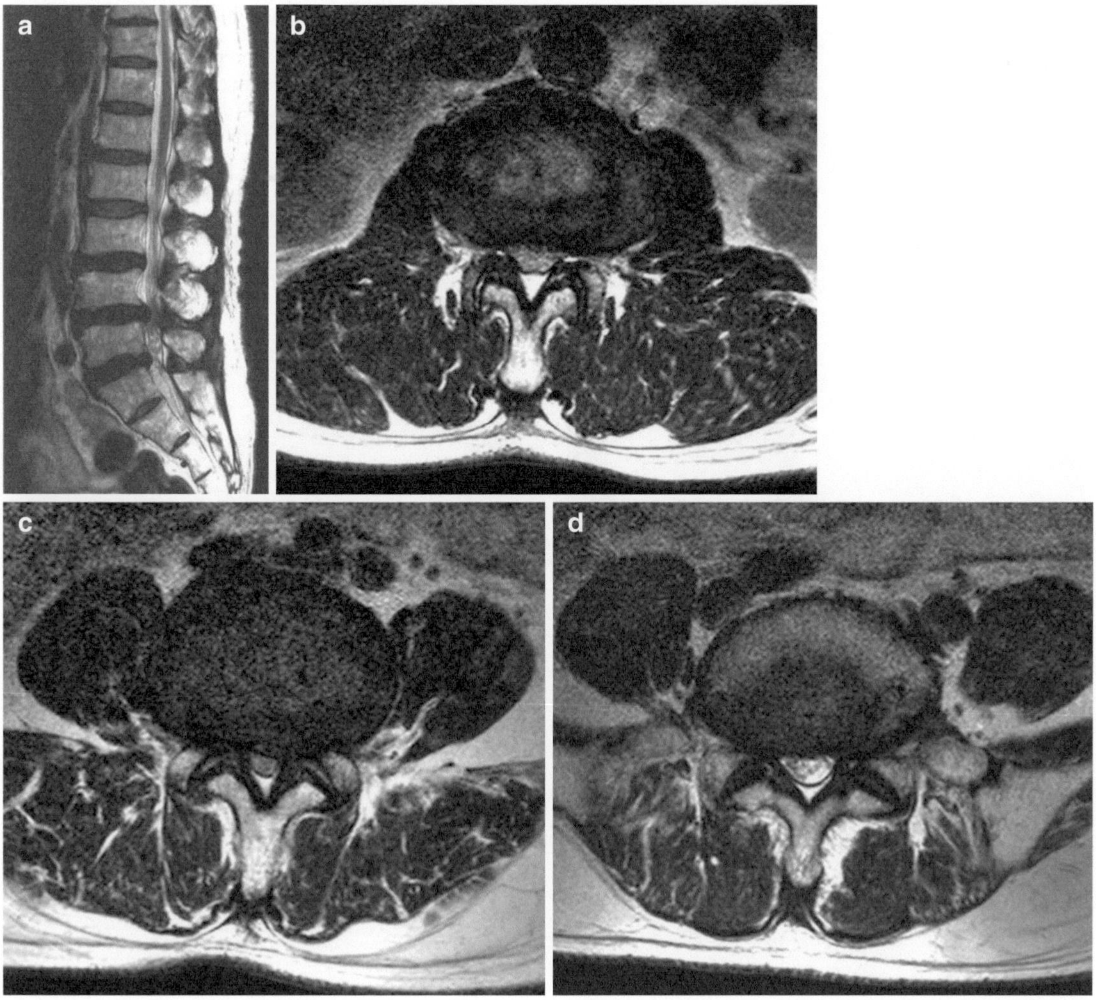

Fig. 5.30 Lumbar central canal stenosis
In the MR T2-enhanced coronal image (**a**), various degrees of central canal stenosis are observed from L2/3 to L5/S1. In the T2-enhanced axial image, at the L2/3 site (**b**), some nerve roots within the dural sac appear as one, and some appear separately, indicating moderate stenosis. At the L4/5 site (**c**), all nerve roots within the dural sac appear bundled together, indicating severe stenosis. At the L5/S1 site (**d**), the cerebrospinal fluid part in front of the cauda equina within the dura mater is not clearly visible, but each nerve root appears separately, indicating mild stenosis

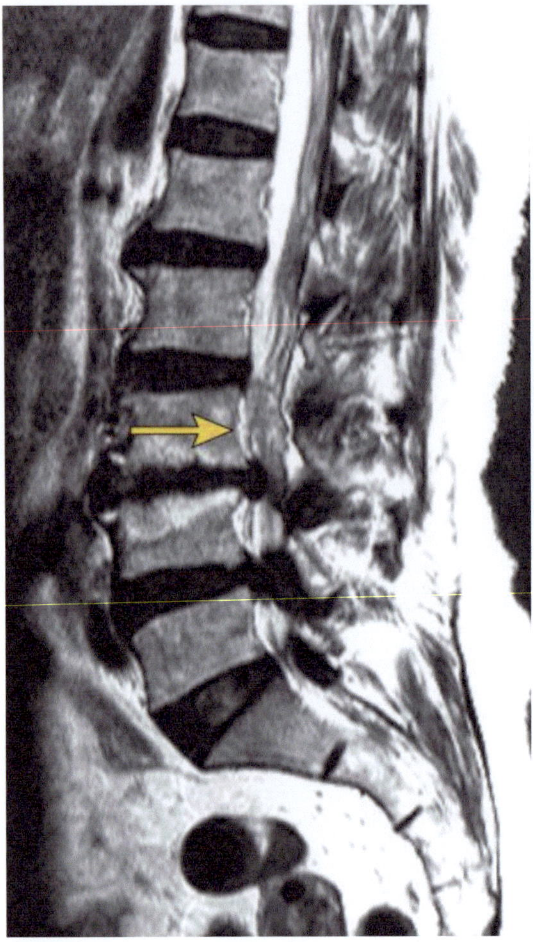

Fig. 5.31 Lumbar central canal stenosis
Central canal stenosis is observed at L3/4, L4/5, and the nerve root within the dural sac at the L3 vertebral body level can be seen to be twisted and stretched (arrow). Due to the central canal stenosis, the cauda equina nerve roots are continuously compressed, and the flow of cerebrospinal fluid causes the nerve roots to roll upwards, stretching the nerve roots of the proximal compression parts

Table 5.8 Grades of lumbar spine foraminal stenosis

Mild foraminal stenosis (grade 1)	Perineural fat obliteration in the two opposing directions (vertical or transverse). No evidence of morphologic change
Moderate foraminal stenosis (grade 2)	Perineural fat obliteration surrounding the nerve root in the four directions without morphologic change, in both vertical and transverse directions
Severe foraminal stenosis (grade 3)	Nerve root collapse or morphological change

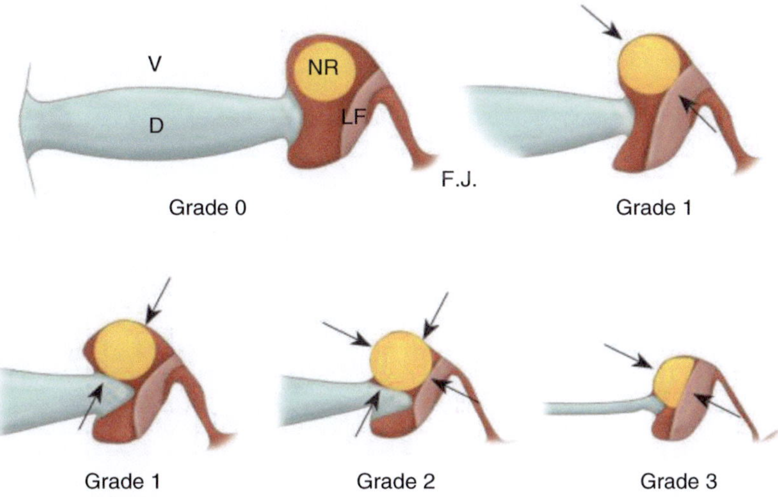

Fig. 5.32 Grade of lumbar foraminal stenosis
If the degree of fat tissue loss around the nerve root is observed in the opposing directions (up-down or front-back), it is considered neural foraminal. The diagnosis was made of stenosis, and if there is a loss of adipose tissue around the nerve root in one direction only (up-down or front-back), it is considered mild (grade 1), and if there is a loss of adipose tissue around the nerve root in two or more directions, it is considered moderate (grade 2). Also, even if the adipose tissue is not completely lost, if the nerve root is compressed and flattened, it is classified as severe (grade 3)

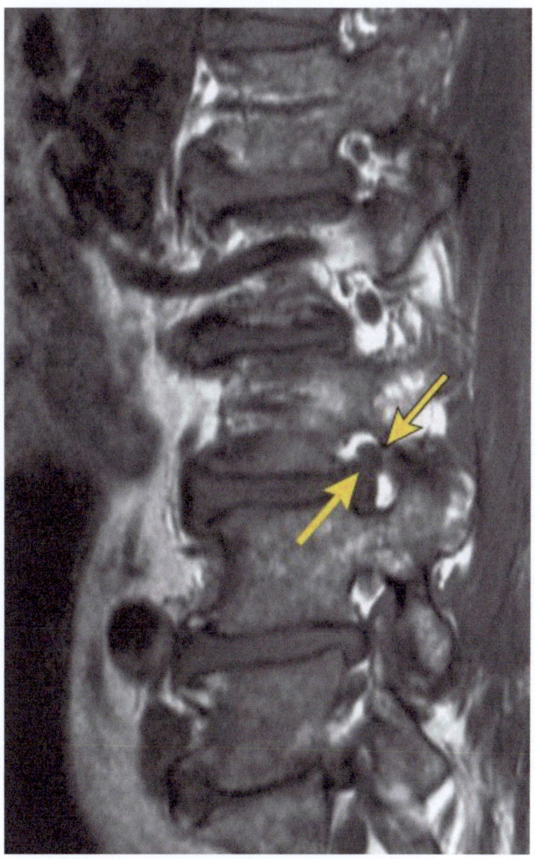

Fig. 5.33 Mild lumbar foraminal stenosis (grade 1)
The adipose tissue around the nerve root of the L3/4 neural foramen appears to be lost in the front lower and back upper directions (arrow), so it can be diagnosed as foraminal stenosis, and since the adipose tissue around the nerve root is lost in only one direction, it is mild

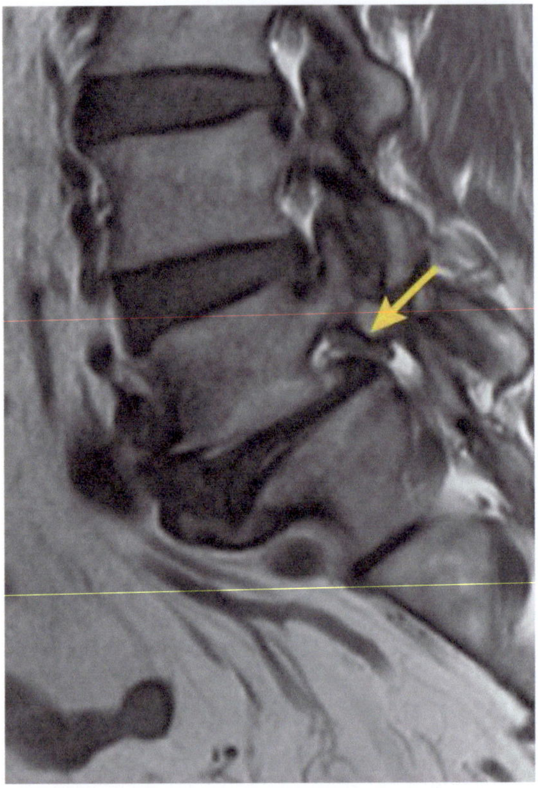

Fig. 5.34 Severe lumbar foraminal stenosis (grade 3)
There is spondylolisthesis due to spondylolysis at L5/S1, and foraminal stenosis is observed due to this. Since the nerve root is compressed and flattened (arrow), it is severe (grade 3) foraminal stenosis

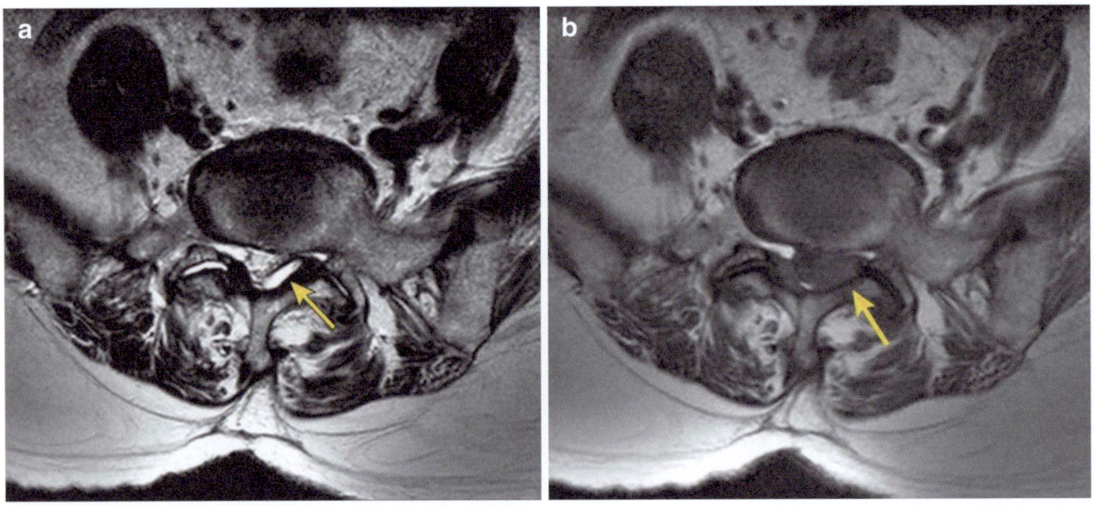

Fig. 5.35 Facet joint synovial cyst
Due to degenerative changes in the facet joint, joint effusion leaks into the surrounding space, showing a mass shape, and this is called a synovial cyst of facet joint origin (arrow)

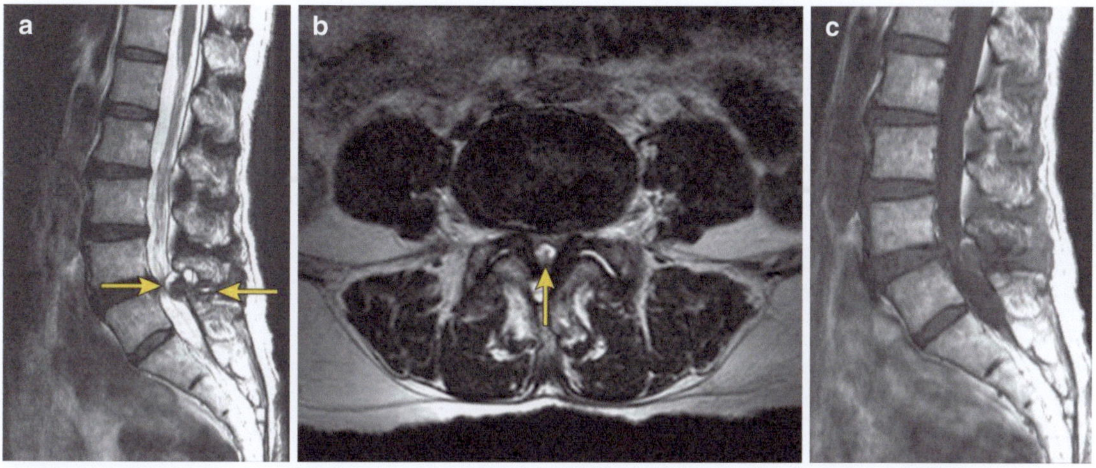

Fig. 5.36 Baastrup's phenomenon
The spinous process can enlarge due to degenerative changes in the spinous process and interspinous ligament, and pseudoarthrosis and burs can form in the interspinous ligament (arrow). Such degenerative changes in the spinous process and interspinous ligament are called Baastrup's phenomenon

5.2 Thoracic Spine

5.2.1 Anatomy

The thoracic spine shows different anatomical features from the lumbar spine or cervical spine, and degenerative changes are rare.

The thoracic spine consists of 12 segments, and 12 pairs of ribs are attached to each side (Fig. 5.37). The thoracic spine closer to the cervical spine has a similar shape to the cervical spine, but the closer to the lumbar spine, the more it resembles the lumbar spine. The first and second thoracic spines have a flat anterior surface. The third thoracic spine is the smallest among the thoracic spines, and the anterior surface is convex. From the fourth thoracic spine downwards, the vertebral body gradually enlarges. The pedicles of the thoracic spine, unlike those of the cervical or lumbar spine, run parallel to each other front and back (Fig. 5.37). The pedicles of the thoracic spine also increase in size as they go down. The joint surface with the ribs is formed on the outer surface of the pedicle. Therefore, the upper surface of the pedicle in the thoracic spine is convex or flat upwards. The lower surface of the pedicle is very concave and has a deep groove. As a result, the neural foramen in the thoracic spine is located at the lower back of the vertebral body.

The lamina of the thoracic spine is thick. The superior articular process is located upwards from the connection between the vertebral body and the pedicle, showing a flat joint surface, facing the posterior surface. The inferior articular process is located downwards from the lamina, with a joint surface facing forward (Fig. 5.37). Therefore, the facet joint surface in the thoracic spine is located on the coronal surface, and due to these anatomical characteristics, degenerative spondylolisthesis or retrolisthesis is very rare compared to the lumbar spine. The transverse process of the thoracic spine is located posteriorly and laterally from the boundary between the pedicle and the lamina. The transverse process of the thoracic spine is longest at the first thoracic spine, and it gets smaller as it goes down, and it is almost non-existent at the twelfth thoracic spine [1, 2, 30].

5.2.2 DISH

Diffuse idiopathic skeletal hyperostosis (DISH) is a chronic bone-forming change that invades the spine and extra-spinal skeleton, mainly causing

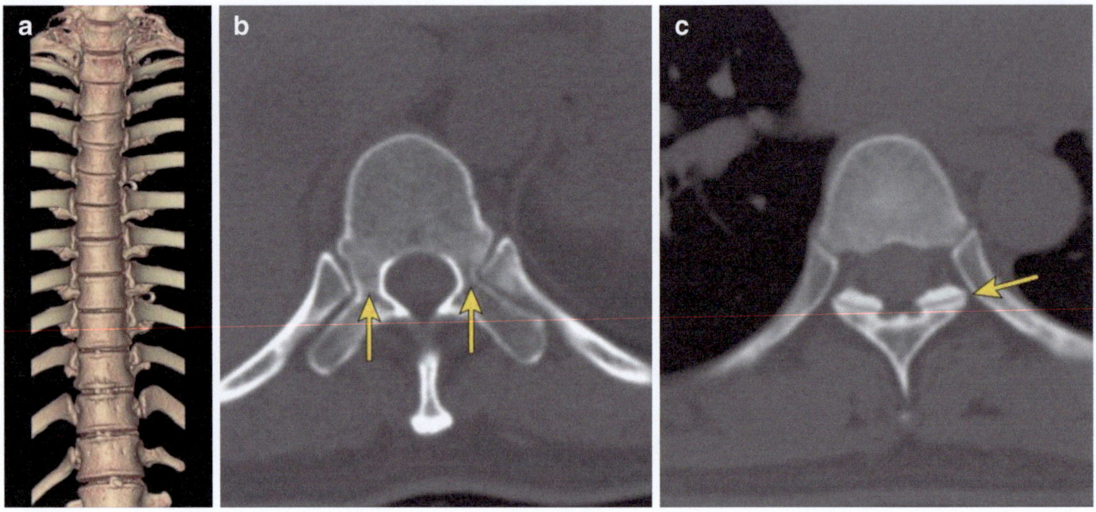

Fig. 5.37 Thoracic spine CT
The thoracic spine consists of 12 segments, with 12 pairs of ribs attached to each side. The vertebral body of the thoracic spine gets larger as it goes down from the 4th thoracic spine (**a**). The pedicle of the thoracic spine runs parallel front and back (**b**, arrow). The facet joint surface of the thoracic spine is located on the coronal plane (**c**, arrow)

bone formation in ligaments or tendons. It appears.

Although the cause of DISH is still unknown, it can be considered a special form of degenerative change as it is prevalent in old age. It primarily affects the thoracic spine, but the cervical spine and lumbar spine can also be affected. The diagnostic criteria are calcification or ossification of the spine outside the vertebral body, affecting four or more consecutive vertebral bodies, maintaining the height of the intervertebral disc, and no abnormalities in both SI joints (Table 5.9) [3].

DISH mainly occurs between the 7th and 11th thoracic spine. In DISH, lateral calcification and ossification of the vertebral body appear (Fig. 5.38). This ossification shows various thicknesses. In DISH, ossification can also occur in ligaments or tendons other than the ossification of the vertebral body. In particular, ossification of the posterior longitudinal ligament (OPLL) in the cervical spine can often be accompanied, and symptoms due to spinal cord compression can occur in such cervical OPLL, which can be the most problematic clinically in DISH patients. Ossification can also occur in ligaments of the pelvis, heel, foot, elbow, hand, knee, etc., osteophytes around the joints, and ossification at the tendon attachment site.

Table 5.9 Diagnostic criteria for DISH

1. Presence of flowing calcification and ossification along the anterolateral aspect of at least four contiguous vertebral bodies, with or without associated localized, pointed excrescences at the intervening vertebral body-intervertebral disc junctions
2. Relative preservation of intervertebral disc height in the involved vertebral segment and the absence of extensive radiographic changes of "degenerative" disc disease, including vacuum phenomenon and vertebral body marginal sclerosis. A cervical central canal stenosis

Diagnoses that need to be differentiated from DISH are degenerative spinal changes and ankylosing spondylitis. In degenerative spinal changes, the intervertebral disc space narrows, vacuum changes appear in the intervertebral disc, and changes such as bone hardening in the adjacent vertebral body appear. Also, in DISH, the point of differentiation is that ligament ossification is in continuous spinal segments, and there is bone formation in other ligaments or tendons. The syndesmophyte of ankylosing spondylitis is

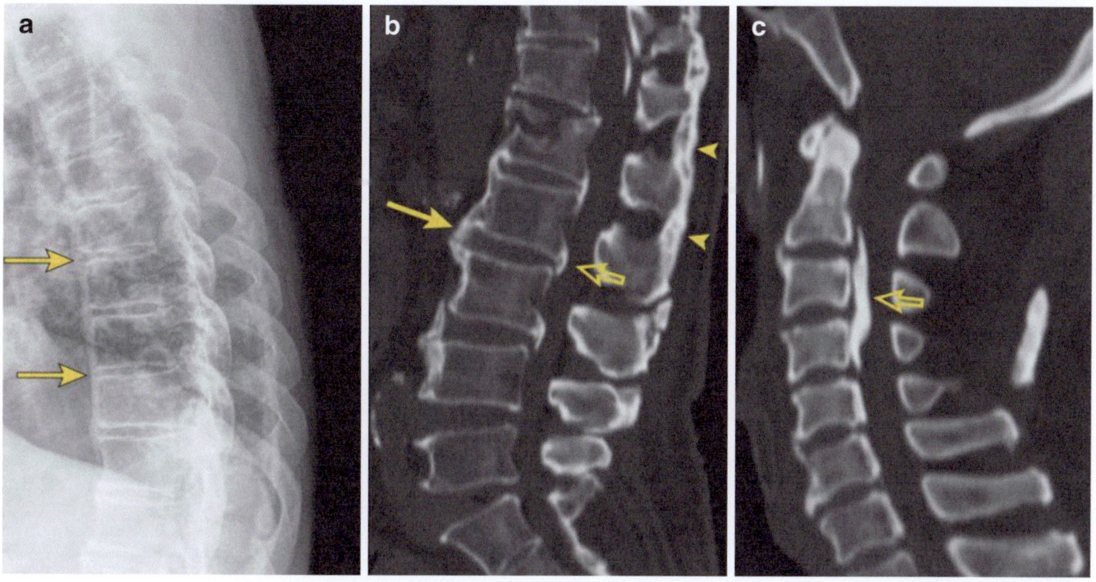

Fig. 5.38 DISH (diffuse idiopathic skeletal hyperostosis)
On a simple X-ray (**a**), osteophytes connecting the first half of the thoracic spine vertebral body are observed (arrow). On lumbar CT (**b**), thoracic spine and lumbar Osteophytes connecting the first half of the vertebral body to the spine are observed (arrow), and Ossificatin of posterior longitudinal ligament (OPLL) is also observed (empty arrow), ossification is also present in the supraspinous ligament (arrowhead). Lumbar 1 vertebral body and thoracic spine 11 and 12 spinous processes is accompanied by a fracture. Cervical spine CT (**c**) shows OPLL (empty arrow)

thin and located along the boundary of the disc, but in DISH, the ossification is larger and thicker and is located further from the intervertebral disc. In DISH, findings suggesting sacroiliitis such as irregular changes in the SI joint should not be observed [3].

5.2.3 Ossification of Ligamentum Flavum

Ossification of the ligamentum flavum is a representative ligament ossification disease that can cause symptoms in the spine along with OPLL. It is prevalent in Far East Asians like Koreans or Japanese.

Ossification of the ligamentum flavum occurs in the thoracic spine, and this ossification of the ligamentum flavum can compress the spinal cord from the back and cause myelopathy. Since this ossification of the ligamentum flavum is often observed at the junction of the thoracic spine and lumbar spine, it is necessary to carefully observe the lower part of the thoracic spine that is also photographed when interpreting lumbar spine MR images. Since the relationship with the spinal cord cannot be accurately known only by the MR coronal plane, the axial plane should be photographed to understand the relationship with the spinal cord. On MR, if the hypertrophied ligamentum flavum shows a sharp attachment, the possibility of ossification of the ligamentum flavum is high. For an accurate diagnosis, it is necessary to confirm ossification on CT (Fig. 5.39).

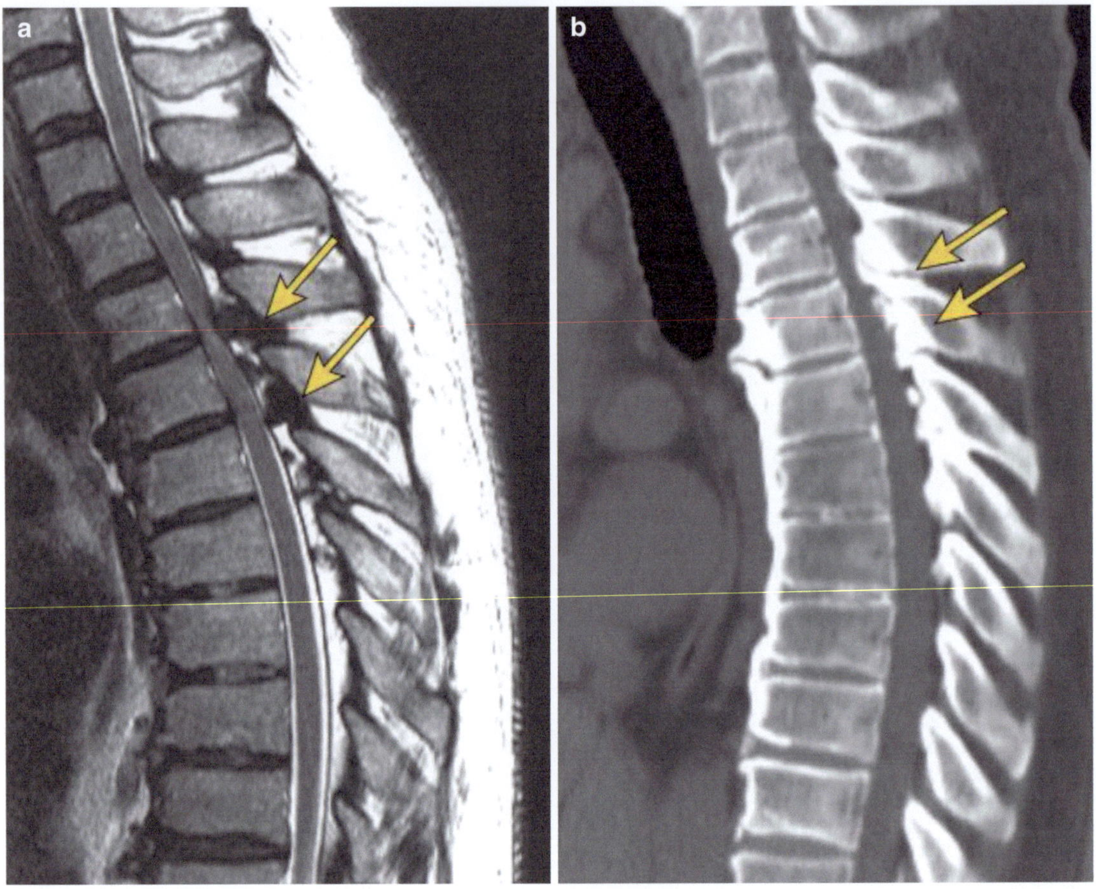

Fig. 5.39 Ligamentum flavum ossification
On the MR T2-enhanced image of the cervical spine, central canal stenosis findings are observed between the 4/5 and 5/6 of the cervical spine due to swelling of the intervertebral disc and buckling of the ligamentum flavum (**a**). The buckling of the ligamentum flavum between the 5/6 of the cervical spine (arrow) is not due to the posterior ligamentum flavum, so it disappears by only increasing the height of the intervertebral disc by removing the swollen intervertebral disc in front through surgery (**b**, arrow)

5.3 Cervical Spine

5.3.1 Anatomy

The cervical spine is composed of a total of 7 vertebral segments, and there are pairs of joints on both the front and back sides from the 2nd to the 7th cervical spine. On the front side, there is a joint of Luschka located behind the vertebral body, and on the back side, there are facet joints on both sides.

The vertebral body of the cervical spine increases in size as it goes down, and the left-right length becomes larger than the front-back. The upper surface of the vertebral body is concave, and the lower surface is convex. Unlike the thoracolumbar spine, the cervical spine has an uncinate process in the posterior direction of the vertebral body, which is a protruding part upwards forming a joint with the upper vertebral body, called the uncovertebral joint or joint of Luschka (Fig. 5.40). The joint of Luschka is a joint-shaped structure created by the curvature of the vertebral body, which is different from the actual joint. Clinically, the term uncovertebral joint is used more than the term joint of Luschka. In the cervical spine, the pedicle is located at the back of the vertebral body and is small, connected to the lateral mass on the outside (Fig. 5.40). The lateral mass is a structure only in

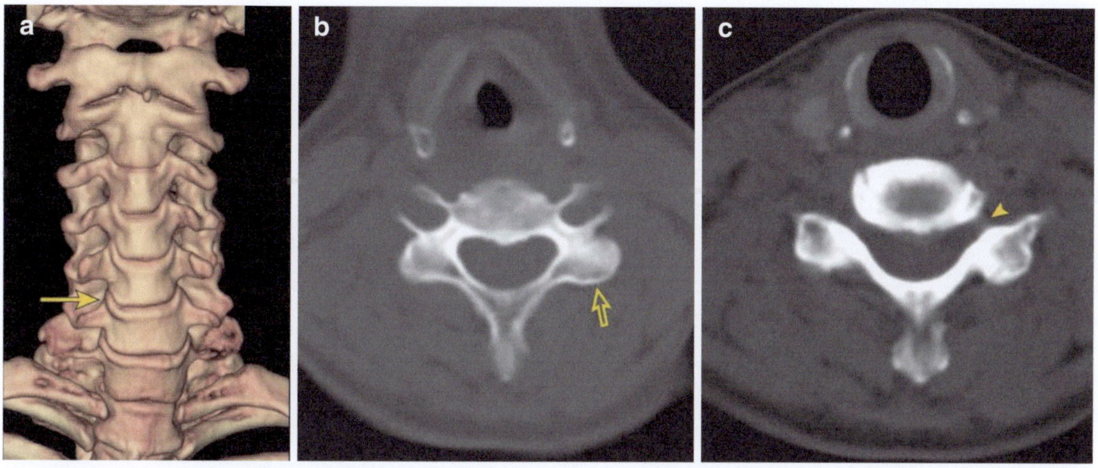

Fig. 5.40 Cervical spine CT
Cervical spine has an uncinate process posteriorly and superiorly to the vertebral body, which protrudes upward and forms an uncovertebal joint with the upper vertebral body (**a**, arrow). In the cervical spine, the pedicle is located posteriorly at the back of the vertebral body, is small, and extends outward It is connected to the lateral mass (empty arrow) (**b**). The neural foramen (arrowhead) of the cervical spine is located anteriorly between the intervertebral disc and uncovertebral disc. The posterolateral part of the joint is bordered by the pedicle above and below, and the superior articular process behind (**c**)

the cervical spine, forming upper and lower joints through the facet joint. There is a lamina from the lateral mass to the posterior medial side, and there is a spinous process at the back where the two laminae meet. The spinous process in the cervical spine is usually bifid in shape [1, 2, 30, 31].

The neural foramen of the cervical spine is a part where the nerve root exits, which is clinically very important. The neural foramen of the cervical spine is bounded by the intervertebral disc and the posterior lateral part of the uncovertebral joint in front, the pedicle above and below, and the superior articular process in the back (Fig. 5.40). Therefore, in the cervical spine, the nerve root exits right in front of the facet joint, right behind the uncovertebral joint. In the cervical spine, degenerative changes cause the uncovertebral joint to form osteophytes toward the neural foramen, compressing the nerve root, which is the most common cause of nerve root compression in the cervical spine.

The intervertebral disc of the cervical spine, unlike the lumbar spine, has almost no annulus fibrosus in the back part. Therefore, the posterior fissure of the intervertebral disc in the cervical spine should be seen as a fissure of the nucleus pulposus itself rather than a rupture of the annulus fibrosus.

5.3.2 Cervical Spondylotic Myelopathy

Degenerative changes in the cervical spine can cause central canal stenosis. The spinal abnormalities that appear due to the compression of the spinal cord by this degenerative change-induced central canal stenosis are clinically called cervical spondylotic myelopathy (CSM) [34]. Hyperreflexia or gait disorder are characteristic clinical findings of CSM. Since CSM is a diagnostic term that includes clinical symptoms, it is unreasonable to describe it as CSM when interpreting images. Therefore, in the image interpretation text, the presence or absence of central canal stenosis, which is the cause of CSM, and the presence or absence of compressive myelopathy appearing as signal intensity due to compression within the spinal cord are mentioned.

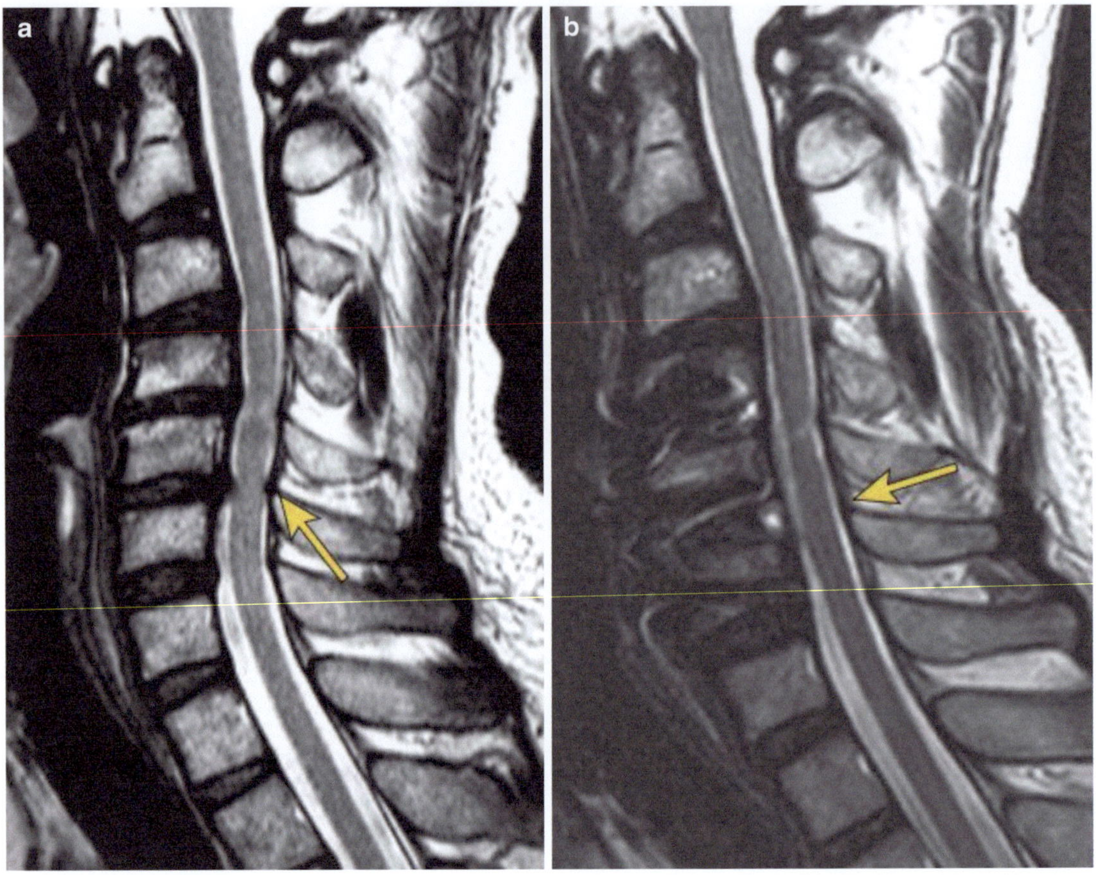

Fig. 5.41 Cervical central canal stenosis
Cervical spine MR T2-weighted image showed swelling of the intervertebral disc and buckling of the ligamentum flavum in the 4th/5th cervical spine
Central canal stenosis is observed in spine 5/6 (**a**). Cervical
The buckling (arrow) of the ligamentum flavum in spine 5/6 is not ligamentum flavum thickening, so the front swollen intervertebral disc was surgically removed
It disappears even if you remove it and increase the height of the intervertebral disc (**b**, arrow)

The main cause of central canal stenosis causing CSM is bulging due to degenerative changes in the intervertebral disc and buckling of the ligamentum flavum. Unlike the lumbar spine, in the cervical spine, the ligamentum flavum is rather than becoming thicker, it is common for the intervertebral disc to buckle and protrude forward due to a decrease in height. Therefore, in the cervical spine, it is often possible to see the buckling of the posterior ligamentum flavum disappear and the pressure on the front and back of the spine disappear simultaneously by surgically removing the bulging intervertebral disc from the front and only increasing the height of the intervertebral disc (Fig. 5.41). In the cervical spine, osteophytes originating from the vertebral body or OPLL are more common than in other spinal segments, and these are also major causes of central canal stenosis (Fig. 5.42). Also, like in the lumbar spine, degenerative spondylolisthesis or retrolisthesis can occur in the cervical spine, and these alignment disorders also cause central canal stenosis.

Unlike the lumbar spine, the spinal cord is located in the central canal in the cervical spine, so it is possible to see high signal shadows in T2-enhanced images within the spinal cord due to spinal cord compression caused by central

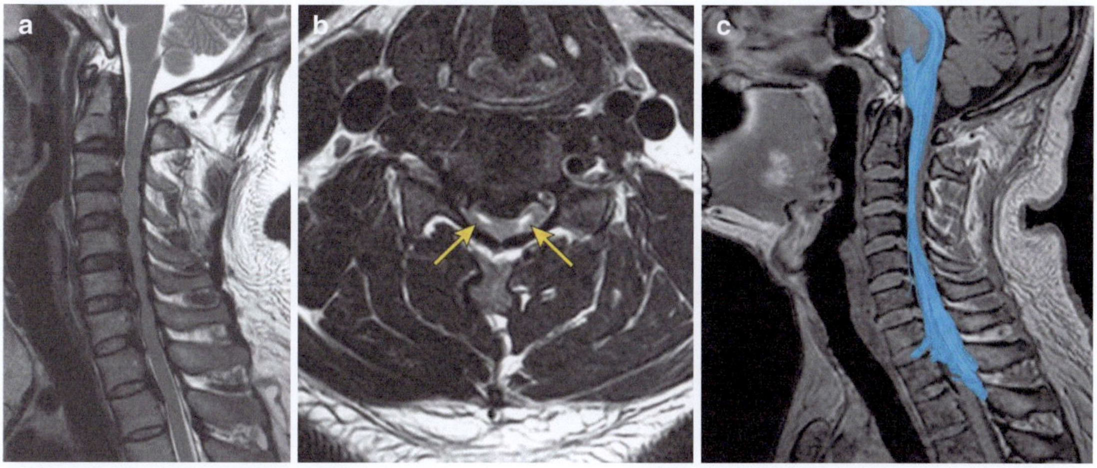

Fig. 5.42 Cervical central canal stenosis
There is central canal stenosis due to OPLL on MR T2-weighted image (**a**). Due to spinal cord compression caused by central canal stenosis on T2-weighted axial image. High-signal shadows are visible on T2-weighted images within the spinal cord (arrow), a finding suggestive of "compressive myelopathy" (**b**). Figure (**c**) is the diffusion tensor It is a tractography implemented in video , and is in the research phase for clinical application in patients with cervical spine stenosis

canal stenosis, and if such findings are observed, it can be interpreted as "compressive myelopathy" on MR images (Fig. 5.42) [34, 35]. Compressive myelopathy can be divided into a diffuse pattern, discrete focal pattern, and fuzzy focal pattern in cross-section, and among these, the fuzzy focal pattern has the worst prognosis [28]. Compressive myelopathy sometimes accompanies severe signal changes along the spinal cord, which can be mistaken for myelitis or spinal cord tumors, so caution is required. In this case, the high signal shadow in the fusiform shape of the spinal cord suggests compressive myelopathy [29].

The diagnostic criteria and grades for central canal stenosis of the cervical spine are as follows. If the loss of cerebrospinal fluid is more than 50% compared to the adjacent normal part and there is no deformation of the spinal cord, it is grade 1, if there is deformation of the spinal cord but no high signal intensity in T2-enhanced images, it is grade 2, and if there is a change in high signal intensity within the spinal cord, it is grade 3 (Table 5.10, Fig. 5.43) [36].

Table 5.10 Diagnostic criteria and grades for cervical spine central canal stenosis

Grade 0	Absence of central canal stenosis
Grade 1	Near complete obliteration of subarachnoid space, including obliteration of the arbitrary subarachnoid space exceeding 50% without any sign of cord deformity
Grade 2	Central canal stenosis with cord deformity but absent spinal cord signal change
Grade 3	Presence of spinal cord signal change near the compressed level on T2-weighted images

5.3.3 Cervical Spondylotic Radiculopathy

Clinically, the condition where symptoms appear due to the compression of the nerve root by degenerative changes in the cervical spine is called cervical spondylotic radiculopathy (CSR). Typically, patients complain of pain radiating to the arm or numbness.

As mentioned earlier, foraminal stenosis often occurs in the cervical spine due to osteophytes from the uncovertebral joint. This foraminal ste-

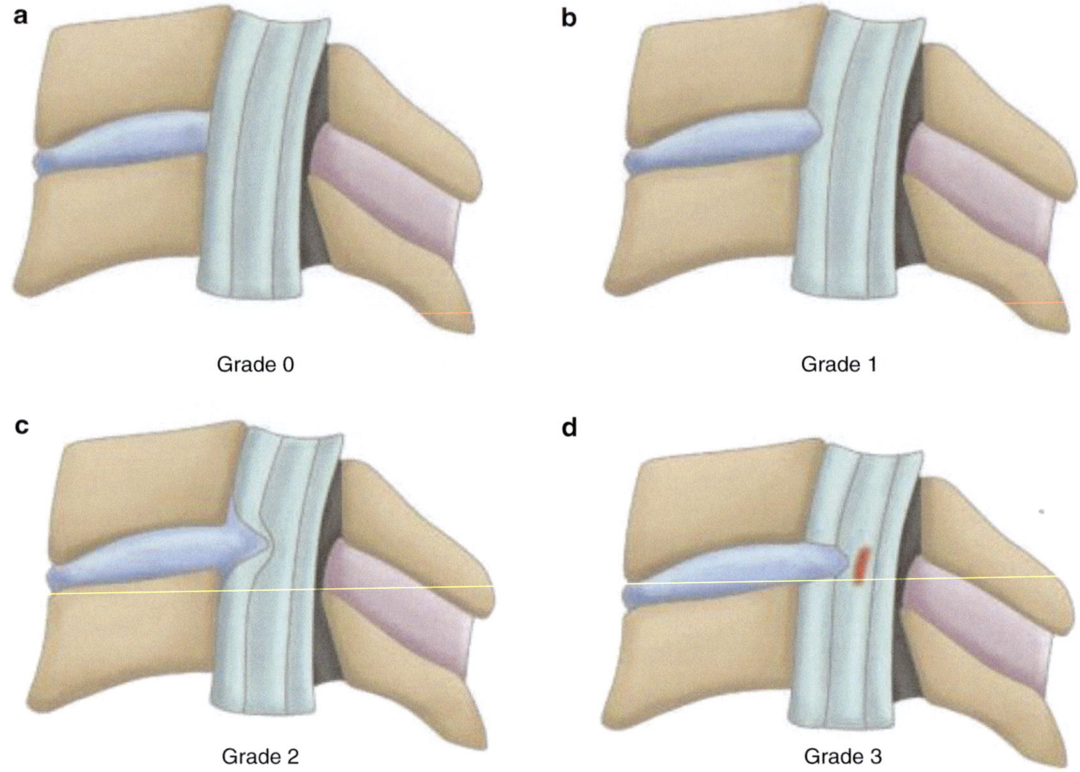

Fig. 5.43 Grade of cervical central canal stenosis
If the loss of cerebrospinal fluid is more than 50% compared to the adjacent normal part and there is no deformation of the spinal cord, it is classified as grade 1, if there is deformation of the spinal cord but no high signal intensity in the spinal cord on T2-weighted images, it is grade 2, and if there is a change in high signal intensity in the spinal cord, it is classified as grade 3

nosis can be easily observed on general X-ray images. On the anteroposterior view of a general X-ray, osteophytes growing laterally from the uncovertebral joint can be observed, and on the oblique view, osteophytes from the uncovertebral joint growing toward the neural foramen can be observed (Fig. 5.44) [2, 3, 37]. On the lateral view, a double line can be observed at the bottom of the vertebral body due to osteophytes. The neural foramen of the cervical spine is oriented anterolaterally, so it is difficult to know about foraminal stenosis from MR sagittal images, unlike the lumbar spine, and the presence of foraminal stenosis is determined on the axial plane (Fig. 5.44).

In addition to osteophytes from the uncovertebral joint, osteophytes originating from the facet joint and thickening due to degenerative changes in the facet joint can also cause foraminal stenosis.

The criteria for diagnosing cervical foraminal stenosis are as follows. On the axial plane, the anterior-posterior length of the neural foramen lateral nerve root, or the length between the posterior of the vertebral artery and the anterior of the superior articular process, is used as a reference. If the anterior-posterior length of the narrowest part of the neural foramen is even slightly narrow, it is diagnosed as foraminal stenosis. If it is narrowed by <50%, it is diagnosed as non-severe foraminal stenosis (grade 1), and if it is narrowed by more than 50%, it is diagnosed as severe foraminal stenosis (grade 2) (Fig. 5.45).

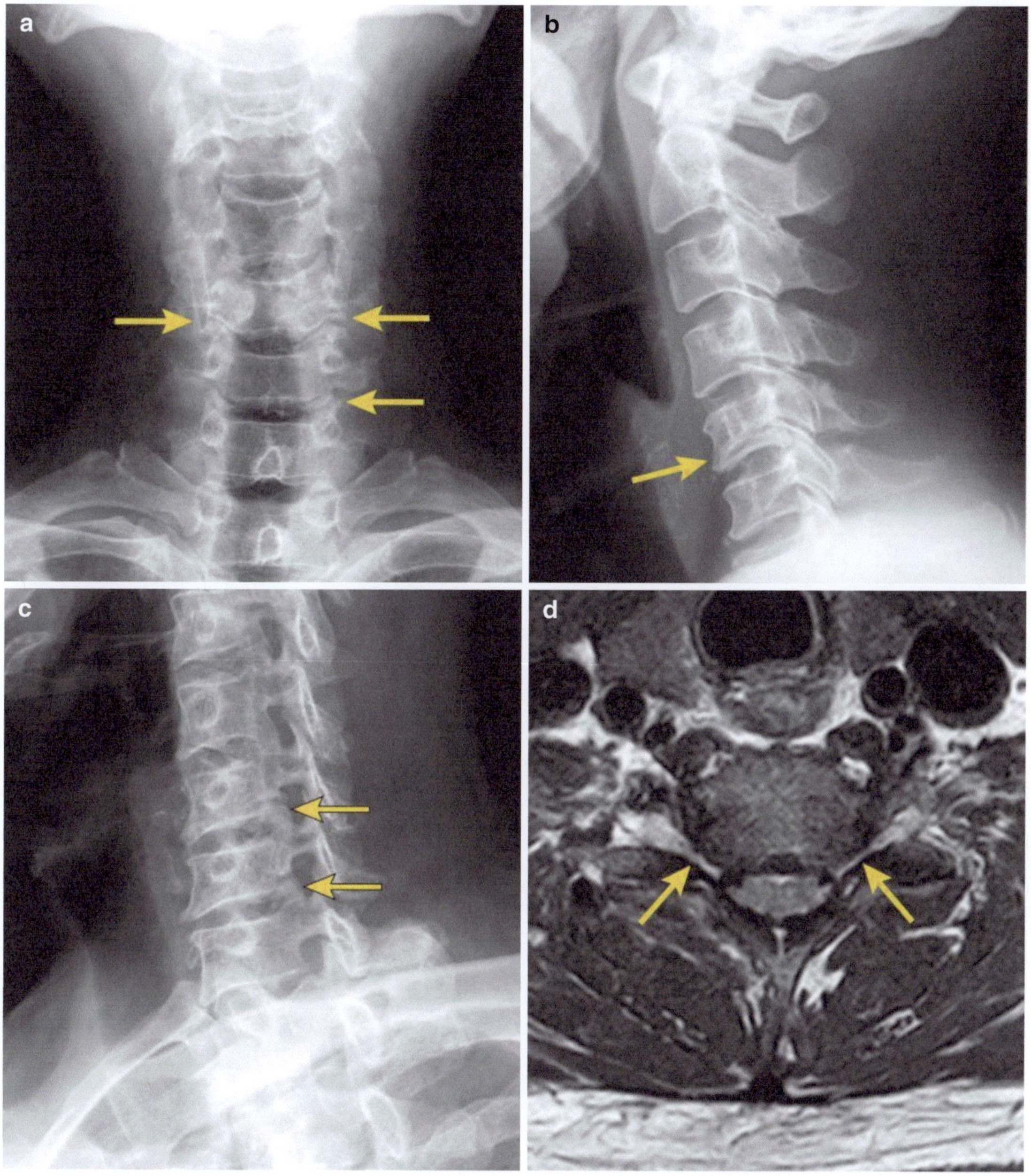

Fig. 5.44 Cervical foraminal stenosis
On the anterior-posterior view of the general X-ray (**a**), osteophytes (arrows) growing laterally from the uncovertebral joint are observed on both sides of the cervical spine 5/6 and on the left side of the cervical spine 6/7. On the lateral view (**b**), a line caused by osteophytes is seen separated from the lower cortex of the vertebral body at the bottom of the cervical spine 5 vertebral body, and a double line (arrow) is observed. If an oblique image is taken (**c**), osteophytes of the uncovertebral joint growing toward the left neural foramen of the cervical spine 5/6 and cervical spine 6/7 can be observed (arrow). On the MR T2-weighted axial image (**d**), bilateral neural foramen stenosis findings due to osteophytes at the cervical spine 5/6 are observed (arrow)

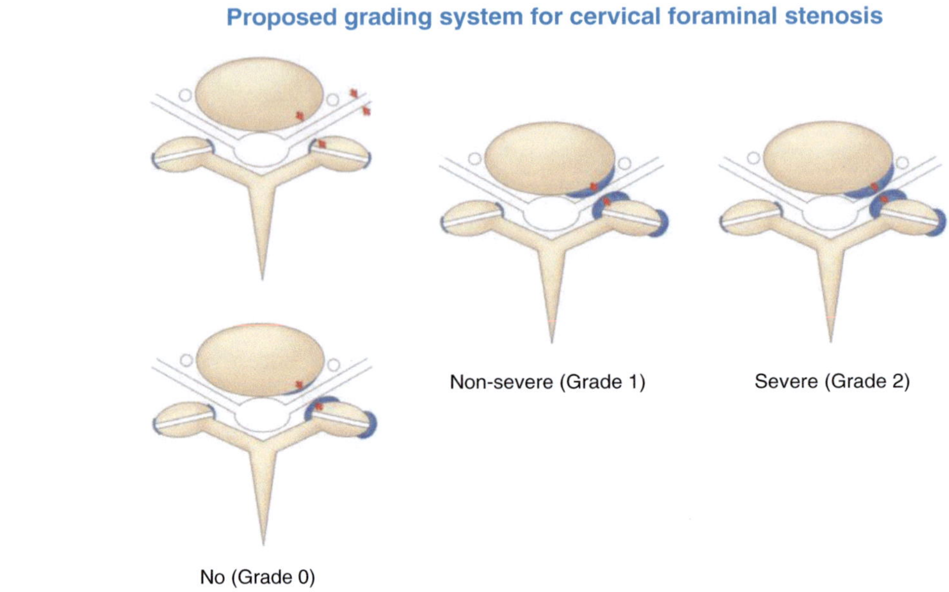

Fig. 5.45 Proposed grading system for cervical foraminal stenosis
The criteria for diagnosing cervical spine neural foramen stenosis are as follows. If the anterior-posterior length of the narrowest part of the neural foramen is slightly narrowed based on the anterior-posterior length of the lateral nerve root of the neural foramen on the axial plane, or the length between the posterior surface of the vertebral artery and the anterior surface of the superior articular process, it is diagnosed as foraminal stenosis. If it is narrowed by <50%, it is diagnosed as non-severe foraminal stenosis (grade 1), and if it is narrowed by more than 50%, it is diagnosed as severe foraminal stenosis (grade 2)

5.3.4 Disc Herniation

In the cervical spine, unlike the lumbar spine, osteophyte formation is common and nerve root compression often occurs due to osteophyte formation, which is sometimes referred to as a "hard disc." In contrast, cases caused by displacement of the intervertebral disc itself are sometimes referred to as "soft disc herniation" [3].

T1-weighted images or oblique echo field T2-weighted images are helpful in distinguishing between osteophytes and intervertebral discs. On T1-weighted images, osteophytes typically show low signal shadows, similar to adjacent cortical bone. In contrast, the displaced intervertebral disc shows a shadow similar to the adjacent intervertebral disc and a slightly higher shadow than the adjacent cortical bone [38]. Also, on oblique echo field T2-weighted images, the intervertebral disc shows a high signal shadow, so in disc herniation, the displaced intervertebral disc shows a high signal shadow, but osteophytes show a low signal shadow (Fig. 5.46). Also, CT imaging can distinguish between osteophytes and intervertebral discs. In some cases, disc herniation and osteophytes are observed together, suggesting chronic disc herniation.

Unlike the lumbar spine, there is no established terminology for disc herniation in the cervical spine. However, it was only mentioned that the disc nomenclature system announced in the lumbar spine can also be used in the cervical spine and thoracic spine [12, 26].

5.3.5 Ossification of Posterior Longitudinal Ligament (OPLL)

OPLL is a disease in which ossification appears in the posterior longitudinal ligament that connects the back of the vertebral body vertically, and it most commonly occurs in the cervical

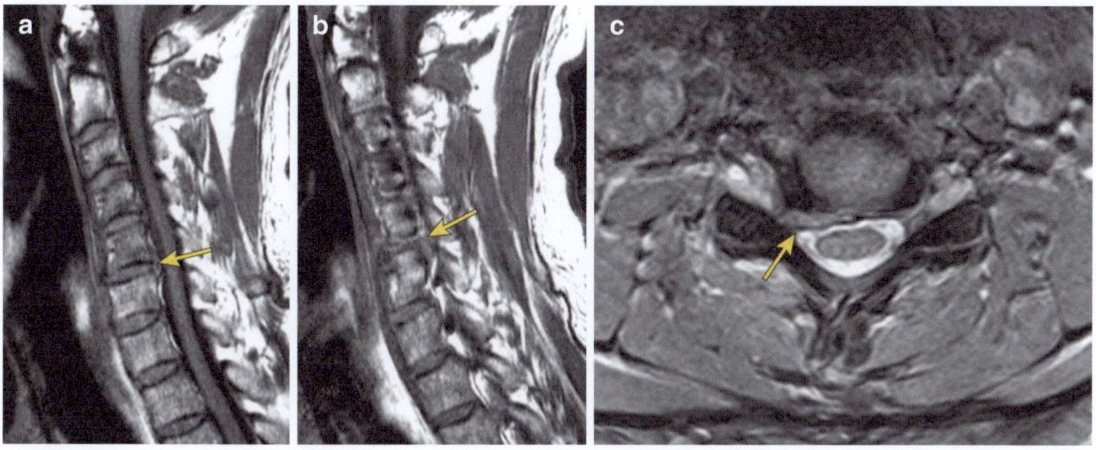

Fig. 5.46 Cervical soft disc herniation
In the T1-enhanced images (**a**, **b**), the protruded intervertebral disc at the cervical spine 5/6 shows a similar shade to the adjacent intervertebral disc, and a slightly higher shade than the adjacent cortical bone (arrow), so it can be distinguished from osteophytes. Also, in the oblique echo field T2-enhanced image (**c**), the protruded intervertebral disc shows a high signal shade (arrow)

spine. OPLL is a disease that is common in East Asians, and its cause is not yet clearly known. OPLL is common in DISH patients [3].

OPLL in the cervical spine can cause myelopathy due to spinal cord compression. It can be diagnosed by confirming a bone fragment running vertically on the lateral view of a general radiograph, distinguishable from the posterior wall of the vertebral body. If the lateral view of the general radiograph is not properly taken, the misaligned posterior wall of the vertebral body can be mistaken for OPLL. On the lateral view of a general radiograph, OPLL can be divided into the following four types: continuous, segmental, mixed, or other type (localized or circumscribed type) (Table 5.11, Fig. 5.47) [39].

Table 5.11 OPLL classification based on lateral radiograph

Continuous type	A long lesion extending over several vertebral bodies
Segmental type	One or several separate lesions behind the vertebral bodies
Mixed type	A combination of continuous and segmental types
Other type (localized or circumscribed type)	The lesion mainly located posterior to a disc space

Fig. 5.47 Four types of ossified posterior longitudinal ligament (OPLL)
On a general lateral radiograph, OPLL can be divided into the following four types: continuous, segmental, mixed, or other type (localized or circumscribed type)

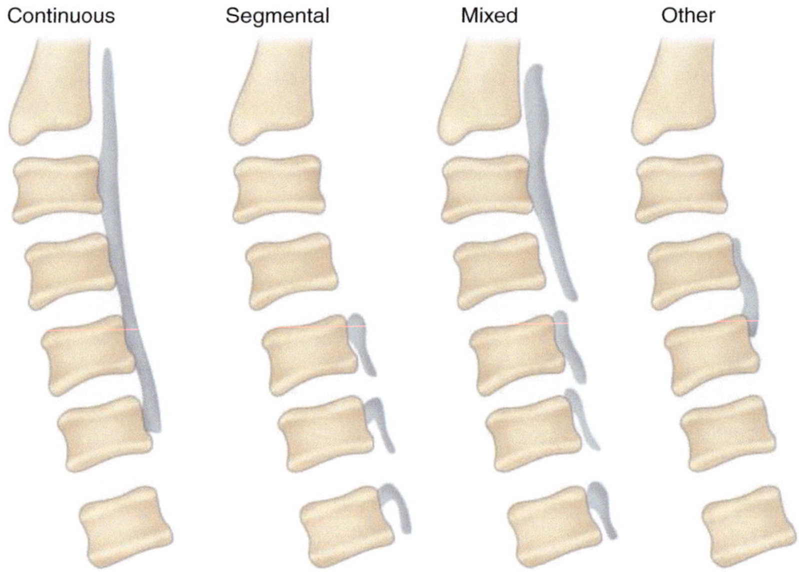

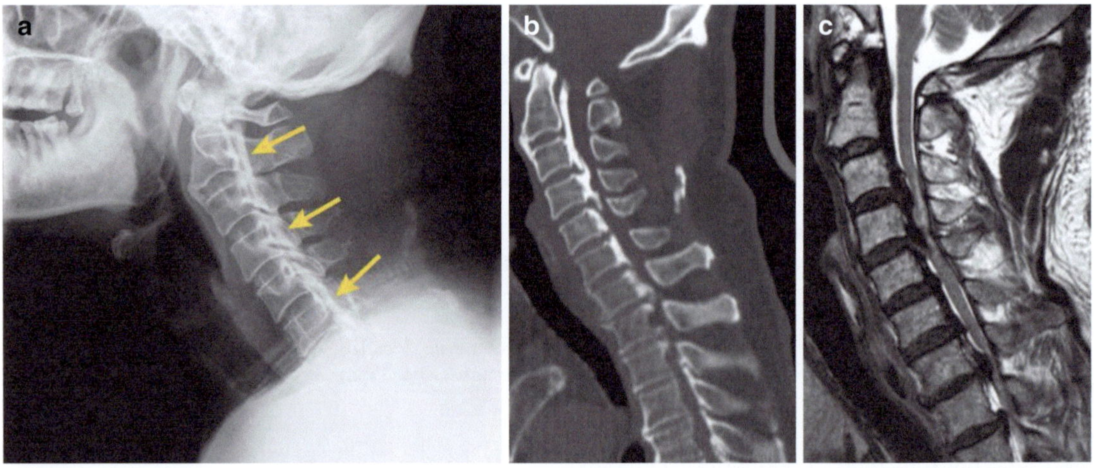

Fig. 5.48 Ossified posterior longitudinal ligament (OPLL)
On a general lateral radiograph (**a**), you can see the bone fragments running vertically up and down, distinguished from the back wall of the vertebral body across the entire cervical spine (arrow). On the CT image (**b**), OPLL is observed throughout the cervical spine, corresponding to the mixed type among the four types. In the MR T2-enhanced image (**c**), spinal cord compression associated with ossification of the posterior longitudinal ligament is observed

CT imaging allows for accurate observation of OPLL. In the case of OPLL, ossification can also occur in the adjacent dura mater, and special care is required during surgery in such cases. If dural ossification is accompanied, there is a high risk of spinal cord injury along with dural damage if OPLL is forcibly removed. It is difficult to directly confirm dural ossification from imaging findings, but as an indirect finding, OPLL may appear as a double layer on CT. The possibility of accompanying dural ossification is high in such cases (Fig. 5.48) [40].

On MR images, it is difficult to distinguish between hypertrophy of the posterior longitudi-

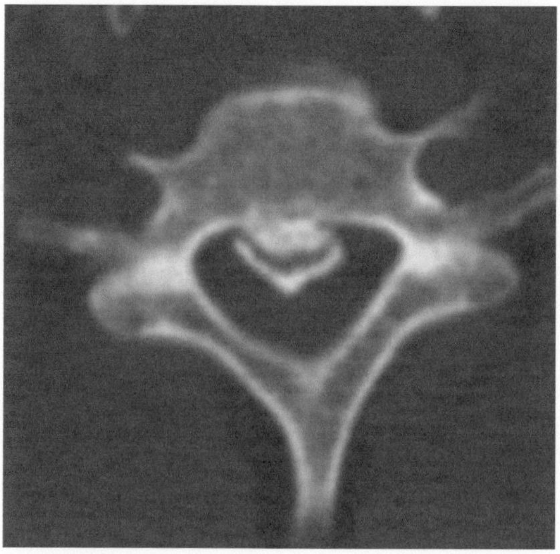

Fig. 5.49 Double layered OPLL
On the CT axial image, if OPLL appears in two layers, it is a finding that can be well accompanied by dural ossification

nal ligament and ossification of the posterior longitudinal ligament unless fatty bone marrow appears within the OPLL. However, the degree of accompanying spinal compression and changes in signal intensity within the spinal cord can be diagnosed with MR (Fig. 5.49). OPLL can appear segmentally, form multiple layers, and can only appear on the posterior surface of the vertebral body across multiple segments.

Bibliography

1. Devereaux MW. Anatomy and examination of the spine. Neurol Clin. 2007;25:331–51.
2. Naidich TP, Castillo M, Cha S, Raubaud C, Smirniotopoulos J, Kollias S, et al. Imaging of the spine. Philadelphia: Elsevier-Saunders; 2011. p. 45–184.
3. Resnick D, Kransdorf M. Bone and joint imaging. 3rd ed. Philadelphia: Elsevier-Saunders; 2005. p. 394–424.
4. Aprill C, Bogduk N. Volvo Award Winner: high intensity zone: a diagnostic sign of painful lumbar disc on MRI. Br J Radiol. 1992;65:361–9.
5. Fagan A. ISSLS prize winner: the innervation of the intervertebral disc: a quantitative analysis. Spine. 2003;28:2570–6.
6. Nizard RS, Wybier M, Laredo JD. Radiologic assessment of lumbar intervertebral instability and degenerative spondylolisthesis. Radiol Clin N Am. 2001;39:55–71.
7. Castellvi AE, Goldstein LA, Chan DP. Lumbosacral transitional vertebrae and their relationship with lumbar extradural defects. Spine (Phila Pa 1976). 1984;9:493–5.
8. O'Driscoll CM, Irwin A, Saifuddin A. Variations in morphology of the lumbosacral junction on sagittal MRI: correlation with plain radiography. Skeletal Radiol. 1996;25:225–30.
9. Carrino JA, Campell PD Jr, Lin DC, Morrison WB, Schweitzer ME, Flanders AE, et al. Effect of spinal segment variants on numbering vertebral levels at lumbar MR imaging. Radiology. 2011;259(1):196–202.
10. Pfirrmann CW, Metzdorf A, Zanetti M, et al. Magnetic resonance classification of lumbar intervertebral disc degeneration. Spine. 2001;26:1873–8.
11. Malfair D, Beall DP. Imaging the degenerative disease of the lumbar spine. Magn Reson Imaging Clin N Am. 2007;17:221–8.
12. Fardon DF, Milette PC, Combined Task Forces of the North American Spine Society, American Society of Spine Radiology, and American Society of Neuroradiology. Nomenclature and classification of lumbar disc pathology. Recommendations of the Combined Task Forces of the North American Spine Society, American Society of Spine Radiology, and American Society of Neuroradiology. Spine. 2001;26(5):E93–113.
13. Costello RF, Beall DP. Nomenclature and standard reporting terminology of intervertebral disc herniation. Magn Reson Imaging Clin N Am. 2007;17:167–74.
14. Knutsson F. The vacuum phenomenon in the intervertebral discs. Acta Radiol. 1942;23:173.
15. Resnick D, Niwayama G, Guerra J Jr, et al. Spinal vacuum phenomena: anatomical study and review. Radiology. 1981;139:141.
16. Modic MT, Steinberg PM, Ross JS, et al. Degenerative disk disease: assessment of changes in vertebral body marrow with MR imaging. Radiology. 1988;166:193–9.
17. Crock HV. Internal disc disruption. A challenge to disc prolapse fifty years on. Spine. 1986;11:650–3.
18. Schwarzer AC, Derby R, Bogduk N, et al. The prevalence and clinical features of internal disc disruption in patients with chronic "low back pain". Spine. 1995;20:878–1883.
19. Bogduk N, editor. Practice guidelines for spinal diagnostic & treatment procedure. International Spine Intervention Society; 2004.
20. Merskey H, Bogduk N, editors. Classification of chronic pain. Descriptions of chronic pain syndromes and definitions of pain terms. 2nd ed. Seattle, WA: IASP Press; 1994. p. 180–1.
21. Roberts S, Eisenstein SM, Menage J, Evans EH, Ashton IK. Mechanoreceptors in intervertebral discs: morphology, distribution, and neuropeptides. Spine. 1995;20:2645–51.

22. Johnson WE, Evans H, Menage J, Eisenstein SM, El Haj A, Roberts S. Immunohistochemical detection of Schwann cells in innervated and vascularized human intervertebral discs. Spine. 2001;26:2550–7.
23. Slipman CW, Patel RK, Zhang L, et al. Side of symptomatic annular fissure and site of low back pain: is there a correlation? Spine. 2001;26:E165–9.
24. Carragee EJ, Paragioudakis SJ, Khurana S. Lumbar high-intensity zone and discography in subjects without low back problems. Spine. 2000;25:2987–92.
25. Mathis JM, Golovac S. Image-guided spine interventions. 2nd ed. New York: Springer; 2010. p. 107–46.
26. Fardon DF, Williams AL, Dohring EJ, Reed Murtagh F, Gabriel SL, Rothman GK, Sze. Lumbar disc nomenclature: version 2.0. Recommendations of the combined task forces of the North American Spine Society, the American Society of Spine Radiology and the American Society of Neuroradiology. Spine J. 2014;14:2525–45.
27. Panjabi M. The stabilizing system of the spine. Part II: Neutral zone and instability hypothesis. J Spinal Disord. 1992;5:390.
28. You JY, Lee JW, Lee E, Lee GY, Yeom JS, Kang HS. MR classification system based on axial images for cervical compressive myelopathy. Radiology. 2015;276(2):553–61.
29. Bae YJ, Lee JW, Park KS, et al. Compressive myelopathy: magnetic resonance imaging findings simulating idiopathic acute transverse myelopathy. Skeletal Radiol. 2013;42:793–802.
30. Frymoyer JW, Wiesel SW. The adult and pediatric spine. 3rd ed. Philadelphia: Lippincott Williams and Wilkins; 2004. p. 899–944.
31. Goethem JV, Hauwe LVD, Parizel PM. Spinal imaging. In: Diagnostic imaging of the spine and spinal cord. Berlin, Heidelberg: Springer-Verlag; 2007. p. 109–254.
32. Sirvanci M, Bhatia M, Caniyusufoglu KA, Duran C, Tezer M, Ozturk C, et al. Degenerative lumbar spinal stenosis: correlation with Oswestry Disability Index and MR imaging. Eur Spine J. 2008;17:679–89.
33. Guen YL, Joon WL, Hee SC, Kyoung-Jin O, Heung SK. A new grading system of lumbar central canal stenosis on MRI: an easy and reliable method. Skeletal Radiol. 2011;40:1033–9.
34. Naderi S, Ozgen S, Pamir MN, Ozek MM, Erzen C. Cervical spondylotic myelopathy: surgical results and factors affecting prognosis. Neurosurgery. 1998;43(1):43–9.
35. Lee JW, Kim JH, Park JB, Park KW, Yeom JS, Lee GY, Kang HS. Diffusion tensor imaging and fiber tractography in cervical compressive myelopathy: preliminary results. Skeletal Radiol. 2011;40:1543–51.
36. Kang Y, Lee JW, Koh YH, Hur S, Kim SJ, Chai JW, Kang HS. New MRI grading system for the cervical canal stenosis. AJNR Am J Neuroradiol. 2011;197:W1–7.
37. Ross JS, Moore KR, Shas LM, Bord B, Crim J. Diagnostic imaging: spine. 2nd ed. Amirsys; 2010.
38. Kang HS, Lee JW, Kwon JW. Radiology illustrated: Spine. Springer; 2014.
39. Hirabayashi K, Miyakawa J, Satomi K, Maruyama T, Wakano K. Operative results and postoperative progression of ossification among patients with ossification of cervical posterior longitudinal ligament. Spine (Phila Pa 1976). 1981;6:354–64.
40. Hida K, Iwasaki Y, Koyanagi I, Abe H. Bone window computed tomography for detection of dural defect associated with cervical ossified posterior longitudinal ligament. Neurol Med Chir (Tokyo). 1997;37:173–5. discussion 175–176

Infectious Spondylitis

6

Wan Tae Kim

Infectious diseases of the spine can cause damage by invading the vertebral body, intervertebral disc, perispinal soft tissue, and epidural space, and clinically, it can be difficult to distinguish from degenerative changes, inflammatory diseases, and spinal tumors. Despite the development of antibiotic therapy today, spinal infections are not decreasing and are rather increasing due to drug abuse, HIV infection, aging, widespread misuse of antibiotics, and increased use of steroids and immunosuppressants. Spinal infections are caused by bacteria, tuberculosis, and fungi. It is caused by various pathogens such as parasites, and each disease shows different clinical courses and prognoses, so it is important to understand characteristic findings and make accurate differential diagnoses.

6.1 Pyogenic Spondylitis

6.1.1 Incidence

Pyogenic spondylitis is a relatively rare disease, currently accounting for 2–4% of all musculoskeletal infections. The incidence is higher in men than in women at a ratio of 1.5:1–3:1, and it can occur at all ages, but it mainly occurs between the ages of 40 and 60. Pyogenic spondylitis most commonly affects the lumbar spine, followed by the thoracic and cervical spine [1, 2].

The incidence of pyogenic spondylitis is steadily increasing, and the reasons include an aging population, intravenous drug abuse, AIDS, reactivation of latent infections, overuse of antibiotics, drug-resistant pathogens, new pathogens, and worsening socio-economic conditions. Other factors include malnutrition, immune damage, chronic steroid use, diabetes, malignant tumors, chronic alcoholism, renal failure, and an increase in spinal surgery.

6.1.2 Pathogens

The most common pathogen of pyogenic spondylitis is *Staphylococcus aureus*, which accounts for 60–90% of spinal infections, and other causes include Streptococcus, Pneumococcus, Enterococcus, *Escherichia coli*, Klebsiella, Salmonella, and *Pseudomonas aeruginosa*. In particular, the frequency of Streptococcus is increasing in patients with endocarditis and colon polyps, and the frequency of Klebsiella and *P. aeruginosa* is increasing in intravenous drug abusers.

Pyogenic spondylitis often follows an infection in another part of the body, and the most common primary site is a urinary tract infection, but also includes inflammatory bowel disease, otitis media, tooth extraction, contaminated intravenous needle, sepsis, abortion, cellulitis, fasciitis, subcutaneous abscess, or pyomyositis.

W. T. Kim (✉)
Department of Radiology, Veterans Health Service Medical Center, Seoul, Republic of Korea

© The Author(s), under exclusive license to Springer Nature Singapore Pte Ltd. 2025

H. S. Kang, J. W. Lee (eds.), *Spinal Imaging*, https://doi.org/10.1007/978-981-95-1386-4_6

6.1.3 Pathogenesis and Pathology

The route of infection is primarily due to hematogenous spread from other parts of the body, and it occurs more often through arteries than veins. This is because the first site to be invaded is the subchondral area of the vertebral body adjacent to the intervertebral disc, and it is also proven that the general infection of the vertebral body coincides with the distribution of the spinal artery [3]. Infection through the vein occurs through Batson's venous plexus, which is a vein adjacent to the spine with lower pressure than the veins in the pelvis and lacks intravascular valves, allowing for retrograde flow. It is known that reflux can occur, making it easy for infections or tumors in the pelvis spread to the vertebral body.

Infections of the vertebral body through arteries or veins initially invade the cartilage under the front of the vertebral body adjacent to the intervertebral disc, soon destroying the vertebral endplate and spreading to the intervertebral disc. As the infection progresses, it spreads to adjacent vertebral bodies and the destruction of the intervertebral disc and the narrowing of the intervertebral disc space occur. If the infection continues to spread, inflammatory tissue spreads under the ligament, causing erosion in front of the vertebral body, or inflammation spreads to the surrounding soft tissue of the spine through the anterior longitudinal ligament (Fig. 6.1).

In children, because fetal blood vessels remain in the intervertebral disc, blood supply occurs, so the causative bacteria can directly spread to the intervertebral disc, and discitis can occur first.

In addition to hematogenous spread, spinal puncture, discography, steroid injections for the diagnosis and treatment of pain, and direct infection after surgery can also be the cause.

6.1.4 Clinical Symptoms

Patients mainly complain of gradually progressing pain over several months or years, and lethargy, fever, loss of appetite, muscle spasms, stiffness, rigidity, weakness, fatigue, difficulty swallowing, weight loss, and night sweats may appear. Generally, exercise can exacerbate the pain of spinal infection, and rest can alleviate the pain [4].

Physical examination often shows findings of local tenderness, subcostal mass, and increased thoracic kyphosis. Neurological examination may show signs of nerve root compression including radiculopathy, meningeal irritation symptoms, and neurological deficits such as lower extremity weakness, reflex loss, and paraplegia. Neurological deficits vary depending on the site and extent of the infection, the type and toxicity of the causative substance, and the body's ability to include or resist the infection. Collapse

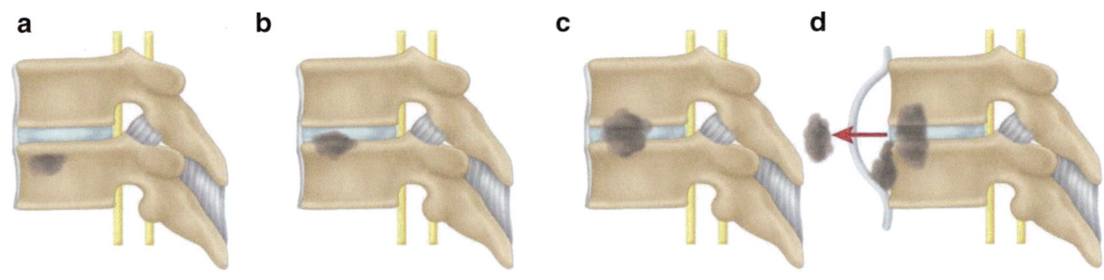

Fig. 6.1 Sequential stages of infectious spondylitis (**a**) In the early stages of infection, the anterior subchondral area of the vertebral body adjacent to the intervertebral disc is first invaded. (**b**) The infection destroys the vertebral endplate and spreads to the intervertebral disc. (**c**) As the infection progresses, it extends to the adjacent vertebral body, resulting in destruction of the intervertebral disc and narrowing of the disc space. (**d**) If the infection continues to spread, inflammatory tissue extends to the subligamentous region, causing anterior vertebral osteophytes or inflammation spreading to the surrounding soft tissues through the anterior longitudinal ligament (arrow)

of the vertebral body and epidural inflammatory tissue compress the neural structures and block their blood supply, damaging the function of the spinal cord or causing spinal cord infarction. Cervical spondylitis can progress forward to cause esophageal disorders and pharyngeal abscesses and sinusitis. Thoracic spondylitis can cause sinusitis, empyema, and pericarditis. Lumbar spondylitis can cause peritonitis and subdiaphragmatic abscess. Untreated infections can lead to permanent spinal deformities such as wedge-shaped vertebral body deformity, gibbus deformity, and scoliosis. Severe infections can cause permanent neurological deficits such as paraplegia and quadriplegia. If the infection spreads to the psoas muscle, temporary or permanent hip joint contracture may occur [5]. Chronic spinal infection can present a more confusing clinical picture, generally characterized by less severe pain. Limb paralysis may gradually progress, accompanied by signs and symptoms of spinal and cauda equina compression, but fever may not be present [1].

6.1.5 Clinical Examination and Diagnostic Methods

Infectious spondylitis requires accurate diagnosis as it can leave serious sequelae if not treated appropriately early on, and identification of the causative organism is essential for appropriate treatment. The diagnosis of infectious spondylitis relies on physical examination, blood tests, and blood cultures, followed by imaging diagnosis, with confirmation by bacteriological or histological examination. The positive rate of bacterial culture in surgical biopsy is reported to be about 50–90%.

Laboratory tests often show an increase in white blood cell count, but in children or the elderly, especially in patients with reduced immunity and in cases of infection with tuberculosis or parasites, the white blood cell count may not increase [6].

The most useful blood tests are erythrocyte sedimentation rate (ESR) and C-reactive protein (CRP), which increase in about 73–90% of cases. However, these test values can also increase in pregnancy, tumors, granulomatous diseases, and may be normal in infections with low virulence of the strain. If the body temperature rises above 39 degrees, a blood culture test is necessary, and it shows positive in less than 25% of cases [1]. According to the known 50% rule in pyogenic spondylitis, symptoms lasting for more than 3 months, increased ESR, fever, increased white blood cell count, etc., are reported to occur in only about 50% of patients.

6.1.6 Imaging Diagnosis

(1) Plain Radiography.

Pyogenic spondylitis most commonly occurs in the lumbar spine, with typical findings being abnormalities in one intervertebral disc and two adjacent vertebral bodies. The vertebral body and intervertebral disc are the most commonly involved sites, but the posterior structures of the spine, the epidural space, and the soft tissues around the spine can also be primarily or secondarily involved.

In the early stages of spinal infection, plain radiography usually appears normal, as it typically appears normal for 2–3 weeks after infection, so the sensitivity and specificity of plain radiography in diagnosing spondylitis are very low. Around 1–2 weeks after infection, only signs of decreased density around the endplate can be seen, and between 3–6 weeks, erosion of the endplate and narrowing of the intervertebral disc space can be seen. After 8 weeks, progressive narrowing of the intervertebral disc space, destruction of the vertebral body, and bone hardening due to new bone formation can be seen.

In the case of hematogenous spread, the area commonly first invaded is the subchondral area of the vertebral body adjacent to the intervertebral disc, followed by the invasion of the intervertebral disc. When the intervertebral disc is invaded, the height of the disc decreases, and the boundary of the vertebral endplate becomes irregular, which may only

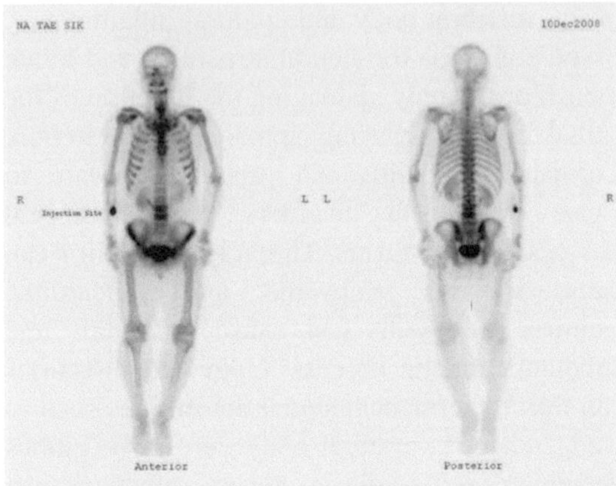

Fig. 6.2 99mTc-MDP bone scan of a patient with pyogenic spondylitis
The uptake of the radionuclide along the vertebral endplate of the third and fourth vertebrae where the infection is present appears in a sandwich-like shape

be a minor change, but it becomes more distinct as the infection progresses, and osteolytic areas also appear in the adjacent vertebral body. Depending on the type of bacteria, it is known that definite bone destruction can be observed at least 8 weeks after infection. If the intervertebral disc is destroyed and the gap narrows and osteolytic areas are visible, pyogenic spondylitis should be considered first. Usually, after about 10–12 weeks, the regeneration process appears as bone sclerosis, and other findings such as new bone formation, osteophytosis, spinal stenosis, spinal scoliosis, spinal spondylolisthesis, and bony ankylosis can also appear [7].

(2) Nuclear Medicine Examination.
Nuclear medicine examination can quickly determine the presence and location of infection. 99mTc-MDP bone scan is non-specific in diagnosing infection because it increases shadow non-specifically in cases where bone metabolism is hyperactive, such as bone infection, bone tumor, and fracture, and its disadvantage is its low resolution. 67Ga scan reacts specifically to inflammatory cells, so it can diagnose earlier than 99mTc-MDP bone scan and can increase specificity and sensitivity. It can help find the source of infection because it increases shadow as a positive reaction in other infected areas, and the imaging findings increase the intake of radioactive isotopes along the vertebral endplate, looking like a sandwich (Fig. 6.2). 67Ga scan normalizes faster than 99mTc-MDP bone scan after infection treatment, so it helps track the treatment process [8]. 111Indium leukocyte bone scan has lower sensitivity in diagnosing spinal infection, but it can more clearly determine peripheral soft tissue infection.

(3) CT.
Although the diagnostic value of CT in infectious spondylitis has decreased with the advent of MRI, it is a useful test method that can observe bone destruction of the spine and spread to surrounding soft tissues. CT findings of pyogenic spondylitis include disc herniation and destruction, loss of perivertebral fat layer, and soft tissue abscess. Perivertebral abscesses that have invaded the psoas muscle can be clearly diagnosed by performing a contrast-enhanced examination. Above all, CT is excellent in evaluating bone destruction, and it is very useful in performing an auxiliary role in the diagnosis and evaluation of spondylitis using coronal and sagittal reconstructed images. Also, in some cases, CT follow-up examination is very useful in infectious spondylitis. It is also used to evaluate the degree of healing of spondylitis. Tissue biopsy or aspiration from the spine is usually performed under fluoroscopy or CT guidance, and CT is particularly useful when the lesion is in the sacrum or upper spine. Because it can accurately guide the needle to the inflammatory lesions of the bone destruction site or the soft tissue around the spine, CT is more widely used to confirm bacteria by performing tissue biopsy or aspiration in infectious spondylitis, and it can also be used to guide the catheter in percutaneous drainage of abscesses in the soft tissue around the spine.

(4) MRI.
In the diagnosis of spondylitis, MRI is a highly sensitive (96%), specific (94%), and accurate (92%) imaging method, with excellent contrast between tissues, making it the most sensitive to detect infections, and easy

to identify the invaded range. Therefore, MRI can be considered the optimal imaging method for evaluating bone marrow and soft tissue invasion around the spine, and the spinal canal and spinal cord in infectious diseases of the spine [6].

When an infection occurs in the vertebral body, the earliest change is the accumulation of extracellular fluid in the bone marrow, which appears as a signal intensity change in the bone marrow on MRI before bone destruction changes occur. As a result, it shows low signal intensity on T1-weighted images and high signal intensity on T2-weighted images, with changes on T1-weighted images being more reliable. T2-weighted images may not clearly show the change in high signal intensity due to increased extracellular fluid because the bone marrow fat appears as high signal intensity on fast spin echo images (Fig. 6.3). However, using fat suppression imaging

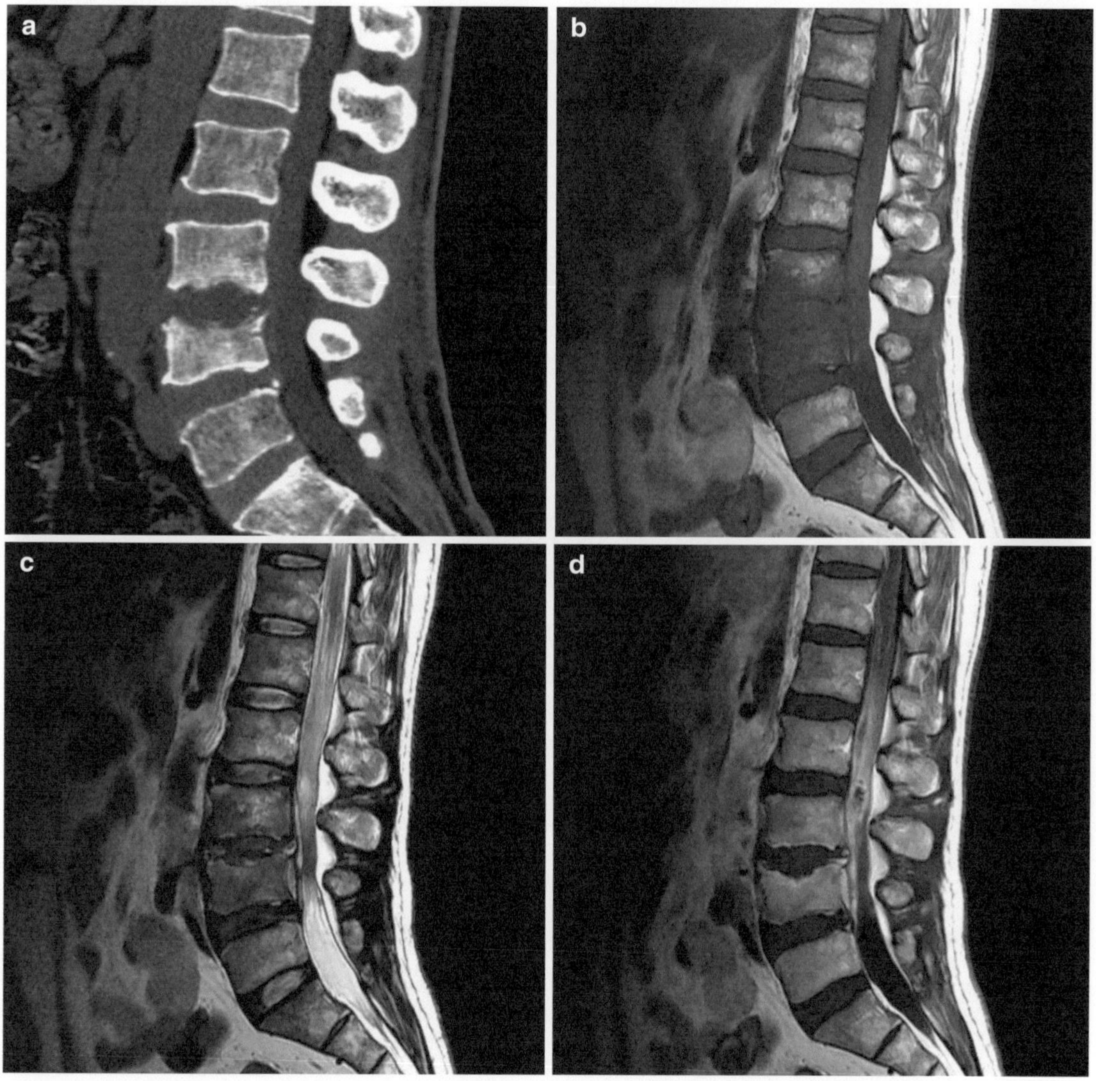

Fig. 6.3 Pyogenic spondylitis in a 55-year-old man
On lumbar CT, osteophyte formation and bone destruction around the intervertebral disc of the third and fourth vertebrae are observed. On lumbar MR, involvement of the vertebral body, intervertebral disc, and surrounding soft tissues is observed, and a phlegmon that enhances minimally in the anterior epidural space is observed on contrast-enhanced images. Axial CT image (**a**), axial MR T1-weighted image (**b**), T2-weighted image (**c**), contrast-enhanced T1-weighted image (**d**)

techniques like STIR, abnormal high signal intensity can be clearly identified [9]. As the infection progresses, the boundary of the vertebral disc disappears and the height of the intervertebral disc decreases with increased signal intensity on T2-weighted images, indicating that the infection has invaded the intervertebral disc. When the adjacent vertebral disc is destroyed across the intervertebral disc and the signal intensity of the vertebral body changes, it shows the typical findings of pyogenic spondylitis that invades two consecutive vertebral bodies and the intervertebral disc in between (Fig. 6.4). However, there are many cases where diagnosis is difficult because there are non-typical findings similar to tuberculous spondylitis, such as only one vertebral body being invaded, or the intervertebral disc in between is normal while the adjacent vertebral bodies are invaded [4, 10].

MRI allows for a very accurate assessment of the spread of inflammation to the soft tissues around the spine, which is very important in determining the treatment plan for spondylitis. Especially, soft tissue changes in the epidural space may appear as phlegmon or abscess formed by granulation tissue. Since an abscess is an indication for surgical treatment, it is important to distinguish between phlegmon and abscess. Contrast-enhanced examination obtained after intravenous injection of gadolinium contrast agent is very useful in more accurately assessing inflammatory changes in these soft tissues [7]. After contrast enhance-

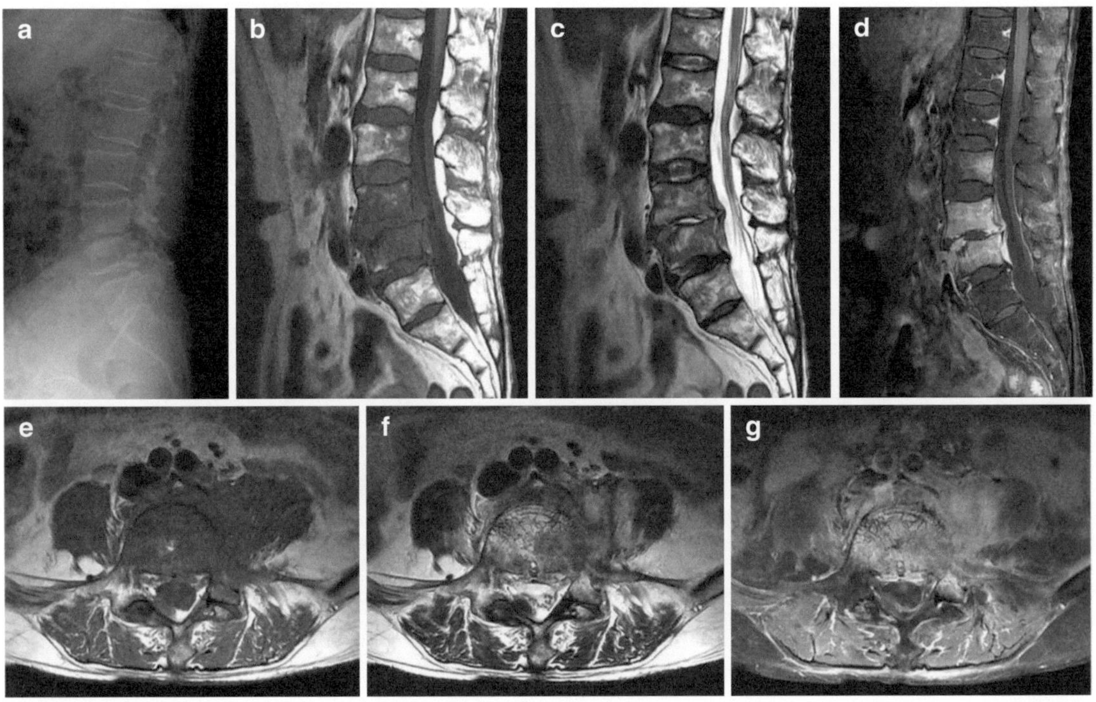

Fig. 6.4 Pyogenic spondylitis in a 72-year-old man
On plain radiography, the intervertebral disc space of the fourth and fifth vertebrae is narrowed, and osteophyte formation of the vertebral endplate is observed. On lumbar MR, osteomyelitis of the fourth and fifth lumbar vertebrae, involvement of the intervertebral disc, osteophyte formation of the anterior vertebral endplate, and a perivertebral mass showing minimal enhancement are observed. Findings of infection enhancing in connection with the Batson venous plexus in the posterior body of the third lumbar vertebra are observed. Lateral plain radiograph (**a**), axial MR T1-weighted image (**b**), T2-weighted image (**c**), contrast-enhanced T1-weighted image (**d**), axial T1-weighted image (**e**), T2-weighted image (**f**), contrast-enhanced T1-weighted image (**g**)

ment, cellulitis shows almost uniform enhancement, while abscesses in the epidural space do not enhance in the liquefied center and show enhancement on the periphery. The liquefied center often requires surgical drainage because it has no blood flow and cannot be reached by antibiotics injected intravenously.

Pyogenic spondylitis involves fewer vertebrae compared to tuberculous spondylitis, rarely forms masses around the spine, and the formed masses themselves are small and usually enhance minimally, not only that, but they also invade surrounding tissues by digging in, these findings help in differentiation (Fig. 6.5). Pyogenic infections show a characteristic pattern of spreading by destroying surrounding soft tissues because they have proteolytic enzymes [11]. Most pyogenic spondylitis enhances minimally, but depending on the toxicity of the bacteria and the body's response, it can also show peripheral enhancement similar to tuberculosis [12].

MRI can also be used to assess treatment progress in patients with pyogenic spondylitis, with a decrease in the size of soft tissue inflammation, fatty infiltration in the bone marrow, and a decrease in enhancement being MRI findings that indicate healing of infectious spondylitis. The first response to appear is a decrease in the size of the inflammatory soft tissue, and a definite finding suggesting healing, although it appears late, is fatty infiltration, which is observed as a high

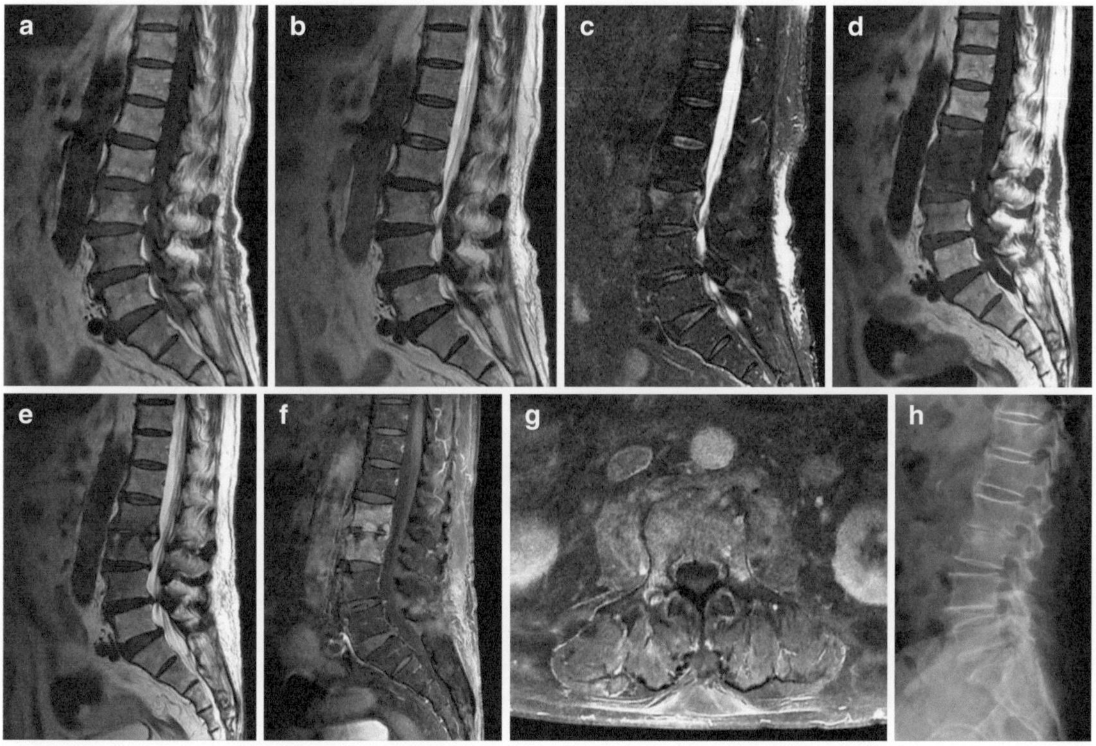

Fig. 6.5 Pyogenic spondylitis in a 79-year-old man Initial MR images (**a–c**) show osteomyelitis invading the upper endplate of the third lumbar vertebra, with the intervertebral disc preserved. Sagittal T1-weighted image (**a**), T2-weighted image (**b**), T2 fat-suppressed image (**c**). Follow-up MR images (**d–f**) show sclerosis of the vertebral endplate, increased signal intensity of the intervertebral disc, and narrowing of the intervertebral disc space, with minimal enhancement of the perivertebral mass after contrast enhancement. Plain radiographs also show sclerosis of the second and third lumbar vertebrae and significant narrowing of the intervertebral disc space. Follow-up sagittal T1-weighted image (**d**), T2-weighted image (**e**), contrast-enhanced T1-weighted image (**f**), axial contrast-enhanced T1-weighted image (**g**), and lateral plain radiograph (**h**)

signal intensity periphery around the spine on T1-weighted images [13, 14].

6.1.7 Treatment

The primary goal of treating pyogenic spondylitis is to eradicate the infection, and secondary goals include preventing and treating spinal instability that can occur with the infection, preventing or treating neurological symptoms, and preventing and treating spinal deformities. The best method is to administer antibiotics that are sensitive to the causative bacteria confirmed through biopsy or blood culture, but while waiting for the test results, broad-spectrum antibiotics are started and the antibiotics are changed according to the sensitivity test once the causative bacteria are confirmed. The timing of antibiotic administration is through intravenous injection for 6 weeks, and then switched to oral administration. The treatment effect of antibiotic administration can be judged using the erythrocyte sedimentation rate test and C-reactive protein test methods, 67Ga scan, and MRI.

In cases where there is no response despite appropriate antibiotic administration, or when bone destruction is severe, in cases where spinal deformities have occurred or prevention is needed, or when there are findings of neurological paralysis or abscess formation, surgical treatment can be considered.

6.2 Epidural Abscess

6.2.1 Incidence

Spinal epidural abscess is an emergency condition with high morbidity and mortality rates, and although it is a relatively rare disease, its prevalence is continuously increasing [15]. Diabetes, intravenous drug abuse, chronic renal failure, excessive alcohol consumption, immunodeficiency, and local steroid injections are important risk factors for epidural abscess. The increase in complex procedures using devices and percutaneous spinal procedures can also be a cause. There is no clear evidence of genetic or racial differences in epidural abscesses. Epidural abscesses can be seen in all age groups, but are relatively common in the 50 s and 60 s. Patients may show mechanical compression or ischemic damage to the spinal cord, and surgery should be considered when there is compression of the nerves or spinal cord, gradual neurological damage, or persistent severe pain.

6.2.2 Causative Organism

The most common strain is Staphylococcus, accounting for 62–67%, of which about 12% are antibiotic-resistant bacteria (methicillin-resistant *Staphylococcus aureus*). Mycobacterium tuberculosis is the next most common at 25%, and others include Streptococcus, *E. coli*, Pseudomonas, Bacillus, *Serratia marcescens*, etc. [16].

6.2.3 Mechanism of Occurrence

The main route of infection is hematogenous spread from an infection source outside the vertebral body, and direct spread of the infection or spread from adjacent infections can occur. Hematogenously originated abscesses are usually located posterior to the dura and often accompany facet joint infections. The sites of occurrence are the lower thoracic (50%), lumbar (35%), and cervical (14%) in order [17]. Overall, there are many abscesses due to spread from the vertebral body and intervertebral discs, so the frequency of abscesses occurring anterior to the dura is about 4 times higher than posterior to the dura. The distribution of abscesses is often across multiple segments rather than confined to one segment and can exist across the entire spinal canal. About 15% of epidural abscesses are due to postoperative infections, and some are due to epidural procedures such as epidural anesthesia.

6.2.4 Clinical Symptoms

The typical clinical symptoms are severe back pain and rapid neurological symptoms.

In cases of acute infection, typical signs such as localized back pain, fever, and progressing neurological symptoms can appear, but it is rare for all these symptoms to appear at once. Also, there are no clinical symptoms unique to this disease, so in about 50% of cases, it can progress from initial paralysis to complete paralysis. The speed of paralysis is characterized by being very fast, and in some cases, it progresses to complete paralysis in about 72 to 96 hours. In children, there may be systemic symptoms such as irritability and abdominal pain.

6.2.5 Clinical tests and diagnostic methods

Generally, blood tests are known to be less credible for diagnosis, but an increase in erythrocyte sedimentation rate or C-reactive protein is very useful and most patients show increased findings. Blood culture tests show a positive response in about 60%.

6.2.6 Imaging diagnosis

(1) Simple shooting.
Simple shooting hardly helps in the early detection of epidural infections of the spine. However, it can help diagnose if intervertebral discitis is accompanied.

(1) CT.
CT can help prove epidural and perispinal expansion of the abscess and associated vertebral lesions. Myelography, which injects contrast medium into the spinal canal, can well show the location of the abscess and the correlation between the abscess and the spinal cord, but spinal puncture required for the procedure can spread the infection to previously uninfected areas, so it is desirable not to use it if infection is suspected.

(2) MRI.
MRI is the best imaging diagnostic method from the initial stage of spinal epidural infection, and it is known to be 90–100% sensitive to the diagnosis of spinal epidural infection and abscess [16, 18]. MRI quickly and accurately locates the lesion, defines the range of the lesion, and helps plan and monitor treatment. The typical MRI findings of an epidural abscess are low signal intensity on T1-weighted images, high signal intensity on T2-weighted images, and peripheral enhancement on gadolinium-enhanced images of epidural soft tissue masses (Fig. 6.6). The advantages of MRI include the ability to know the range of the abscess and the degree of spinal cord compression, and the status of infection of surrounding tissues such as spondylitis and discitis [15].

6.2.7 Treatment

Treatment should be performed urgently and requires rapid decompression and drainage and long-term administration of antibiotics. If neurological symptoms occur, emergency surgery is required [19].

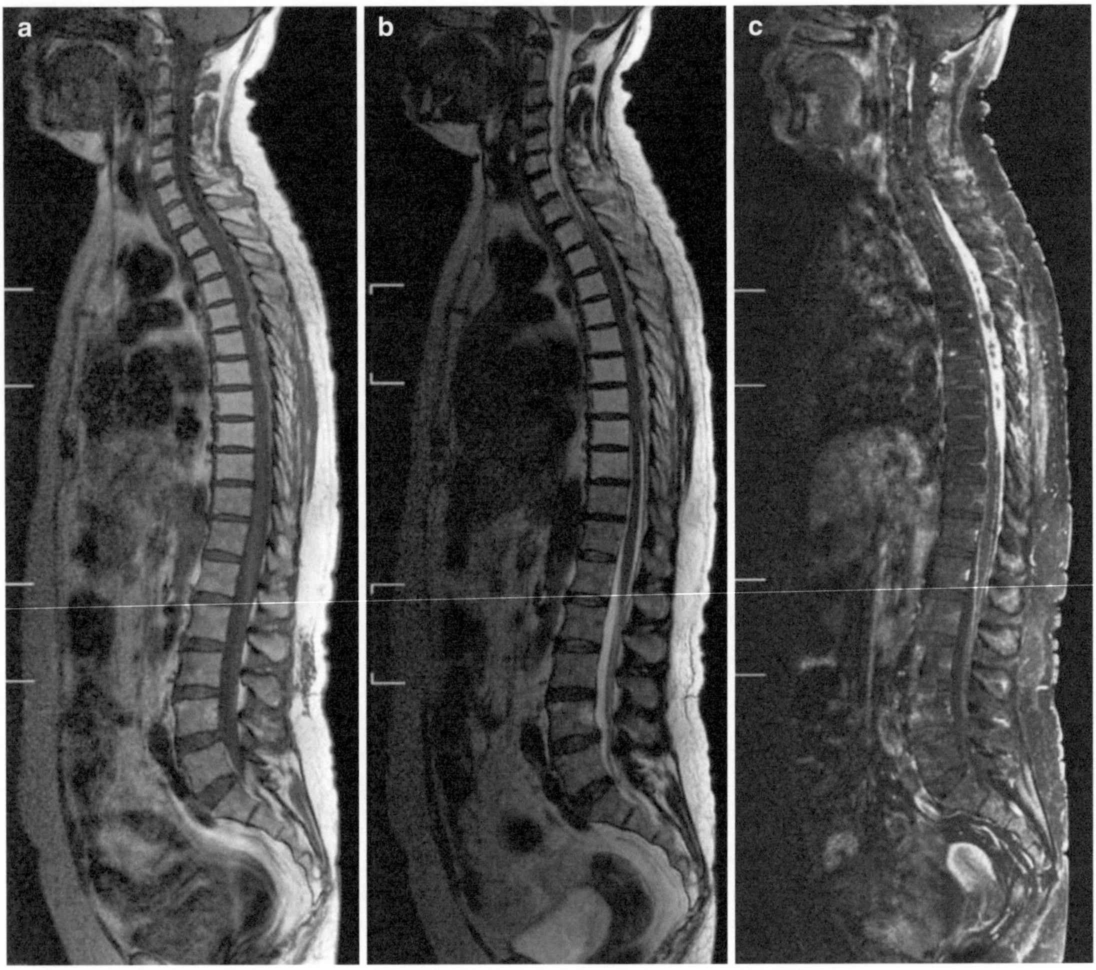

Fig. 6.6 Epidural abscess in a 60-year-old woman
A patient with an epidural abscess that occurred after epidural catheter insertion, showing a soft tissue mass in the epidural space with peripheral enhancement on thoracic MR. MR sagittal T1-weighted image (**a**), T2-weighted image (**b**), contrast-enhanced T1-weighted image (**c**)

6.3 Tuberculous Spondylitis

6.3.1 Incidence

Skeletal tuberculosis accounts for about 2–3% of all tuberculosis, and about 50% of these occur in the spine. Tuberculous spondylitis is most common in the upper lumbar and lower thoracic spine, but also occurs in the cervical and sacral spine, and the frequency of thoracic involvement is higher compared to pyogenic spondylitis.

Looking at the age of onset, while the incidence of tuberculosis in children under 10 is decreasing, the incidence in adults is increasing. This is due to the development of preventive medicine such as BCG vaccination in childhood and the advancement of diagnostic technology, which has reduced the chance of infection in children, while the reactivation of latent bacteria and secondary infections have increased the frequency in adults. The distribution of tuberculosis infection between men and women is known to be similar.

6.3.2 Causative Agent

The main causative agent is Mycobacterium tuberculosis, and recently, infections caused by atypical mycobacteria are also on the rise. Tuberculosis bacteria are weakly toxic, causing inflammation to progress slowly and forming large abscesses around the spine, which is characterized by early necrosis pathologically.

6.3.3 Mechanism of Occurrence

Spinal tuberculosis is mainly transmitted hematogenously, and some are infected directly from surrounding organs. Most tuberculous spondylitis begins in the form of tuberculous endarteritis near the spinal disc in the front part of the vertebral body, and as it progresses, it spreads along the anterior or posterior longitudinal ligament, or the inflammation invades the adjacent intervertebral disc through the subchondral endplate (Fig. 6.7).

Tuberculous spondylitis can be divided into peridiscal infection and central infection. First, peridiscal infection appears in the upper and lower vertebral bodies centered on the intervertebral disc due to the characteristics of the spinal segmental vessels, accounting for more than 50%. It erodes the cartilaginous endplate, resulting in narrowing of the intervertebral disc space. Next, central infection appears throughout the vertebral body, showing a lot of vertebral body deformation. The anterior invasion of the infection starts under the anterior longitudinal ligament, lifts the periosteum, causes circulatory disorders, and forms necrosis and abscesses (Fig. 6.8). In this case, the amount of bone destruction is small, so the deformation is less. Compared to pyogenic spondylitis, there is almost no fever, pain, or abscess, the progression is gradual, the abscess formation is clear, and the new bone formation is less in imaging studies, and because the intervertebral disc is preserved initially, the phenomenon of narrowing of the intervertebral disc space appears late.

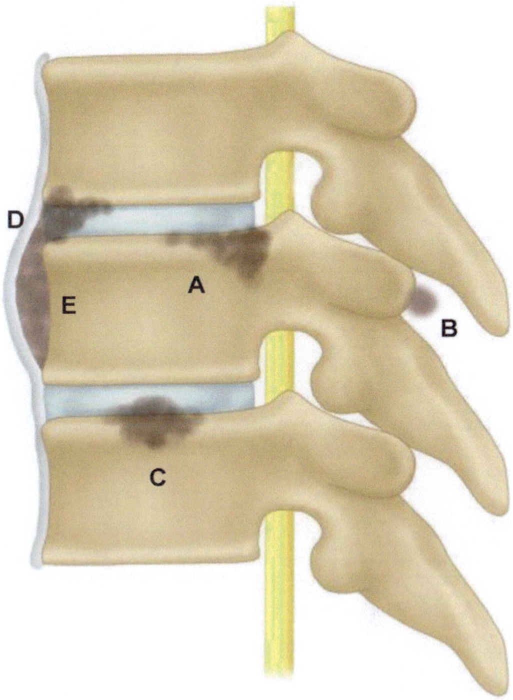

Fig. 6.7 Site of occurrence of tuberculous spondylitis Tuberculous lesions mainly appear confined to the vertebral body (**a**) or can rarely occur in the posterior structures (**b**). Infections that invade the intervertebral disc (**c**) or spread anteriorly to the vertebral body (**d**) are also common. The downward spread of inflammation causes sclerosis in front of the vertebral body (**e**)

6.3.4 Clinical Symptoms

Tuberculosis infection shows symptoms gradually over several months to years. Symptoms are very diverse, making clinical diagnosis difficult, mainly showing systemic symptoms such as weight loss, fatigue, intermittent fever, and locally showing spinal pain, tenderness, muscle tension, muscle weakness, decreased range of motion, palpation of spinal abscess, neurological symptoms, and spinal deformities. In particular, if diagnosis is delayed, severe deformities of the spine may occur. Therefore, it is very important to make an accurate diagnosis early. Also, tuberculous spondylitis shows more paralysis than pyogenic spondylitis, which is due to the frequent invasion of the neural arch, and it is known that

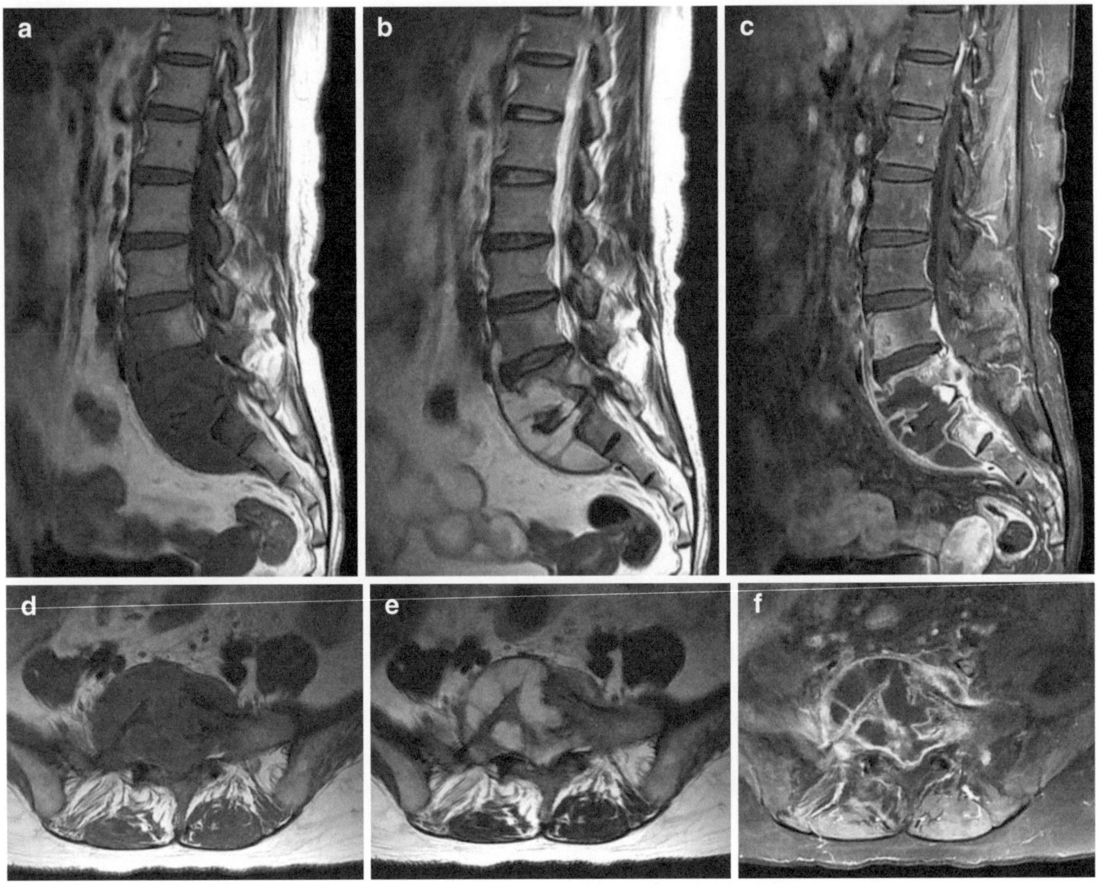

Fig. 6.8 Tuberculous spondylitis in a 67-year-old woman MR images show osteomyelitis invading from the fourth lumbar vertebra to the first sacral vertebra, with a large perivertebral abscess showing thin peripheral enhancement. MR sagittal T1-weighted image (**a**), T2-weighted image (**b**), contrast-enhanced T1-weighted image (**c**), axial T1-weighted image (**d**), T2-weighted image (**e**), contrast-enhanced T1-weighted image (**f**)

the frequency of early paralysis is about 5 times higher than that of delayed paralysis.

6.3.5 Clinical Examination and Diagnostic Methods

Blood tests show an increase in erythrocyte sedimentation rate and C-reactive protein. The tuberculin skin reaction test may be positive but is nonspecific.

Traditional slaughter methods or bacterial cultures have the disadvantage of low probability of positivity and taking a lot of time, but recently, direct testing is possible using the polymerase chain reaction method, and the selection of antibiotics that react to bacteria is also possible within 2-3 hours. The typical nodules seen in tuberculosis infection consist of a central necrotic area surrounded by epithelioid histiocytes. Langerhans type giant cells are scattered among these histiocytes, and a border of mixed chronic inflammatory cells exists around them. If these findings are seen, a pathological diagnosis can be made.

6.3.6 Imaging diagnosis

(1) Simple shooting.

In the early stages of infection, decreased opacity of the vertebral body, irregularity of the endplate, narrowing of the intervertebral disc space, increased soft tissue opacity around the spine, and destruction of the interosseous endplate are observed. In the later stages, findings such as spinal kyphosis, scoliosis, and vertebral fusion are seen. The typical finding is the collapse occurring at the front of two adjacent vertebral bodies and the destruction of the intervertebral disc. Gibbus deformity can also be seen due to the destruction of the anterior vertebral body along with the preservation of the posterior spinal structures [20]. Scalloping can be seen from the front of the vertebral body, but bone membrane reaction or bone sclerosis is not well seen. Recently, there are many cases showing atypical findings, the frequency of cervical tuberculous spondylitis is increasing, there are many reports of posterior invasion, multiple vertebral bodies are seen to be invaded, the intervertebral disc is preserved, and there are many cases where bone sclerosis is seen. Soft tissue masses typically show calcification. Perispinal abscesses can appear as psoas-shaped masses on both sides of the spine on simple radiographs. These perispinal abscesses appear as irregular or tear-shaped calcifications as they are treated.

(2) Nuclear medicine examination.
An increase in opacity can be seen on a 99mTc-MDP bone scan, but it is nonspecific. A hypersensitive 67Ga scan can be performed for inflammation.

(3) CT.
Through a CT scan, the extent of vertebral body destruction, the extent of the abscess, and the destruction of the posterior bone can be seen. It can be seen in detail. In particular, CT is superior to MRI in confirming calcification [21].

In the early stages of infection, erosion or bone destruction areas is not clear, so coronal and sagittal reconstructed CT images can show these changes well. In more chronic diseases, CT typically shows clear bone lysis and extensive destruction of the vertebral endplate, as well as subperiosteal lesions and sclerosis of the bone margin.

In patients with tuberculous spondylitis, calcified perispinal masses and irregular, thickened edge enhancement are almost characteristic findings of tuberculosis.

Percutaneous biopsy and abscess drainage can be performed under CT guidance (Fig. 6.9).

(4) MRI.
In patients with tuberculous spondylitis, MRI allows easy identification of perispinal abscesses, intraosseous abscesses, spinal canal or nerve root involvement, and posterior element involvement. Characteristic MRI findings have been reported as various degrees of cortical bone destruction, intraosseous abscesses with peripheral enhancement, large perispinal abscesses, clear invasion of perispinal soft tissues, subliga-

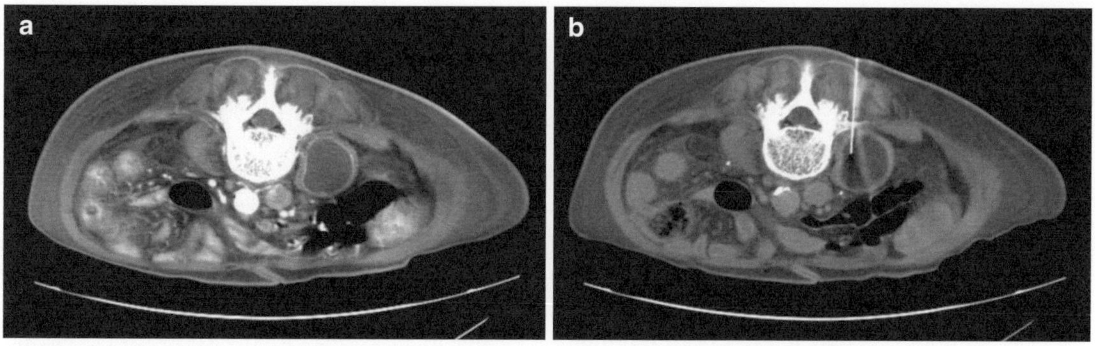

Fig. 6.9 Percutaneous drainage under CT guidance in a patient with tuberculous spondylitis
Contrast-enhanced CT (**a**) shows an abscess with peripheral enhancement in the psoas muscle. Aspiration and drainage of the abscess were performed under CT guidance (**b**)

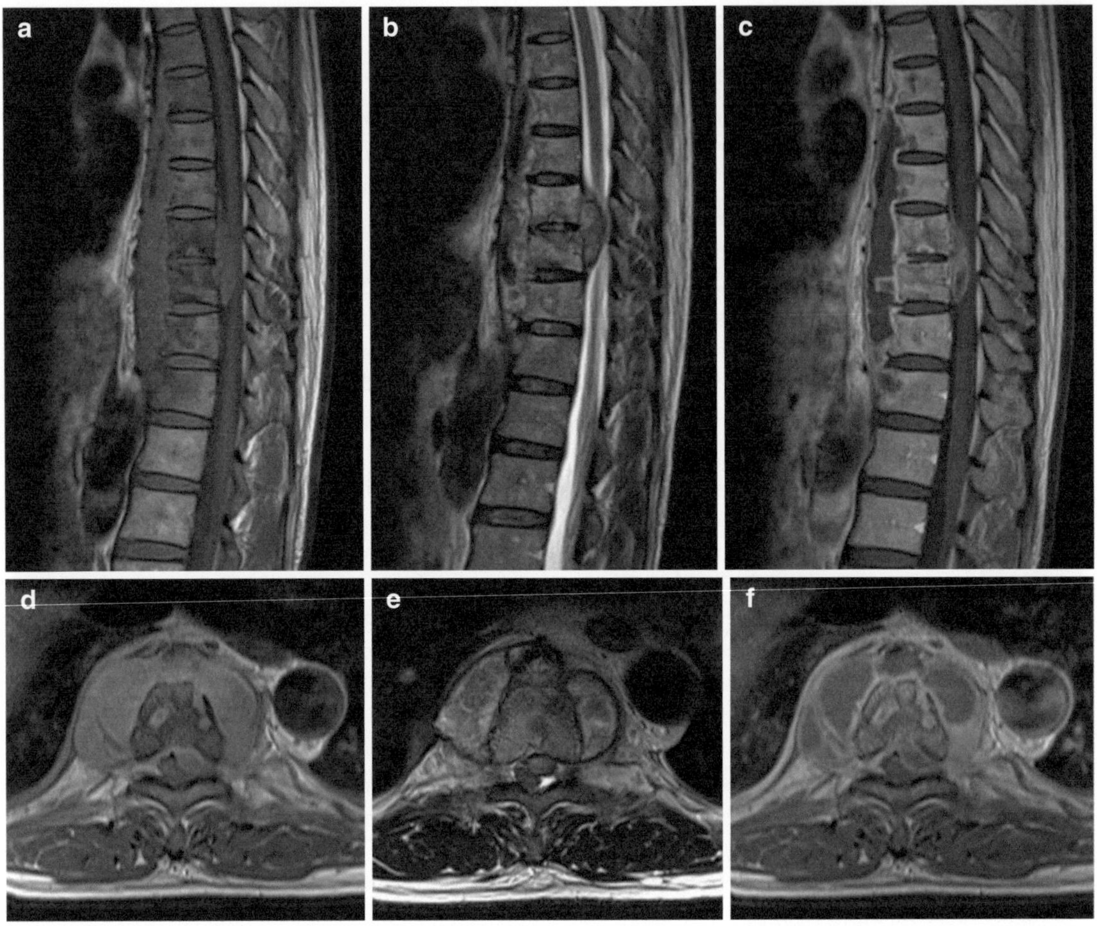

Fig. 6.10 Tuberculous spondylitis in a 60-year-old man On thoracic MR, a large perivertebral abscess showing subligamentous extension along the anterior longitudinal ligament of the lower thoracic spine and adjacent osteomyelitis and bone marrow edema of the lower thoracic spine are observed. Also, an epidural abscess is observed at the back of the spine, and thin rim enhancement is observed after contrast enhancement. Sagittal T1-weighted image (**a**), T2-weighted image (**b**), contrast-enhanced T1-weighted image (**c**), axial T1-weighted image (**d**), T2-weighted image (**e**), contrast-enhanced T1-weighted image (**f**)

mentous extension of inflammatory tissue, and relatively preserved intervertebral discs (Fig. 6.10) [22]. The reason why the intervertebral disc is preserved for a long time can be explained by the fact that there are no proteolytic enzymes, so the cartilage of the spinal disc is maintained and the invasion of the intervertebral disc occurs late. Tuberculous spondylitis can spread to posterior structures such as the pedicle, lamina, transverse process, spinous process, and has been reported in about 5% to 24% of spinal tuberculosis. This involvement of posterior structures shows a higher frequency than pyogenic spondylitis. In tuberculous spondylitis, it can invade more vertebral bodies than pyogenic, and skip lesions can occur that invade distant vertebral bodies with normal vertebral bodies in between, and the frequency of such skip lesions is known to be about 4% of spinal tuberculosis. For this reason, in cases where tuberculous spondylitis is suspected, imaging should be performed including as wide a range of the spine as possible so as not to miss distant foci (Fig. 6.11). As the inflammation progresses, characteristic gibbus deformities occur along with spinal kyphosis and scoliosis due to vertebral body

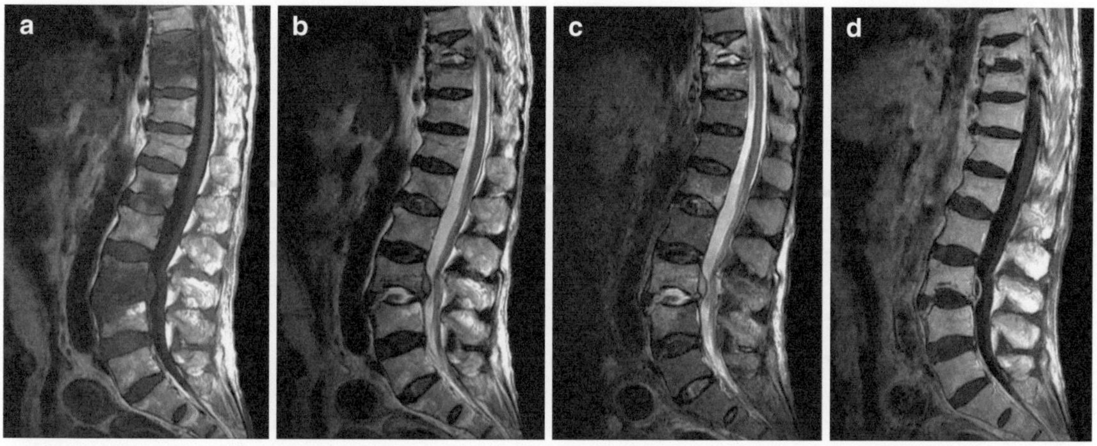

Fig. 6.11 Tuberculous spondylitis in an 84-year-old man Osteomyelitis involving multiple vertebral bodies in the lower thoracic and lumbar spine is observed, with skip lesions involving distant vertebral bodies with normal vertebral bodies in between. Sagittal T1-weighted image (**a**), T2-weighted image (**b**), T2 STIR image (**c**), contrast-enhanced T1-weighted image (**d**)

destruction and collapse, and ankylosis of the vertebral body can also occur during the healing process [20, 21].

The MRI findings of the mass formed around the spine can help differentiate between tuberculous spondylitis and pyogenic spondylitis. In the case of tuberculous spondylitis, the frequency of mass formation is high and the size of the mass is large, and the perispinal abscess does not have proteolytic enzymes. Therefore, it tends to grow by pushing rather than destroying structures such as the anterior longitudinal ligament or the aorta. On the other hand, pyogenic spondylitis often invades around vessels such as the aorta and vena cava as the inflammatory tissue penetrates the ligament. Post-contrast MRI images are particularly useful in characterizing tuberculous spondylitis, showing relatively thin rim enhancement of abscesses in bone and soft tissue [12, 23]. Epidural spread or meningeal involvement is also well observed after contrast enhancement. The thick and irregular rim enhancement of the abscess wall and the uncertain boundary of the spread of inflammation around the spine suggest pyogenic spondylitis, but there are reports that minimal contrast enhancement can occur in active inflammatory tissue areas during contrast enhancement in tuberculous spondylitis [12, 24]. Pyogenic spondylitis is usually treated with antibiotics alone, but tuberculous spondylitis often requires surgical treatment and different anti-tuberculosis treatments than general antibiotics, so it is very important to distinguish these two [13].

6.4 Fungal Spondylitis

6.4.1 Incidence

The incidence of fungal infections has been increasing in recent years, but fungal infections of the spine are relatively rare. Fungal infections mainly occur as opportunistic infections in immunocompromised patients, and fungal infections of the spine mainly appear as discitis or osteomyelitis.

6.4.2 Causative Organism

Candida species are the most common causative organisms, followed by Aspergillus [25, 26].

6.4.3 Mechanism of Occurrence

Spinal involvement generally occurs as a result of hematogenous or direct spread from an initial lung infection [25, 26].

Fungal infections cause a variety of inflammatory responses, from granuloma formation in chronic inflammation to abscess formation.

6.4.4 Clinical Symptoms

Fungal spondylitis is very similar to the clinical manifestations of other spondylitis. Fungal spondylitis is mainly found in AIDS patients, immunosuppressed patients, and patients receiving long-term steroid and chemotherapy. There are times when it is difficult to distinguish fungal infection from spinal metastasis of a tumor, in which case clinical findings and histological findings are important.

6.4.5 Imaging Diagnosis

(1) Plain Radiography.
The imaging features of spinal fungal infection are similar to tuberculosis. They invade the anterior vertebral body, preserve the disc, and sometimes form large perivertebral abscesses. Fungal infections can rarely invade the posterior elements and adjacent ribs [27].

(2) CT.
CT can define the extent of the disease and help in differential diagnosis. In contrast to pyogenic spondylitis, fungal spondylitis often preserves the disc. Also, while tumors that invade the spine typically show complete bone destruction, fungal spondylitis can form cavities and sequestra in the spine [27].

(3) MRI.
The MRI findings of fungal spondylitis differ from those of pyogenic infection, and it does not show high signal intensity in the vertebral body and intervertebral disc on T2-weighted images, or it shows lower high signal intensity than expected. Also, in fungal spondylitis, the intranuclear cleft of the intervertebral disc can be preserved. These changes in signal intensity are often explained by the decreased inflammatory response in immunocompromised patients [26]. Fungal spondylitis can sometimes manifest without invading the intervertebral disc, and in such cases, the MRI findings may appear similar to those of tuberculous spondylitis.

Candida spondylitis can occur simultaneously or later due to disseminated candidiasis, often appearing as a granuloma without disc involvement [28]. As spondylitis progresses, disc destruction is accompanied in 50% of cases, and perispinal abscesses are associated (Fig. 6.12). Compared to tuberculous spondylitis, the size of the perispinal abscess is smaller, and skip lesions or subligamentous extension of inflammation are rare [29].

Aspergillus infection typically affects one or more vertebrae. Typical imaging findings include disc swelling with protrusion of the annulus fibrosus, enhancement of the anterior or posterior longitudinal ligament, and enhancement of the subligamentous space without disc enhancement. Aspergillus infection can cause vertebral body collapse, form epidural abscesses, or cause direct spinal cord infection. Also, Aspergillus spondylitis can invade multiple vertebral bodies like tuberculous spondylitis, showing skip lesions or subligamentous extension of inflammation, a sawtooth appearance of the vertebral endplate, or low signal intensity under the cartilage on T2-weighted images (Fig. 6.13) [30].

In immunocompromised patients, when spondylitis involving the vertebral body and intervertebral disc occurs, the possibility of fungal spondylitis should be considered in addition to pyogenic or tuberculous spondylitis.

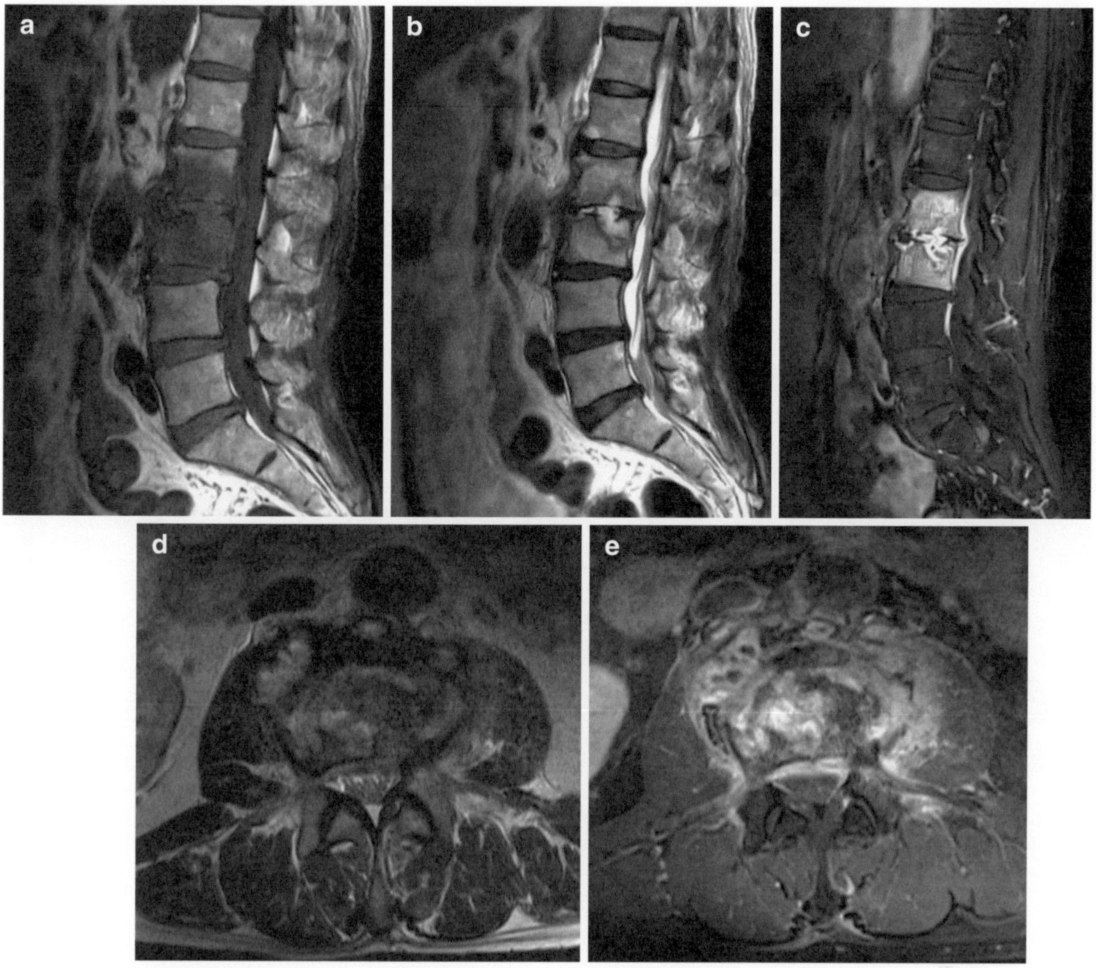

Fig. 6.12 Candida spondylitis in a 73-year-old man
On MR, signal intensity changes due to osteomyelitis of the second and third lumbar vertebrae are seen, and end-plate edema and intervertebral disc destruction are observed. On contrast-enhanced images, there is clear enhancement of the marrow along with inflammatory findings extending to the intervertebral disc. On axial images, a small perivertebral abscess is observed. Sagittal T1-weighted image (**a**), T2-weighted image (**b**), contrast-enhanced T1-weighted image (**c**), axial T2-weighted image (**d**), contrast-enhanced T1-weighted image (**e**)

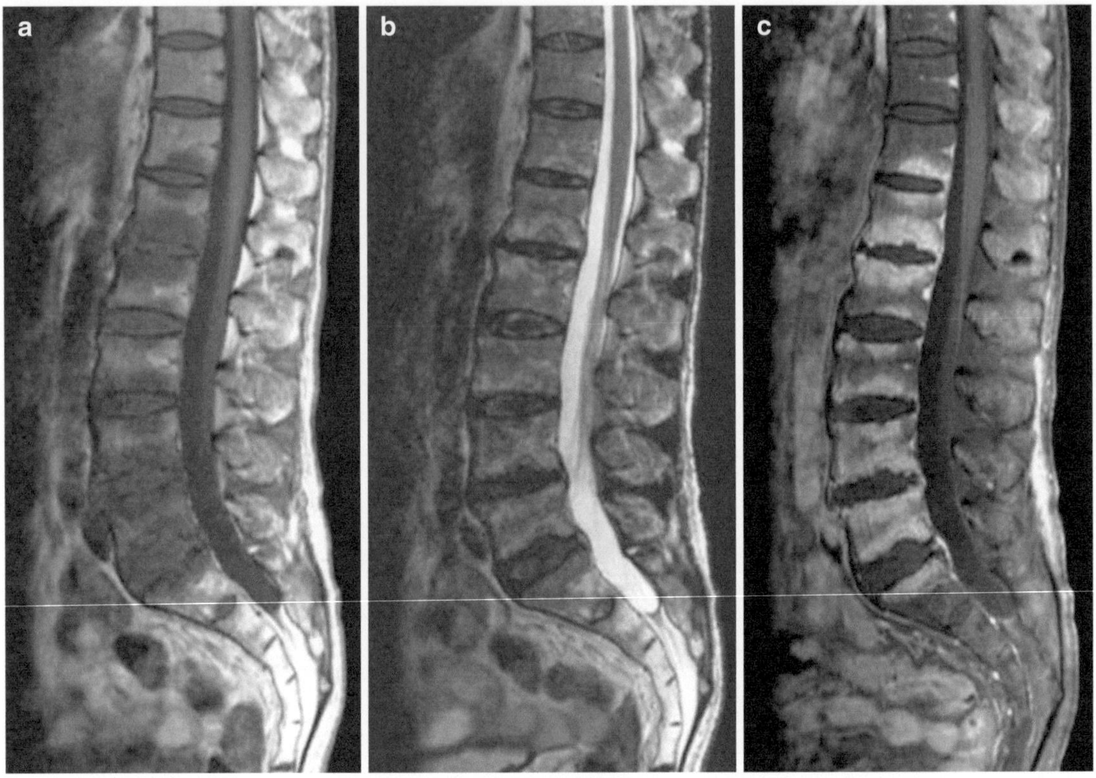

Fig. 6.13 Aspergillus spondylitis in a 66-year-old man Osteomyelitis involving the entire lumbar region and endplate edema are observed, and the intranuclear cleft of the intervertebral disc is preserved. Sagittal T1-weighted image (**a**), T2-weighted image (**b**), contrast-enhanced T1-weighted image (**c**)

6.5 Brucella Spondylitis

6.5.1 Incidence

Brucellosis is a zoonotic infectious disease caused by Brucella bacteria, commonly occurring in dairy farmers, farmers, slaughterhouse workers, and veterinarians in developing countries [31]. Brucellosis is known to be endemic in the Mediterranean and Middle East regions, and in Korea, it continues to occur in people related to livestock farming. Most cases of brucellosis in Korea occur through direct contact with infected livestock, with a significantly higher proportion of adult males. It mainly occurs in those over 50 years old [32].

Complications of brucellosis often include musculoskeletal disorders such as peripheral arthritis, spondylitis, and sacroiliac arthritis, among which spondylitis is the most serious and common complication [33].

Brucella spondylitis most commonly occurs in the lumbar spine, followed by the thoracic and cervical spine. It usually occurs in a single vertebra and very rarely in multiple vertebrae.

6.5.2 Causative Agent

Brucella bacteria, gram-negative coccobacilli, are classified into six species depending on the host they mainly invade. Among them, Brucella melitensis (goats, sheep), Brucella abortus (cattle), Brucella suis (pigs), and Brucella canis (dogs) are known to cause human brucellosis.

While Brucella melitensis accounts for the majority of human brucellosis worldwide,

Brucella abortus is known to be the cause of human brucellosis epidemic in Korea [32].

6.5.3 Mechanism of Occurrence

Direct transmission between humans is rare, and it is transmitted to humans by consuming dairy products obtained from infected animals without sterilization, through direct contact with highly infectious by-products such as the placenta of infected animals, or by inhaling infectious substances through the respiratory system [31]. Considering that Brucella, once entered into the human body, mainly proliferates in the reticuloendothelial system, the risk of human infection increases when consuming raw liver or spleen of cattle.

The most common site of primary infection in the human body is the musculoskeletal system, and spinal involvement typically appears in the subacute and chronic stages of brucellosis [33]. Brucella spondylitis occurs due to hematogenous dissemination, mostly starting from the superior endplate of the vertebral body. Depending on the toxicity in the human body and the host's immune status, it can spread to the entire spine, intervertebral disc space, and adjacent vertebrae. It can also be accompanied by radiculopathy and localized neuritis. Osteomyelitis or subacute and chronic meningitis with osteomyelitis can occur simultaneously.

6.5.4 Clinical Symptoms

Brucellosis is a systemic infectious disease that can affect all organs and cause various non-specific clinical manifestations [34]. The most common symptom is fever, which is known to persist irregularly for a long time. Following fever, fatigue, sweating, and muscle pain are commonly complained symptoms. Joint pain without arthritis is also common, mainly occurring in joints such as the shoulder, knee, and ankle. The most common organ where complications occur is the gastrointestinal tract, with various digestive symptoms accompanied by loss of appetite, weight loss, nausea, vomiting, and abdominal discomfort. These gastrointestinal symptoms occur in the majority of patients, regardless of the route of infection of brucellosis. When the vertebral body is involved, there may be symptoms of nerve root compression, disc herniation, lower body paralysis, or limb paralysis.

Because the incubation period of the pathogen varies from 4 weeks to 5 months, early diagnosis is difficult, so detailed medical history and exposure investigation are essential for diagnosis [31, 34].

6.5.5 Clinical Examination and Diagnostic Methods

Because the clinical symptoms of brucellosis are diverse and non-specific, it is difficult to diagnose based on clinical findings alone. Confirmation of brucellosis requires the isolation and culture of bacteria from blood or tissue samples, and the sensitivity of blood culture tests varies greatly from 15 to 70% depending on the laboratory [35].

If Brucella bacteria are not isolated from tissue samples, brucellosis can be diagnosed by serological tests. A positive reaction in the standard tube agglutination test (STA) can be used for diagnosis.

Brucella spondylitis can cause dangerous neurological and hematological complications if diagnosis and treatment are delayed, and it is necessary to differentiate it from other diseases that cause infections in the spine, especially tuberculosis.

6.5.6 Imaging Diagnosis

(1) Simple Radiography.
The spondylitis that occurs during Brucella infection is known to most commonly affect the lower lumbar spine. Brucella spondylitis can take the form of a localized lesion or a subacute lesion. Localized Brucella spondylitis mainly appears confined to the anterior

part of the vertebral endplate. Subacute Brucella spondylitis can involve the entire vertebral body, extend the adjacent intervertebral disc, and progress through the endplate and vertebral body around the disc to the extradural space.

The initial findings of Brucella spondylitis are characterized by osteoporosis of the infected vertebrae. About 3 months after the onset of symptoms due to infection, erosive changes appear at the front of the upper endplate of the vertebral body in simple radiographs. Initially, there is little change in the posterior elements of the vertebral body, and the spine mostly maintains its normal shape [36]. In some cases of Brucella spondylitis, a small air shadow may appear between the intervertebral disc and the adjacent upper endplate, which could be a characteristic of ischemia and avascular necrosis of the intervertebral disc adjacent to the infected end. As spondylitis progresses, changes such as a decrease in intervertebral disc height, destruction and patchy sclerosis of the vertebral endplate, and syndesmophytes may appear, and signs of displacement along the vertebral axis or ankylosis of the vertebral body may also be shown. If ankylosis of the vertebral body occurs due to Brucella spondylitis, it can destroy the entire vertebral body and cause intervertebral disc herniation. Despite such extensive lesions, vertebral collapse and scoliosis are known to be relatively rare.

(2) MRI.

Magnetic resonance imaging plays an important role in diagnosis and follow-up observation, being more sensitive than other imaging tests. Bones and soft tissues infected with Brucella show low signal intensity in T1-weighted images and high signal intensity in T2-weighted images. Localized Brucella spondylitis appears as a lesion with abnormal signal intensity in part of the vertebral body, mainly confined to the front of the discovertebral junction. Chronic Brucella spondylitis shows abnormal signal intensity spreading through the adjacent vertebrae and the intervertebral disc in between (Fig. 6.14). The intervertebral disc appears with increased signal intensity in T2-weighted images in the early stages of infection, and may appear similar to disc swelling or disc herniation. As the infection progresses, the height of the intervertebral disc decreases and enhancement is observed. The facet joints of the spine are also often involved. Typical MRI findings of Brucella

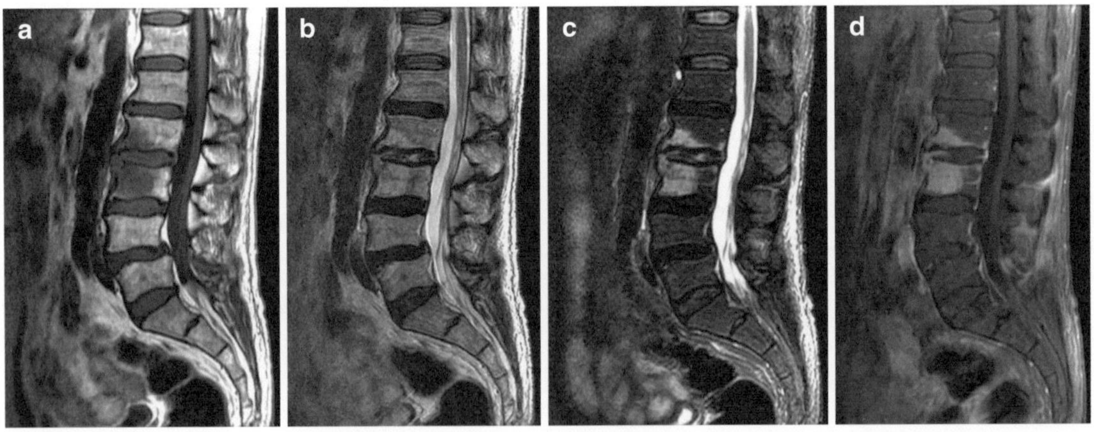

Fig. 6.14 Brucella spondylitis in a 60-year-old man
On lumbar MR, signal intensity changes due to osteomyelitis of the second and third lumbar vertebrae are seen, and endplate edema of the upper endplate of the third lumbar vertebra is accompanied. On contrast-enhanced images, the marrow's inflammation extending to the intervertebral disc along with enhancement is observed. MR sagittal T1-weighted image (**a**), T2-weighted image (**b**), T2 STIR image (**c**), contrast-enhanced T1-weighted image (**d**)

spondylitis appear within 1 month after the onset of clinical symptoms [37, 38]. Infections caused by Brucella bacteria often extend to the extradural space, with increased signal intensity seen in the surrounding muscles and soft tissues, and the boundary between muscle and fat may be lost due to edema or granulation tissue. Paraspinal abscesses have been reported in about 10% of Brucella spondylitis cases, but compared to the 50% of tuberculous spondylitis cases where abscesses are accompanied, the frequency is relatively low, and the size of the abscess is also small [39].

Brucellar spondylitis can also show imaging features of radiculitis, arachnoiditis, and neuritis, especially in lumbar brucellosis, where the peritoneum adjacent to the infected spine can thicken and the lymph nodes around the aorta can enlarge.

6.6 Infectious Spondylitis in Children

In children, the frequency of infectious diseases affecting the spine is somewhat lower than in adults. In children, the intervertebral disc receives direct blood supply, so infection of the intervertebral disc can occur primarily (Fig. 6.15). That is, after bacteremia, the infection can first invade the intervertebral disc through the connected vessels and sequentially invade the adjacent vertebral endplates. In such cases, changes in simple radiography can be very subtle and easily overlooked [40].

The imaging findings of infectious spondylitis in children are not significantly different from those in adults, but in the case of tuberculous spondylitis, it tends to show a wider distribution than when it occurs in adults.

A unique infectious disease of the spine that occurs in children is chronic recurrent multifocal

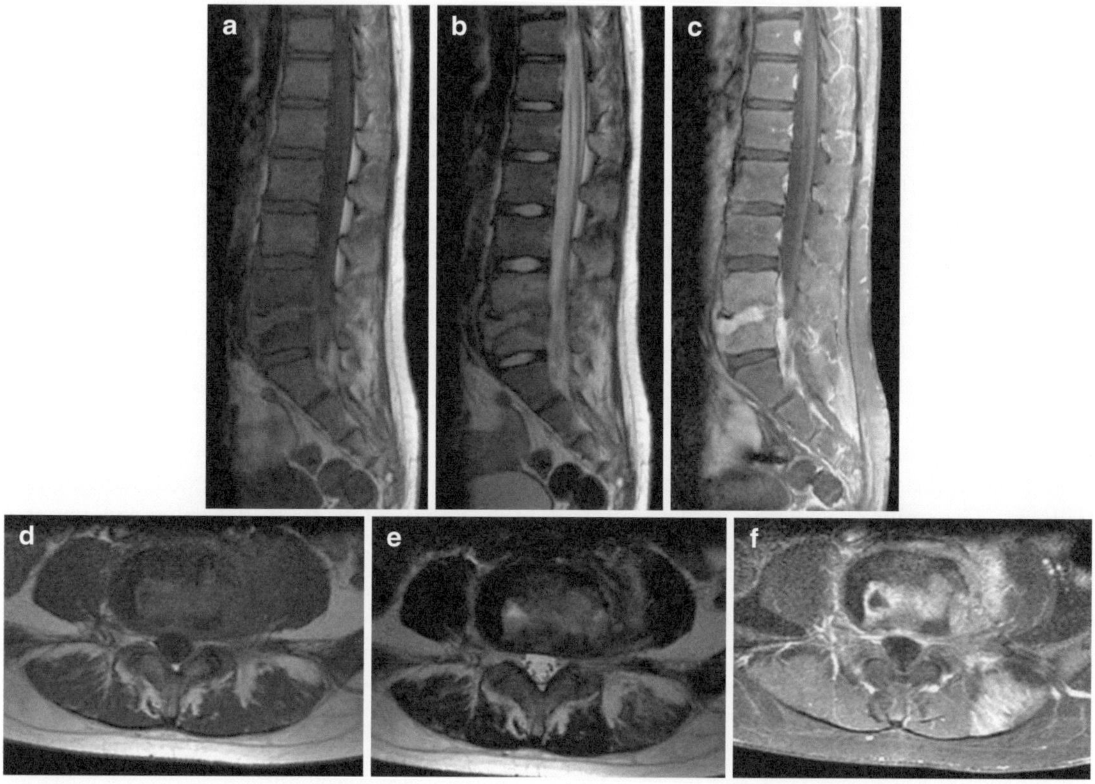

Fig. 6.15 Pyogenic spondylitis in a 13-year-old boy
On lumbar MR, osteomyelitis of the fourth and fifth lumbar vertebrae, intervertebral disc invasion, and phlegmon around the spine showing enhancement and abscess of the spinal disc are observed. MR Sagittal T1-weighted image (**a**), T2-weighted image (**b**), contrast-enhanced T1-weighted image (**c**), axial T1-weighted image (**d**), T2-weighted image (**e**), contrast-enhanced T1-weighted image (**f**)

osteomyelitis, a disease that affects both the spine and the limbs. It is rare to confirm pathogens in bacterial culture, and bacterial culture through tissue biopsy usually does not help in diagnosis. This disease shows symptoms and signs of infection, shows a pattern of repeated improvement and deterioration, and eventually heals, but does not respond to antibiotic treatment, so it is treated with symptomatic therapy [41, 42].

6.7 Differential Diseases

Infectious spondylitis needs to be differentiated from other diseases that show changes in the intervertebral disc and vertebral endplate, and the types of differential diseases to consider vary depending on the progression and spread of infectious spondylitis.

6.7.1 Tumors

In both infectious spondylitis and tumors occurring in the spine, cortical bone and cancellous bone destruction and changes in the surrounding soft tissues of the spine can be observed in images. Generally, metastasis does not invade the intervertebral disc. If the boundary of the vertebral endplate is lost due to intervertebral disc invasion and the adjacent vertebral body is simultaneously invaded, infectious spondylitis should be considered first. Also, the swelling associated with infection tends to obliterate the fat plane of the surrounding soft tissues of the spine, while in bone tumors, the fat plane is maintained or partially lost. Generally, considering all these points, it is not difficult to distinguish between infectious spondylitis and bone tumors. However, tumors can show atypical imaging findings, making it not easy to distinguish from infectious spondylitis, and in cases like chordoma, where the changes in signal intensity of the intervertebral disc and the pattern of soft tissue invasion in T1- and T2-enhanced images are very similar to infectious spondylitis, accurate differential diagnosis can be made by focusing more on the clinical situation and the location of the lesion.

6.7.2 Compression Fracture

There are cases where compression fractures appear similar to infectious spondylitis, making diagnosis difficult. In the case of compression fractures, the main differential point from infectious spondylitis is that the intervertebral disc is not invaded and the vertebral endplate is preserved. However, compression fractures and infections can occur simultaneously, and in such cases, diagnosis is very tricky, so if there is any suspicion of infection, it is advisable to perform a tissue biopsy. If a spinal vacuum echo is seen, it suggests a positive compression fracture, and it can be differentiated from infectious spondylitis. Vacuum echo can be easily confirmed in simple shooting, and in MRI, it shows low signal intensity in T1- and T2-enhanced images.

6.7.3 Degenerative Intervertebral Disc Disease

When the intervertebral disc undergoes degenerative changes, it shows low signal intensity in T2-enhanced images, suggesting disc dehydration, often the height of the disc decreases, and the edge of the vertebral endplate is well preserved. Along with the degenerative changes of the intervertebral disc, the signal intensity of the vertebral endplate can change, and Modic et al. reported three types of changes in the signal intensity of the vertebral endplate [43]. Among them, Modic type 1 lesions showing changes in bone marrow signal intensity of low signal intensity in T1-enhanced images and high signal intensity in T2-enhanced images, and Modic type 3 lesions showing low signal intensity in both T1- and T2-enhanced images can appear similar to infectious spondylitis. However, generally in Modic type 1 lesions, the signal intensity of the intervertebral disc tends to be normal or decreased in T2-enhanced images, and can show a vacuum phenomenon, and does not show inflammatory changes or abscesses in the surrounding spinal soft tissues. Also, the "Claw sign," which shows a linear high signal intensity at the boundary between

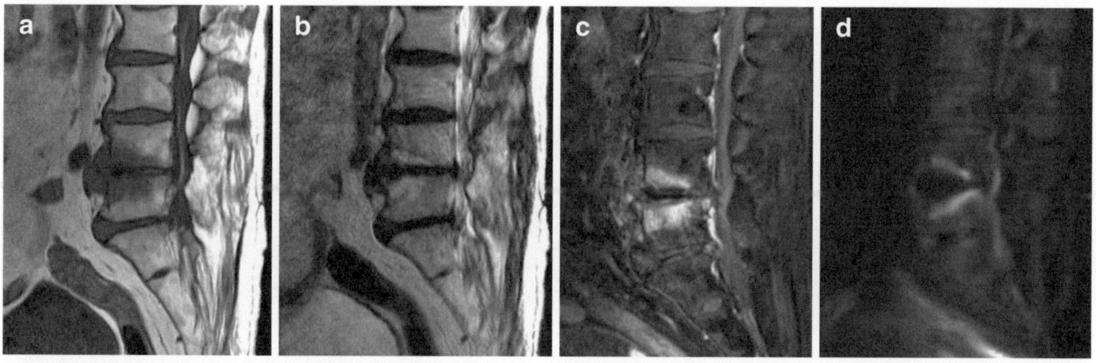

Fig. 6.16 Modic type 1 lesion in a 72-year-old man On lumbar MR, the fourth and fifth lumbar vertebrae show Modic type 1 lesions with low signal intensity on T1-enhanced images and high signal intensity on T2-enhanced images, and vacuum phenomenon of the intervertebral disc is accompanied. Clear enhancement of the bone marrow is seen on the enhanced image, and the Claw sign is observed on the diffusion-enhanced image. MR Sagittal T1-weighted image (**a**), T2-weighted image (**b**), contrast-enhanced T1-weighted image (**c**), diffusion-enhanced image (**d**)

normal and abnormal bone marrow in diffusion-weighted MR images, is known as a characteristic finding of Modic type 1 lesions (Fig. 6.16) [44]. If the vertebral endplate shows severe destruction, the possibility of infectious spondylitis is high.

6.7.4 Schmorl's Node

Schmorl's node refers to the formation of a node when the intervertebral disc escapes into the vertebral body from a weakened part of the vertebral endplate, and occasionally, changes in signal intensity showing bone marrow edema or inflammatory form around the node can be seen. At this time, contrast enhancement can be observed in the intervertebral disc, and these imaging findings can cause confusion with infectious spondylitis (Fig. 6.17). T1-enhanced images are helpful for accurate diagnosis. It is important to recognize the escape through the spinal disc of the intervertebral disc. Unlike infectious spondylitis, abnormalities occur only on one side of the vertebral body adjacent to the intervertebral disc, and it is important to distinguish the relatively clear concentric bone marrow swelling centered on the node.

6.7.5 Ankylosing Spondylitis

In ankylosing spondylitis, erosion can occur in the central and transitional spinal discs, and in this case, it may look similar to infectious spondylitis, causing confusion in diagnosis. Typically, in ankylosing spondylitis, there is sclerotic change around the bone erosion, and the spinal disc is well maintained in areas other than bone erosion. However, in advanced ankylosing spondylitis, all spinal discs are destroyed, but in such cases, syndesmophytosis, squaring of the vertebral body, fusion of the apophyseal joint, etc. are accompanied, so it is not difficult to distinguish from infectious spondylitis. Ankylosing spondylitis often causes osteoporosis, and if spinal fusion progresses here, the risk of fracture increases. Fractures mainly appear as horizontal fractures that include the vertebral body and posterior structures near the thoracolumbar or thoracic junction. There are often cases where the discovery is delayed after the occurrence of a fracture and union is not properly formed, and as a result, a pseudo-joint is formed, which is called an Andersson lesion. In simple radiography, bone erosion and hardening appear centered on the fracture, so it looks similar to infectious spondylitis and needs to be distinguished. In MRI, it can

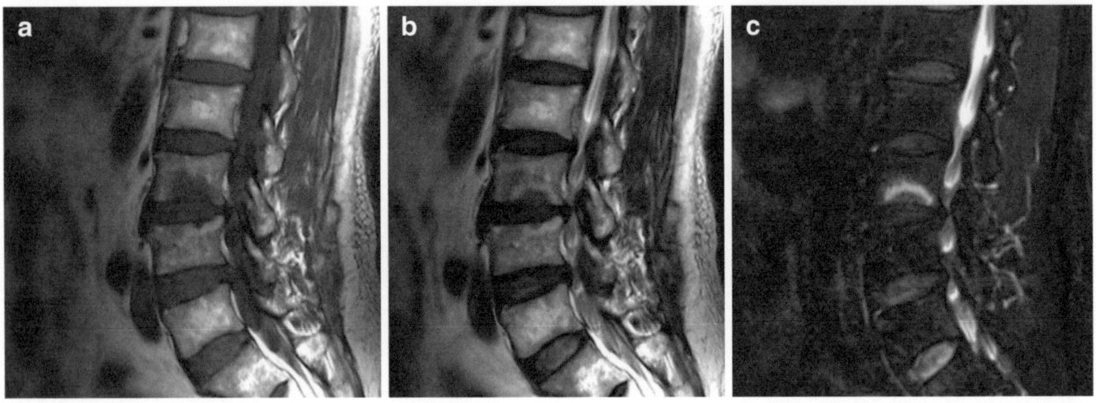

Fig. 6.17 Acute Schmorl's node in a 73-year-old man- There is a defect in the lower endplate of the third lumbar vertebra, and changes in signal intensity due to surrounding bone marrow edema are observed. MR sagittal T1-enhanced image (**a**), T2-enhanced image (**b**), fat-suppressed T2-enhanced image (**c**)

be distinguished from infectious spondylitis by invading both the vertebral body and the posterior structures, and not seeing an abscess around the spine.

6.7.6 Neuropathic Arthritis

Spinal neuropathic osteoarthritis is a very rare disease that invades and destroys the intervertebral disc, adjacent vertebral body, and facet joint. The spine is invaded in 6–12% of patients diagnosed with neuropathic arthritis. Initially, it is similar to degenerative disc disease, but the progression is fast, so it is difficult to distinguish from infectious spondylitis as the destruction of the intervertebral disc and spinal disc progresses. In MRI, the signal intensity and contrast enhancement shape, erosion of the spinal disc, and soft tissue mass formation around the spine are similar to infectious spondylitis. There are also reports that it shows relatively low signal intensity compared to the high signal intensity seen in the intervertebral disc and bone marrow during infection on T2-weighted images. Vacuum phenomenon of the intervertebral disc, anterior displacement, facet arthrosis, joint destruction, and bone debris are known to be useful findings in distinguishing spinal neuropathic arthritis from infectious spondylitis [45].

Bibliography

1. DeSanto J, Ross JS. Spine infection/inflammation. Radiol Clin North Am. 2011;49:105–27.
2. Quinones-Hinojosa A, Jun P, Jacobs R, Rosenberg WS, Weinstein PR. General principles in the medical and surgical management of spinal infections: a multidisciplinary approach. Neurosurg Focus. 2004;17:E1.
3. Ratcliffe JF. The arterial anatomy of the developing human dorsal and lumbar vertebral body. A microarteriographic study. J Anat. 1981;133:625–38.
4. Hong SH, Choi JY, Lee JW, Kim NR, Choi JA, Kang HS. MR imaging assessment of the spine: infection or an imitation? Radiographics. 2009;29:599–612.
5. Cottle L, Riordan T. Infectious spondylodiscitis. J Infect. 2008;56:401–12.
6. Tali ET, Gultekin S. Infections of the spinal column. In: Naidich TP, editor. Imaging of the spine. Philadelphia, PA: Saunders/Elsevier; 2011. p. 407–34.
7. Rothman SL. The diagnosis of infections of the spine by modern imaging techniques. Orthop Clin North Am. 1996;27:15–31.
8. Lisbona R, Derbekyan V, Novales-Diaz J, Veksler A. Gallium-67 scintigraphy in tuberculous and nontuberculous infectious spondylitis. J Nucl Med. 1993;34:853–9.
9. Carragee EJ. The clinical use of magnetic resonance imaging in pyogenic vertebral osteomyelitis. Spine (Phila Pa 1976). 1997;22:780–5.
10. Ledermann HP, Schweitzer ME, Morrison WB, Carrino JA. MR imaging findings in spinal infections: rules or myths? Radiology. 2003;228:506–14.
11. Jinkins JR, Bazan C 3rd, Xiong L. MR of disc protrusion engendered by infectious spondylitis. J Comput Assist Tomogr. 1996;20:715–8.
12. Jung NY, Jee WH, Ha KY, Park CK, Byun JY. Discrimination of tuberculous spondylitis from

pyogenic spondylitis on MRI. AJR Am J Roentgenol. 2004;182:1405–10.
13. Gouliamos AD, Kehagias DT, Lahanis S, Athanassopoulou AA, Moulopoulou ES, Kalovidouris AA, et al. MR imaging of tuberculous vertebral osteomyelitis: pictorial review. Eur Radiol. 2001;11:575–9.
14. Gillams AR, Chaddha B, Carter AP. MR appearances of the temporal evolution and resolution of infectious spondylitis. AJR Am J Roentgenol. 1996;166:903–7.
15. Numaguchi Y, Rigamonti D, Rothman MI, Sato S, Mihara F, Sadato N. Spinal epidural abscess: evaluation with gadolinium-enhanced MR imaging. Radiographics. 1993;13:545–59. discussion 559-560
16. Rigamonti D, Liem L, Sampath P, Knoller N, Namaguchi Y, Schreibman DL, et al. Spinal epidural abscess: contemporary trends in etiology, evaluation, and management. Surg Neurol. 1999;52:189–96. discussion 197
17. Tang HJ, Lin HJ, Liu YC, Li CM. Spinal epidural abscess--experience with 46 patients and evaluation of prognostic factors. J Infect. 2002;45:76–81.
18. Lury K, Smith JK, Castillo M. Imaging of spinal infections. Semin Roentgenol. 2006;41:363–79.
19. Siddiq F, Chowfin A, Tight R, Sahmoun AE, Smego RA Jr. Medical vs surgical management of spinal epidural abscess. Arch Intern Med. 2004;164:2409–12.
20. Almeida A. Tuberculosis of the spine and spinal cord. Eur J Radiol. 2005;55:193–201.
21. Shanley DJ. Tuberculosis of the spine: imaging features. AJR Am J Roentgenol. 1995;164:659–64.
22. Moore SL, Rafii M. Imaging of musculoskeletal and spinal tuberculosis. Radiol Clin North Am. 2001;39:329–42.
23. Chang MC, Wu HT, Lee CH, Liu CL, Chen TH. Tuberculous spondylitis and pyogenic spondylitis: comparative magnetic resonance imaging features. Spine (Phila Pa 1976). 2006;31:782–8.
24. De Backer AI, Mortele KJ, Vanschoubroeck IJ, Deeren D, Vanhoenacker FM, De Keulenaer BL, et al. Tuberculosis of the spine: CT and MR imaging features. JBR-BTR. 2005;88:92–7.
25. Chhem RK, Wang S, Jaovisidha S, Schmit P, Friedman L, Bureau NJ, et al. Imaging of fungal, viral, and parasitic musculoskeletal and spinal diseases. Radiol Clin North Am. 2001;39:357–78.
26. Williams RL, Fukui MB, Meltzer CC, Swarnkar A, Johnson DW, Welch W. Fungal spinal osteomyelitis in the immunocompromised patient: MR findings in three cases. AJNR Am J Neuroradiol. 1999;20:381–5.
27. Kim CW, Perry A, Currier B, Yaszemski M, Garfin SR. Fungal infections of the spine. Clin Orthop Relat Res. 2006;444:92–9.
28. Munk PL, Lee MJ, Poon PY, O'Connell JX, Coupland DB, Janzen DL, et al. Candida osteomyelitis and disc space infection of the lumbar spine. Skeletal Radiol. 1997;26:42–6.
29. Lee SW, Lee SH, Chung HW, Kim MJ, Seo MJ, Shin MJ. Candida spondylitis: comparison of MRI findings with bacterial and tuberculous causes. AJR Am J Roentgenol. 2013;201:872–7.
30. Kwon JW, Hong SH, Choi SH, Yoon YC, Lee SH. MRI findings of Aspergillus spondylitis. AJR Am J Roentgenol. 2011;197:W919–23.
31. Pappas G, Akritidis N, Bosilkovski M, Tsianos E. Brucellosis. N Engl J Med. 2005;352:2325–36.
32. Korea Center for Disease Control and Prevention. Current situation of human brucellosis in Korea, Oct 2002-2005. CDMR. 2006;17:1–7.
33. Lim KB, Kwak YG, Kim DY, Kim YS, Kim JA. Back pain secondary to Brucella spondylitis in the lumbar region. Ann Rehabil Med. 2012;36:282–6.
34. Young EJ. An overview of human brucellosis. Clin Infect Dis. 1995;21:283–9.
35. Memish Z, Mah MW, Al Mahmoud S, Al Shaalan M, Khan MY. Brucella bacteraemia: clinical and laboratory observations in 160 patients. J Infect. 2000;40:59–63.
36. Namiduru M, Karaoglan I, Gursoy S, Bayazit N, Sirikci A. Brucellosis of the spine: evaluation of the clinical, laboratory, and radiological findings of 14 patients. Rheumatol Int. 2004;24:125–9.
37. Solera J, Lozano E, Martínez-Alfaro E, Espinosa A, Castillejos ML, Abad L. Brucellar spondylitis: review of 35 cases and literature survey. Clin Infect Dis. 1999;29:1440–9.
38. Ozaksoy D, Yucesoy K, Yucesoy M, Kovanlikaya I, Yuce A, Naderi S. Brucellar spondylitis: MRI findings. Eur Spine J. 2001;10:529–33.
39. Sharif HS, Aideyan OA, Clark DC, et al. Brucellar and tuberculous spondylitis: comparative imaging features. Radiology. 1989;171:419–25.
40. Heller RM, Szalay EA, Green NE, Horev GD, Kirchner SD. Disc space infection in children: magnetic resonance imaging. Radiol Clin North Am. 1988;26:207–9.
41. Ranson M. Imaging of pediatric musculoskeletal infection. Semin Musculoskelet Radiol. 2009;13:277–99.
42. Khanna G, Sato TS, Ferguson P. Imaging of chronic recurrent multifocal osteomyelitis. Radiographics. 2009;29:1159–77.
43. Modic MT, Masaryk TJ, Ross JS, Carter JR. Imaging of degenerative disk disease. Radiology. 1988;168:177–86.
44. Patel KB, Poplawski MM, Pawha PS, Naidich TP, Tanenbaum LN. Diffusion-weighted MRI "claw sign" improves differentiation of infectious from degenerative modic type 1 signal changes of the spine. AJNR Am J Neuroradiol. 2014;35:1647–52.
45. Wagner SC, Schweitzer ME, Morrison WB, Przybylski GJ, Parker L. Can imaging findings help differentiate spinal neuropathic arthropathy from disk space infection? Initial experience. Radiology. 2000;214:693–9.

7 Spondyloarthritis

Seunghun Lee

7.1 Introduction/Overview of Spondyloarthritis

Spondyloarthritis (SpA) is a chronic inflammatory rheumatic disease characterized by sacroiliitis and spondylitis, mainly manifesting as oligoarthritis in the lower limbs, enthesitis, etc. It is more common in young men, has a high expression rate of HLA-B27 antigen, and does not find rheumatoid factor in the blood. Joint involvement can be monoarticular, oligoarticular, or polyarticular. Often accompanying uveitis, psoriasis, and inflammatory bowel disease are considered extra-articular symptoms.

Spondyloarthritis can be classified into ankylosing spondylitis (AS), psoriatic arthritis (PsA), reactive arthritis (ReA), inflammatory bowel disease-associated arthritis (enteropathic spondyloarthritis), juvenile-onset spondyloarthritis, undifferentiated SpA, etc., based on clinical features. According to the classification of the Assessment of SpondyloArthritis international Society (ASAS), it is divided into axial SpA (aSpA) that mainly affects the SI joint, spine, thoracic cage, and peripheral SpA (pSpA) that mainly affects the extremities. Axial SpA includes not only the radiographic stage where sacroiliitis is clearly visible in simple radiography but also non-radiographic aSpA that is not visible. Ankylosing spondylitis corresponds to the radiographic stage of aSpA, and psoriatic arthritis, reactive arthritis, inflammatory bowel disease-associated arthritis, etc., usually correspond to peripheral SpA.

S. Lee (✉)
Department of Radiology, Hanyang University College of Medicine, Seoul, Republic of Korea
e-mail: radsh@hanyang.ac.kr

7.1.1 Classification Criteria of Spondyloarthritis

The classification criteria were created not for diagnosis but for epidemiology and research. The first classification criteria related to spondyloarthritis were created in 1961 for ankylosing spondylitis. These criteria have been revised several times and are still in use as the Modified New York Criteria (1984) (Table 7.1) [1], which is currently used as the standard for ankylosing spondylitis [2]. The radiological changes of the SI joint are as shown in Table 7.2.

In the 1990s, the Amor criteria and the diagnostic criteria of the European Spondyloarthropathy Study Group (ESSG) were proposed as classification criteria for the entire group of spondyloarthritis diseases, including ankylosing spondylitis (Table 7.3).

Unlike the modified New York criteria for ankylosing spondylitis, these criteria made it possible to classify spondyloarthritis patients more comprehensively by including various features of spondyloarthritis in the classification criteria, and were used until the new classifica-

© The Author(s), under exclusive license to Springer Nature Singapore Pte Ltd. 2025

H. S. Kang, J. W. Lee (eds.), *Spinal Imaging*, https://doi.org/10.1007/978-981-95-1386-4_7

Table 7.1 Modified New York Classification criteria for AS (1984)

1. Clinical criteria: (a) Low back pain and stiffness for more than 3 months, which improves with exercise, but is not relieved by rest (b) Limitation of motion of the lumbar spine in both the sagittal and frontal planes (c) Limitation of chest expansion relative to normal values correlated for age and sex
2. Radiological criterion: Sacroiliitis grade 2 bilaterally or grade 3–4 unilaterally
—Definite AS if the radiological criterion is associated with at least one clinical criterion.

van der Linden S, Valkenburg HA, Cats A. Arthritis Rheum. 1984;27:361–368

Table 7.2 Grading of radiographic changes in the SI joint

Grade	
0	Normal
1	Suspicious changes
2	Minimal abnormality—small localized areas with erosion or sclerosis, without alteration in the joint width
3	Unequivocal abnormality—moderate or advanced sacroiliitis with one or more of the following; erosions, evidence of sclerosis, widening, narrowing, or partial ankylosis
4	Severe abnormality—total ankylosis

Data from Bennett PH, Wood PHN(eds). Population studies of the rheumatic diseases. Amsterdam, Excerpta Medica Foundation. International Congress Series No.148, 1963:456

Table 7.3 Classification criteria for spondyloarthropathy by ESSG

Two major criteria	Sub-items
1. Inflammatory back pain	1. In case of family history
2. Synovitis (asymmetric, mainly in the lower limbs)	2. Psoriasis
	3. Inflammatory bowel disease
	4. History of urethritis, cervicitis, or acute diarrhea within a month of arthritis onset
	5. Alternating buttock pain
	6. Enthesopathy
	7. Sacroiliitis (radiological evidence)

Note: If there is one of the inflammatory spinal pain or synovitis on the left, and one or more of the detailed items on the right, it can be diagnosed as spondyloarthritis

tion criteria of ASAS came out [2]. With the introduction of MRI and anti-TNF agents in the 2000s, new concepts were introduced in the diagnosis and treatment of spondyloarthritis. In MRI, inflammation was found early in the form of subchondral bone marrow edema before radiological changes appeared in simple imaging of the SI joint, and anti-TNF agents showed excellent effects in spondyloarthritis, especially in early disease patients. Therefore, there was an increased interest in early disease before radiological changes appear in spondyloarthritis, and the need for new classification criteria that overcome the limitations of existing classification criteria increased.

The Assessment of SpondyloArthritis international Society (ASAS) proposed new criteria by dividing spondyloarthritis into axial spondyloarthritis (aSpA) (Table 7.4) and peripheral spondyloarthritis (pSpA) (Table 7.5) based on two major symptoms, spinal and peripheral symptoms. The ASAS aSpA classification criteria included various clinical features of spondyloarthritis, MRI findings of the sacroiliac joint, and HLA B27 results in the criteria, covering the entire range of axial diseases. In particular, the new criteria of ASAS included non-radiographic aSpA, which was excluded from the classification criteria of ankylosing spondylitis [2].

7.1.2 Clinical Findings of Spondyloarthritis

7.1.2.1 Clinical Symptoms

(1) Prevalence

The prevalence of spondyloarthritis varies by ethnicity, and this difference is directly related to the prevalence of HLA-B27. In the West, the prevalence of ankylosing spondylitis is known to be 0.1–0.4%, and the prevalence of spondyloarthritis is reported to be higher, usually 0.3–2.5% [2]. A recent meta-analysis on the global prevalence of ankylosing spondylitis was based on 36 studies that met the conditions, with 238 per 100,000 in Europe and 167 per 100,000 in Asia. In North America, there are 319 cases per 100,000

Table 7.4 ASAS aSpA classification criteria

When the following are satisfied in patients with back pain lasting more than 3 months that started before the age of 45	
If there is sacroiliitis on imaging and one or more features of spondyloarthritis or if HLA-B27 is positive and there are two or more features of spondyloarthritis	
Features of spondyloarthritis • Inflammatory back pain • Arthritis • Enthesitis (heel) • Dactylitis • Uveitis • Psoriasis • Crohn's disease/colitis • Good response to NSAIDs • Family history • HLA-B27 positive • Increased CRP	Sacroiliitis on imaging • Active sacroiliitis on MRI • Confirmed sacroiliitis on plain X-ray

Rheumatology, Beommoon Education 2nd Edition

Table 7.5 ASAS pSpA classification criteria

When arthritis, enthesitis, or dactylitis is present, and the following are satisfied	
One or more of the following features of spondyloarthritis	Or two or more of the following features of spondyloarthritis
Uveitis Psoriasis Crohn's disease/colitis Preceding infection HLA-B27 Sacroiliitis on imaging	Arthritis Enthesitis Dactylitis History of inflammatory back pain Family history

people, in South America, there are 102 cases per 100,000 people, and in Africa, there are 74 cases per 100,000 people [3].

(2) Symptoms

The main musculoskeletal symptoms of spondyloarthritis are inflammation caused by spondylitis and sacroiliitis, chronic back pain, peripheral arthritis, enthesitis, dactylitis, etc. Often, it is accompanied by non-musculoskeletal symptoms such as psoriasis, oral ulcers, uveitis, and inflammatory bowel disease that invade the skin, mucous membranes, eyes, or intestinal mucosa. Chronic back pain is the most important symptom in aSpA patients and needs to be distinguished from mechanical back pain. ASAS defines it as inflammatory back pain if it satisfies four or more of the following five items:

- Chronic back pain in those under 40 years of age
- Gradually occurring (insidious onset) chronic back pain
- Chronic back pain that improves with exercise
- Chronic back pain that does not improve with rest
- Chronic back pain that is severe at night and improves upon waking

Inflammatory back pain usually shows rapid improvement within 24-48 h with anti-inflammatory doses of non-steroidal anti-inflammatory drugs (NSAIDs). Peripheral arthritis of spondyloarthritis often occurs in the lower extremities, especially the knees and ankles. Arthritis is asymmetrical and occurs acutely in 1–3 joints. Enthesis is the part where ligaments, tendons, joint capsules, and fascia attach to the bone, and inflammation in this area is called enthesitis, which is one of the important features of spondyloarthritis. Enthesitis of the Achilles tendon or plantar fascia at the tuberosity of the calcaneus is the most common, and this area has pain and tenderness, accompanied by swelling. Enthesitis also occurs in the hip bone, elbow, shoulder, sternum, and posterior spinal joints. Dactylitis is a general swelling of the fingers or toes, also known as sausage digit. It mainly occurs due to inflammation of the flexor tendon, tendon sheath, and surrounding soft tissues and often accompanies psoriasis [4]. Spondyloarthritis has a family history, and not only spondyloarthritis but also uveitis, psoriasis, or inflammatory bowel disease are found in first- or second-degree relatives.

(3) Laboratory findings

The HLA-B27 gene is the most important genetic risk factor for axial aSpA and is known as one of the genes with the strongest association with common human diseases. It is found in up to 70% of patients with spondyloarthritis, and in ankylosing spondylitis, it is higher, found in over 90%. The HLA-B27 test is commonly performed when spondyloarthritis is suspected, but it is not diagnostic because it is positive in about 6–8% of the normal population. However, if spondyloarthritis is not confirmed on imaging, in situations where it is not, it becomes an important factor in diagnosing spondyloarthritis. The erythrocyte sedimentation rate (ESR) and C-reactive protein (CRP) must be included in the test in situations where spondyloarthritis is suspected. It is known that the increase in C-reactive protein is observed in about 40% of axial spondyloarthritis [5]. Therefore, the normal level of C-reactive protein cannot rule out the possibility of axial spondyloarthritis. In patients who have already been diagnosed with axial spondyloarthritis, C-reactive protein is used as a tool to measure disease activity [6].

7.1.3 Imaging Findings of Axial spondyloarthritis

The imaging diagnosis of axial spondyloarthritis (aSpA) is mainly performed through plain radiography, MRI, bone scan, and CT, and the diagnosis using ultrasound is limited (Fig. 7.1).

7.1.3.1 Plain Radiography Findings

Plain radiography, which has been used since the 1930s for diagnosis and staging in patients suspected of having ankylosing spondylitis, was mainly performed in the SI joint and spine, and only chronic bony changes appearing as sequelae of inflammation can be found. Therefore, plain radiography is not suitable for early diagnosis of axial spondyloarthritis, but is merely a method of

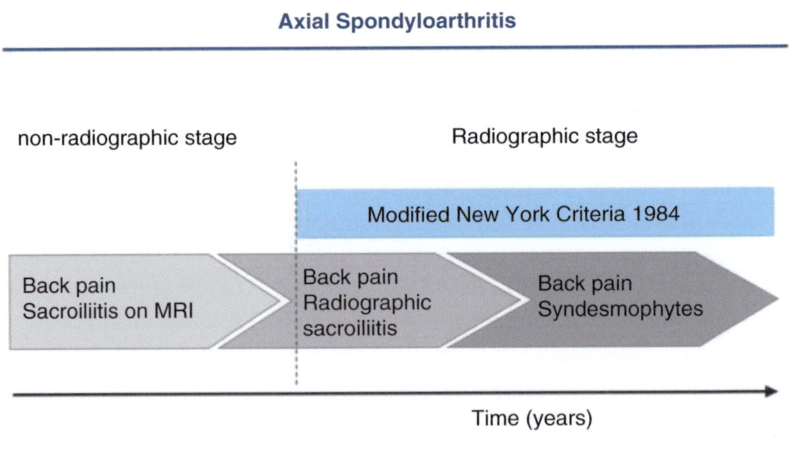

Fig. 7.1 Stages of axial spondyloarthritis (https://www.asas-group.org/education/asas-slide-library/)

choice for finding chronic bone changes. Nevertheless, in cases where axial spondyloarthritis is suspected, it is recommended to always consider performing AP view of pelvis radiography, and it is good to include both hip joints, which are relatively frequently invaded, in the shooting range [7]. Radiological findings of axial spondyloarthritis that can be seen in plain radiography of the sacroiliac joint include sclerosis, erosions, changes in joint width, or ankylosis, and based on these findings, radiological changes in sacroiliac arthritis can be graded (Table 7.2). To diagnose radiological sacroiliac arthritis, it is sufficient if it is grade 2 or higher on both sides or grade 3 or higher on one side. Plain radiography of the spine is not generally necessary for the diagnosis of axial spondyloarthritis, but in patients who have already been diagnosed with axial spondyloarthritis, the AP view and lateral view of the cervical spine and lumbar spine are taken to evaluate the presence or absence of findings such as squaring, erosion, sclerosis, and syndesmophyte, and are used to evaluate the severity of the disease (Fig. 7.2). Of course, changes in the thoracic spine are often seen, but the thoracic spine is not routinely examined and evaluated because it overlaps with surrounding tissues. It is very rare to see syndesmophyte in the spine when the changes in radiological arthritis in the SI joint are not clear. However, when it is difficult to determine the presence or absence of radiological arthritis in the SI joint, the presence of syndesmophyte in the spine can help in the diagnosis of axial spondyloarthritis.

7.1.3.2 MRI Findings

MR imaging is useful for observing both acute active inflammation and chronic structural changes in the SI joint. Especially, according to the ASAS criteria announced in 2009, in the classification criteria for spondyloarthritis, MR imaging findings showing active inflammation of the sacroiliac joint, which is not clearly visible in simple radiography, have been added (Table 7.4) [8].

(1) Imaging findings of acute active sacroiliitis and chronic sacroiliitis

The magnetic resonance imaging technique for evaluating sacroiliitis primarily uses the oblique coronal scan obtained parallel to the axis of the sacrum as the basic plane and additionally obtains oblique axial scans or axial scans. The required oblique coronal

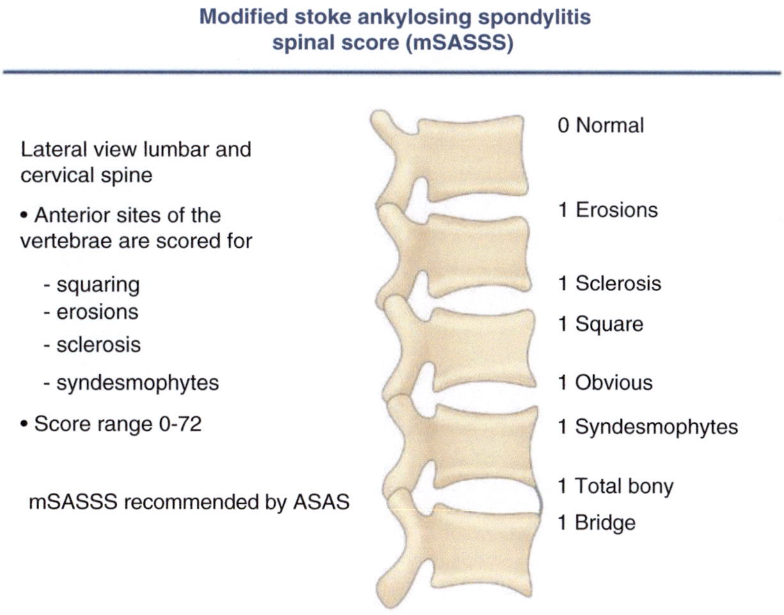

Fig. 7.2 Modified Stoke Ankylosing Spondylitis Spinal Score (mSASSS)

scan varies by hospital, but mainly determines the activity of the lesion through STIR or fat-suppressed T2-weighted images, and determines the fat deposition in the periarticular bone marrow and the presence of bony erosion through T1-weighted images or fat-suppressed T1-weighted images or T2-weighted images [9–12]. In some cases, fat-suppressed contrast-enhanced T1-weighted images are performed to determine the presence or absence of enthesitis or synovitis [13]. Compared to other imaging techniques, magnetic resonance imaging characteristically shows acute active inflammatory lesions such as subchondral bone marrow edema, osteitis, enthesitis, and synovitis of the SI joint, so it can diagnose sacroiliitis early before morphological changes such as bony erosion or bone hardening appear in simple radiography or CT, and can also diagnose chronic morphological changes such as bony erosion, periarticular fat deposition, subchondral sclerosis, and ankylosis [9–12]. Bone marrow edema or osteitis appears as low signal intensity on T1-weighted images and high signal intensity on fat-suppressed T2-weighted images or STIR and shows enhancement on fat-suppressed contrast-enhanced T1-weighted images, which is the most important criterion for determining the activity of sacroiliitis (Fig. 7.3) [13]. Bone marrow edema usually appears bilaterally and symmetrically and is well seen in the lower and posterior 1/3 of the joint [13]. Synovitis appears as low or moderate signal intensity on T1-weighted images with loss of normal cartilage signal intensity and appears as various degrees of high signal intensity on fat-suppressed T2-weighted images or STIR, and shows linear or dot-like enhancement in contrast enhancement (Fig. 7.4). Differentiating synovitis from joint fluid can be difficult on STIR, and in this case, synovitis can be differentiated by using fat-suppressed contrast-enhanced T1 weighted images [13]. Synovitis shows similar signal intensity to synovitis and enhancement on fat-suppressed contrast-enhanced T1-weighted images (Fig. 7.5). Enthesitis seen in the posterior superior 1/3 of the SI joint also shows high signal intensity on fat-suppressed T2-weighted images and STIR and is enhanced on contrast-enhanced T1- weighted images (Fig. 7.6). In particular, it is defined as non-radiographic aSpA when there is subchondral bone marrow edema or osteitis showing enhancement in magnetic resonance imaging findings, which is not diagnosed in radiographic images such as simple radiography or CT (Figs. 7.1, and 7.3). Subchondral sclerosis appears as a low signal intensity on all magnetic resonance images, appearing thicker than the surrounding cortical bone, and the

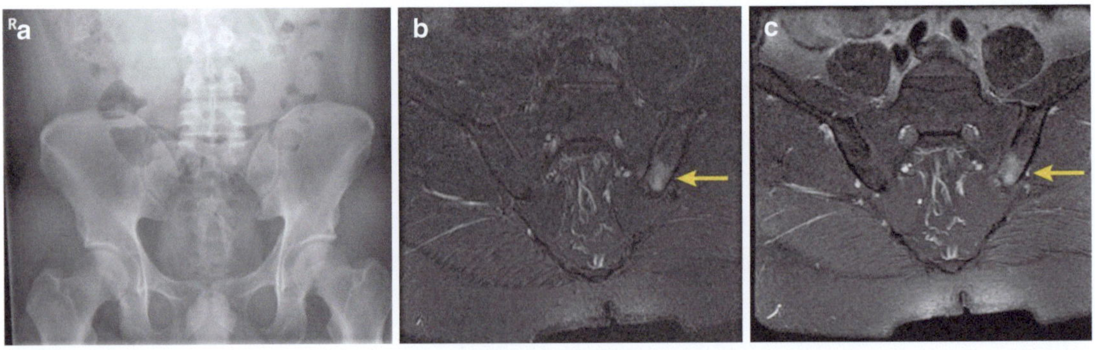

Fig. 7.3 Example of non-radiographic aSpA. (**a**) No clear sacroiliitis is seen in the simple radiograph of the pelvis. (**b**) Coronal oblique STIR image shows subchondral bone marrow edema in the left ilium (arrow) (**c**) There is a lesion with good contrast enhancement (arrow)

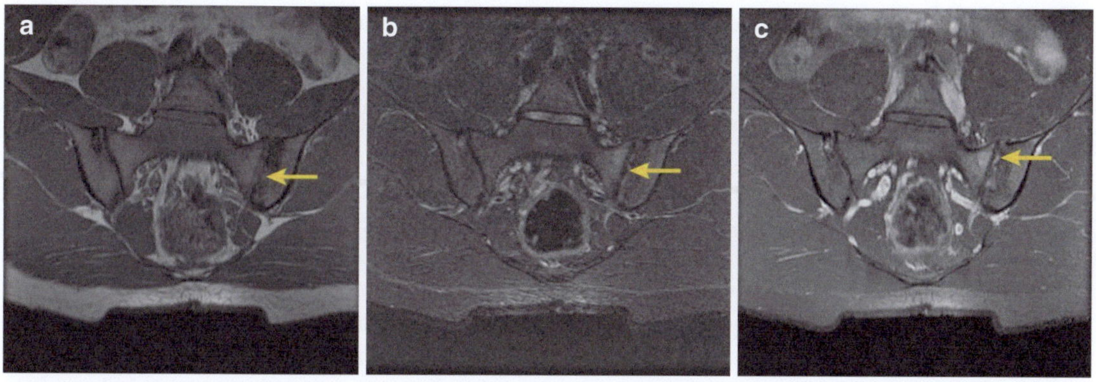

Fig. 7.4 (**a**) Oblique coronal T1-weighted image. (**b**) Oblique coronal STIR image. (**c**) Oblique coronal, fat-suppressed Gd-enhancement images show focal erosion, sclerosis, and synovitis (arrow) in the left SI joint

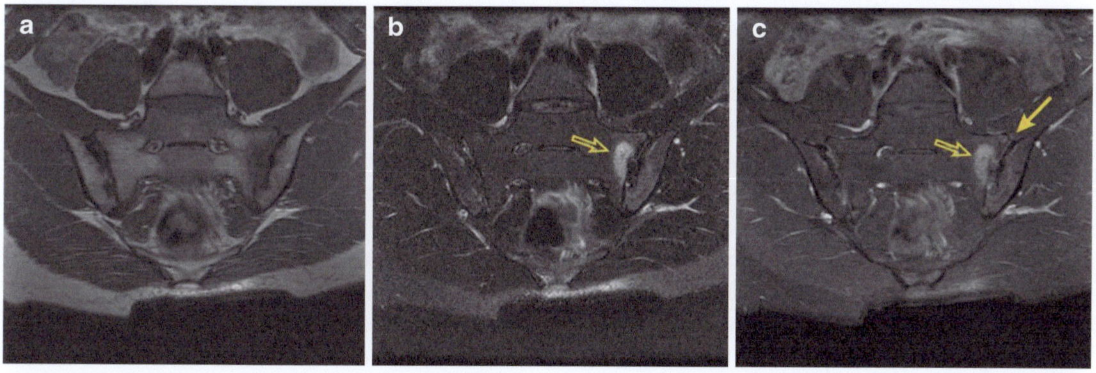

Fig. 7.5 (**a**) Oblique coronal T1-weighted image, (**b**) Oblique coronal fat-suppressed T2-weighted image, (**c**) Oblique coronal, fat-suppressed Gd-enhancement images show focal capsulitis (arrow) in front of the left SI joint, and active inflammation (empty arrow) in the left SI joint

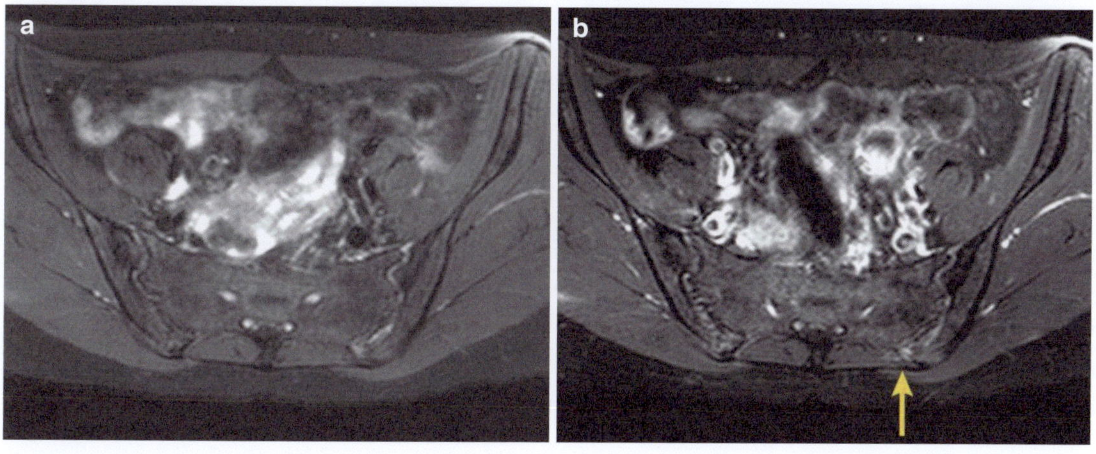

Fig. 7.6 (**a**) Axial STIR image. (**b**) Axial fat-suppressed Gd-enhancement images show focal enthesitis (arrow) toward the left SI joint

cortical bone marrow interface is not clearly visible (Fig. 7.4). Bony erosion first appears in the long bone, and the bony cortex is not maintained, showing an irregular defect shape of the subchondral bone of the joint surface, appearing as low signal intensity on T1-weighted images, and high signal intensity on fat-suppressed T2-weighted images or STIR (Fig. 7.4). Periarticular fat deposition appears adjacent to bony erosion and is associated with chronic bony erosion (Fig. 7.7).

(2) Imaging findings of acute active spondyloarthritis and chronic spondyloarthritis
The magnetic resonance imaging technique for evaluating spondyloarthritis of the spine includes sagittal T1-weighted images and fat-suppressed T2-weighted images, and fat-suppressed contrast-enhanced T1-weighted images are more sensitive in detecting acute inflammation and are used to differentiate from infectious diseases. Axial images are useful for viewing lesions of the facet joint, costovertebral joint, costotransverse joint, etc. Acute active inflammation in the spine is observed in the vertebral body, discovertebral junction, facet joint, costovertebral joint, costotransverse joint, atlantoaxial joint, and attachment sites of the posterior spinal ligament, initially prominent changes in the thoracolumbar and lumbosacral junction, and as it progresses, it appears as changes in the entire spine (Fig. 7.8). Inflammation of the vertebral body is osteitis of the edge of the vertebral body where the outer fiber of the annulus fibrosus attaches and enthesitis of the anterior longitudinal ligament, posterior longitudinal ligament, mainly prominent in the upper and lower corners and the front. It is known to commonly appear at the thoracolumbar junction rather than the lower lumbar spine, and in the acute phase, it shows low signal intensity on T1-weighted images and high signal intensity on fat-suppressed T2-weighted images or STIR due to bone marrow edema. As osteitis progresses for a long time and reaches the healing process, bone marrow edema disappears and is converted to fatty bone marrow, so it shows high signal intensity on T1-weighted images and low signal intensity on fat-suppressed T2-weighted images or STIR (Fig. 7.9). Discal spondylodiscitis initially appears as bony erosion of the vertebral endplate and surrounding bone marrow edema with a

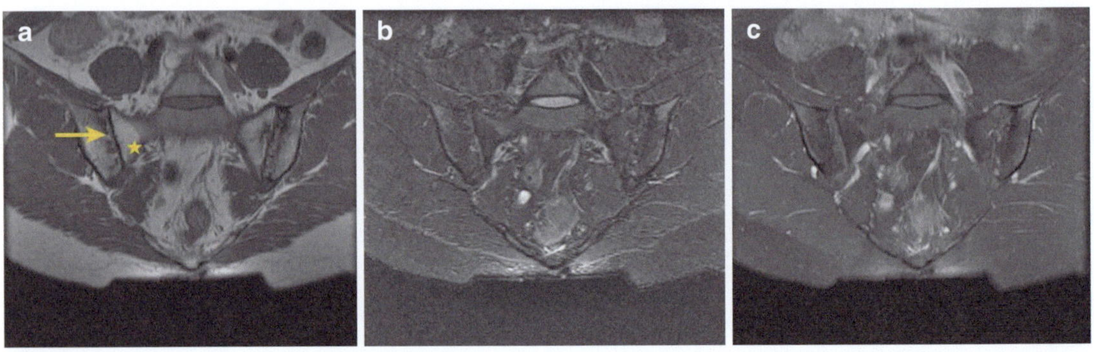

Fig. 7.7 (**a**) Oblique coronal T1-weighted image. (**b**) Oblique coronal fat-suppressed T2-weighted image. (**c**) Oblique coronal, fat-suppressed Gd-enhancement images show focal erosion, sclerosis (arrow), and abnormal fat deposition (asterisk) in the right SI joint

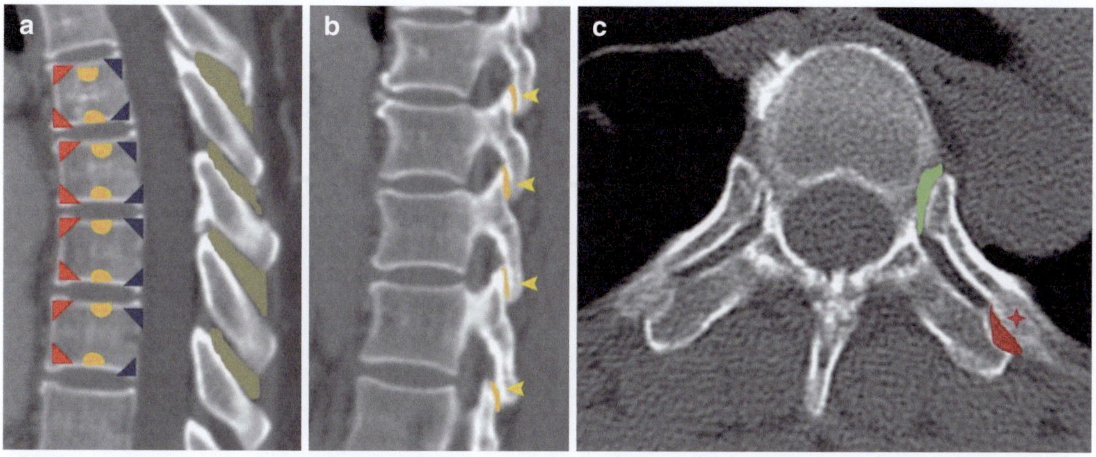

Fig. 7.8 Sagittal reconstruction images (**a**, **b**) of the thoracic spine and axial image (**c**). SpA invades the corners (triangles) of the vertebral body, discovertebral junction (semi-circular), facet joint (empty arrow), costovertebral joint (arrowhead), and costovertebral joint (asterisk)

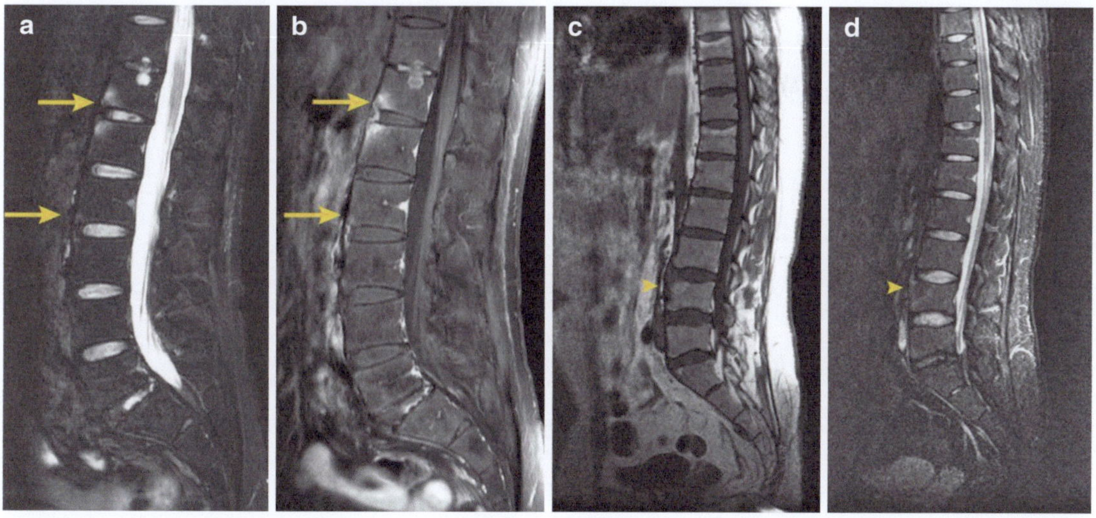

Fig. 7.9 Sequence of sagittal T2-weighted image, fat-suppressed Gd-enhancement T1-weighted image and T1-weighted image, fat-suppressed Gd-enhancement T1-weighted image. (**a**, **b**) pictures show the findings of spondylitis showing acute bone marrow edema, and (**c**, **d**) pictures are examples of findings converted to fatty marrow

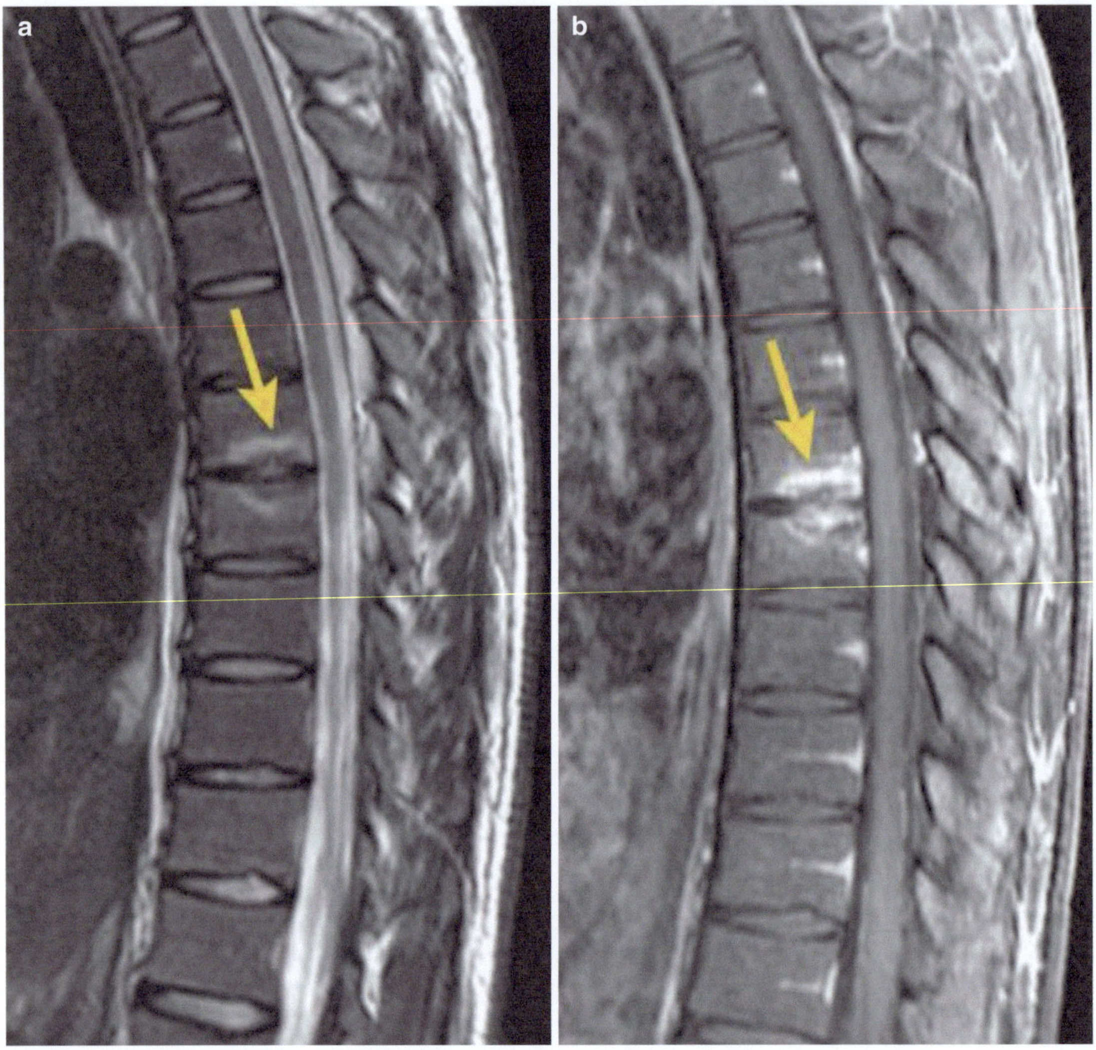

Fig. 7.10 Sequence of sagittal T2-weighted image, fat-suppressed Gd-enhancement T1-weighted image
Findings of endplate erosion at the discovertebral junction and surrounding bone marrow edema (arrow) are visible

hemispheric appearance in the upper and lower parts centered on the intervertebral disc, also called an inflammatory Andersson lesion (Fig. 7.10). Acute active inflammation of the facet joint, costovertebral joint, costotransverse joint, etc. can be seen as joint effusion, marginal bone marrow edema, synovitis, etc. (Fig. 7.11), and as it progresses to chronic, it shows findings such as periarticular fat deposition, bony erosion, syndesmophyte, ankylosis, etc. The enthesitis findings of the supraspinous ligament and interspinous ligament appear as peripheral bone marrow edema and osteitis, and when chronic, they show a characteristic dagger sign in the lumbar spine due to ossification of the ligament (Fig. 7.12).

(3) Other imaging techniques

Bone scintigraphy has been used for decades to detect active inflammation in patients with spondyloarthritis. However, bone scintigraphy is the finding of increased intake at the

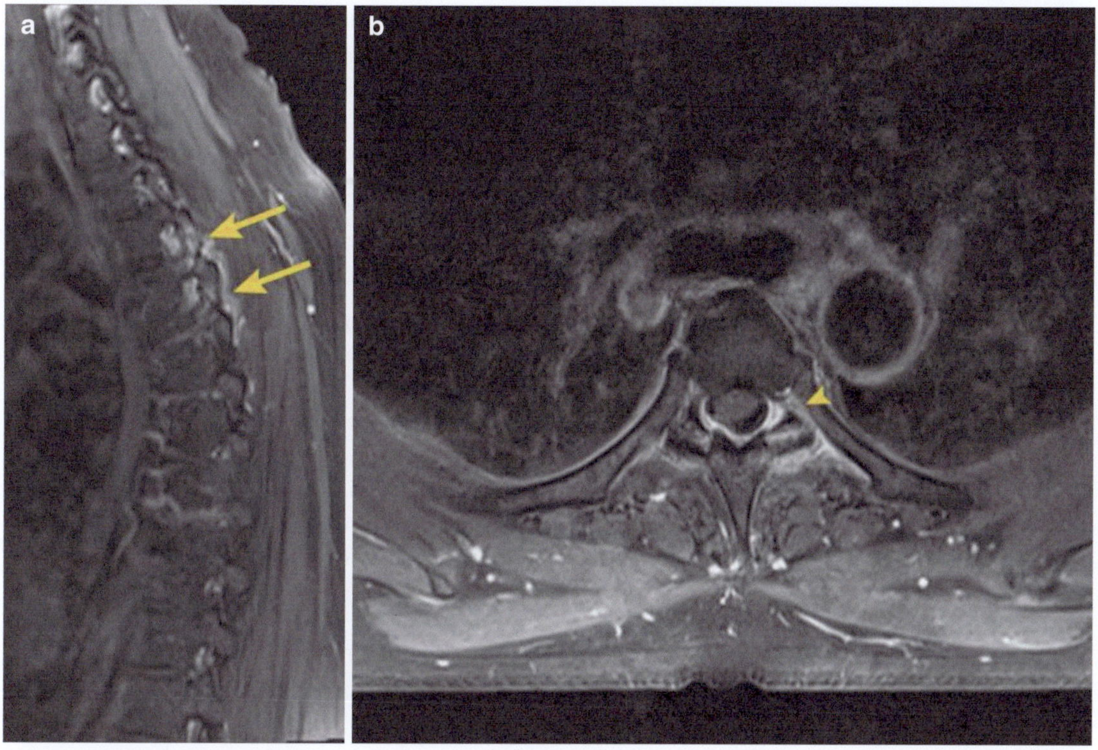

Fig. 7.11 Inflammation showing contrast enhancement at the facet joints (arrow) and costovertebral joint (arrowhead) is visible in the fat-suppressed Gd-enhancement T1-weighted images

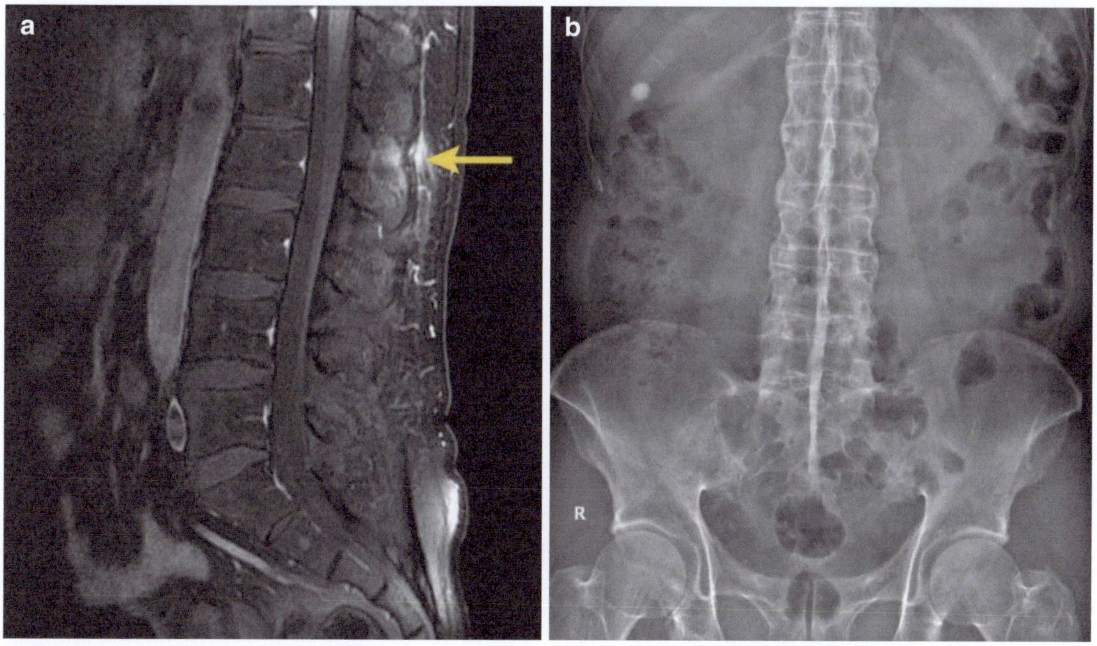

Fig. 7.12 Findings of enthesitis (arrow) at the attachment of the L1–2 interspinous and supraspinous ligament are visible, and if it progresses, a dagger sign appears as if the spinous processes are attached as seen on the right in the plain radiograph

inflammation site is too nonspecific, so recently MRI is replacing the role of scintigraphy in diagnosis and management [14].

Chronic bone changes are more advantageous for CT in detection, but the amount of radiation exposure compared to other imaging tests should be considered. Also, CT cannot detect active inflammation and cannot find fat deposition in the bone marrow caused by chronic inflammatory changes, but MRI can. Also, in aSpA, plain radiography is the first imaging test performed when a spinal fracture is suspected, but if it is not found in plain radiography, CT must be taken. In conclusion, CT can provide additional information about chronic structural changes in the SI joint or spine in patients suspected of spondyloarthritis when plain radiography is a negative finding, and MRI is difficult to take, and bone scintigraphy or ultrasound is not recommended for the diagnosis of axial spondyloarthritis [7].

7.1.4 Imaging Findings of Peripheral Spondyloarthritis (Peripheral SpA, pSpA)

The peripheral joint involvement of spondyloarthritis appears as enthesitis, arthritis, and dactylitis and will be explained in detail in the imaging findings of each disease to be explained in the introduction/discussion. To diagnose peripheral SpA, it can be helpful to find peripheral enthesitis that can support the diagnosis of spondyloarthritis through ultrasound or MRI, and peripheral arthritis, tenosynovitis, and bursitis can be detected using ultrasound or MRI [7]. To measure the disease activity of peripheral arthritis, ultrasound and MRI can help detect tenosynovitis and enthesitis, just like at the time of diagnosis, and provide additional information about clinical and biochemical evaluations. The decision on when to repeat ultrasound and MRI varies depending on the clinical situation. High frequency color/power Doppler tests are sufficient to detect inflammation, and the use of ultrasound contrast agents is not necessary [7].

In clinical situations, plain radiography is recommended for monitoring structural damage caused by peripheral arthritis, and it is known that MRI and/or US can provide additional information [7].

7.1.5 Pathogenesis and Etiology of Spondyloarthritis

The characteristic pathological findings of spondyloarthritis are enthesitis and bone destruction and formation. In enthesitis lesions, immune cells such as T cells, B cells, bone marrow-derived macrophages, osteoclasts, and cells related to neovascularization are observed. The inflammation of spondyloarthritis is presumed to progress by activating these various cells under genetic influences represented by HLA-B27, secreting various cytokines in response to environmental factors such as bacteria and mechanical stress. Another unique pathology of spondyloarthritis, bone formation, goes through endochondral bone formation, where mesenchymal cells first differentiate into chondrocytes and then ossification occurs. Bone formation is bone morphogenic protein (BMP) or it is presumed to be regulated through the wingless (Wnt) pathway. Unlike rheumatoid arthritis, where inflammation and bone destruction (structural damage) are paired, the connection between inflammation and bone formation in spondyloarthritis is still controversial [2].

7.2 Specific/General Discussion on Spondyloarthritis

7.2.1 Ankylosing Spondylitis

7.2.1.1 Diagnostic Criteria

Ankylosing spondylitis (AS) is a disease with an unknown cause, which chronically progresses as an inflammatory, self-limited condition that affects the synovial joint, cartilaginous joint, and bone attachment sites of tendons or ligaments. It primarily affects the axial skeleton and characteristically invades the SI joint bilaterally and symmetrically first [15–18]. The typical invasion order starts from the SI joint, then affects the thoracolumbar, lumbosacral area, and as the disease becomes chronic, it affects the middle part of the lumbar spine, upper thoracic spine, and cervical spine. It also affects the large joints of the limbs such as the hip, shoulder, and knee joint, as well as the hands, wrists, and feet (Fig. 7.13). The most commonly used criteria for diagnosing AS is the Modified New York Criteria (Table 7.1) [1]. It consists of three clinical signs and two radiological findings, and if one or more clinical signs and one radiological abnormality are satisfied, a diagnosis can be made.

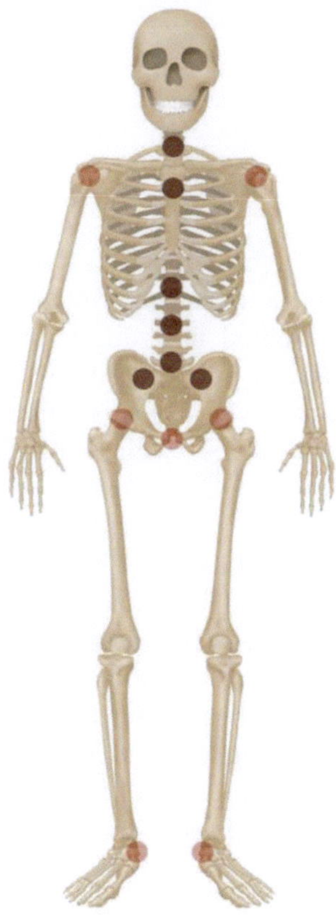

Fig. 7.13 Sites of AS invasion
The typical invasion sequence starts from the SI joint and invades the thoracolumbar, lumbosacral junction, and as the disease becomes chronic, it invades the middle part of the lumbar spine, upper thoracic spine, and cervical spine, and other large joints of the limbs including the hip joint, shoulder joint, and also invades the hands, wrists, and feet (ÿ indicates more common invasion sites, ÿ indicates less common invasion sites)

7.2.1.2 Clinical Findings and Laboratory Findings

The age of onset for AS is 15–35 years old, and the male-to-female ratio is about 4–10:1, occurring more frequently in men. Symptoms usually begin in late adolescence or early adulthood, and it is rare for them to start after the age of 40. Clinical symptoms can be divided into joint symptoms and extra-articular symptoms, and joint symptoms can be further classified into spondylitis, peripheral arthritis, and symptoms caused by enthesitis [15, 16]. The most common initial symptom in patients is lower back pain, which is severe in the morning, improves with exercise, and does not improve with rest, showing the pattern of inflammatory back pain. Hip pain alternates between unilateral and bilateral, and as the disease progresses, bilateral pain persists. Local tenderness and pressure pain in the SI joint area can be prominent in the early stages of the disease, and clinical symptoms may be mild or completely absent when bony ankylosis of the SI joint occurs. Cases showing changes in the spine without findings of sacroiliitis are very rare, less than 3%, so sacroiliitis is a very important finding in the diagnosis of AS. Sacroiliitis almost always appears in the early stages of the disease, and initially, it can show asymmetric and unilateral lesions, but after progression, it shows bilateral lesions in 90% of cases. In the lumbar spine, there is muscle spasm, tenderness, and proximal atrophy around the spine, and in the thoracic spine, thoracic expansion is reduced and kyphotic curvature is exaggerated, making it difficult to look forward.

Peripheral joint symptoms are observed in about 10–20% in the early stages and can progress up to about 50%. It appears that the most commonly affected peripheral joints are the hip and shoulder joints. The characteristic feature is inflammation of the attachment of ligaments or tendons to the bone, with frequent pain and tenderness at the attachment of the Achilles tendon, the plantar fascia, the iliac crest, the femoral greater trochanter, the ischial tuberosity, and other areas.

Other symptoms and signs include uveitis (about 20%), heart disease (cardiomegaly, conduction disorders, pericarditis, etc.), and lung involvement (fibrosis and cavities in the upper lobes). In laboratory findings, rheumatoid factor is negative and ESR, CRP, etc. increase during the active phase of the disease. The HLA-B27 antigen is positive in about 6–8% of normal people, but in AS patients, it appears positive in 90% [15, 16].

7.2.1.3 Imaging Findings of AS: Centered on the SI Joint

Anatomically, the SI joint is a synovial joint between the sacrum and ilium, surrounded by a fibrous capsule, with the upper 1/3 of the joint connected by ligaments and only the lower 2/3 forming a synovial joint. The cartilage of the sacral joint surface is thicker than that of the ilium, so when a lesion occurs in the sacroiliac joint, the ilium side shows more severe findings initially. In AS, sacroiliitis is difficult to diagnose clinically, and the period between the onset of clinical symptoms and the appearance of sacroiliitis on radiological examination can range from several months to several years.

(1) Plain radiography
The diagnosis of AS is determined by clinical findings, laboratory findings, and radiological findings, but in the first 5 years after the onset of clinical symptoms of sacroiliitis, no abnormalities can be found on plain radiography, so plain radiography may not help in the diagnosis of early AS. Sacroiliitis almost always appears early in the disease, initially showing asymmetrical and unilateral lesions, but after progression, it shows bilateral and symmetrical lesions in 90% (Fig. 7.14). Radiological findings of sacroiliitis invade the ilium side more than the sacral side, the synovial joint of the anterior lower part more than the ligament part of the posterior upper part, and eventually invade the entire area.

It is essential for diagnosis to confirm abnormalities in both SI joints on radiography along with typical clinical findings [15–19]. Sacroiliitis is also a key element of the Modified New York Criteria, the grading system is described in Table 7.2, and it looks like Fig. 7.15 on plain radiography.

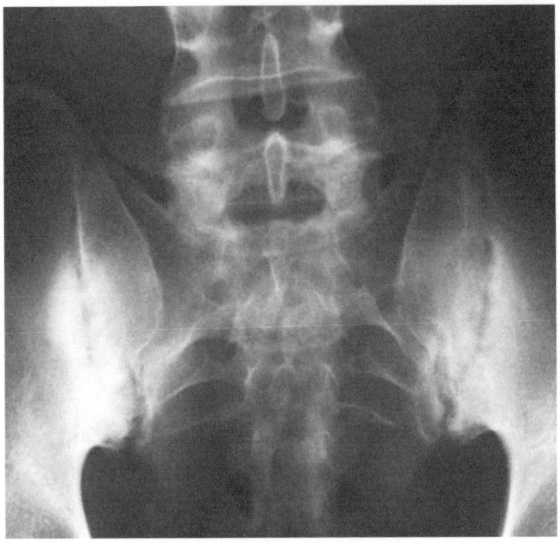

Fig. 7.14 Plain radiographic findings of AS sacroiliitis In the pelvis AP view, relatively symmetrical bony erosion, subchondral bony sclerosis, and joint space narrowing are seen in bilateral sacroiliitis

(2) Bone scan
In early AS, the bone scan shows an increase in the uptake of radioactive isotopes due to increased blood flow due to inflammatory reactions, but generally, the sensitivity and specificity are low, so it is difficult to make an early diagnosis with this method alone [15, 19].

(3) CT
In the early stages of AS, when the SI joint is involved, due to its complex structure, There are many cases where it is difficult to diagnose with simple shooting alone. CT shows bony erosion, bony sclerosis, and joint space better than simple shooting, which is useful for early diagnosis of AS sacroiliitis [15, 19]. CT findings of sacroiliitis include uneven bony sclerosis on the sacral side, localized narrowing of the joint space, and bony erosion (Fig. 7.16). However, in the early stages of the disease, an MRI examination is needed before morphological changes such as bony erosion and bony sclerosis appear.

(4) MRI
The MRI findings of AS are the same as the description of the MRI findings of axial spondyloarthritis.

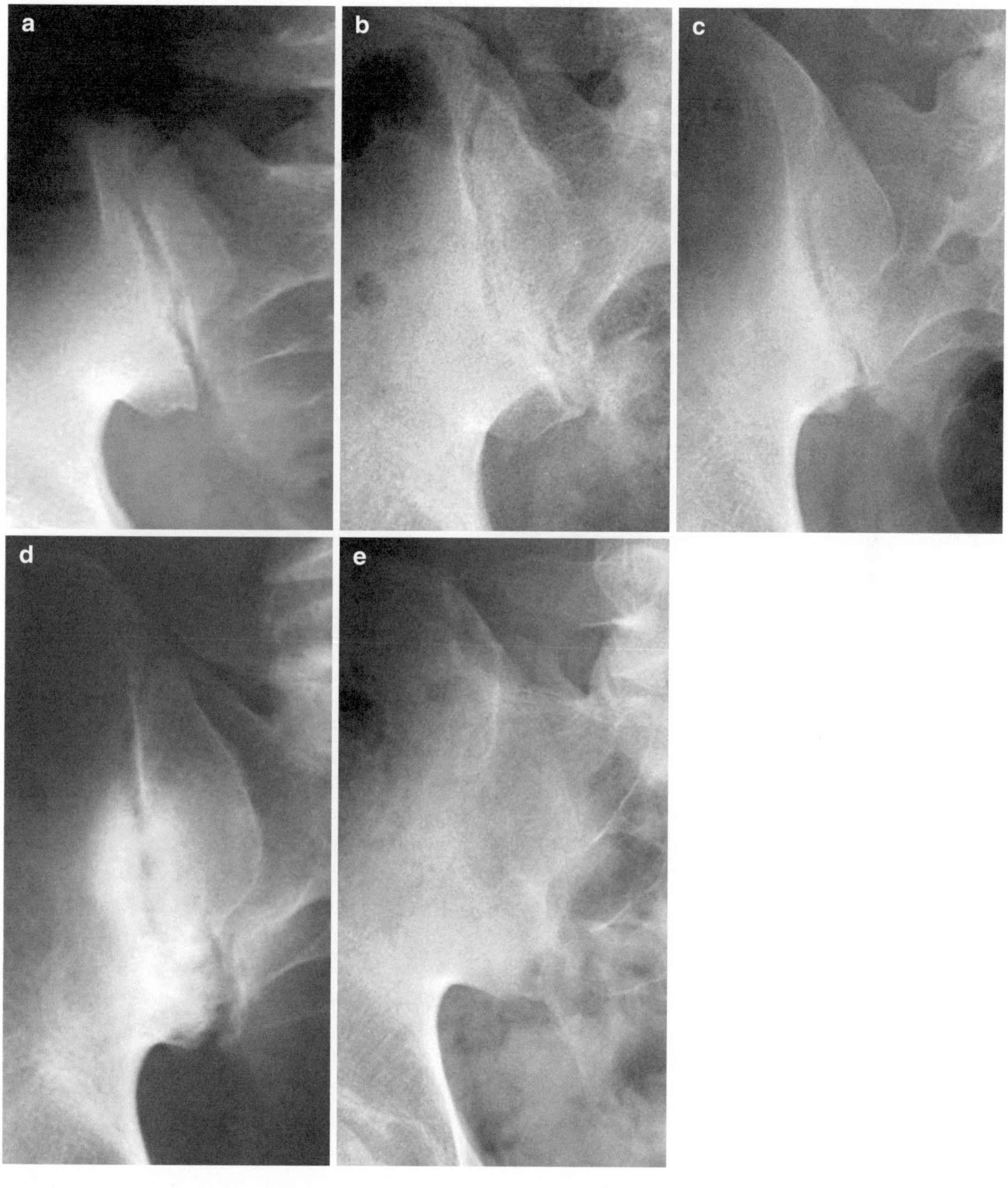

Fig. 7.15 Radiologic grading of AS sacroiliitis. (**a**) Grade 0, (**b**) Grade 1, (**c**) Grade 2, (**d**) Grade 3, (**e**) Grade 4

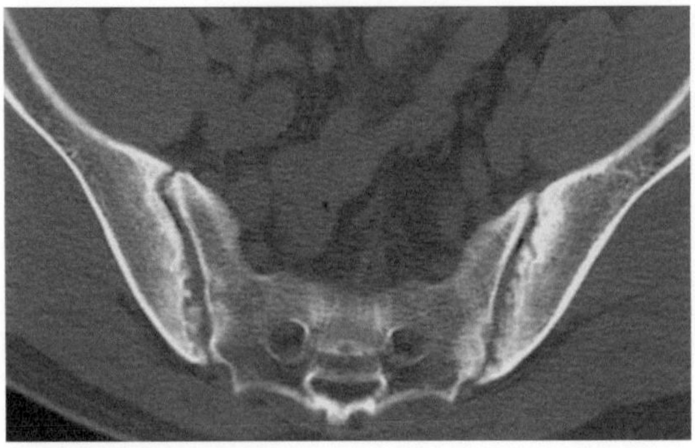

Fig. 7.16 CT findings of AS sacroiliitis
In the axial CT, relatively symmetrical bony erosion and subchondral sclerosis are seen in bilateral sacroiliac joints, and these findings are more severe in the ilium than in the sacrum. Bony erosion is fused together, showing an increase in joint space

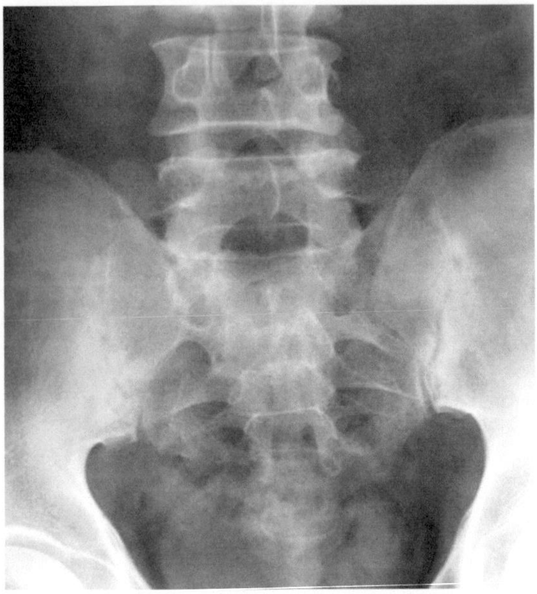

Fig. 7.17 Differential diagnosis of AS sacroiliitis: psoriatic arthritis
In the pelvic frontal view, asymmetric bony erosion, subchondral sclerosis, and joint space narrowing are seen in bilateral sacroiliac joints. If the sacroiliac joints are invaded unilaterally or asymmetrically bilaterally, the possibility of psoriatic arthritis or reactive arthritis/Reiter's syndrome is high

(5) Differential diagnosis: centered on the SI joint

① Seronegative spondyloarthritis

In AS or inflammatory bowel disease-related arthritis, the SI joint is typically bilaterally and symmetrically invaded, but psoriatic arthritis and reactive arthritis show asymmetric invasion in about 50%. If the SI joint shows bilateral and symmetrical sacroiliitis or complete bone fusion, the possibility of AS is high, and if it invades unilaterally or the SI joint is invaded asymmetrically on both sides, the possibility of psoriatic arthritis or reactive arthritis is high (Fig. 7.17) [15, 16].

② Rheumatoid arthritis

Unlike AS, which shows characteristic clinical and radiological findings of the SI joint, rheumatoid arthritis is relatively rare and clinically shows mild findings. In rheumatoid arthritis, the SI joint is invaded asymmetrically or unilaterally and shows shallow bony erosion (superficial erosion), and bony sclerosis is absent or minimal. On the other hand, AS invades the sacroiliac joint bilaterally and symmetrically, shows deep bony erosion (deep erosion) and moderate or more bony sclerosis, and commonly shows extensive bony ankylosis in advanced cases. The presence or absence of HLA-B27 antigen and rheumatoid factor is also important in distinguishing the two diseases, and AS does not accompany rheumatoid nodules [15, 16].

③ Infectious arthritis

Pyogenic arthritis primarily invades unilaterally, destruction of the synovial membrane, articular cartilage, and subchondral bone comes early, and changes in the surrounding soft tissues such as periosteal osteomyelitis, surrounding soft tissue swelling, abscess, and edema are severe (Fig. 7.18). In the case of tuberculosis, the destruction of bone and

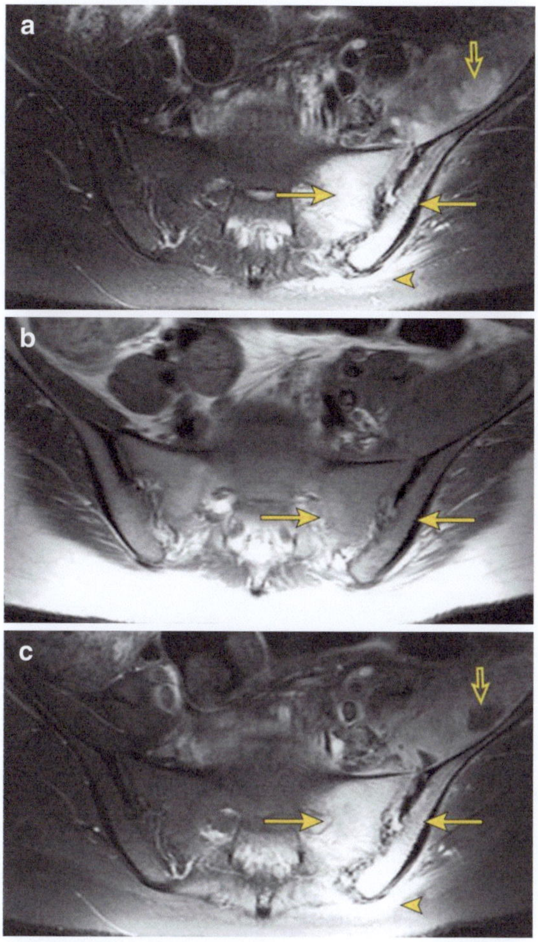

Fig. 7.18 Differential diagnosis of AS sacroiliitis: septic arthritis

There is destruction of the articular cartilage and subchondral bone in the left SI joint. There is bone marrow edema in the adjacent sacrum and ilium (arrow). It forms an abscess, swelling, and small abscess (empty arrow) in the iliacus muscle forward, and it spreads to the buttock fascia area backward (arrowhead). (**a**) Fat-suppressed T2-weighted axial image, (**b**) T1-weighted axial image, (**c**) fat-suppressed contrast-enhanced T1-weighted axial image

cartilage is remarkable compared to AS, and abscesses are seen in the surrounding soft tissues [15, 16].

④ Degenerative arthritis

Degenerative changes in the SI joint can show similar findings to AS on simple shooting. Degenerative arthritis of the SI joint often occurs in the elderly. Degenerative changes are limited to the lower 2/3 of the joint, and the main radiological findings are loss of joint space, subchondral bony sclerosis, and formation of anterior marginal osteophytes (Fig. 7.19) [15, 16].

⑤ Other diseases

Hyperparathyroidism, osteitis condensans ilii (OCI) invades the SI joint bilaterally and symmetrically, just like AS. In hyperparathyroidism, subchondral absorption mainly occurs symmetrically on both sides of the ilium, but there are no findings of narrowed joint space or severely irregular joint surfaces. OCI shows well-defined triangular bony sclerosis around the ilium of the SI joint, and the SI joint shows normal findings (Fig. 7.20) [15, 16].

7.2.1.4 Imaging Findings of AS: Centered on the Spine

(1) Simple shooting

In AS, changes in the spine are observed at the discovertebral junction, facet joint, costovertebral junction, posterior ligamentous attachment, atlantoaxial joint, etc. Initially, changes are distinct at the thoracolumbar junction and lumbosacral junction, but as it progresses, changes appear throughout the entire spine.

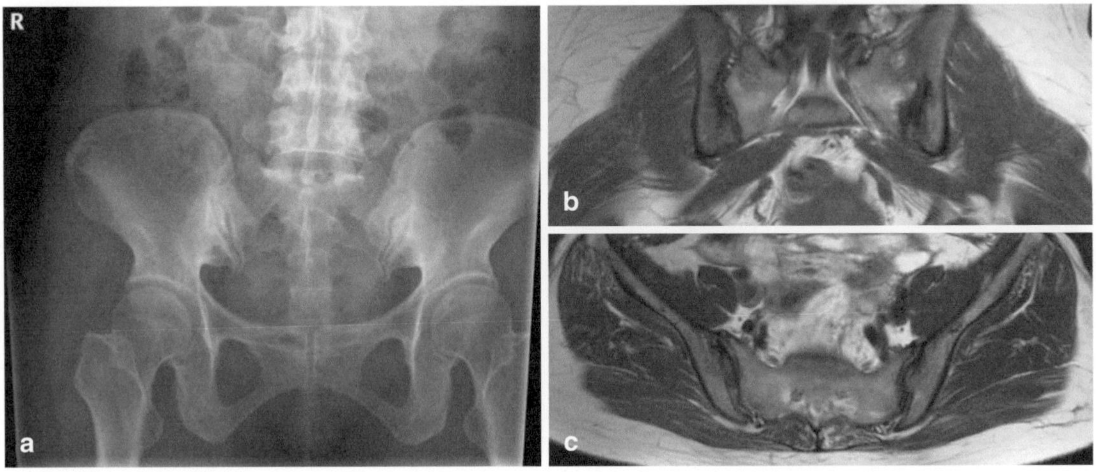

Fig. 7.19 Findings of sacroiliitis in degenerative arthritis
On plain radiography, cortical irregularity and slight sclerosis are seen along both SI joints (**a**). In MR images (**b**) and (**c**), there are low signal intensity lesions appearing as sclerosis and irregularity along both SI joints

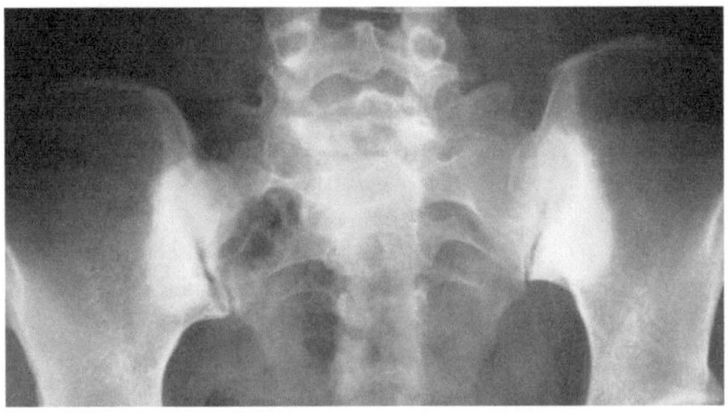

Fig. 7.20 Differential diagnosis of sacroiliitis in AS: osteitis condensans ilii
On the pelvic frontal view, triangular bone sclerosis with good boundaries is seen on the iliac side of both SI joints, and the SI joint shows relatively normal findings

① Discovertebral junction area
Lesions in the discovertebral junction area include osteitis, syndesmophyte, erosion and destruction of the discovertebral junction area, and discal calcification [6, 12, 15, 16, 18].

(a) Osteitis
The initial changes cause osteitis at the corners of the upper and lower front of the vertebral body where the outer fiber of the annulus fibrosus attaches, causing local bony erosion (focal erosion, Romanus lesion). This is one of the important findings that occur early in AS. As bone erosion caused by osteitis heals, transient reactive sclerosis, shiny corner sign appears in the adjacent area (Fig. 7.21). It is formed at the corners of the upper and lower front of the vertebral body. As new bone formation appears, the concavity of the front of the vertebral body disappears, making the vertebral body look square (squaring) in lateral simple shooting [20].
(b) Syndesmophyte
Inflammatory ossification of the outer fiber of the annulus fibrosus forms syndesmophytes, which gradually progress

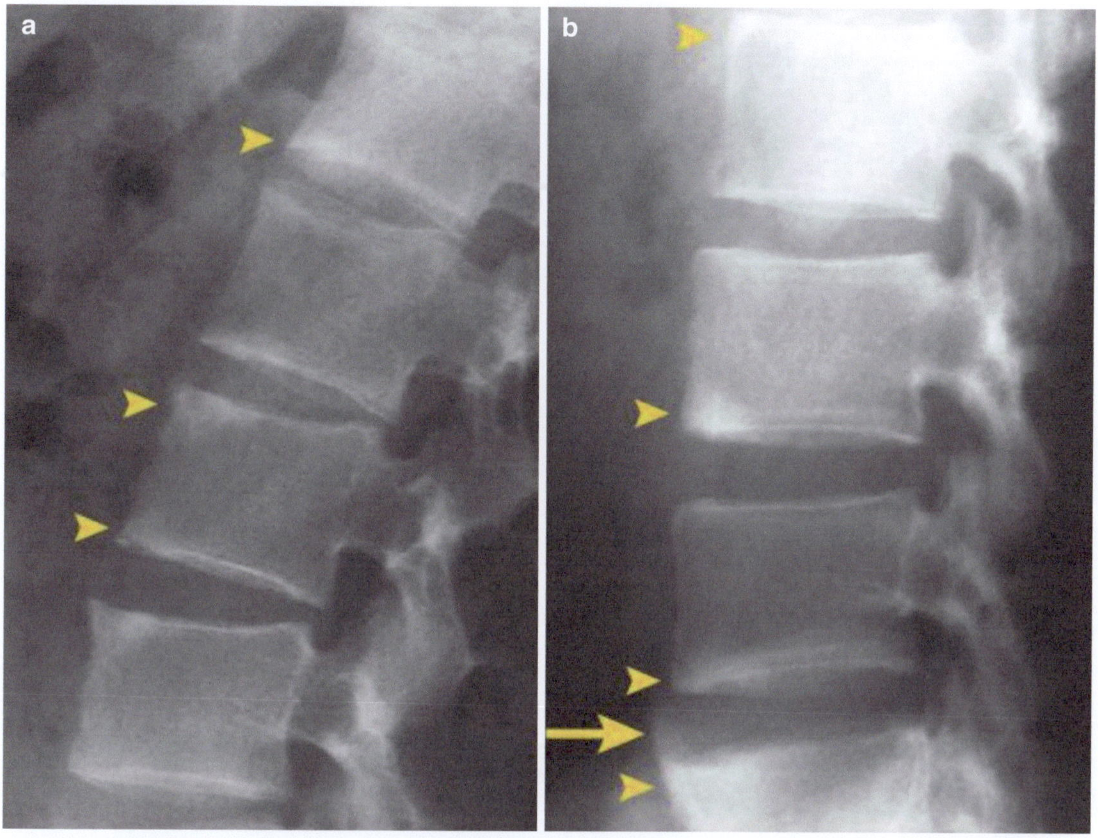

Fig. 7.21 Vertebral osteitis in AS. (**a**) On the lumbar lateral view, bony erosion romanus lesion and surrounding reactive sclerosis are seen on the anterior surface of the vertebral body (arrowhead). The concavity of the anterior surface of the vertebral body disappears and the vertebral body appears square (squaring sign). (**b**) On the lumbar lateral view, reactive sclerosis is seen on the corner of the anterior surface of the vertebral body (arrowhead) (shiny corner sign), and a syndesmophyte is partially formed in the lower lumbar (arrow)

along the edge of the intervertebral disc in a vertical direction, connecting several upper and lower vertebral bodies to show a characteristic bamboo spine (Fig. 7.22).

(c) Erosion and destruction of the discovertebral junction area

Erosion and destruction of the discovertebral junction area can be classified into three major categories. Localized central discovertebral lesions are observed not only in AS but also in non-AS cases, showing Schmorl's or cartilaginous nodes in the center of the discovertebral junction area. Localized peripheral discovertebral lesions occur when bone defects occur in the anterior or posterior of the discovertebral junction area, which may be associated with intervertebral disc damage, kyphosis, Schmorl's node formation, enthesitis, etc. And extensive central and peripheral discovertebral lesions show extensive bone destruction and bony sclerosis in the entire discovertebral junction area, indicating significantly advanced AS (Fig. 7.23). Erosion and destruction of the discovertebral junction are either inflammatory lesions inherent in the disease (inflammatory Andersson lesion) or pseudoarthrosis (non-inflammatory Andersson lesion) that occurs after a fracture. In these cases, they look similar to tumors, neurogenic arthritis, infec-

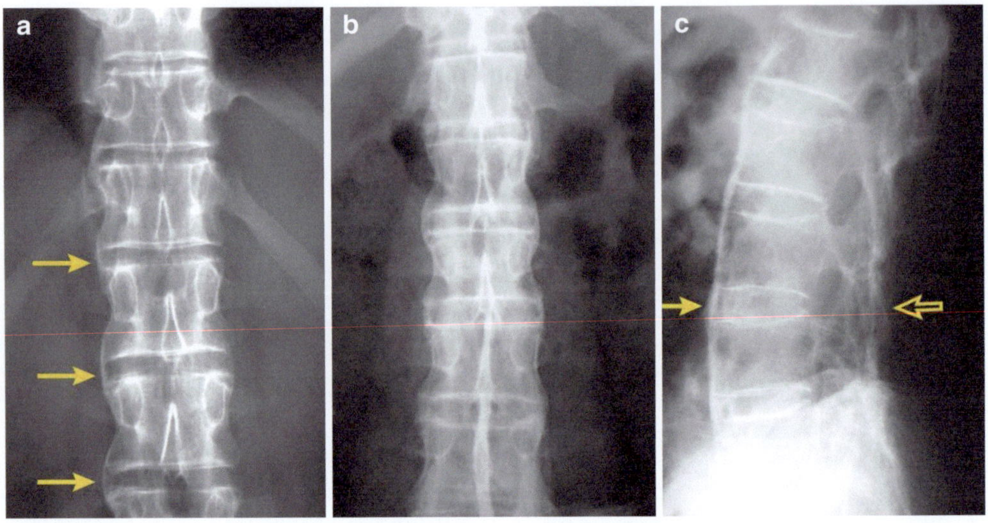

Fig. 7.22 Syndesmophyte in ankylosing spondylitis (3 different patients). (**a**) On the lumbar frontal view, the syndesmophyte is formed vertically along the edge of the intervertebral disc and is located within the boundary of the vertebral body, which is a marginal syndesmophyte (arrow). (**b**) In advanced cases, multiple syndesmophytes connect several upper and lower vertebral bodies, showing a characteristic bamboo spine. (**c**) On the lumbar lateral view, the syndesmophyte is formed vertically along the edge of the intervertebral disc (arrow) and is accompanied by bone fusion of the facet joint (empty arrow)

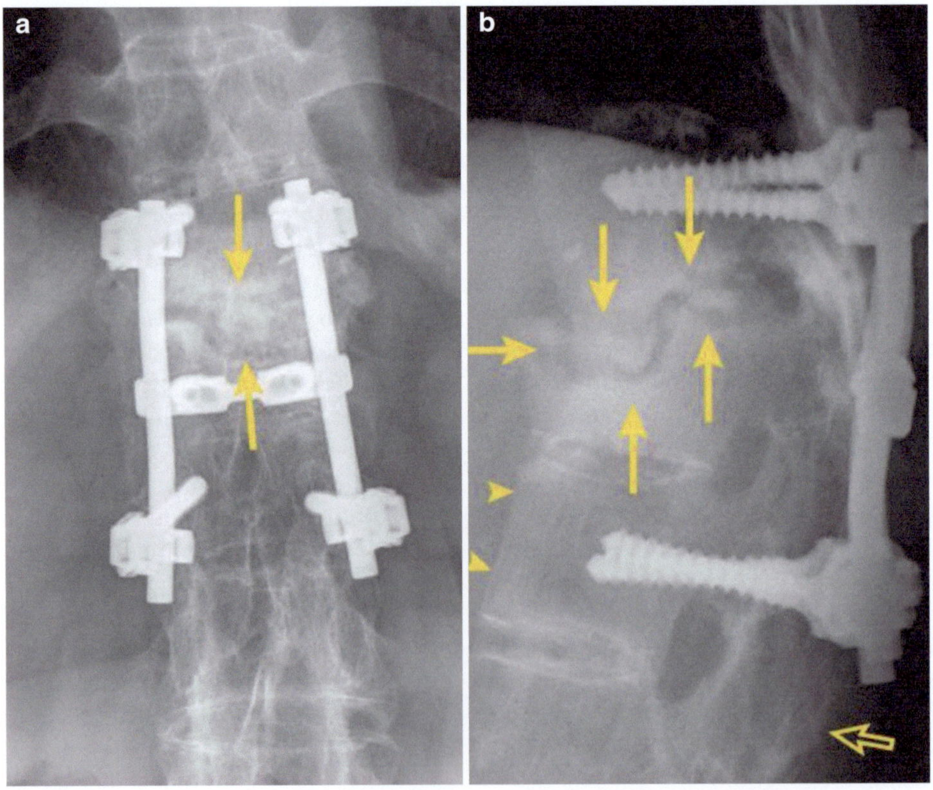

Fig. 7.23 Pseudoarthrosis (Andersson lesion) in ankylosing spondylitis
On the thoracolumbar frontal and lateral views, there is extensive bone resorption and bone sclerosis due to bony erosion and bone destruction at the T12–L1 site of the thoracolumbar junction (arrow). On the lateral view, the vertebral body appears squaring (arrowhead) and there is bone fusion of the facet joint (empty arrow)

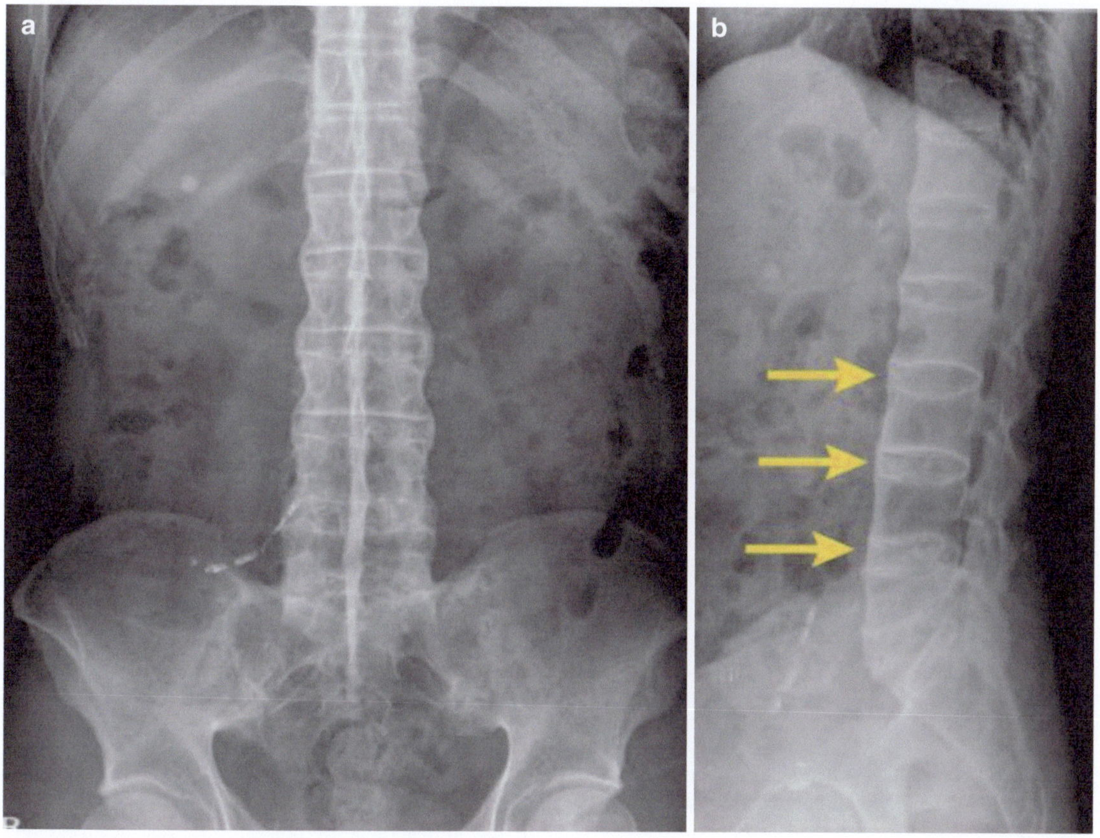

Fig. 7.24 Discal calcification and osteoporosis in advanced AS

tious arthritis, etc., so differential diagnosis is absolutely necessary, and MRI helps in their differential diagnosis.

(d) Discal calcification

Calcification in a circular or linear form appears in one or more intervertebral discs and is prominently observed due to osteoporosis of the surrounding vertebral bodies (Fig. 7.24).

② Apophyseal joint, facet joint

Facet joint lesions are characterized by indistinct bony erosion, subchondral bony sclerosis, joint space narrowing, and bony union, which can be well observed in lumbar oblique view radiography and cervical lateral view radiography. However, in the thoracic spine, these simple radiographs may not be sufficient, and CT may be necessary for observation. In AS, bony fusion of the facet joint is very prominent in the cervical spine. In this case, hypoplasia of the vertebral body and intervertebral disc, which appears during juvenile rheumatoid arthritis, is not accompanied and shows normal vertebral body and intervertebral disc (Fig. 7.25). In the lumbar spine, ossification of the ligaments results in characteristic radiological findings such as the dagger sign and trolley track sign (Fig. 7.26). The dagger sign represents a hardened vertical line in the center of the lumbar frontal photo due to ossification of the supraspinous ligaments and interspinous ligaments, and the trolley track sign represents three hardened vertical lines in the lumbar frontal photo due to ossification of the supraspinous ligaments, interspinous ligaments, and facet joint.

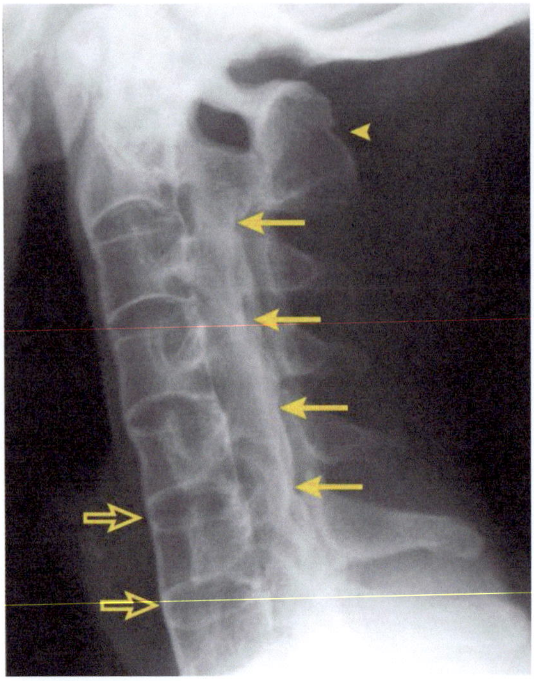

Fig. 7.25 Bone fusion of the facet joint in ankylosing spondylitis
In the lateral cervical spine image, complete bony fusion of the facet joint is seen throughout the entire cervical region (arrow), and there is a syndesmophyte on the vertebral body (empty arrow). There is bony fusion on the spinous process between the first and second cervical vertebrae (arrowhead). Unlike Juvenile RA, the size of the vertebral body and intervertebral disc is relatively normal

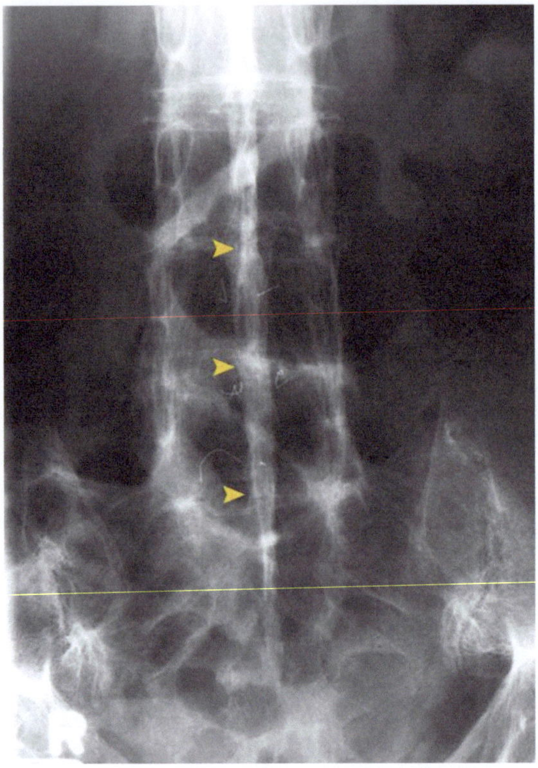

Fig. 7.26 Dagger sign of ankylosing spondylitis
In the lumbar anterior image, a vertical sclerotic line appears like a dagger in the center due to ossification of the supraspinous ligament and interspinous ligament (arrowhead)

③ Atlantoaxial joint

In AS, the involvement of the atlantoaxial joint appears in the form of atlantoaxial subluxation (AAS) and atlantoaxial ankylosis (AAA). AAS is a common finding in rheumatoid arthritis, usually reported to be involved in 12–33% of cases, but in some cases, it has been reported to be found in 86% of RA patients. AAS is also a relatively common finding in AS, usually reported in 2–6.7% of cases, and in some cases, it has been reported to be found in 21% of AS. Recent studies have reported that when the standard for AAS is considered to be 3 mm or more, AAS was observed in about 14.1% of patients with AS, and the risk of AAS increases as the disease activity increases, as evidenced by a high CRP level that does not respond to NSAID/DMRAD when peripheral arthritis is present. AAA, although less frequent than AAS, is another finding that often appears in long-standing AS patients [21].

(2) Magnetic Resonance Imaging (MRI)

MRI can detect early osteitis of the thoracolumbar vertebral body and determine the active state by detecting bone marrow edema, and characteristic MRI findings make the diagnosis of AS possible [6]. It can also diagnose complications such as traumatic spinal injury, cauda equina syndrome, and spinal stenosis.

The characteristic early MRI findings of AS involving the thoracolumbar vertebral body are osteitis occurring at the corners and

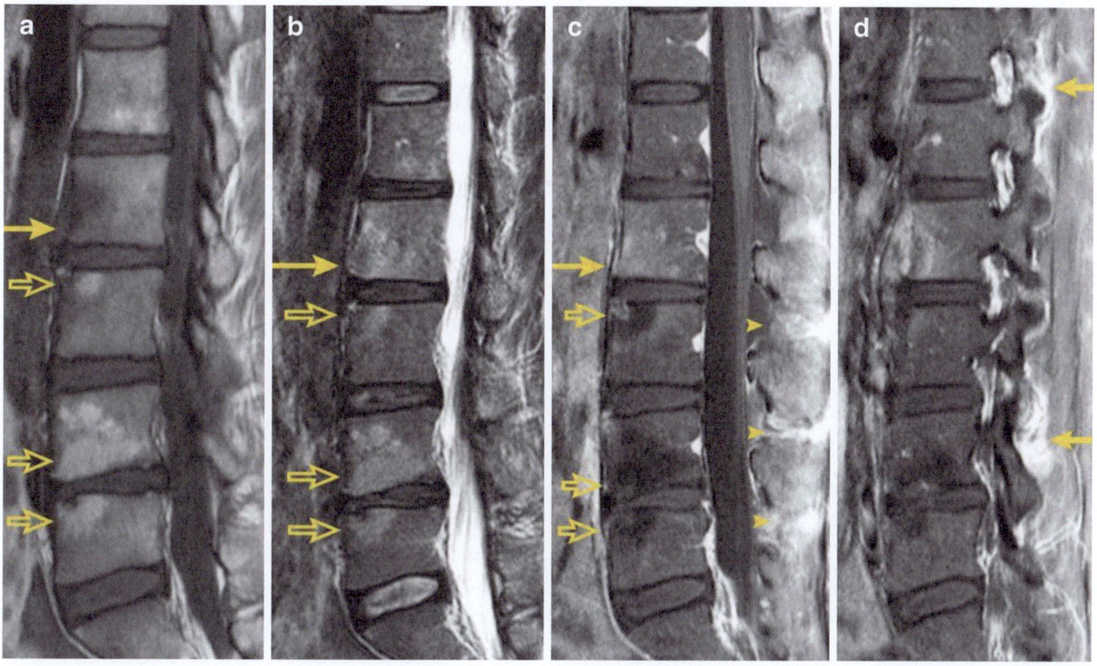

Fig. 7.27 MRI findings of vertebral osteitis in ankylosing spondylitis
In the sagittal T1 (**a**) and T2 (**b**) enhanced images, there is active vertebral osteitis (arrow) with bone marrow edema in the lower anterior part of the second lumbar vertebra, and chronic vertebral osteitis (empty arrow) with fat deposition in the upper anterior part of the third and fifth lumbar vertebrae, and the lower anterior part of the fourth lumbar vertebra. Depending on the affected area in the same patient, the progression of osteitis can vary, and both low signal intensity and high signal intensity can appear in T1-enhanced images. In the fat-suppressed contrast-enhanced T1-enhanced image (**c**), enhancement between the spinous processes indicates enthesitis (arrowhead). In the fat-suppressed contrast-enhanced T1-enhanced image (**d**), enhancement in the facet joint between the twelfth thoracic and first lumbar vertebrae, and between the third and fourth lumbar vertebrae, suggests active arthritis (thick arrow)

front of the vertebral body, which is more commonly observed at the thoracolumbar junction than the lower lumbar spine. Initially, due to peripheral bone marrow edema, low signal intensity is observed in T1-weighted images. The fat-suppressed T2-weighted images or STIR show high signal intensity (Fig. 7.27). As osteitis progresses and reaches the healing process, bone marrow edema disappears and is converted to fatty marrow, so it shows high signal intensity in T1-weighted images and low signal intensity in fat-suppressed T2-weighted images. If the degree of osteitis progression varies depending on the site of invasion in the same patient, low signal intensity and high signal intensity can appear together in T1-weighted images [12]. According to recent reports, the "'MR corner sign" is a reliable finding in AS, and it is suggested to actively examine it if this finding is seen. The signal intensity changes of the bone marrow seen in degenerative disc disease, which should be differentiated, are more commonly observed in the lower lumbar spine and mostly appear parallel from front to back along the disc. Traumatic fractures and stress fractures can occur in the spine of patients with advanced AS. Fractures can occur even with minor trauma, and accurate diagnosis using CT and MRI is essential because they are unstable fractures that can cause serious problems such as spinal cord injury (Fig. 7.28). Carrot stick fractures are common in the cervical and thoracolumbar junctions, most of which invade the disc and

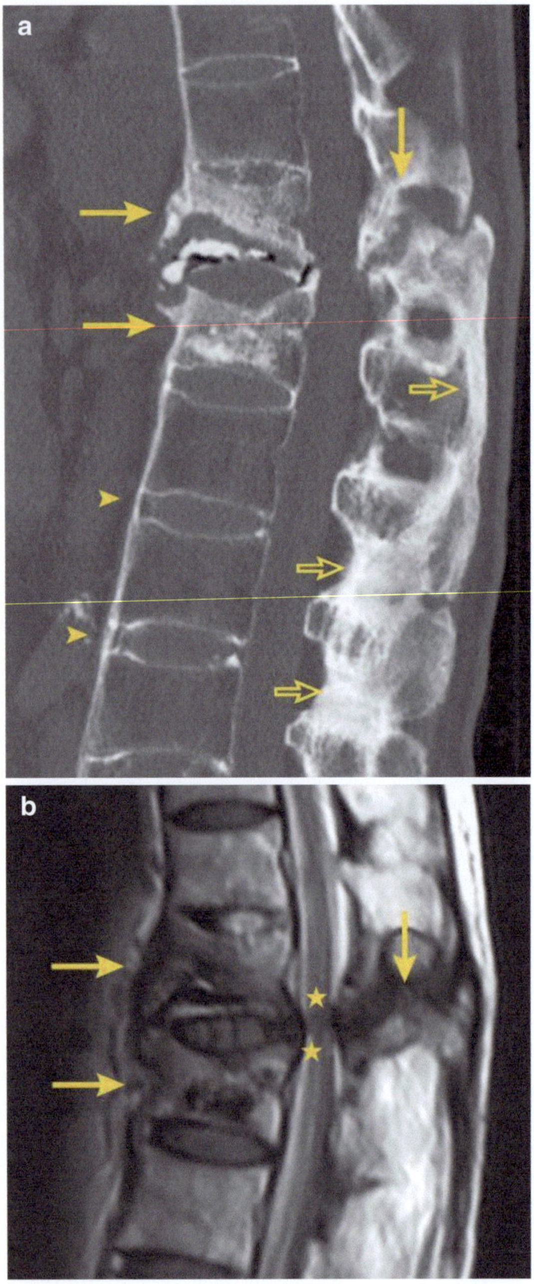

Fig. 7.28 CT and MRI findings of vertebral fractures in AS. (**a**) In the sagittal CT, there is a fracture in the T12–L1 vertebral body, and a fracture line extending to the posterior spine is observed (arrow). The vertebral body shows bone sclerosis and bone resorption, and the disc interval is widened, suggesting pseudoarthrosis. Syndesmophytes are formed vertically along the edge of the intervertebral disc (arrowhead), and there is ossification of the supraspinal ligament and interspinal ligaments (empty arrow). (**b**) In the same patient's sagittal T2-enhanced image, there is a fracture in the vertebral body, and a fracture line extending to the posterior spine is observed (arrow). Spinal stenosis is shown due to pseudoarthrosis (asterisk)

have many hyperextension injuries, but occasionally there are hyperflexion injuries. An important fact is that traumatic spinal cord injuries often occur regardless of the presence or absence of spinal fractures because the rigid spine cannot properly absorb external shocks. MRI examination is essential to evaluate the presence or absence of spinal cord injury in these patients. A rare complication in patients with advanced AS is cauda equina syndrome, where MRI can find expansion of the dural sac, arachnoid diverticula, and bony erosion of the lamina. The frequency of spinal stenosis is high in AS patients due to ossification of the facet joint, spinal ligaments, and discs, which can be well evaluated by CT, and MRI also helps evaluate spinal stenosis.

(3) Differential diagnosis: centered on the spine
① Other seronegative spondyloarthritis: paravertebral ossification

Paravertebral ossification seen in psoriatic arthritis and reactive arthritis is common in the thoracic spine, rough and thick, and asymmetric, and it is distinguished from the symmetrical syndesmophyte located at the edge of the spine observed in AS (Fig. 7.29) [15, 16]. Osteitis with bony sclerosis at the corners of the upper and lower front of the vertebral body, and the vertebral body appearing square are similar to AS, but bone union findings of the facet joint are rare compared to AS or inflammatory bowel disease arthritis. Bony erosion of the odontoid process and subluxation of the atlantoaxial joint observed in AS are also observed in psoriatic arthritis and reactive arthritis, but severe cervical involvement is not seen. In AS, the observed osteoarthritis of the cervical facet joint is also observed in juvenile rheumatoid arthritis, but in AS, it shows normal-sized vertebral bodies and intervertebral discs, whereas in juvenile rheumatoid arthritis, it shows a decrease in the formation of vertebral bodies and intervertebral discs [15, 16].
② Diffuse idiopathic skeletal hyperostosis (DISH): flowing anterolateral ossification

DISH (diffuse idiopathic skeletal hyperostosis) is a disease that occurs in the elderly and mainly invades the lower cervical and

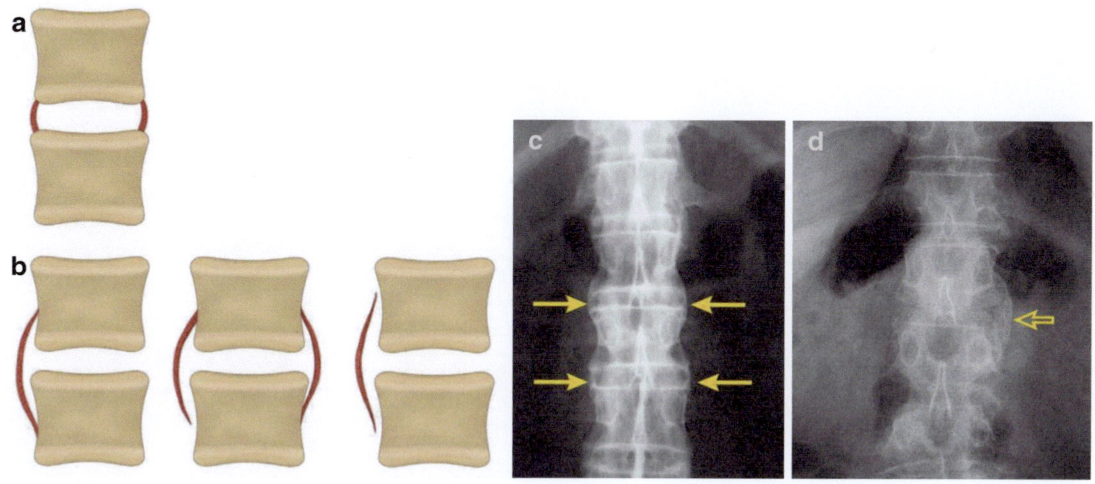

Fig. 7.29 Differentiation of syndesmophyte: marginal versus non-marginal syndesmophyte. (**a**) Schematic diagram of marginal syndesmophyte, which is observed in AS, spinal involvement of inflammatory bowel disease. (**b**) Schematic diagram of non-marginal syndesmophyte, which is observed in psoriatic arthritis, reactive arthritis/ Reiter's syndrome. (**c**) Marginal syndesmophyte of ankylosing spondylitis (arrow). (**d**) Non-marginal syndesmophyte of psoriatic arthritis (empty arrow)

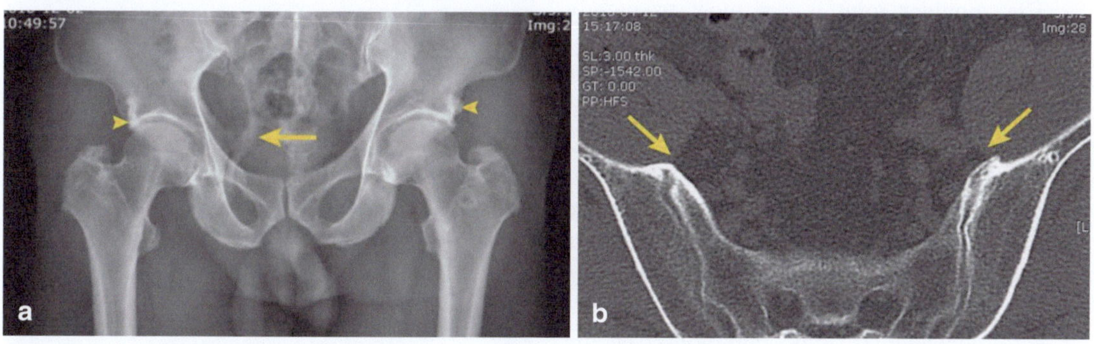

Fig. 7.30 Findings shown in plain radiography and CT images when DISH invades the pelvic bones
In simple shooting photos, heterotopic ossification (arrow) is seen along both anterior inferior iliac spines (arrowhead) and the right sacrotuberous ligament, and in the axial CT image, osseous bridges (arrow) are seen in front of both SI joints. No distinct sacroiliitis is seen in both SI joints in the visible area

thoracic spine, characterized by ossification of the ligaments around the spine. It forms characteristic irregular and thick ossification around the spine on the front of the vertebral body, which is formed separately from the vertebral body. Also, the intervertebral disc space is maintained, there is no invasion of the spine's facet joint, and there are findings of para-articular bridging due to bone formation on the anterior, anterosuperior, anteroinferior articular margins of the SI joint (Fig. 7.30) [15, 16].

③ Spondylosis deformans: osteophyte

It shows a triangular outgrowth due to hyperostosis at the attachment site of the annulus fibrosus [15, 16].

7.2.1.5 Imaging Findings of AS: Centered on Peripheral Joints

In patients with long-standing AS, radiological findings of peripheral joint abnormalities are observed in more than 50% of cases, mainly in the hip joint, shoulder joint, and foot.

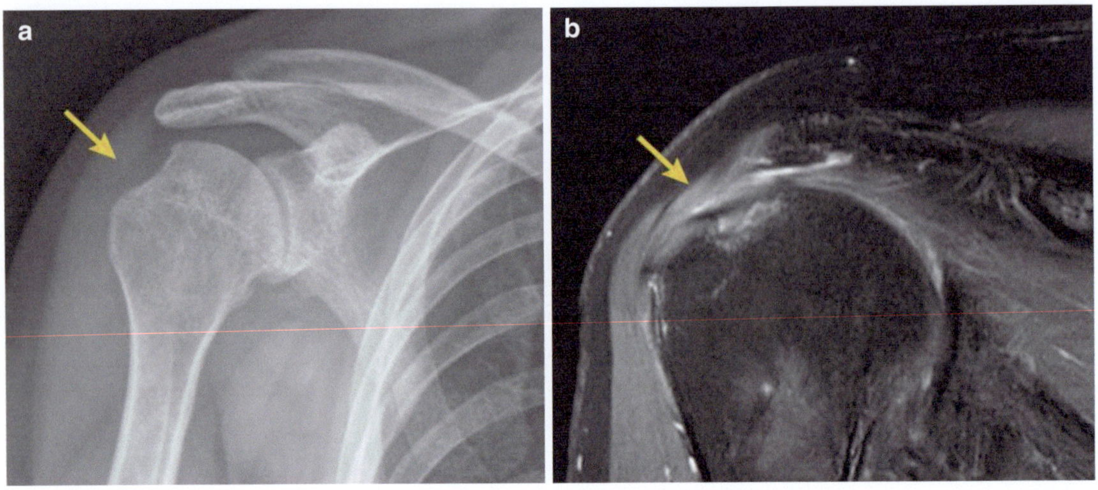

Fig. 7.31 Hatchet sign that can appear when AS invades the shoulder joint
It is a finding that appears as a large erosion on the superolateral aspect of the right humeral head, looking like the blade of an axe

(1) Shoulder joint
The shoulder joint is the most frequently invaded site in patients with long-standing AS and is more common bilaterally. It shows findings such as osteoporosis, diffuse joint space loss, and bony erosion of the superolateral humeral head, which look similar to rheumatoid arthritis. In some patients, the entire outside of the humeral head is destroyed, which is called a hatchet sign (Fig. 7.31). Also, bone destruction of the acromioclavicular joint commonly occurs bilaterally, which is the same as the findings seen in rheumatoid arthritis. Increased joint space of the acromioclavicular joint due to bone resorption of the proximal clavicle can also occur in rheumatoid arthritis, infection, hyperparathyroidism, trauma, etc. [15, 16].

(2) Hand and wrist joints
While the involvement of the elbow is relatively rare, asymmetrical abnormalities in the small joints of the hand and wrist are not uncommon. Periarticular soft tissue swelling, periarticular osteoporosis, joint space narrowing, and bony erosion are observed [15, 16].

(3) Hip joint and pelvis
Clinically and radiologically, the involvement of the hip joint is an important feature of AS, showing bilateral (93%) and symmetrical (73%) distribution, and uniform joint space loss and osteophytes formation are characteristic (Fig. 7.32). Initial findings include osteophytes on the lateral side of the femoral head, which progress to form collar osteophytes around the femoral neck. Subsequently, due to the diffuse loss of joint space, the femoral causes axial migration of

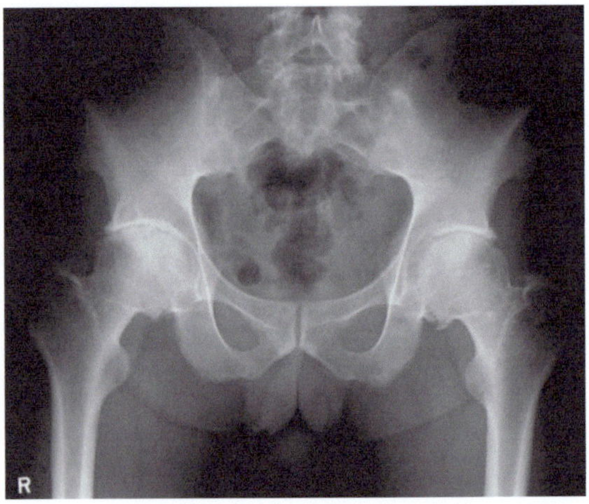

Fig. 7.32 Hip arthritis of AS
In the pelvic frontal photo, there is bone fusion in both SI joints and relatively symmetrical uniform joint space loss and osteophyte formation in both hip joints. The tendon attachment site of the ischial tuberosity shows an irregular beard shape due to inflammation and periostitis

the head, eventually leading to protrusio acetabuli in the pelvis. Diffuse decrease in joint space and formation of osteophytes are characteristic findings in hip disease in AS patients, but they are also observed in CPPD, Paget's disease, etc. In RA, bilateral and symmetrical involvement and diffuse, uniform loss of joint space are characteristic, with less prominent formation of osteophytes. This is a difference from AS, but in long-standing RA, secondary degenerative changes can also show osteophytes. Intra-articular ankylosis is also a complication of hip involvement in AS. In AS patients who have undergone arthroplasty, heterotopic ossification can be seen around the joint. In osteoarthritis, it involves one or both sides, and the upper or inner side narrows asymmetrically, showing osteophytes in the femur and acetabulum. The marginal area of the pelvis becomes irregular, and this whiskering is due to inflammation and periostitis at the attachment site of the tendon to the bone (Fig. 7.33). This whiskering appears on the iliac crests, femoral greater trochanters, ischial tuberosity, etc. Also, bony erosion, bony sclerosis, and joint stiffness can occur in the symphysis pubis (Fig. 7.34) [15, 16].

(4) In knee joint about 30% of long-standing AS, radiological findings appear in the knee joint, typically showing bilateral and symmetrical changes in the three compartments. Findings include joint fluid, osteoporosis, decreased joint space, marginal area bony erosion, subchondral bone cysts, and periarticular periostitis [15, 16].

(5) Ankle joint, foot, calcaneus changes in the ankle are rare, and in the foot, bilateral symmetrical or asymmetrical changes occur in the metatarsophalangeal joint (MTP joint), first tarsometatarsal joint (1st TMT joint), and interphalangeal joint (IP joint) of the big toe. Findings include soft tissue swelling, diffuse loss of joint space, bony erosion and adjacent bony proliferation, periostitis of the phalanx and metatarsal bone, and intra-articular ankylosis. It shows fibular deviation of the toes due to subluxation of the MTP

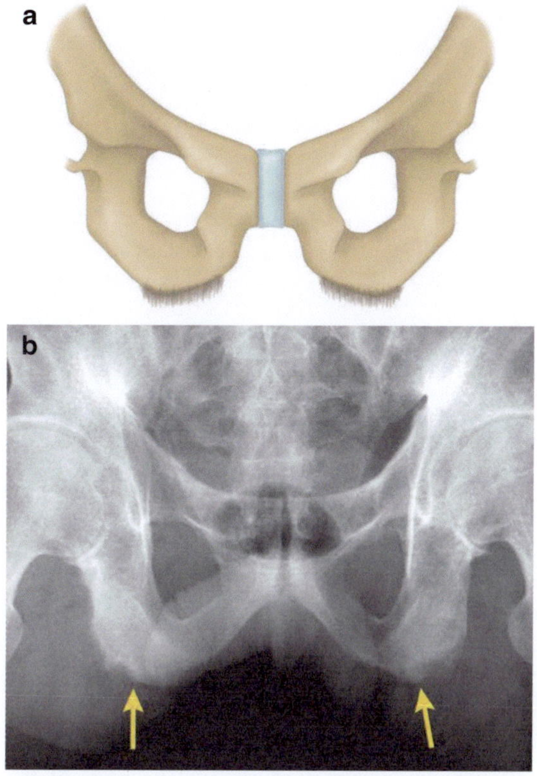

Fig. 7.33 AS's enthesitis: ischial tuberosity. (**a**) This is a schematic diagram showing irregular beard-shaped enthesitis caused by inflammation and periostitis at the tendon attachment site of the ischial tuberosity. (**b**) In the pelvic frontal photo, the tendon attachment site of the ischial tuberosity shows an irregular beard-shaped enthesitis (arrow)

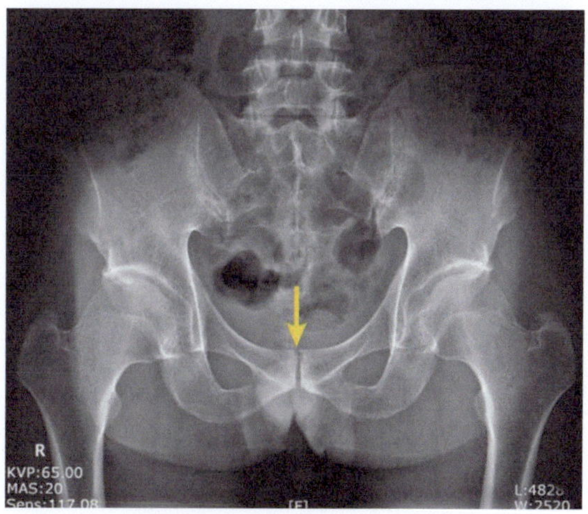

Fig. 7.34 Changes in AS symphysis pubis
A photo with distinct sacroiliitis findings in both SI joints, showing erosion (arrow) in the symphysis pubis

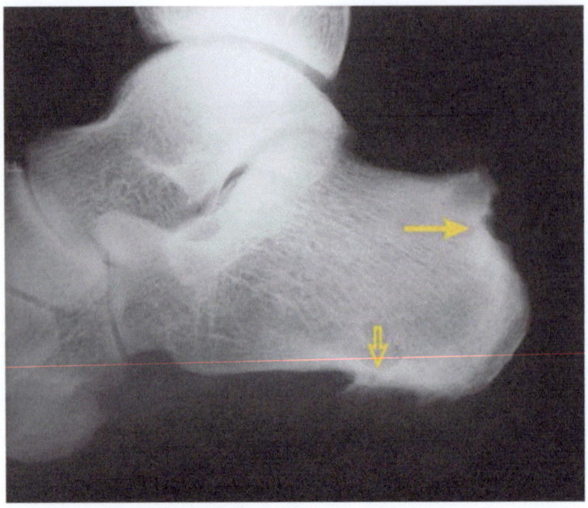

Fig. 7.35 AS's enthesitis: calcaneus
In the lateral photo of the calcaneus, it shows a bony erosion (arrow)8 associated with retrocalcaneal bursitis in the posterior superior of the calcaneus. It shows an enthesophyte at the attachment site of the plantar fascia (empty arrow). This finding is similar to the enthesitis of other seronegative spondyloarthropathies

joint, which is less frequent than RA but appears severe. Radiological findings of the calcaneus are common with plantar calcaneal enthesophytes of the calcaneus and are associated with retrocalcaneal bursitis, soft tissue swelling, bony erosion of the posterior superior part of the calcaneus, and frequent findings of Achilles tendon non-posterior (Fig. 7.35). In RA, shallow bony erosion and well-defined enthesophytes are seen, whereas in AS, as in psoriatic arthritis and reactive arthritis, significant bony erosion, peripheral bony sclerosis, and poorly defined enthesophytes at the ligament attachment site are seen [15, 16]. In AS patients, MRI findings of the ankle and foot include increased joint fluid in the ankle joint, soft tissue edema, bone marrow edema, and bony erosion, acute or chronic in the hindfoot. Achilles tendonitis, para-articular enthesophyte, enthesophyte at the attachment site of the Achilles tendon and plantar fascia, plantar fasciitis, retrocalcaneal bursitis, bony erosion in the midfoot, decreased joint space and subchondral bony sclerosis, soft tissue swelling, and bone marrow edema are observed.

(6) Temporomandibular joint
In AS, bony erosion appears on the condyle of the mandible, and MRI is useful for evaluation [15].

7.2.1.6 Comorbidities of AS

AS can be accompanied by RA, DISH, inflammatory bowel disease, etc.

(1) Rheumatoid arthritis
Rheumatoid arthritis and AS can coexist, typically in young men where AS occurs at a young age and rheumatoid arthritis occurs when it becomes inactive. The clinical and radiological findings of both diseases appear together, and if a patient with rheumatoid arthritis shows extensive SI joint and thoracic vertebral abnormalities, it suggests the possibility of coexisting AS [15].
(2) DISH
In elderly people with long-standing AS, AS and DISH can coexist. In this case, the characteristics of AS such as bone fusion of both SI joints, syndesmophyte and narrowing and bone fusion of the facet joint, and the characteristics of DISH such as irregular and thick paravertebral ossification along the anterior margin of the spine, especially the thoracic spine, are seen simultaneously [15].
(3) Inflammatory Bowel Disease-Associated Arthritis
Ulcerative colitis, Crohn's disease, and other inflammatory bowel diseases and AS can coexist in some patients. The activity of bowel disease is not correlated with the activity of the spine or SI joint [15].

7.2.2 Psoriatic Arthritis

(1) Clinical findings and laboratory findings
Psoriatic arthritis appears in 2–6% of psoriasis patients, with similar incidence in men and women and often starts between the ages of 20 and 50. The severity and duration of skin disease are not related to the onset of arthritis, and usually arthritis occurs after skin lesions, but changes in nails are more

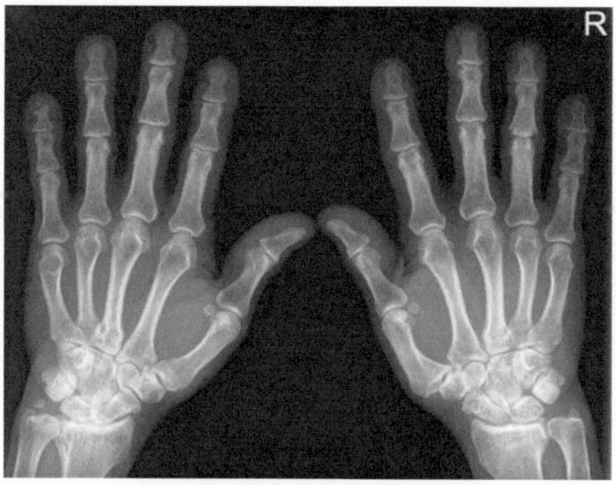

Fig. 7.36 Sausage digit, finger of a psoriasis patient

related to changes in joints. However, in about 15% of patients, arthritis appears before skin lesions, so it is important to diagnose psoriatic arthritis in imaging tests. The commonly involved joints are the IP joint, MCP joint of the hand, and the IP joint, MTP joint of the foot, and the SI joint and spine are also involved in 20–40%. If there is redness, soft tissue swelling, and pain around the DIP joint, or if asymmetric involvement is confined to one entire finger due to tenosynovitis, the entire swollen finger is called a sausage digit (Fig. 7.36).

In laboratory findings, rheumatoid factor is negative, ESR or CRP is normal or increased during the acute phase, and often shows an increase in serum uric acid. HLA-B27 antigen appears positive in up to 75% of patients with sacroiliac joint involvement, and in approximately 30% of cases with only peripheral joint involvement [15, 16].

(2) Imaging findings of psoriatic arthritis

Psoriatic arthritis typically affects the synovial joint, cartilaginous joint, trunk, and limb skeleton, particularly at the ligament and tendon attachment sites of the bones, and characteristically shows asymmetrical involvement. It commonly affects the PIP joint, DIP joint, MCP/MTP joints of the hands and feet, and the involvement of the distal phalangeal tuft and calcaneus is also characteristic. In the early stages of psoriatic arthritis, radiological findings may be normal. The general radiological findings can be summarized as follows [15, 16].

(1) Common findings of psoriatic arthritis

(a) Soft tissue swelling

Soft tissue swelling can be seen earliest. Soft tissue swelling can be observed in a fusiform shape in the tissues around the joint, or one finger can show a sausage-like swelling.

(b) Normal bone density

Psoriatic arthritis shows normal bone density. The presence of osteoporosis cannot completely rule out the diagnosis of psoriatic arthritis, but it is not a common finding in psoriatic arthritis. The absence of osteoporosis in psoriatic arthritis is useful for differentiating it from rheumatoid arthritis.

(c) Joint space narrowing or widening

In large joints such as the knee, ankle, elbow, and hip joint, the joint space shows diffuse reduction, but in small joints such as fingers and toes, the joint space can be significantly widened due to severe bone destruction in the marginal area and subchondral bone.

(d) Bony erosion and tapered bone ends

In psoriatic arthritis, bony erosion is prominent, and initially, bony erosion in the joint marginal area is dominant, but as it progresses, the central part is also affected. In small joints of the hands and feet, the characteristic "pencil-and-cup" shape is shown due to bone destruction at the head of the phalanx.

(e) Bone proliferation and fluffy periostitis

Bone proliferation is a characteristic finding of psoriatic arthritis, as in other seronegative spondyloarthropathies. In the hands and feet of patients with psoriatic arthritis, periostitis is not common in the diaphyses and metaphyses of the bones, and these changes can occur early in the disease and are often associated with peripheral soft tissue swelling. Characteristically, fluffy and spiculated periostitis is seen around the ligament and tendon attachment sites or around the marginal area bony erosion, and the characteristic "mouse ear" shape is shown due to the marginal area bony erosion and surrounding fluffy periostitis. Also, the entire phalanx appears thick due to endosteal periostitis, also known as ivory phalanx, especially observed in terminal phalanges. Bone proliferation occurs at the attachment sites of ligaments or tendons, and on the posterior and inferior surfaces of the calcaneus, femoral trochanters, ischial tuberosities, medial and lateral malleoli, ulnar olecranon, anterior surface of patella and radial. It appears on the tuberosity of the femur, distal condyles, proximal part of the tibia, etc.

(f) Intra-articular bony ankylosis
Intra-articular bony ankylosis can be observed in large joints, but it is particularly noticeable in the IP joints of the hands and feet. The findings of intra-articular bony ankylosis can also be observed in rheumatoid arthritis, erosive osteoarthritis, infectious arthritis, etc., but it is an important radiological finding of seronegative spondyloarthritis.

(g) Terminal bone resorption (tuft resorption)
Bone resorption at the end of the distal phalanx of the hands and feet is a characteristic finding of psoriatic arthritis, and the nails of the affected fingers are almost always involved.

(h) Malalignment and subluxation
Deformities of the hands and feet can also be observed in some cases of psoriatic arthritis. It shows arthritis mutilans with ulnar deviation of the MCP joint and fibular deviation of the MTP joint. Swan-neck deformity and boutonniere deformity are not as common as rheumatoid arthritis.

(2) Imaging findings of psoriatic arthritis by site

(a) Hand and wrist
Destructive arthritis of the DIP joint of the hand is a well-known finding of psoriatic arthritis, showing bilateral symmetrical or asymmetrical or unilateral involvement, and the adjacent PIP joint is also involved. Often, all three joints (DIP, PIP, and MCP joint) of one finger are involved, suggesting psoriatic arthritis (Fig. 7.37). Initial bony erosion appears in the marginal area of the joint and progresses to the central part. The characteristic "mouse ear" shape is shown due to marginal area bony erosion and surrounding fluffy periostitis (Fig. 7.38). Other important findings include soft tissue swelling, normal bone density, joint space narrowing and intra-articular bony ankylosis, "pencil and cup" shape, and terminal bone resorption (Fig. 7.39). Changes in joint space in the hand are common, and initially, the joint space widens due to bony erosion and intra-articular fibrous tissue deposition. About 15% of psoriatic arthritis can show intra-articular bony ankylosis. Abnormalities of the wrist in psoriatic

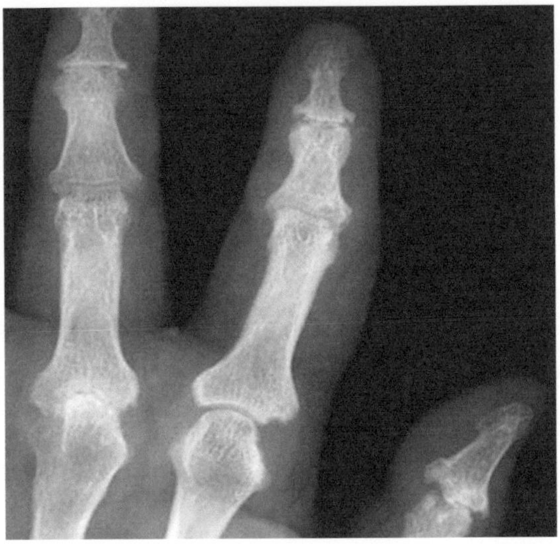

Fig. 7.37 Radiographic findings of the finger in psoriatic arthritis
The thumb and middle finger show a sausage-like swelling and a decrease in the IP joint, MCP joint. However, there is no significant periarticular osteopenia. The interphalangeal joint of the thumb also shows marginal area bony erosion, surrounding osteogenesis, and a decrease in joint space. The absence of periarticular osteoporosis in the DIP joint is a rare finding in rheumatoid arthritis

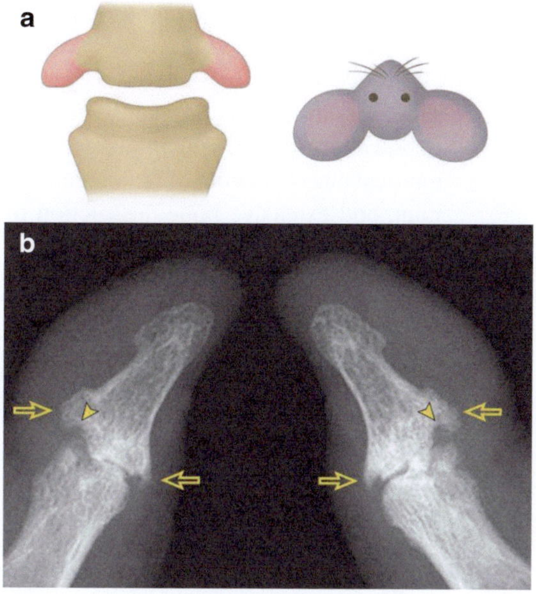

Fig. 7.38 Radiographic findings of the finger in psoriatic arthritis: bony erosion and periostitis. (**a**) Mouse ear schematic. (**b**) The IP joint of both thumbs shows a characteristic "mouse ear" shape due to marginal area bony erosion (arrowhead) and surrounding osteogenesis due to periostitis (empty arrow). The osteogenesis finding due to periostitis is rare in rheumatoid arthritis

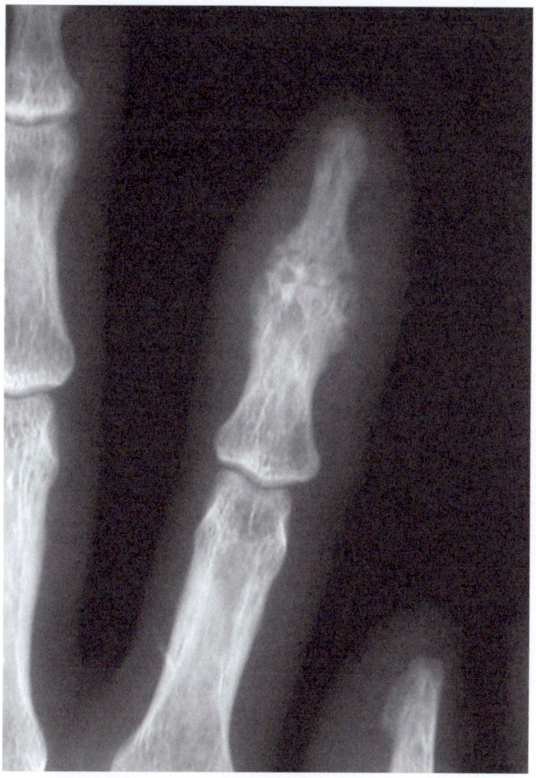

Fig. 7.39 Radiographic findings of the finger in psoriatic arthritis
Soft tissue swelling, bony erosion, and periosteal proliferation around the DIP joint of the lobster claw finger, and joint ankylosis are observed. However, there is no periarticular osteoporosis

arthritis are not as frequent as the fingers [15, 16, 18].

(b) Forefoot
The forefoot is also commonly involved in psoriatic arthritis, with bilateral asymmetrical changes in the MTP joint and IP joint, and extensive bone destruction of the thumb IP joint is a characteristic finding (Fig. 7.40). Common radiological findings include soft tissue swelling, normal bone density, bony erosion and fluffy periostitis, increased joint space, and bone resorption in the metatarsal head and distal phalanx tuft (Fig. 7.41). It also shows an ivory phalanx with dense bone shadow in the terminal phalanx of the thumb. In advanced cases, it shows arthritis mutilans with fibular deviation of the MTP joint (Fig. 7.42) [15, 16, 18].

(c) Calcaneus
Similar to other seronegative spondyloarthropathies, bony erosion, bony sclerosis around the attachment sites of the Achilles tendon and plantar fascia on the posterior and inferior surfaces of the calcaneus, and indistinct enthesophytes at the ligament attachment sites are observed (Fig. 7.43) [15, 16].

In patients with psoriatic arthritis, MRI findings of the ankle joint and foot show Achilles tendinitis or peritendinitis, retrocalcaneal bursitis, increased joint fluid in the ankle joint, soft tissue swelling, bone marrow edema, periarticular enthesophyte, enthesophytes at the attachment sites of the Achilles tendon and plantar fascia, and plantar fasciitis.

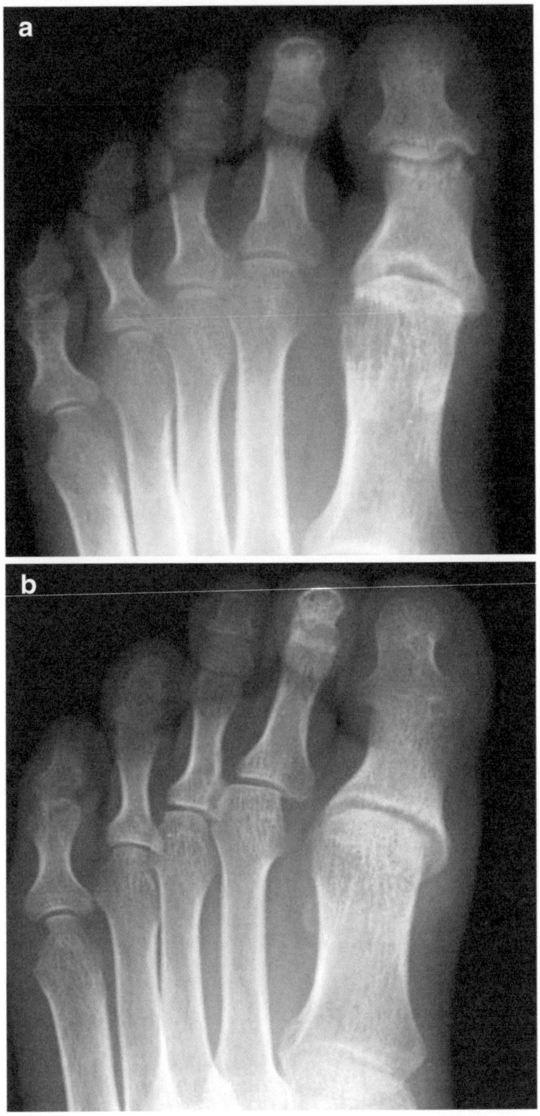

Fig. 7.40 Radiographic findings of the forefoot in psoriatic arthritis. (**a**) Bony erosion and periosteal proliferation are observed in the IP joint and MIP joint of the big toe. There is bony erosion in the head of the fifth metatarsal. (**b**) Two years later, bony ankylosis is found in the interphalangeal joints of the big toe and the second toe in the follow-up examination

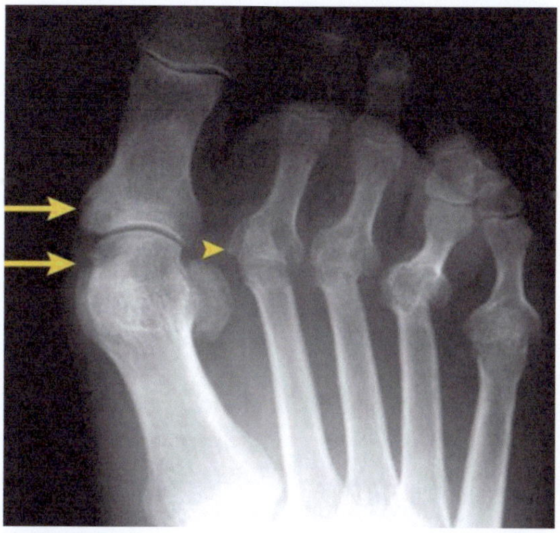

Fig. 7.41 Radiographic findings of the forefoot in psoriatic arthritis
Bony erosion and periosteal proliferation are observed in the MIP joint of the big toe (arrow). Partial dislocation to the fibular side is present in the remaining MIP joints (arrowhead). The absence of significant periarticular osteoporosis is a difference from rheumatoid arthritis

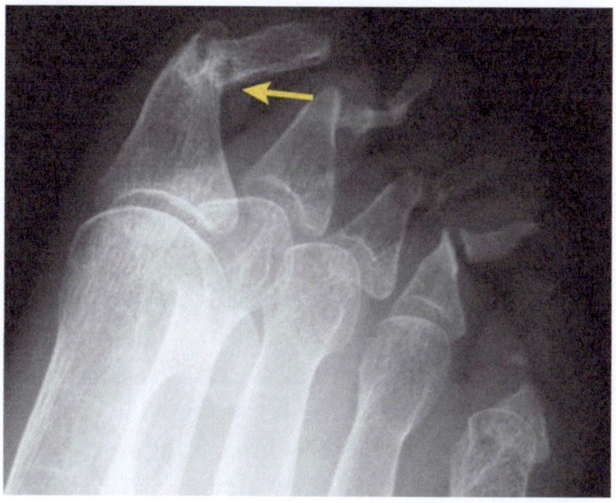

Fig. 7.42 Radiographic findings of the forefoot in psoriatic arthritis: arthritis mutilans
There is mutilating arthritis with severe bone destruction and bone fragment displacement in the PIP interphalangeal joints. There is a "pencil and cup" deformation in the interphalangeal joint of the big toe (arrow), and bone ankylosis in the PIP joints from the second to the fourth

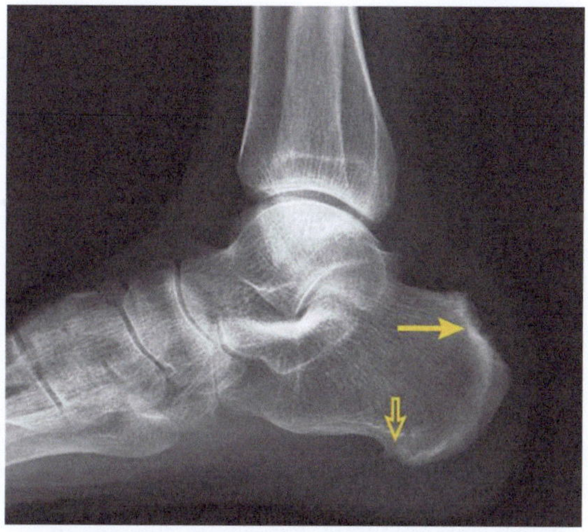

Fig. 7.43 Enthesopathy in psoriatic arthritis: calcaneus
In the lateral view of the ankle joint, soft tissue swelling related to retrocalcaneal bursitis, and bony erosion in the posterior direction of the calcaneus are observed (arrow). Enthesopathic changes are also seen at the attachment site of the plantar fascia (empty arrow). These findings are similar to those of enthesopathy in other seronegative spondyloarthropathies

(d) Sacroiliac joint
Changes in the SI joint on radiographic examination are seen in about 10–25% of patients with moderate to severe psoriatic skin disease, and involvement of the SI joint is seen in 30–50% of patients with psoriatic arthritis. Bilateral asymmetrical involvement of the SI joint is the most common finding, but bilateral symmetrical involvement or unilateral involvement can also be seen (Fig. 7.17). Findings of SI joint changes in psoriatic arthritis include bony erosion, bony sclerosis, and expansion of the joint space. However, reduction of the joint space or bony ankylosis is less than in the case of AS [15, 16, 18].

(e) Spine
Findings when the spine is involved include thick, rough, asymmetrical non-marginal syndesmophytes on the one side of the spine (Fig. 7.29) and atlanto-axial subluxation [15, 16, 18]. On the other hand, involvement of the facet joint (facet joint) is observed at a much lower frequency. The thick, rough, asymmetrical syndesmophytes observed in psoriatic arthritis can appear early before changes in the SI joint or peripheral joints are seen. About 35–75% of psoriatic arthritis can show cervical abnormalities, but severe changes in the cervical spine are not seen.

(3) Differential diagnosis

(a) Other seronegative spondyloarthropathies
Seronegative spondyloarthropathy typically shows soft tissue swelling without osteoporosis when the synovial joint is involved, and bony erosion, bone proliferation, and joint space abnormalities. The distribution of the affected joint sites varies, with psoriatic arthritis showing asymmetrical polyarticular disease involving the upper and lower extremities, especially the IP joint of the hands and feet, and the MTP joint of the foot. In contrast, reactive arthritis is characterized by a low frequency of axial skeleton involvement, rare involvement of the upper extremities, and asymmetrical involvement of the lower extremity joints.

AS or inflammatory bowel disease typically shows bilateral and symmetrical involvement of the SI joint, but psoriatic arthritis and reactive arthritis show bilateral involvement in about 50% and asymmetrical involvement. If the SI joint shows bilateral and symmetrical SI joint or complete bone fusion, the likelihood of AS is high, and if it invades unilaterally or bilaterally but asymmetrically, the SI joint is involved. The possibility of psoriatic arthritis or reactive arthritis is high (Fig. 7.17).

The paravertebral ossification seen in psoriatic arthritis and reactive arthritis often occurs in the thoracic spine, is rough and thick, and is asymmetrical, originating away from the edges of the vertebral body and intervertebral disc, distinguishing it from the symmetrical syndesmophyte located at the edge of the spine observed in AS or inflammatory diseases (Fig. 7.29). Also, in psoriatic spondylitis and reactive arthritis, the osteitis of the anterior vertebral body and the square appearance of the vertebral body, which are observed in AS, are relatively rare. Findings of narrowing, sclerosis, and bony ankylosis of the facet joint (facet joint) may also be observed, but they are much less observed than in AS [15, 16].

(b) Rheumatoid arthritis
The distribution of involved joints in the limb skeleton of some patients with psoriatic arthritis is similar to that of rheumatoid arthritis, but the extensive involvement and asymmetrical involvement of the DIP joints are helpful in differentiation. In psoriatic arthritis, severe marginal area and central bony erosion, bony ankylosis, osteoproliferation, and periostitis, and terminal osteolysis are observed without osteoporosis. In contrast, rheumatoid arthritis shows pannus formation, periarticular osteoporosis, marginal area bony erosion, slight decrease in joint space, fibrous bony ankylosis, and the involved areas are almost all joints of the hand, especially the MCP joint and PIP joint. However, DIP joint involvement is rare in rheumatoid arthritis, both clinically and radiologically. Spinal involvement in rheumatoid arthritis shows severe cervical involvement (atlantoaxial subluxation), while the thoracic spine is mildly or not involved and paravertebral ossification is not observed [15, 16].

7.2.3 Reactive Arthritis

7.2.3.1 Clinical Findings and Laboratory Findings

Reactive arthritis became known when Hans Reiter reported a case of urethritis, conjunctivitis, and arthritis in a patient with hemorrhagic dysentery. Subsequent studies on reactive arthritis reported that gastrointestinal infections caused by Shigella, Salmonella, Campylobacter, or genitourinary infections caused by Chlamydia are related to reactive arthritis. Reactive arthritis closely related to HLA-B27 antigen was first reported in arthritis related to Yersinia enteritis. Although it did not meet the conditions of urethritis or conjunctivitis, etc. of reactive arthritis, it had various similar properties. Today, aseptic arthritis that occurs 2–4 weeks after gastrointestinal, genitourinary, or respiratory infections is defined as reactive arthritis. About 75% of patients with reactive arthritis are positive for HLA-B27 antigen, and it is classified as seronegative spondyloarthritis due to clinical similarities with AS, psoriatic arthritis, etc. The mechanism of arthritis caused by infection is not yet clear. When analyzing joint fluid, the causative bacteria are not detected, and considering the presence of bacterial antigens, antibodies against them, and inflammatory cells, it is thought to be the result of synovitis caused by a type of immune response. It can manifest acutely or chronically, and cases lasting more than 6–12 months are considered chronic [15, 16, 18].

In laboratory findings, rheumatoid factor is negative, ESR and CRP are normal or increased during the acute phase, and HLA-B27 antigen is positive in more than 75%. The findings of synovial fluid biopsy show inflammation and significant pannus formation is rare.

7.2.3.2 Imaging Findings of Reactive Arthritis

(1) General findings of reactive arthritis

In about 60–80% of reactive arthritis, radiological findings are normal in the early stages of the disease. The main sites of occurrence are small joints of the foot, calcaneus, ankle joint, and knee joint in the lower extremities, and SI joint, spine, and symphysis pubis, manubriosternal joint in the axial skeleton. Radiological findings show soft tissue swelling, periarticular osteoporosis, uniform decrease in joint space, bony erosion, and osteomyelitis. Soft tissue swelling is related to joint effusion, periarticular edema, and inflammation of the tendon and bursa. Local periarticular osteoporosis is accompanied in the acute phase of arthritis, and osteoporosis decreases if the joint disease recurs or persists for a long time. Loss of joint space is more frequently observed in small joints of the foot than in the knee and ankle joints. Bony erosion of the joint is observed in the trunk skeleton and limb skeleton, starting in the transitional part of the joint in the early stage and later invading the subchondral bone. The bone proliferation seen in reactive arthritis is a characteristic of all seronegative spondyloarthropathies and is an important finding that helps distinguish it from rheumatoid arthritis. In reactive arthritis, fluffy periostitis is not uncommonly observed in the metacarpal bones, metatarsal bones, phalangeal shafts, malleolar region, and knee joint. Also, enthesitis findings accompanied by bony erosion and periostitis are seen in the posterior and inferior surfaces of the calcaneus where the Achilles tendon and plantar fascia attach, ischial tuberosities, femoral trochanters, etc. Intra-articular bony ankylosis of reactive arthritis is observed in small joints of the hands and feet, but this finding is observed at a much lower frequency than in AS or psoriatic arthritis. In reactive arthritis, calcification or ossification of the tendon can also be seen [15, 16, 18].

(2) Site-specific imaging findings of reactive arthritis

(a) Foot

Reactive arthritis particularly invades the MTP joint and IP joint of the big toe asymmetrically and shows soft tissue swelling, osteoporosis, loss of joint space, and marginal area bony erosion and surrounding bone proliferation (Fig. 7.44). Bony erosion and bone pro-

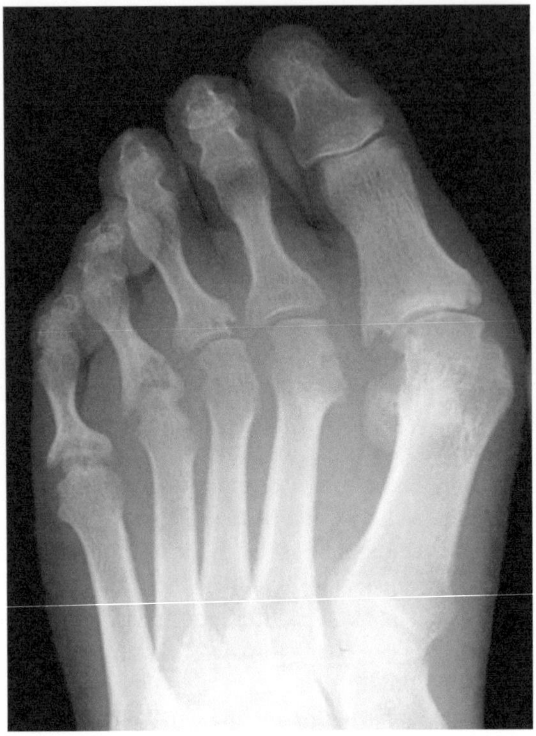

Fig. 7.44 Radiographic findings of the forefoot in reactive arthritis
Marginal area bony erosion, periosteal proliferation, and joint space narrowing are observed in all MIP joints including the big toe. The difference from rheumatoid arthritis is that there is bone proliferation without significant periarticular osteoporosis

liferation are also observed in the sesamoid bone. Bone periosteal reaction can be seen in the metatarsal shaft, and unlike other seronegative spondyloarthropathies, periarticular osteoporosis can be seen. In MRI, tenosynovitis of the tibialis posterior muscle, flexor hallucis longus muscle, flexor digitorum longus muscle is a characteristic finding of reactive arthritis [15, 16, 18].

(b) Calcaneus

Changes in the calcaneus are observed from the rear and the sole of the foot, and simultaneous invasion is frequent, observed in about 25–50%. It shows local bony erosion in the posterior superior part of the calcaneus related to retrocalcaneal bursitis and soft tissue swelling. However, retrocalcaneal bursitis occurs not only in reactive arthritis but also in rheumatoid arthritis, AS, and psoriatic arthritis. Reactive arthritis often shows tendinitis accompanied by Achilles tendon inflammation, but enthesitis at the attachment site of the Achilles tendon is rare compared to AS or psoriatic arthritis.

In cases where the boundary of calcaneus enthesitis is unclear and accompanied by bony sclerosis, it is mainly observed in seronegative spondyloarthritis and is rare in rheumatoid arthritis. Especially in reactive arthritis, it is characterized by significant findings of soft tissue swelling and periostitis in the heel area of the calcaneus and inflammatory enthesitis with unclear boundaries at the plantar fascia attachment site of the calcaneus, but when mature, the boundaries improve and it may be difficult to distinguish from the plantar calcaneal spur observed in normal people [15, 16, 18].

The abnormalities appearing on the sole of the calcaneus show shallow bony erosion and well-defined enthesitis in rheumatoid arthritis, while in AS, psoriatic arthritis, and reactive arthritis, they show significant bony erosion, surrounding bony sclerosis, and enthesitis with unclear boundaries at the ligament attachment site. Bone scans show increased isotope uptake in the rear and sole of the calcaneus. MRI shows findings of plantar fasciitis and tenosynovitis, retrocalcaneal bursitis behind the plantar fascia (Fig. 7.45).

(c) Knee joint

The knee joint always shows synovial fluid and often shows periostitis in the distal metaphyses of the femur. About 10% of long-standing reactive arthritis shows calcification of the medial collateral ligament (MCL) [16].

(d) Hands and wrist joints

In reactive arthritis, unlike psoriatic arthritis, upper limb involvement is rare.

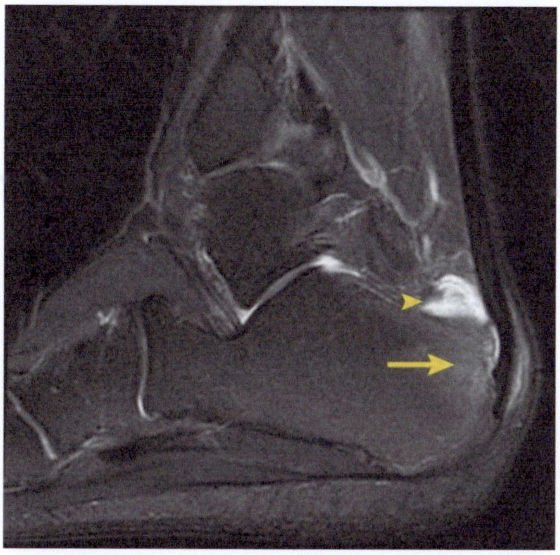

Fig. 7.45 Calcaneal enthesopathy in reactive arthritis: MRI findings
Retrocalcaneal bursitis is present (arrowhead) with adjacent calcaneal bone marrow edema (arrow) and Achilles tendonitis. However, plantar fascia thickening and plantar fasciitis are not accompanied

(e) Sternum and pubic symphysis
In the sternum, periostitis like fluff along with bony erosion is not uncommonly observed, and similar changes also occur in the pubic symphysis [15].

(f) SI joint
Sacroiliitis is common in reactive arthritis, and initially, about 5–10% show abnormalities in the SI joint, but after a few years, about 40–60% show abnormalities. Bilateral asymmetrical changes are typical, and unilateral changes are not uncommon (Fig. 7.46). The pattern of SI joint involvement and joint changes in reactive arthritis are similar to those in psoriatic arthritis [15, 16].

(g) Spine
The frequency of spinal abnormalities in reactive arthritis is lower than in AS or psoriatic arthritis, and paravertebral ossification is observed in about 15%. In reactive arthritis, paravertebral ossification often occurs in the lower thoracic or upper lumbar regions, which is rough and thick and asymmetrical. It is similar

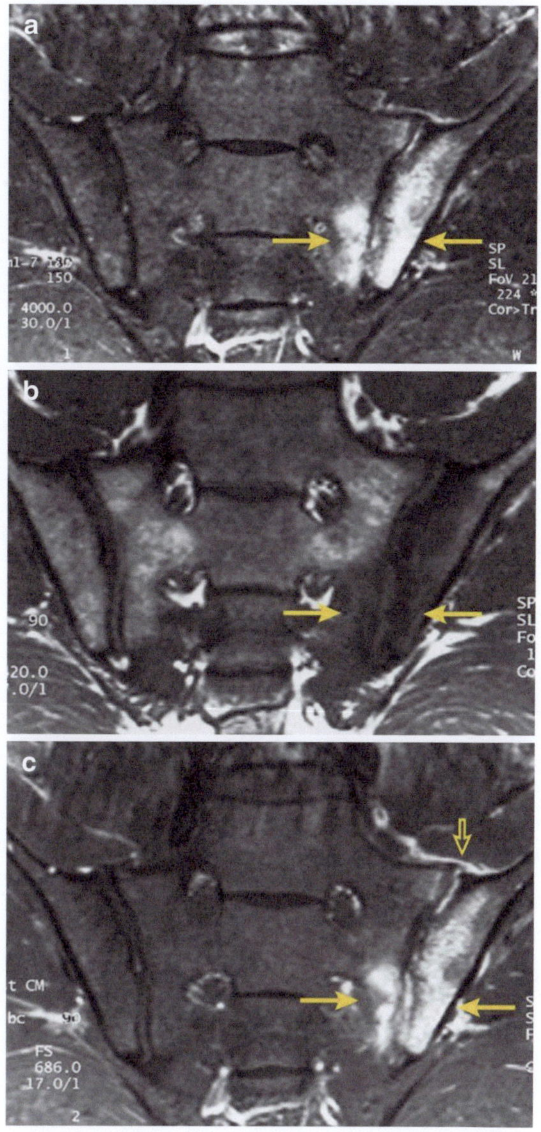

Fig. 7.46 MRI findings of sacroiliac joint arthritis in reactive arthritis: synovitis, bone marrow edema/osteitis, and capsulitis
There is synovitis in the left SI joint, and in the adjacent sacrum and ilium, high signal intensity in the STIR image (**a**), low signal intensity in the T1-enhanced image (**b**), and bone marrow edema/osteitis showing enhancement in the fat-suppressed contrast-enhanced T1-enhanced image (**c**) (arrow). In the fat-suppressed contrast-enhanced T1-nhanced image (**c**), there is accompanying synovitis showing enhancement of the synovium in the left SI joint (empty arrow). On the other hand, the right sacroiliac joint area shows normal findings. These findings suggest ipsilateral active spondylitis, which is distinguished from ankylosing spondylitis that relatively symmetrically invades the sacroiliac joints on both sides

to paravertebral ossification seen in psoriatic arthritis, as it originates from the vertebral body and intervertebral disc, and it is distinguished from the symmetrical syndesmophyte located within the boundaries of the spine observed in AS or inflammatory diseases. Also, in reactive arthritis, the findings of osteitis on the anterior surface of the vertebral body and the vertebral body appearing square, which are observed in AS, are relatively rare, and the findings of narrowing, hardening, and bone fusion of the facet joint can also be seen, but they are observed at a much lower frequency than AS [15, 16].

(3) Differential Diagnosis

Except for the more common cervical involvement in psoriatic arthritis when the SI joint and spine are involved, the findings of psoriatic arthritis and reactive arthritis are similar. However, unlike psoriatic arthritis, reactive arthritis has a lower frequency of involvement in the trunk skeleton and is rare in the upper extremities, and the characteristic finding is the asymmetrical involvement of the lower extremity joints. By considering the distribution pattern of the SI joint, the presence or absence of bony ankylosis, the presence or absence of osteitis on the anterior surface of the vertebral body, the involvement and presence or absence of bony ankylosis of the facet joint, and the shape of paravertebral ossification, it can be differentiated from AS [15, 16].

7.2.4 Inflammatory Bowel Disease-Associated Arthritis (Enteropathic Spondyloarthritis)

7.2.4.1 Clinical Findings and Laboratory Findings

It is known that enteropathic arthritis occurs in about 15% of patients with inflammatory bowel disease. The most common causes of enteropathic arthritis are ulcerative colitis and Crohn's disease, with ulcerative colitis being more common. Other causes include Whipple's disease and infectious enteritis. Both the extremities and the axial skeleton can be involved, and while peripheral arthritis is closely related to the activity of inflammatory bowel disease, spondylitis or spinal disease is not related to the activity of inflammatory bowel disease. Spinal involvement can precede or follow bowel disease.

The clinical symptoms due to musculoskeletal involvement are joint pain and effusion. The most commonly involved joints are the knees, ankles, elbows, and wrists, which improve spontaneously within 1–3 months, and there is no permanent damage to the peripheral joints. The involvement of the trunk skeleton is similar to the findings of AS, but the frequency of AS is 20 times higher than in normal people. In ulcerative colitis and Crohn's disease, cases with bilateral sacroiliitis without spinal involvement are about 4 times more common than cases with sacroiliitis and spondylitis together. Laboratory findings are negative for rheumatoid factor, and HLA-B27 is positive in about 10–12% [15, 16].

7.2.4.2 Imaging Findings of Inflammatory Bowel Disease-Associated Arthritis

Often, abnormalities in the spine and SI joint are discovered incidentally during small bowel or colon imaging. The radiological findings are similar to those of AS.

(a) SI joint

Radiologically, bilateral and symmetrical sacroiliitis is characteristic and the most common finding, showing bony erosion, bony sclerosis, and changes in joint space (Fig. 7.47). In the later stages, bony ankylosis of the SI joint occurs. The pattern of SI joint involvement is similar to AS. If the SI joint shows bilateral and symmetrical sacroiliitis or complete bony fusion, the possibility of AS or inflammatory bowel disease-associated arthritis is high, and if it invades unilaterally or the SI joint is invaded asym-

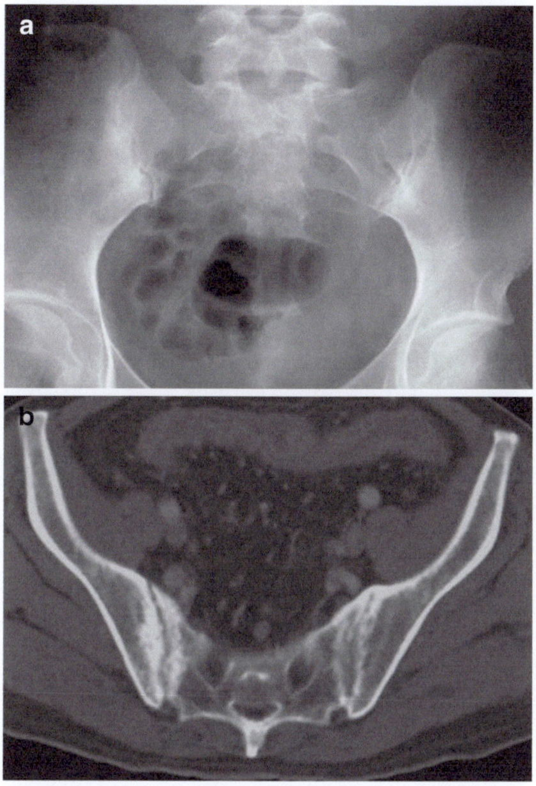

Fig. 7.47 Sacroiliac arthritis of ulcerative colitis (UC)
A. In the pelvic frontal photo, there is relatively symmetrical bony erosion, subchondral sclerosis, and joint space narrowing in both sacroiliac joints. B. In the axial CT, there is relatively symmetrical sacroiliac arthritis in both sacroiliac joints and findings of intra-abdominal ulcerative colitis are seen. The pattern of sacroiliac joint involvement in ulcerative colitis is similar to AS, making it difficult to distinguish between the two

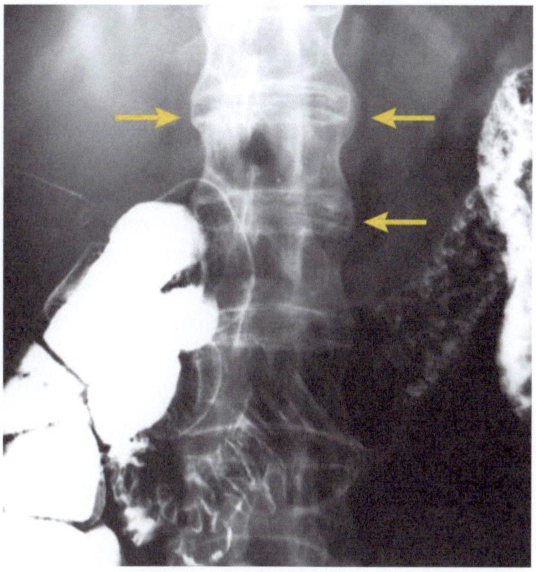

Fig. 7.48 Syndesmophyte of UC
In the lumbar frontal photo, syndesmophyte is formed vertically along the edge of the intervertebral disc, forming thin ossification within the boundary of the vertebral body (arrow). This finding is similar to the findings seen in ankylosing spondylitis. Colon contrast photo shows UC findings

metrically bilaterally, the possibility of psoriatic arthritis or reactive arthritis is high [15, 16].

(b) Spine
Osteitis accompanied by bony sclerosis at the corners of the upper and lower front of the vertebral body, the vertebral body appears square, and findings of bony ankylosis of the facet joint are observed. Inflammatory ossification of the outer fiber of the annulus fibrosus forms a syndesmophyte located symmetrically at the edge of the spine, gradually progressing to connect several upper and lower vertebral bodies, showing a characteristic bamboo shape (Fig. 7.48). This finding is similar to the findings observed in AS and is distinguished from the asymmetric, rough, thick, and paravertebral ossification that occurs away from the vertebral body and intervertebral disc seen in psoriatic arthritis and reactive arthritis [15, 16].

(c) Peripheral joints
Radiological findings in the peripheral joints of ulcerative colitis and Crohn's disease are nonspecific and often show soft tissue swelling and periarticular osteoporosis, and findings of bony erosion or narrowing of the joint space are rare. In the metaphyses-diaphyses area of long bones such as the radius, ulna, tibia, and fibula, bilateral linear periosteal new bone formation can be seen, which may indicate hypertrophic osteoarthropathy [15, 16].

7.2.5 Undifferentiated Spondyloarthritis

This is a diagnosis for cases that satisfy the ESSG classification criteria (Table 7.3) but do not belong to a specific form of disease such as AS, psoriatic arthritis, reactive arthritis, inflammatory bowel disease-associated arthritis, etc. It is known as the largest subgroup among spondyloarthritis, and studies on clinical aspects, treatment response, prognosis, etc. are ongoing. Unlike AS, the incidence is similar in men and women and the age of onset is wider, but onset after 55 years of age is rare. The most common initial symptoms are peripheral arthritis, back pain, and enthesitis in order, and the frequency of HLA-B27 antigen is 6–78%, showing a very wide range in various studies.

Bibliography

1. van der Linden S, Valkenburg HA, Cats A. Evaluation of diagnostic criteria for ankylosing spondylitis: a proposal for modification of the New York criteria. Arthritis Rheum. 1984;27:361–8.
2. Baek Han-Ju. Overview of Spondyloarthritis. In: Korean Rheumatism Association. Rheumatology, 2nd ed. Beommun Education 2018, pp. 227-232
3. Dean LE, Jones GT, MacDonald AG, Downham C, Sturrock RD, Macfarlane GJ. Rheumatology. 2014;53(4):650–7.
4. Inman R, Sieper J. Oxford textbook of axial spondyloarthritis. Oxford University Press; 2016. p. 19–28.
5. Rudwaleit M, van der Heijde D, Landewé R, Listing J, Akkoc N, Brandt J, et al. The development of Assessment of spondyloarthritis international Society classification criteria for axial spondyloarthritis (part II): validation and final selection. Ann Rheum Dis. 2009;68:777–83.
6. van der Heijde D, Lie E, Kvien TK, Sieper J, Van den Bosch F, Listing J, et al. ASDAS, a highly discriminatory ASAS-endorsed disease activity score in patients with ankylosing spondylitis. Ann Rheum Dis. 2009;68(12):1811–8.
7. Mandl P, Navarro-Compán V, Terslev L, Aegerter P, van der Heijde D, D'Agostino MA, et al. EULAR recommendations for the use of imaging in the diagnosis and management of spondyloarthritis in clinical practice. Ann Rheum Dis. 2015;74:1327–39.
8. Lee S. MRI features of axial spondyloarthritis and differential diagnosis: focusing on the spine and sacroiliac joint. J Rheumatic Dis. 2014;21(3):54–65.
9. Jee WH, McCauley TR, Lee SH, Kim SH, Im SA, Ha KY. Sacroiliitis in patients with ankylosing spondylitis: association of MR findings with disease activity. Magn Reson Imaging. 2004;22:245–50.
10. Rudwaleit M, Jurik AG, Hermann KG, Landewe R, van der Hiejde D, Braliakos X, et al. Defining active sacroiliitis on magnetic resonance imaging (MRI) for classification of axial spondyloarthritis: a consensual approach by the ASAS/OMERACT MRI group. Ann Rheum Dis. 2009;68:1520–7.
11. Bredella MA, Steinbach LS, Morgan S, Ward M, Diavis JC. MRI of the sacroiliac joints in patients with moderate to severe ankylosing spondylitis. Am J Roentgenol. 2006;187:1420–6.
12. Lacout A, Rousselin B, Pelage JP. CT and MRI of spine and sacroiliac involvement in spondyloarthritis. Am J Roentgenol. 2008;191:1016–23.
13. Sieper J, Rudwaleit M, Baraliakos X, Brandt J, Braun J, Burgos-Vargas R, et al. The Assessment of SpondyloArthritis international Society (ASAS) handbook: a guide to assess spondyloarthritis. Ann Rheum Dis. 2009;68(Suppl. 2):ii1–44.
14. Song IH, Carrasco-Fernández J, Rudwaleit M, Sieper J. The diagnostic value of scintigraphy in assessing sacroiliitis in ankylosing spondylitis: a systematic literature research. Ann Rheum Dis. 2008;67(11):1535–40.
15. Resnick D, Kransdorf MJ. Bone and Joint Imaging. 3rd ed. Elsevier Saunders; 2005. p. 267–315.
16. Yochum TR, Rowe LJ. Essentials of skeletal radiology. 2nd ed. Williams and Wilkins; 1996. p. 877–910.
17. Braun J, Bollow M, Sieper J. Radiologic diagnosis and pathology of the spondyloarthropathies. Rheum Dis Clin North Am. 1998;24:697–735.
18. Jacobson JA, Girish G, Jiang Y, Resnick D. Radiographic evaluation of arthritis: inflammatory conditions. Radiology. 2008;248:378–89.
19. Guglielmi G, Scalzo G, Cascavilla A, Carotti M, Salaffi F, Grassi W. Imaging of the sacroiliac joint involvement in seronegative spondylarthropathies. Clin Rheumatol. 2009;28:1007–19.
20. Aufdermaur M. Pathogenesis of 'squared bodies in ankylosing spondylitis. Ann Rheumatic Dis. 1989;48:628–31.
21. Lee JS, Lee S, Bang SY, Choi KS, Joo KB, Kim YB, et al. Stages of ankylosing spondylitis. J Rheumatol. 2012;39(12):2321–6.

8 Spinal Trauma

Sungjun Kim

Spinal injuries are generally described in three parts according to the injured area: upper cervical (from the skull base to the second vertebra), lower cervical (from the third to the seventh vertebra), and thoracolumbar. Various classifications have been proposed for each area depending on the type and mechanism of injury, which can suggest prognosis and treatment. Understanding these classifications is essential for determining which areas to focus on in imaging. However, various researchers have proposed different classifications, which can be confusing for beginners as to which classification to use for imaging evaluation. This chapter focuses on learning imaging findings according to the most widely used classifications in clinical practice for spinal injuries.

8.1 Upper Cervical

Upper cervical injury can be defined as an injury to the skull base-atlas-axis complex. Upper cervical injuries are typically classified according to the location of the injury, in the order of dissociation, atlas fracture, atlantoaxial injury, and axis fracture. For convenience of description and understanding, from here on, the skull base/occipital bone will be referred to as C0, the atlas as C1, the axis as C2, and the subsequent vertebrae as C3, C4, C5, C6, C7.

8.1.1 Anatomy and Biomechanics

To properly evaluate the imaging of upper cervical injuries, it is essential to understand the complex anatomy of this area. C0 and C1 are connected by bilateral occipitoatlantal joints. C1 and C2 are connected by bilateral articular processes, and the odontoid process of C2 is located between the anterior neural arch and transverse ligament of C1, acting as the axis of rotation for C1, and the transverse ligament prevents anterior and posterior displacement of C1 (Fig. 8.1).

The occipitoatlantal joint is a shallow ball-in-socket shape, with a shallower feature in the sagittal direction than in the coronal direction, which causes dislocation or displacement to occur anteriorly and posteriorly. Also, in the sagittal direction, the joint surface is round, so a significant part of the neck's flexion-extension occurs at this joint, but in the coronal direction, the joint surface is flat, so this joint is responsible for the neck's rotation.

The contribution to rotation is small (Fig. 8.2). The rotation of the neck mainly occurs at the atlantoaxial joint, with C1 rotating around the odontoid process of C2. The maximum range of flexion-extension, lateral bending, and rotation in the upper cervical spine is reported to be 25°, 5°,

S. Kim (✉)
Department of Radiology, Yonsei University College of Medicine, Seoul, Republic of Korea
e-mail: AGN70@yuhs.ac

© The Author(s), under exclusive license to Springer Nature Singapore Pte Ltd. 2025
H. S. Kang, J. W. Lee (eds.), *Spinal Imaging*, https://doi.org/10.1007/978-981-95-1386-4_8

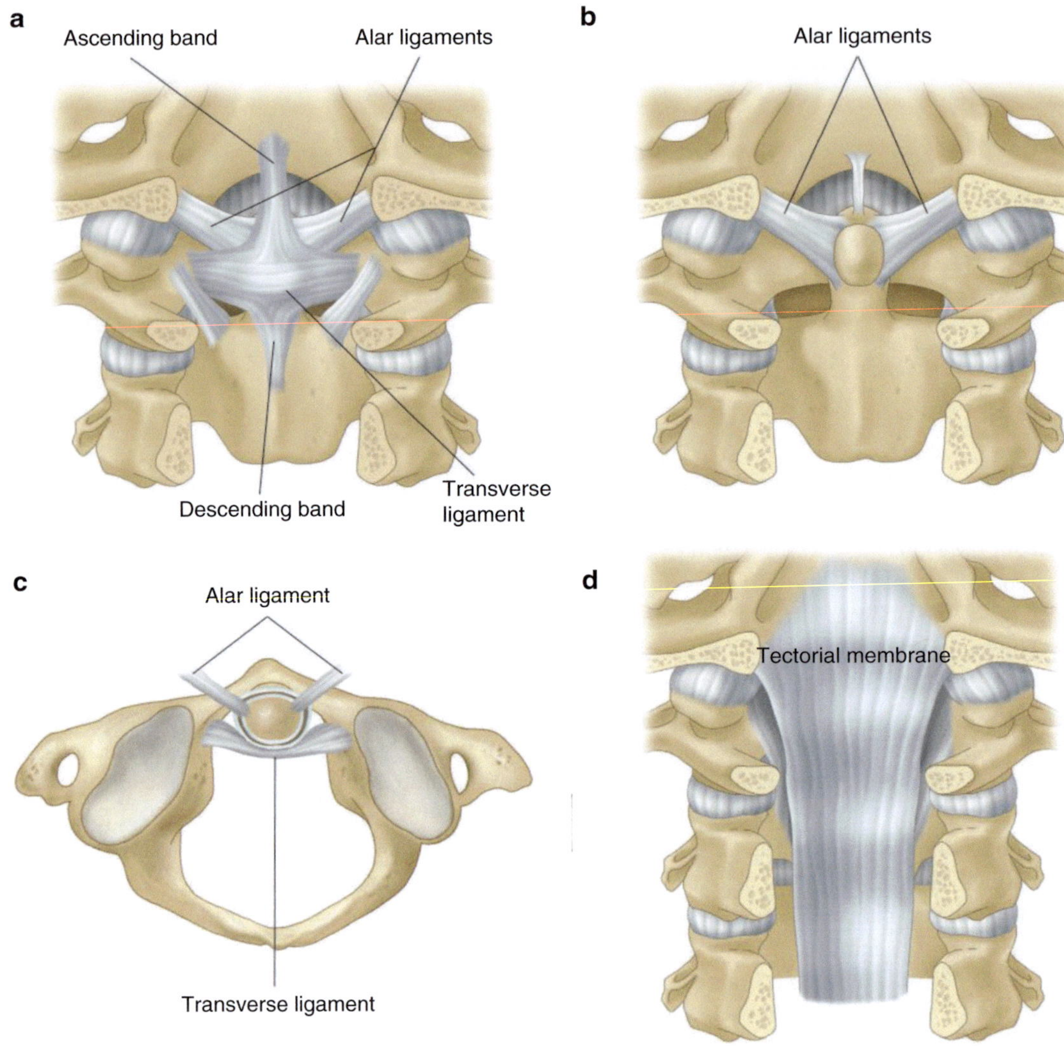

Fig. 8.1 Schematic of the major bone and ligament structures of the upper cervical spine
Schematic view from the back with the atlas and posterior parts of the skull and cervical spine removed (**a**, **b**, **d**) and a schematic view from above of the joint between the atlas and the odontoid process (**c**). The alar ligament forms a pair on each side, connecting the end of the odontoid process and the occipital condyle, limiting the rotation of the skull and atlas. The transverse ligament, combined with the ascending band and descending band, forms the cruciate ligament, which prevents anterior displacement of the skull and atlas from behind the odontoid process. The tectorial membrane is a structure continuous with the posterior longitudinal ligament, covering the posterior surface of the upper vertebra and the aforementioned cruciate ligament and alar ligament, attaching to the occipital bone, and preventing anterior displacement of the occiput and atlas

and 5° between C0 and C1, and 20°, 5°, and 40° between C1 and C2, respectively [1]. Understanding the normal range of motion of the upper cervical spine greatly aids in understanding the imaging of injuries in this area.

The upper cervical spine is supported by a somewhat complex combination of ligaments, which can be broadly divided into the following three groups (Fig. 8.1).

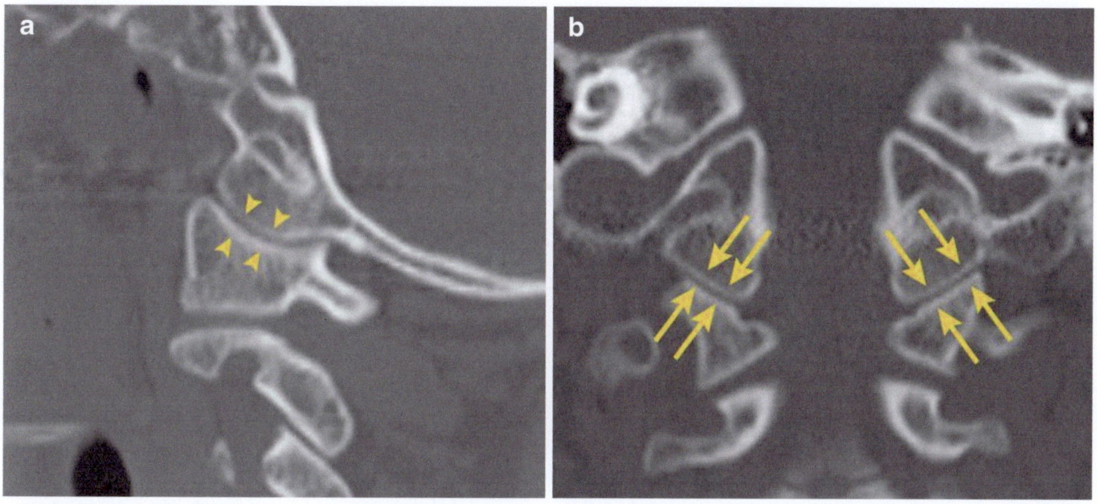

Fig. 8.2 The relationship between the articular surface and joint movement of the occipitoatlantal joint
Sagittal (**a**) and coronal (**b**) reformat CT images of the occipitoatlantal joint. The occipitoatlantal joint is shallow and round in the anterior-posterior direction (arrowhead), and deep and flat in the left-right direction (arrow), allowing more freedom of movement in the flexion direction than in the rotation direction

① The anterior atlantooccipital membrane and posterior atlantooccipital membrane connecting C0 and C1
② The tectorial membrane, two alar ligaments, and apical ligament connecting C1 and C2
③ The cruciate ligament located from C0 to C2

The anterior atlantooccipital membrane and posterior atlantooccipital membrane each connect the front and back of C1 and the foramen magnum. The tectorial membrane is a continuation of the posterior longitudinal ligament, attaching at the most proximal part to the front of the foramen magnum. The alar ligaments are a pair of structures that attach to the ends of the odontoid process and the inside of the occipital condyle. The apical ligament is a ligament that connects the end of the odontoid process and the front of the foramen magnum. The cruciate ligament is a cross-shaped ligament composed of the transverse ligament connecting the medial tubercle of the anterior neural arch of C1 and the ascending band (connected to the front of the foramen magnum) and descending band (connected to the body of C2) that intersect with it (Fig. 8.1).

Among these, the tectorial membrane, alar ligaments, and cruciate ligament play the most important roles in fixing C0–C1–C2 to each other, and the dislocation and dissociation of the upper cervical spine are closely related to the degree of damage to these three structures. The reason why pediatric patients are more vulnerable to injuries in this area is often found in the immature development of these structures [2].

8.1.2 Imaging Findings of Upper Cervical Spine Injuries by Location

8.1.2.1 Occipitoatlantal Dissociation

Occipitoatlantal dissociation is an injury that can only be encountered in a very small number of patients who have survived severe injuries that damage all the supporting ligaments mentioned above. The chance of the patient arriving at the hospital alive is slim, so its imaging is not commonly encountered. It has been reported to occur in 0.67–1% of all acute cervical injuries and 8% of fatal traffic accident patients [1].

The Traynelis classification is mainly used, which describes the injury as anterior displacement (type 1), vertical displacement due to distraction (type 2), or posterior displacement (type 3) depending on the direction in which the occipital bone has been displaced [3]. However, this classification has been criticized for merely describing the injury without suggesting a direction for treatment and for overlooking rotational injuries [2].

For imaging diagnosis, a simple lateral radiograph is first used. However, there can be difficulties in evaluating overlapping structures with simple radiographic images, and because it is not a common injury, it can be overlooked, requiring caution. It can be incidentally discovered in the flexion-extension view performed to evaluate instability at other levels. However, it is a very unstable injury, so if there is a clinical situation where occipitoatlantal dissociation is suspected, taking a flexion-extension image is absolutely contraindicated [1]. There are important simple radiographic findings not only in occipitoatlantal dissociation but also in all cervical injuries. It is necessary to check whether there is swelling in the soft tissue adjacent to the cervical spine in the lateral image. It is necessary to check whether the thickness of the soft tissue has thickened, and typically, if the thickness of the soft tissue in front of the cervical spine exceeds 7 mm at the C2 level, 5 mm at the C3 and C4 levels, 22 mm in adults, and 14 mm in children at the C6 level, it is considered abnormal, and the presence of a hematoma is suspected, indicating a high possibility of serious cervical injury, so care must be taken when handling the patient (refer to Figs. 8.3 and 8.21) [4].

There are various measurement methods for objectifying the diagnosis of occipitoatlantal dissociation, and these measurement methods should apply different reference values in children whose ossification has not yet been completed and adults whose ossification has already been completed. Three commonly used methods are described below (Fig. 8.4).

① Power's ratio: It is a method of evaluating the positional relationship between C0 and C1. The ratio of two measurements is calculated, and the measurement method is described in the explanation of Fig. 8.4. If this value is >1, it is read as abnormal.

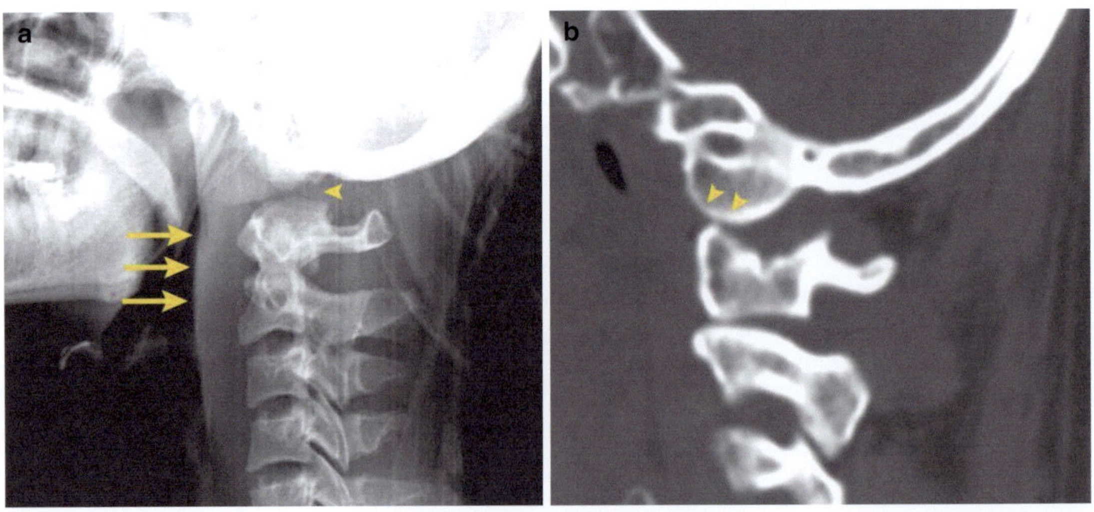

Fig. 8.3 Imaging findings of occipitoatlantal dissociation
(**a**) In the simple radiographic lateral view, the articular process (occipital condyle) of the occipital bone that should be seen above the atlas is not visible, and dissociation between the occipital bone and the atlas is seen (arrowhead). There is a posterior shadow of the soft tissue suggesting a hematoma in the anterior cervical region (arrow). (**b**) In the sagittal reformat CT image, you can see that the occipital condyle is subluxated anteriorly

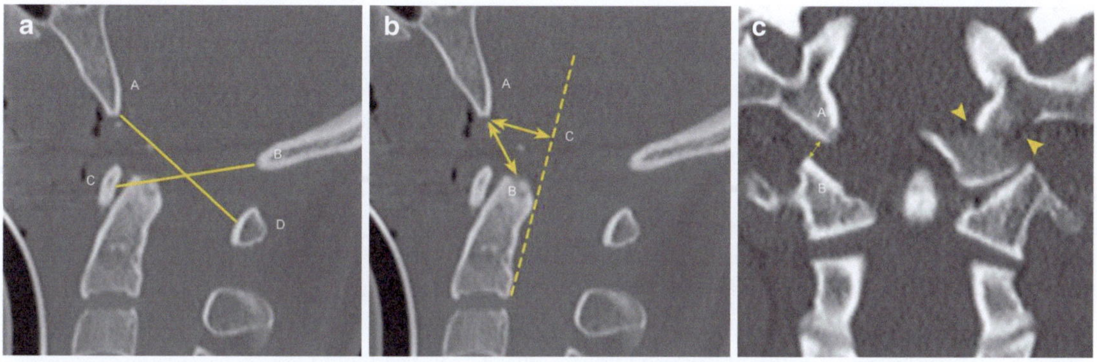

Fig. 8.4 Imaging diagnosis of occipitoatlantal dissociation. Sagittal (**a**, **b**) and coronal (**c**) reformat CT images in normal and abnormal states
A. Power ratio. The ratio of the distance between the basion (**a**) in front of the foramen magnum and the posterior neural arch (**d**) of the atlas to the distance between the opisthion (**b**) behind the foramen magnum and the anterior neural arch (**c**) of the atlas, i.e., AD/BC, is called the power ratio. If the power ratio is >1, it is abnormal. B. Harris method. The distance between the basion (**a**) and the end of the odontoid process (**b**) is called the "basion-dens interval (BDI)," and if this number exceeds 10 mm in those over 13 years old, or 12 mm in those under 13, it is abnormal. The shortest distance between the basion (**a**) and a line parallel to the posterior of the odontoid process (dotted line) is called the "basion-axis interval (BAI)," and if the basion is located more than 12 mm anterior or 4 mm posterior to the dotted line, it is abnormal. The measurement of BDI and BAI together is called the Harris method. C. Measurement of the articular process gap (condylar gap). If the distance between the articular process of the occipital bone (**a**) and the superior articular process of the atlas (**b**) is measured to be more than 4 mm, it is an abnormal finding that requires treatment. Note the accompanying fracture of the left occipital bone articular process in this patient (arrowhead)

② Harris method: It is a method of evaluating the positional relationship between C0 and C2. Two values are measured, the basion-dens interval (BDI) and the basion-axis interval (BAI), and the distance between the front of the foramen magnum (basion) and C2 is measured in the lateral image. The measurement method is described in the explanation of Fig. 8.4. BDI is read as abnormal if it is >10 mm in patients aged 13 and over, and 12 mm in children under 13 [5]. BAI is known to be constant regardless of age, and it is read as abnormal if the basion is located more than 12 mm forward or more than 4 mm backward [6]. These measurements are measured in principle from simple radiographic images of the cervical spine, but according to "The Guide Lines for the Management of Acute Cervical Spine and Spinal Cord Injuries," which has been used since its publication in 2002, if measurement is impossible in simple radiographic images, it is recommended to measure using CT or MRI [7].

③ Condylar gap measurement method: It is to measure the gap between the articular processes of the C0–C1 joint in the coronal reformat image of the CT image (Fig. 8.4), and it does not exceed 2.5 mm in normal, and it is read as a finding requiring treatment if it is >4 mm regardless of children and adults [2, 8, 9].

8.1.2.2 Atlas Fracture

Atlas fractures are not uncommon, accounting for 25% of upper cervical injuries in adults, 3–13% of all cervical injuries, and 1.3–2% of all spinal injuries [10]. Atlas fractures are often collectively referred to as Jefferson fractures, but if we adhere to the classical concept described in the first report, the term Jefferson fracture should only be used for burst fractures. Axial loading is known to be the most common fracture mechanism. Fractures occur at the weakest points, such as the connection between the lateral mass and the neural arch, or directly in the lateral mass where axial loading is transmitted [10].

Various classifications for Atlas fractures have been introduced, but the most commonly cited is the modified version of the classical Jefferson classification by Gheweiler et al. In this classification, type 1 is a fracture only in the posterior neural arch, type 2 is a fracture only in the anterior neural arch, type 3 is a fracture in the anterior neural arch accompanied by fractures in both posterior neural arches, and type 4 is a fracture in the lateral mass (Fig. 8.5). The most common is type 1 injury, followed by type 3 injury. As mentioned above, the classical burst fracture, the Jefferson fracture, should be limited to type 3 injuries [10–12].

The most important thing in evaluating Atlas fractures is whether the fracture is stable or unstable, and the key to this judgment is the status of the transverse ligament. Damage to the transverse ligament is directly related to C1–C2 instability, so when interpreting the instability of an atlas fracture, imaging findings that determine C1–C2 instability should also be interpreted.

The classical radiographic diagnosis for evaluating transverse ligament injury follows the "Spence rule." According to this rule, if the sum of the displaced lengths of both lateral masses of C1 in the open-mouth view exceeds 6.9 mm, it should be diagnosed as a rupture of the transverse ligament (Fig. 8.6) [13]. Also, the atlantodens interval (ADI) is used as a criterion for C1–C2 instability due to transverse ligament injury, which is normal up to 3 mm in adults and up to 5 mm in children where ossification is still in progress and the supporting structures in this area are less developed [1].

However, plain radiographs have limitations as they indirectly assess ligament damage. The only way to directly evaluate ligament damage with imaging is MRI (Fig. 8.7). In a study by Dickman et al., MRI showed very high sensitivity in diagnosing transverse ligament rupture. There are two notable points in this study. First, when the transverse ligament was directly damaged, the injury did not heal with external immobilization alone, but in the case of avulsion fractures at the ligament attachment site, the injury healed with external immobilization. This result is a natural outcome when applying

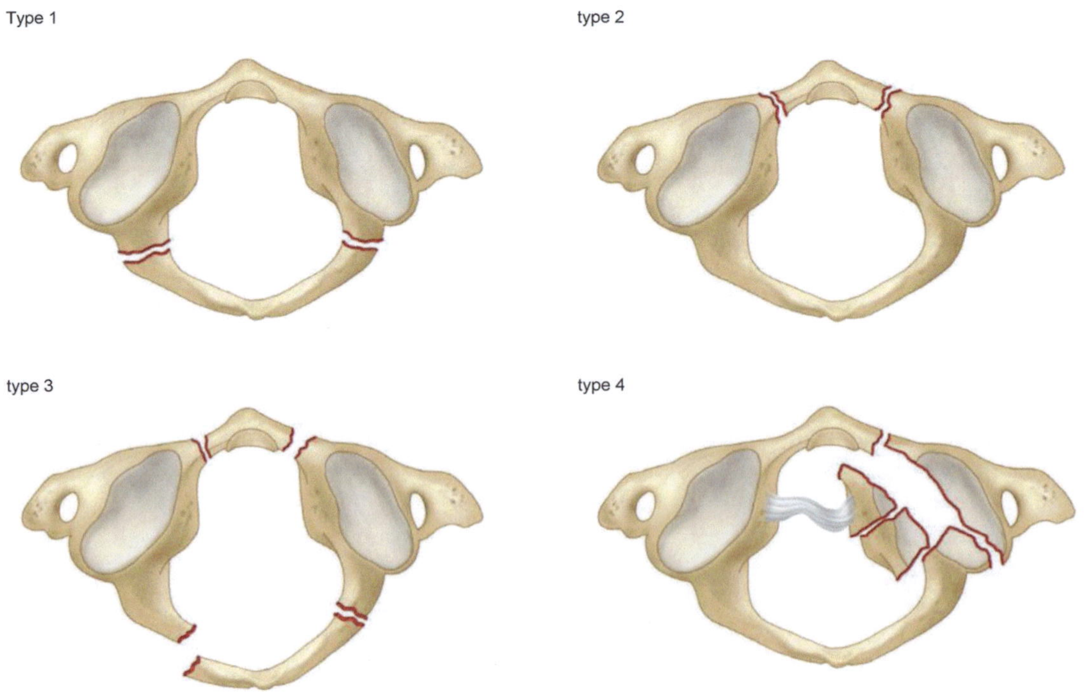

Fig. 8.5 Schematic of the Gheweiler classification (modified Jefferson classification)

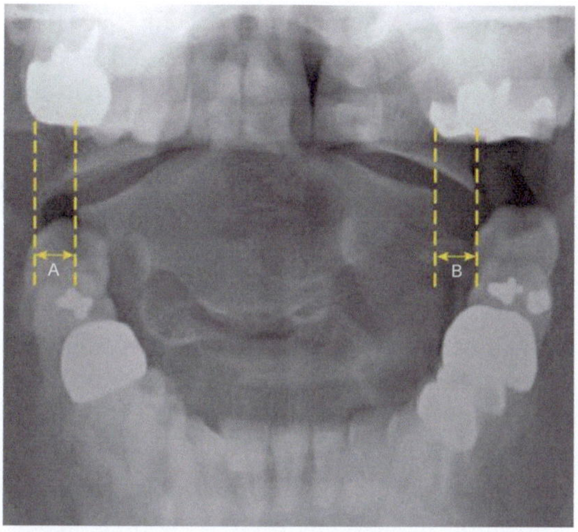

Fig. 8.6 Imaging findings of unstable atlas fracture (Spence's rule)
If the sum of the lengths of the lateral mass of C1 displaced bilaterally or unilaterally (A1B in the image) exceeds 6.9 mm in the open-mouth view, it should be diagnosed as a rupture of the transverse ligament or an avulsion fracture of C1 by the ligament, which means an unstable fracture. This is Spence's rule. In this case, The lateral mass of C1 has shifted to both sides, each showing a displacement of more than 5 mm, for a total displacement of more than 10 mm. This is an example of an unstable atlas fracture

the general principle that bone regeneration is more complete than ligament regeneration. Second, in this study, when only the Spence rule was applied to the target patient group, 61% of the the report suggests that damage to the transverse ligament was not diagnosed in simple radiographs, indicating that there may be limitations in evaluating the stability or instability of atlas fractures with simple radiographs alone [14].

8.1.2.3 Atlantoaxial Instability

When the transverse ligament-alar ligament-apical ligament-facet capsule complex is damaged, C1–C2 instability occurs. Cases of C1–C2 instability caused by trauma are rare because many patients do not survive. It is generally thought to occur when the neck is hyperflexed.

Imaging findings use flexion-extension lateral radiographs. The degree of displacement between C1 and C2 is obtained by measuring the aforementioned ADI. In adults, when all ligaments are not damaged, the displacement is within 3 mm, 3–5 mm when the transverse ligament is damaged, and more than 5 mm when all the afore-

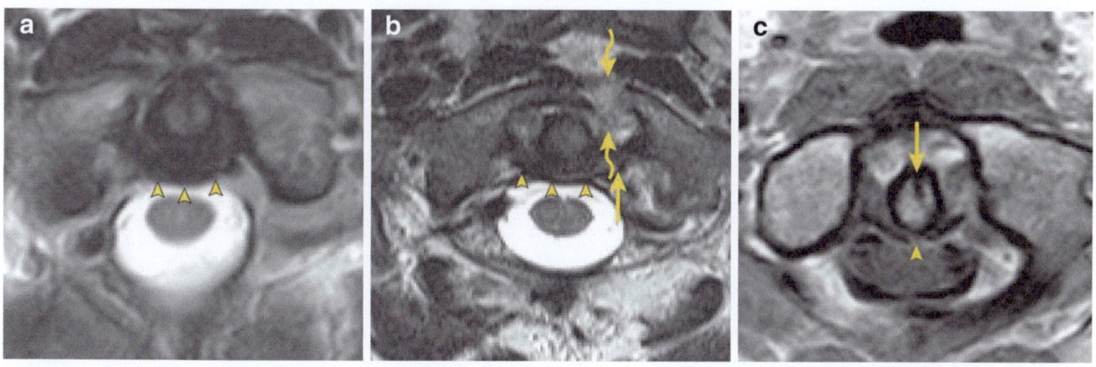

Fig. 8.7 Normal transverse ligament and injury findings in axial MRI images. (**a**) Normal transverse ligament (arrowhead). (**b**) The lateral mass of C1 has an avulsion fracture caused by the transverse ligament (arrow). Note the atlas fracture (curved arrow) associated with the undamaged transverse ligament (arrowhead). A case corresponding to type 4 in the Gheweiler classification. (**c**) The transverse ligament is damaged behind the odontoid process (arrow) (arrowhead)

mentioned ligaments are damaged (Fig. 8.8). In principle, if instability in this area is suspected and there is a possibility of spinal cord injury or swelling, taking flexion-extension images is absolutely contraindicated, but it can be performed if continuous neurological monitoring is possible during the examination [1].

8.1.2.4 Atlantoaxial Rotatory Fixation

Normally, 60% of neck rotation occurs at the C1–C2 joint, about 3–8° at the C0–C1 joint, and the remaining rotation occurs from the third cervical vertebra and below. In other words, the C1–C2 joint is responsible for more than half of neck rotation. According to a report by Pang et al., who studied the relationship between neck rotation and the range of motion between C1 and C2 using CT in children, when the head is rotated 0–23°, C1 rotates alone with C2 fixed, at 24–65° rotation, C1 and C2 rotate together but C1 rotates at a relatively larger angle, and at head rotations exceeding 65°, the angle between C1 and C2 remains around 43° while rotation occurs from the third cervical vertebra and below [15]. The reason why a lot of rotation occurs at C1–C2 is because the shape of the joint is conducive to rotation, but this shape makes it vulnerable to rotational injuries. The condition where the C1–C2 joint is fixed in a rotated state is called atlantoaxial rotatory fixation (hereinafter referred to as AARF). The word "fixation" in this diagnosis is an important concept. It means a "fixed" state of rotation, where it is impossible or limited to rotate in the opposite direction of rotation. This diagnosis is sometimes called "atlantoaxial rotatory subluxation," excluding the concept of "fixation," but since the C1–C2 joint shows a form of dislocation/subluxation even in normal people during rotation, it is more appropriate to include the concept of fixation in the diagnosis [1].

AARF patients show a very characteristic "cock-robin" posture. This refers to a posture where the head is turned to one side due to torticollis and at the same time, the head is tilted to the opposite side of the turned direction (Fig. 8.9). AARF in adults is usually due to severe trauma.

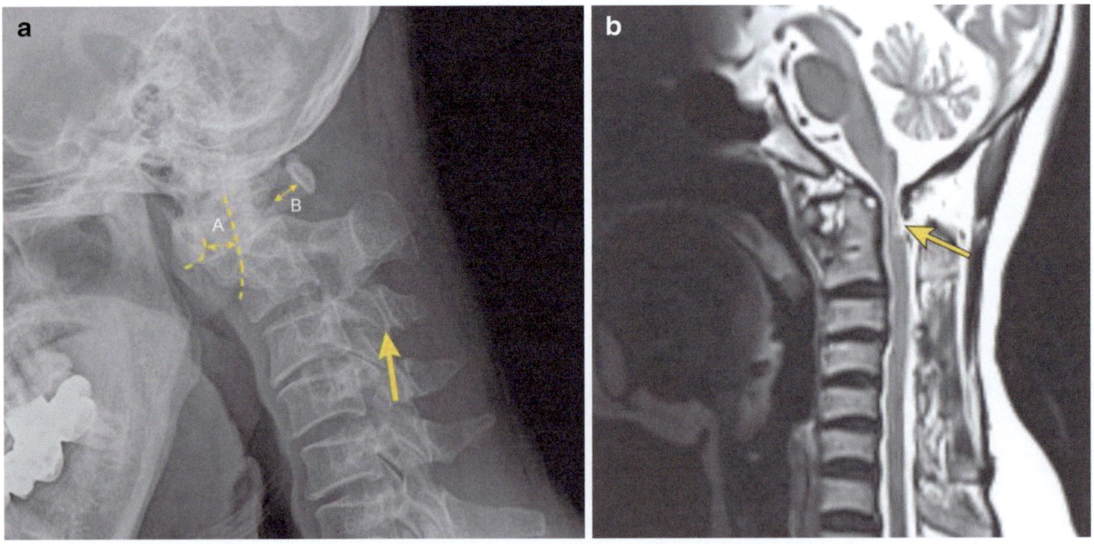

Fig. 8.8 Method of measuring the atlantodens interval (ADI) in simple radiographic lateral images
A. The distance (**a**, double arrows) between the posterior of the anterior neural arch of the atlas (anterior dotted line) and the anterior of the odontoid process of the axis (posterior dotted line) is called the ADI, and if it exceeds 3 mm in adults and 5 mm in children, it is diagnosed as atlas-axis instability. In this case, the ADI (**a**) was measured as 8 mm and diagnosed as atlas-axis instability, and the distance (**b**, double arrows) between the posterior of the odontoid process and the anterior of the posterior neural arch decreased, indicating that the central canal was narrowed due to the anterior displacement of the atlas. B. In the sagittal T2-weighted MRI image of the same patient as in image A, the narrowed central canal and the compressed spinal cord (arrow) can be seen

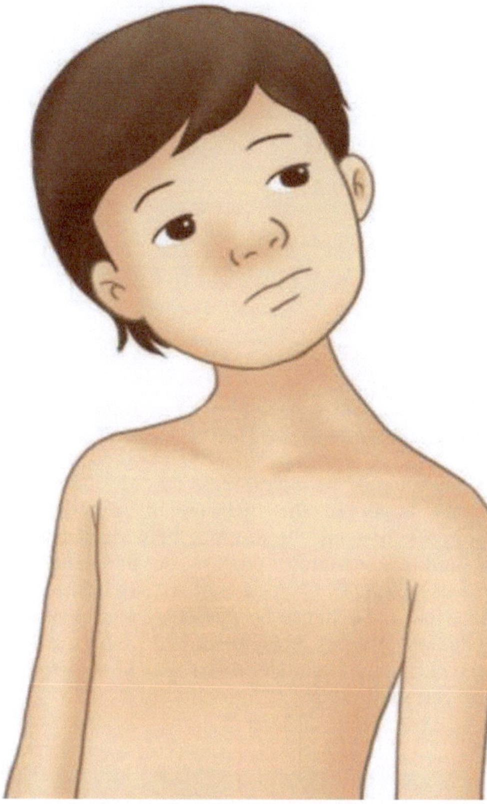

Fig. 8.9 Illustration of the "Cock-robin" posture
A characteristic posture seen in patients with atlantoaxial rotatory fixation. The head is tilted in the opposite direction to which it is turned

It occurs due to dislocation, and it is a very rare injury. On the other hand, in children, it can occur even with very mild trauma, and can also occur due to non-traumatic diseases such as infections. It is said that AARF occurring in children often improves with conservative treatment alone, regardless of the cause [1]. The treatment policy for AARF occurring in children should be determined based on how much reduction occurs when the abnormal rotation occurring in the C1–C2 joint is rotated in the opposite direction. Therefore, not only the diagnosis but also information about the degree of rotation reduction should be obtained from the image [15].

Plain radiographs are the primary diagnostic tool and are evaluated in the open-mouth view. Normally, when an image is obtained with the C1–C2 joint in a neutral position, the bilateral lateral masses of C1 should show a symmetrical shape, and the odontoid process should be located in the exact center between the lateral masses. The bilateral lateral masses of C1 have a long shape front and back, and they are arranged almost parallel to each other, but the distance between the lateral masses is further back than front, so it is not a complete parallel arrangement (Fig. 8.10). If the patient's neck is rotated and fixed and an open-mouth view is obtained, the size and shape of the C1 lateral mass appear asymmetrical, and the odontoid process appears to be skewed to one side. For example, if C1 is rotated to the right, the left lateral mass moves inward and appears larger, and conversely, the right lateral mass moves backward and appears smaller. Also, the front of the left lateral mass moves closer to the odontoid process, so the distance between the odontoid process and the lateral mass appears asymmetrically (the left is smaller than the right) (Fig. 8.10). One thing to note is that these findings can also be seen in normal when the neck is rotated, so the findings of mild AARF and a normal person who took an open-mouth view with the neck rotated can be the same. Therefore, if the above-mentioned abnormalities are seen in the open-mouth view, it is necessary to confirm the clinical information whether it is a patient with a possibility of AARF before making a diagnosis, and if there is a possibility, additional images should be obtained with the neck rotated to both sides to confirm whether the rotation is fixed. Generally, if AARF is suspected from imaging and clinical findings, obtain an open-mouth view with the neck rotated 15° to each side, and if the aforementioned asymmetrical findings persist, it should be diagnosed as AARF. Obtaining CT images in the same way is also a useful method [1, 16]. CT is being used usefully as a method that can measure the rotation angle more objectively and reliably in the diagnosis of AARF (Fig. 8.11). The diagnostic and treatment policy algorithm using CT proposed by Pang et al. is worth studying with interest. In this method, images are obtained by rotating the head in three positions: the direction in which the neck is rotated, the neutral direction, and the opposite direction in which the neck is

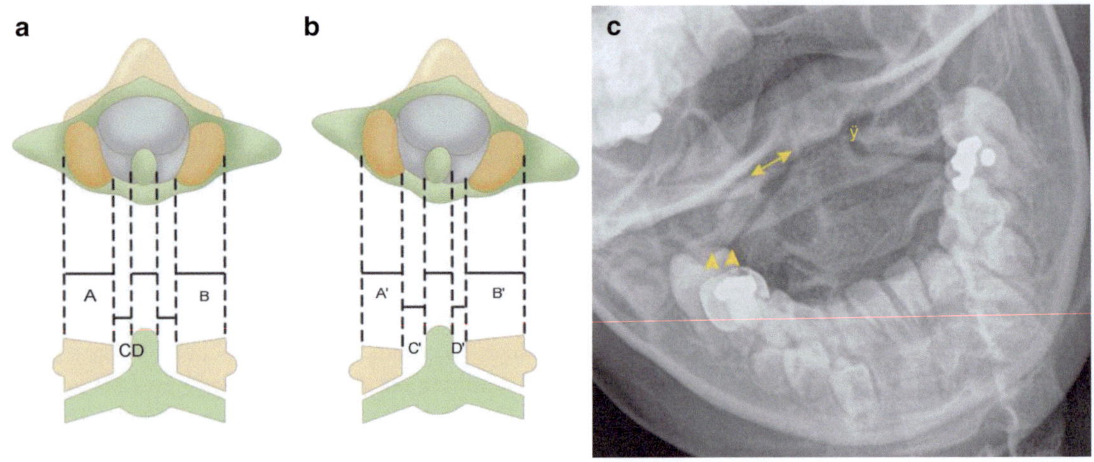

Fig. 8.10 Schematic (**a**, **b**) and case (**c**) for explaining the open-mouth view findings of atlantoaxial rotatory fixation

A. When the atlas-axis joint is in a neutral position (top image), the size of the lateral mass on both sides is symmetrical in the open-mouth view (bottom image) (A 5 B) and the distance between the lateral mass and the odontoid process is also symmetrical (C 5 D). B. When the atlas rotates to one side in the atlas-axis joint (top image), the lateral mass on one side appears relatively larger in the open-mouth view (bottom image) (A9, B9) and the distance between the lateral mass and the odontoid process on the same side decreases (C9, D9). C. A case of AARF. In the open-mouth view, the distance between the lateral mass and the odontoid process is asymmetrical (double arrows, asterisks), and the right lateral mass can be seen to have shifted (arrowhead)

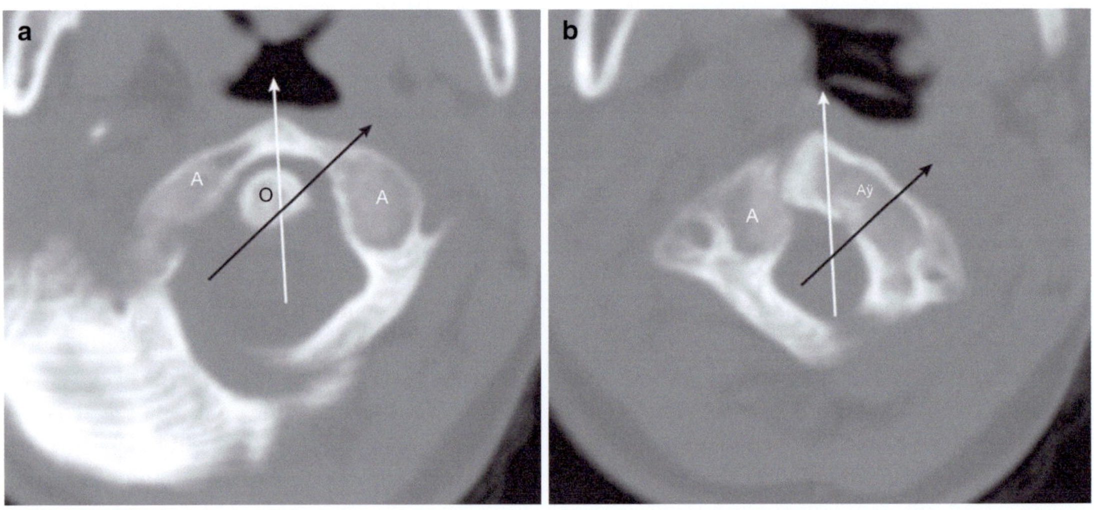

Fig. 8.11 CT findings of atlantoaxial rotatory fixation (AARF)

This is a CT case of an AARF patient whose head is fixed rotated to the right, showing the level of the axial CT image (**a**) where the atlas (A) and odontoid process (O) are visible together, and the axial CT image (**b**) at the axis (A′) level. In both images, the white arrow indicates the frontal direction of the atlas, and the black arrow indicates the frontal direction of the axis, and it can be seen that the atlas is rotated to the right based on the axis. These images are all images taken by rotating the patient's head in the opposite direction of the rotation, and it was possible to confirm the "rotatory fixation" state, which is a non-reduced rotation state, with CT rotated, and in each image, the rotation angle of C1 and C2 based on the neutral line, and the C1–C2 between. The reversibility of C1–C2 rotation is determined by measuring the rotation angle, and it is recommended to determine the treatment policy based on this [15].

The classification of AARF often uses the classification system proposed by Fielding and others, considering the damage to the transverse ligament and alar ligament [1, 17].

Type 1 is the most common form described in the research of Fielding and others, which means a fixed state within the normal range of motion, and is the case where there is no damage to other support structures including the transverse ligament and alar ligament. Type 2 is a form in which AARF shows an ADI of 3–5 mm in width, that is, a form accompanied by anterior displacement of C1, and is the case accompanied by damage to the transverse ligament, and is described as the second most common form. Type 3 is accompanied by anterior displacement of C1 exceeding 5 mm of ADI, and is the case where not only the transverse ligament but also the alar ligament, apical ligament, and C1–C2 facet joint are damaged. Type 4 is described as the rarest form, and is the case where C1 shows posterior displacement due to nonunion of the odontoid process (Fig. 8.12) [17].

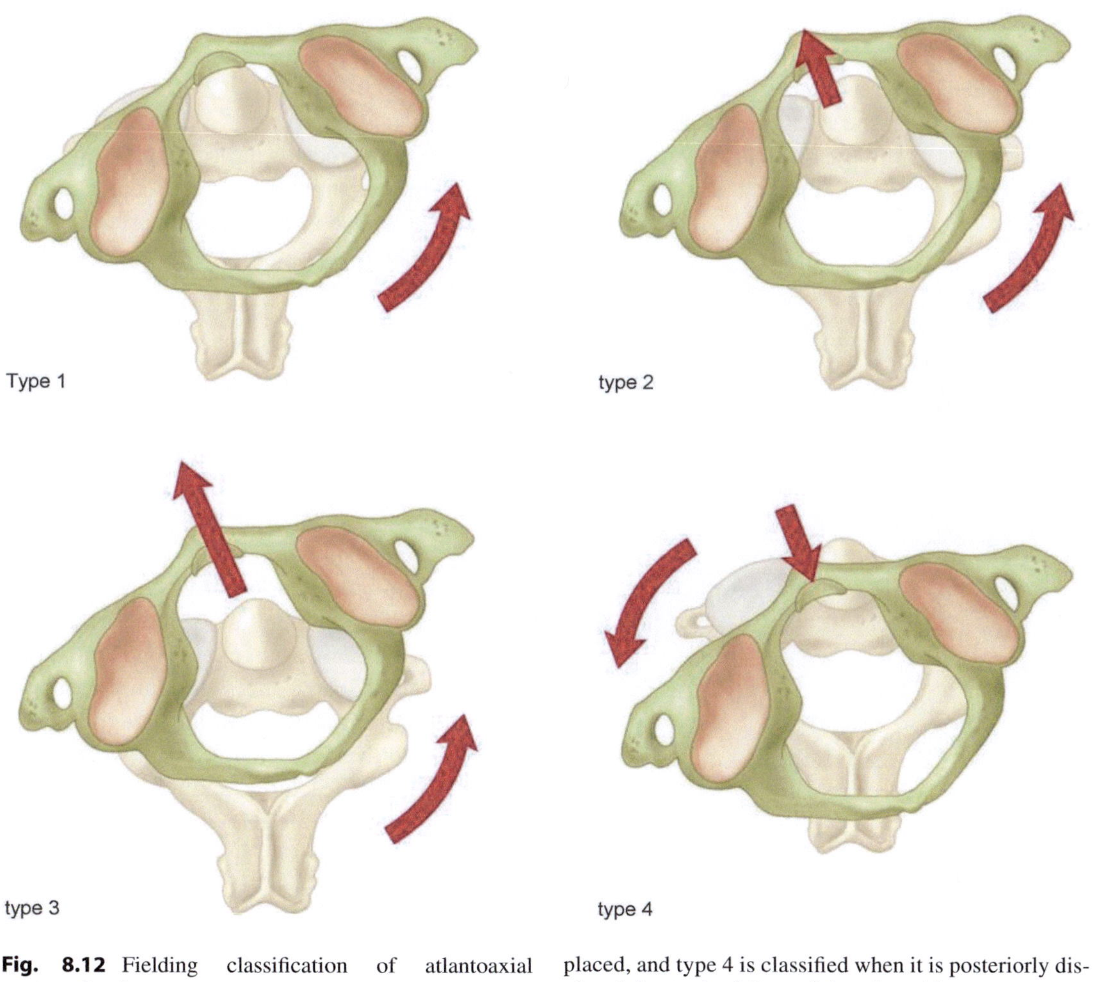

Fig. 8.12 Fielding classification of atlantoaxial rotatory fixation
Type 1 is when the atlas is not anteriorly or posteriorly displaced, type 2 and 3 are when it is anteriorly displaced, and type 4 is classified when it is posteriorly displaced due to the failure of the odontoid process

8.1.2.5 Axis Fracture

Axis fractures account for 20% of all cervical fractures [18]. and are often associated with neurological deficits or acute death. According to a study by Greene and others, out of 1,820 cases of cervical fractures, 340 were axis fractures, and 8.5% of these axis fractures were associated with neurological deficits, and 2.4% were associated with acute death [19]. In this study, it was also reported that out of 340 axis fractures, 199 (59%) were odontoid process fractures, 74 (22%) were hangman's fractures, and the remaining 64 (19%) were axis body fractures. The odontoid process fracture and Hangman's fracture, which show a high frequency and characteristic fracture pattern, are described below [19].

Odontoid Process Fracture

The odontoid process fracture is the most common type of fracture in the axis. Its classification is most widely used as the Anderson classification, which includes the subtype added by Hadley and others in 1988 to the classification proposed by Anderson and D'Alonzo in 1974 [20] (Fig. 8.13). In 2005, Grauer and others proposed a modified classification that added several subtypes according to the treatment policy, but this classification still needs further validation [18, 21], so it will be described according to the Anderson classification here.

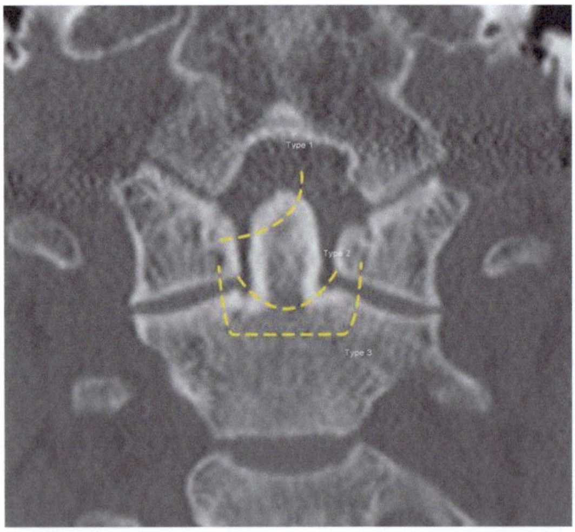

Fig. 8.13 Anderson classification of odontoid process fractures
Type 1 is a very rare oblique fracture at the end of the odontoid process,Type 2 is more common among types 2 and 3. Type 2 occurs at the waist or base of the odontoid process and has the highest frequency of nonunion among the three types, and type 3 is when the fracture of the odontoid process deeply invades the cancellous bone of the axis body, and the frequency of nonunion is lower than type 2

The Anderson classification consists of three basic types and one subtype. Type 1 is a fracture that occurs obliquely at the top of the odontoid process and is thought to be an avulsion fracture by the alar ligament. It is the rarest form among the three types of Anderson classification and is seen in only 1–3% of odontoid process fractures [19, 20]. Type 2 is a fracture of the waist and base of the odontoid process, which is the most common fracture pattern reported with a frequency of about 59% of odontoid process fractures in the study by Greene and others (Fig. 8.14) [19]. The frequency of nonunion in this area is higher compared to types 1 and 3. This is explained by the following three reasons [1].

① The area covered by the transverse ligament can interfere with union due to the ligament getting involved in the fracture surface.
② The frequency is high for the same reason that there is a lot of nonunion of intra-articular fractures due to the presence of a lot of synovial fluid around the odontoid process.
③ The cross-sectional area of the fracture is smaller than that of type 3, so the amount of blood flow delivered to the fracture site is small, reducing the possibility of union.

Type 2A fracture, a subtype of type 2, is a fracture form reported by Hadley et al. It is reported to occur in about 5% of type 2 fractures, referring to comminuted fractures accompanied by small fracture fragments in the anterior or posterior of the fracture site. It has been reported that these are often very unstable fractures compared to general type 2 fractures, and regardless of the direction of the fracture line or the degree of displacement of the fracture fragment, the possibility of nonunion is very high, so it is accepted that fixation through surgical treatment is needed early. Type 3 is when the fracture of the odontoid process deeply invades the cancellous bone area of the axis body, and it has been reported to occur

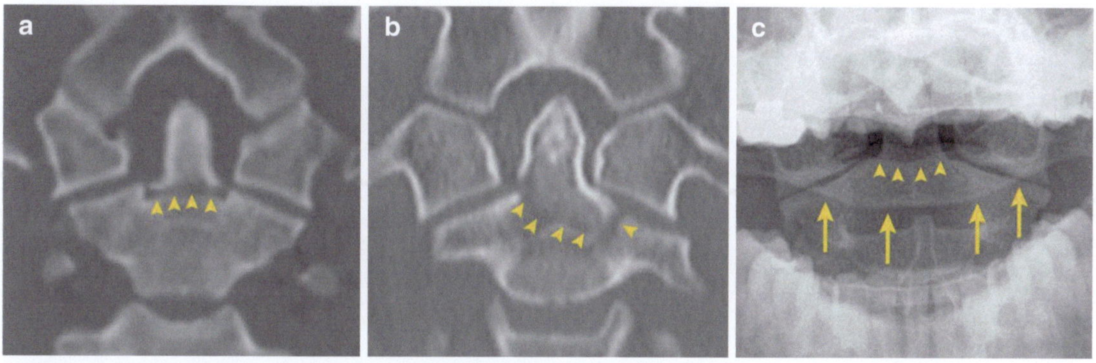

Fig. 8.14 Imaging findings of odontoid process fractures
(**a**) Coronal reformat CT image of Anderson type 2 odontoid process fracture (arrowhead). (**b**) Coronal reformat CT image of Anderson type 3 odontoid process fracture (arrowhead). (**c**) Pitfalls that can be mistaken for the odontoid process in a normal open-mouth view. The line that appears overlapping with the neural arch (arrowhead) of the atlas or the occipital bone (arrow) can be mistaken for a fracture of the odontoid process

at a frequency of about 39–42% of odontoid process fractures. Since the cross-sectional area of the fracture surface is relatively large and the blood supply is abundant, the frequency of nonunion is smaller than that of type 2 (Fig. 8.14).

Odontoid process fractures are primarily evaluated with an open-mouth view and cervical lateral images. In diagnosing odontoid process fractures through an open-mouth view, it should be noted that vertical hypoechoic lines formed by the incisors, soft tissue, the neural arch of C1, the occipital bone, etc., can be mistaken for fractures as they pass through the odontoid process (Fig. 8.14). If these lines cannot be distinguished from fractures, an open-mouth view should be repeated or a CT should be performed. It is important to distinguish between the two common types 2 and 3, which have different prognoses and treatment principles, in the images, but there have been reports of low interobserver and intraobserver agreement in distinguishing these two through simple radiographs, and it has been reported that this discrimination agreement increases when using CT.

Knowledge of the two accessory bones, os odontoideum and ossiculum terminale, is very important in diagnosing fractures of the odontoid process.

The odontoid process begins ossification between 1 and 5 months of gestation, and in newborns, a wide cartilaginous plate is located between this ossification center and the ossification center of the C2 body. In the image, this cartilaginous plate begins to appear as a hypoechoic line at least under the age of 3, and by the age of 8 at the latest, the ossification centers unite and disappear. However, if the hypoechoic line between the odontoid process and the C2 body does not disappear and remains as an accessory bone, it is called os odontoideum, and in this case, it is not easy to distinguish nonunion of fractures through images. The method of distinguishing fractures and os odontoideum when bone fragments are visible is the same as the general method of distinguishing fractures and accessory bones. In order to diagnose a fracture, cortical bone must be visible on the fracture surface of the bone fragment.

It should not be visible, and if the cortical bone completely surrounds the bone fragment, it is interpreted as os odontoideum. There are two main theories about the mechanism of os odontoideum, the congenital hypothesis and the traumatic hypothesis, with the traumatic hypothesis currently gaining more support. As shown in the schematic diagram of Fig. 8.15, the cartilagenous plate between the odontoid process and the axis body is located below the C1–C2 facet joint, so for the congenital hypothesis, i.e., the hypothesis that the ossification center did not fuse for congenital reasons to be supported, the gap between the os odontoideum and the axis body should be

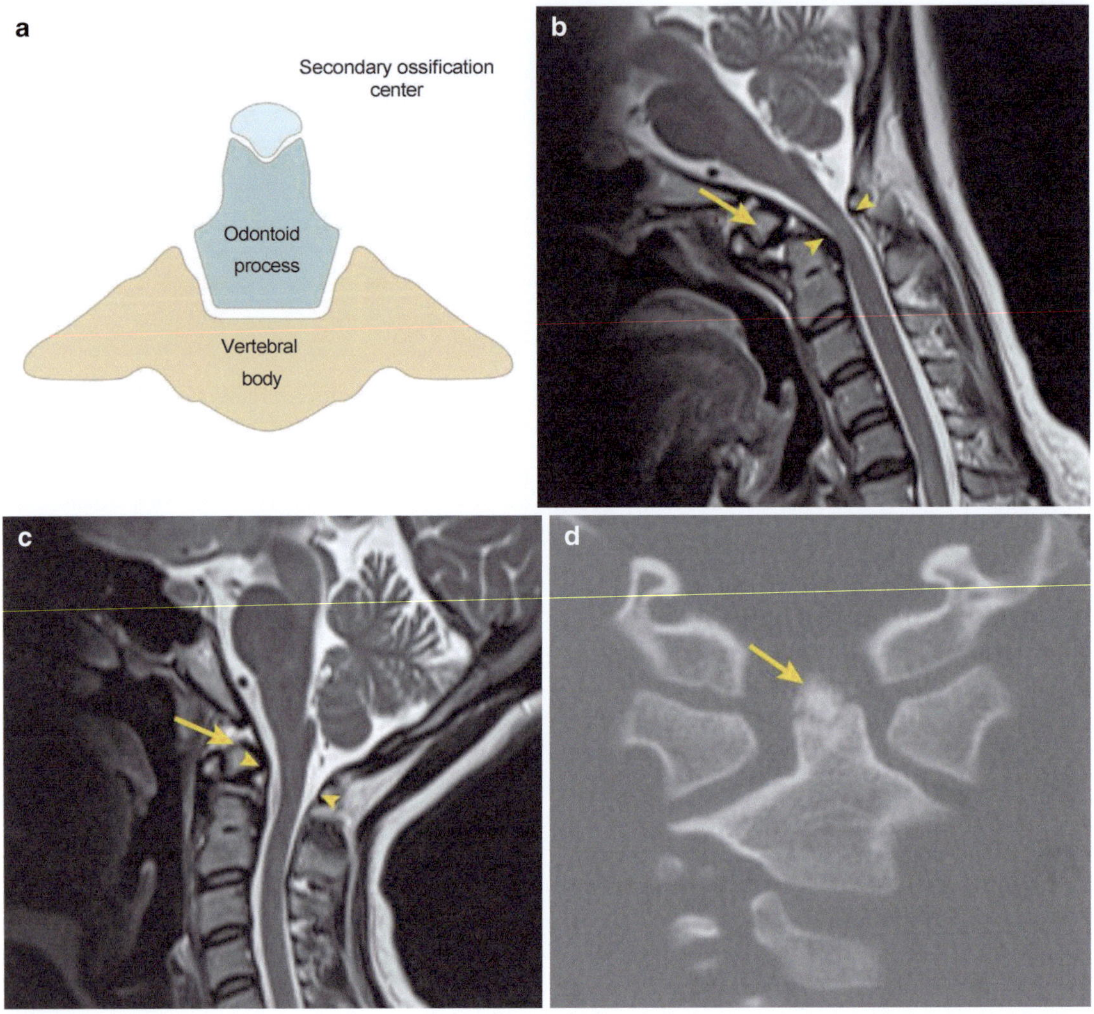

Fig. 8.15 Schematic of the axis' primary ossification center and secondary ossification center, and imaging findings of os odontoideum and ossiculum terminale
(**a**) The odontoid process and the vertebral body originate from different primary ossification centers and usually fuse together between the ages of 3 and 6. As shown in the schematic, the fusion point between the odontoid process and the vertebral body is lower than the typical lower margin of the os odontoideum, so the os odontoideum is between the ossification centers. The congenital theory that it occurs because there is no fusion is losing support. A secondary ossification center occurs at the end of the odontoid process between the ages of 3 and 6 and fuses with the primary ossification center of the odontoid process around the age of 12. The bone fragment that results from this secondary ossification center not fusing with the primary ossification center is called ossiculum terminale. (**b**, **c**) Cases of instability associated with os odontoideum. In the sagittal T2-enhanced images taken in the flexion state (**b**) and extension state (**c**) of the same patient, the os odontoideum (arrow) is visible, and the central canal (central canal, arrowhead) is relatively narrowed in the flexion state than in the extension state, compressing the spinal cord. (**d**) Case of ossiculum terminale. Ossiculum terminale (arrow) incidentally found in the coronal reformat image of the axis

located below the C1–C2 facet joint. However, based on the fact that this gap is usually seen above the facet joint, the traumatic hypothesis is given more weight than the congenital hypothesis (Fig. 8.15a) [22]. Os odontoideum may not cause symptoms, but it is often associated with symptoms such as pain or myelopathy associated with C1–C2 instability. Flexion-extension lateral images are used to evaluate C1–C2 instability, and CT is used when detailed evaluation is needed for surgical planning or when the quality of simple radiographic images is not good. Also,

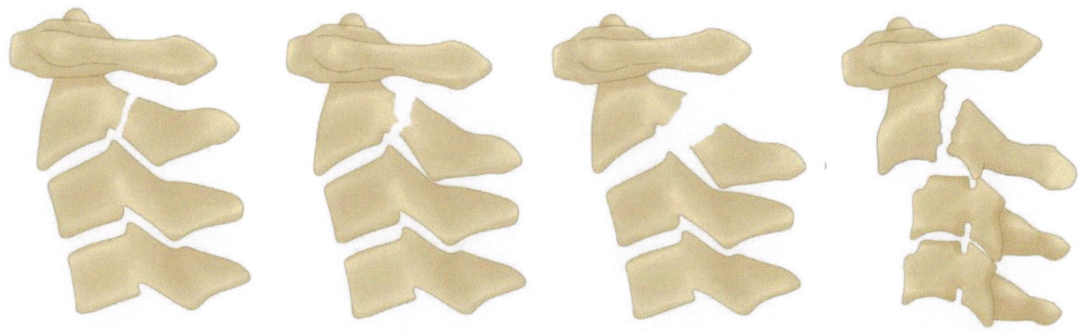

Fig. 8.16 Levine classification of Hangman's fracture Type 1 is when there is <3 mm of displacement at the ismuth fracture site. Type 2 is when there is 3 mm or more of displacement and slight angulation at the ismuth fracture site, and damage to the C2-3 disc and compression fracture of C3 can be accompanied. Type 2A is when there is severe angulation of 15° or more in a state where there is almost no anterior displacement of the vertebral body, accompanied by severe damage to the intervertebral disc. Type 3 is the most unstable case, accompanied by dislocation of the facet joint between C2 and C3, showing facet locking

MRI images should be obtained to evaluate associated myelopathy, etc. (Fig. 8.15b, c) [22].

The end of the odontoid process has a separate secondary ossification center, which is known to start ossification between the ages of 3 and 6 and complete fusion with the odontoid process at the age of 12 (Fig. 8.15a) [23]. The small bone fragment at the end of the odontoid process, which appears as a result of non-fusion, is called ossiculum terminale (Fig. 8.15d), and it is generally thought to have no association with trauma or instability of the upper vertebrae [22].

Hangman's Fracture

Hangman's fracture is the second most common type of axis fracture. It is characterized by a fracture of the pars interarticularis (isthmic portion) of the axis and soft tissue damage between the axis and the third vertebra. Previously, this type of fracture was thought to occur frequently in people who were hanged, hence the name. However, in modern times, there are more reports of fractures caused by traffic accidents related to trauma, and it is also called "traumatic spondylolisthesis of the axis." But since Schneider et al. first used the term "hangman's fracture" for traumatic fractures in 1965, regardless of the mechanism, it tends to be commonly called Hangman's fracture. Fractures at the time of damage in the form of hanging occur due to hyperextension and distraction mechanisms, while most fractures caused by falls or traffic accidents occur due to overextension and compression mechanisms [18].

The morphological classification of Hangman's fracture has been proposed based on the classification by Francis et al. or Effendi et al., and the classification proposed by Levine et al. in 1985 based on Effendi's classification is widely used because it is easy to associate with treatment methods (Fig. 8.16) [1, 24]. Only type 1 is considered a stable fracture, and types 2 and above are considered unstable because there is instability between the axis and the third vertebra. It is considered as an unstable fracture. In the paper where Levine proposed this classification, type 2 fractures were the most common, accounting for more than half of the cases (Fig. 8.17), followed by type 1, type 3, and type 2A in order [1]. However, there is a disagreement on this frequency, with some arguing that type 1 is more common and others arguing that type 2 is more common [19, 25].

8.2 Subaxial Cervical Spine

Subaxial cervical spine injuries are generally defined as injuries from C3 to C7, often referred to as "subaxial cervical spine injury." Subaxial

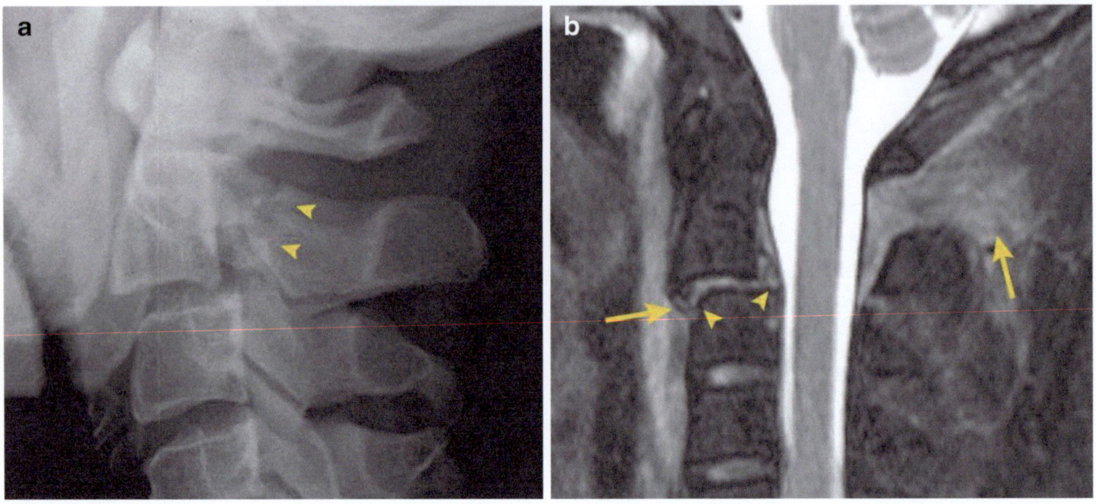

Fig. 8.17 Case of Levine type 2 Hangman's fracture. (**a**) On the lateral simple radiograph, there is a fracture at the ismuth of the axis (arrowhead), and the axis has moved forward. (**b**) On the sagittal fat-suppressed T2-enhanced image, damage to the disc (arrowhead) and swelling of the anterior and posterior ligament complex due to ligament damage (arrow) are visible

cervical spine injuries account for over 65% of all cervical fractures and over 75% of dislocations [26]. Fractures occur most frequently at C6 and C7, and dislocations occur most frequently between C5–C6 and C6–C7 [27]. Understanding the classification of injuries based on anatomical structure and biomechanics is essential for imaging interpretation that helps predict prognosis and treatment policy.

8.2.1 Anatomy and Biomechanics

The subaxial vertebrae from C3 to C7 show a relatively consistent shape. The vertebral body is connected to the lateral mass and lamina through the pedicle on both sides. The transverse process is formed on the anterolateral side of the lateral mass. The vertebral artery foramen is located on the transverse process, through which the vertebral artery passes. Also, the cervical nerve passes over the transverse process (Fig. 8.18a, b). The lateral mass consists of the superior articular process and the inferior articular process, and it appears rhomboid-shaped in lateral plain radiographs or sagittal reformatted CT images. As in the thoracic and lumbar spine, the inferior articular process of the cervical spine is located behind the superior articular process of the vertebra below, arranged like overlapping tiles, supporting the upper cervical spine during neck flexion (Fig. 8.19). The disc between the cervical vertebrae is the most important non-bone structure supporting the cervical spine. In addition to the disc, the anterior longitudinal ligament (ALL), posterior longitudinal ligament (PLL), ligamentum flavum, interspinous ligament, and supraspinous ligament are nonosseous supporting structures. The interspinous ligament and supraspinous ligament are continuous structures that form the nuchal ligament superiorly and attach to the structures of the occipital bone and the posterior-cervical transition area. The facet joint capsule is also an important supporting structure (Fig. 8.18C, D).

Most of the rotation and flexion of the neck occur in the upper cervical spine, but in the subaxial cervical spine, each movement segmentation allows 8–10° degrees of flexion-extension and 3–5 degrees of rotation. However, paradoxically, this flexibility can be a factor that makes cervical spine injuries easily occur due to trauma. Cervical instability can appear in the form of damage to nonosseous structures with almost no

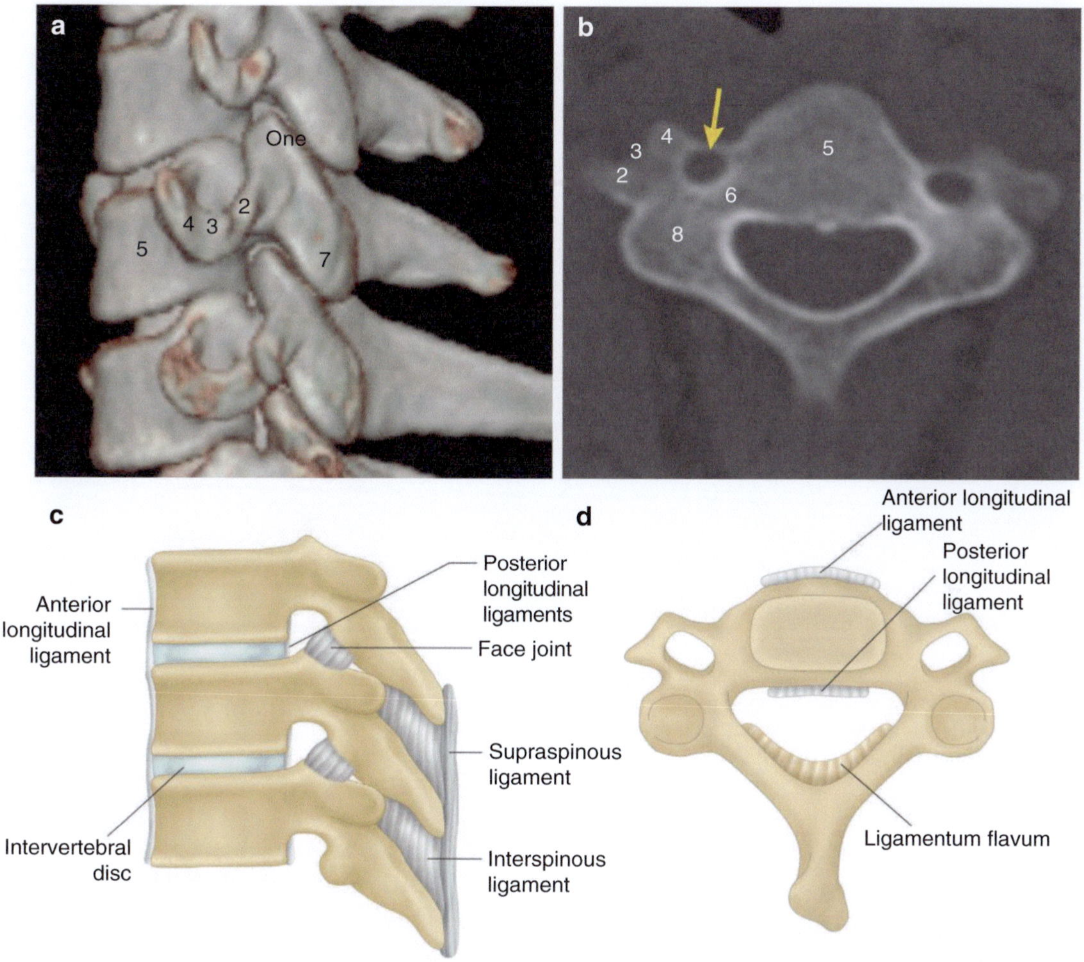

Fig. 8.18 Anatomical diagram of the lower cervical spine
(**a**) Volume rendering CT image of the lower cervical spine viewed from the left side. (**b**) Axial CT image of the lower cervical spine. (**c**) Diagram of the ligament structure of the lower cervical spine viewed from the left side. (**d**) Diagram of the ligament structure of one of the lower cervical vertebrae viewed from above. In Figure (**b**), structures 2, 3, 4 are structures of the transverse process, and the arrow indicates the vertebral artery foramen. The superior articular process and inferior articular process form the lateral mass

cervical bone fractures. In other words, the contribution of nonosseous structures to cervical stability is very large, and even if no fractures are seen, cervical instability due to damage to nonosseous structures can exist, so in all patients suspected of cervical injury, nonosseous structures, the presence of damage should always be considered and evaluated.

The composition of the nonosseous structure of the cervical spine is not significantly different from that of the thoracic spine, except for the presence of the nuchal ligament. However, a close examination of each structure reveals slight differences.

First, the annulus fibrosus of the lower cervical spine is thick at the front and gradually thins as it moves to the back, showing a crescent shape that is very thin at the back of the cervical spine [28]. The thick anterior annulus fibrosus and the fiber arrangement of the ALL follow the direction of the vertebral column, acting as an important support structure that prevents excessive extension of the spine. Since the anterior annulus fibrosus is shorter than the ALL, it is

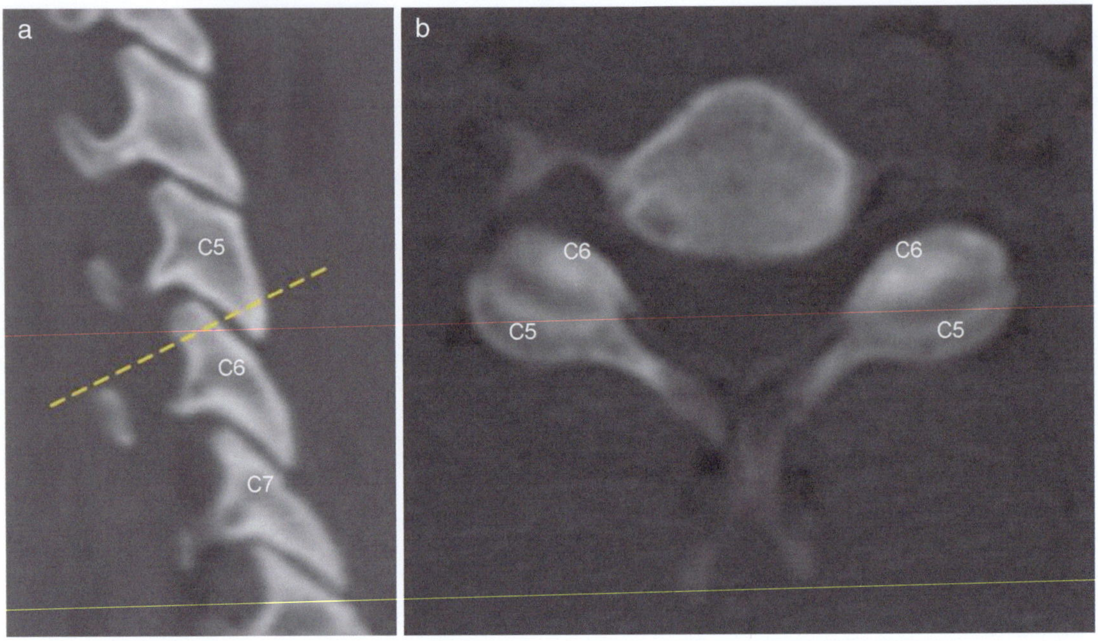

Fig. 8.19 Positional relationship of the articular process of the upper and lower vertebrae in the cervical facet joint Axial image (**b**) obtained at the dotted line level of the sagittal reformat CT image (**a**) of the facet joint. The superior articular process of the lower vertebra is located anterior to the inferior articular process of the upper vertebra

helpful to know that the disc can be damaged first without damage to the ALL in the event of an extension injury, which can sometimes help with image interpretation [29]. The posterior annulus fibrosus is too thin to serve as a support structure during spinal flexion, and instead, the PLL, which has almost the same biomechanical characteristics as the ALL and is wider, plays the role of an important support structure [30]. The facet joint capsule of the cervical spine is very loose compared to the thoracic spine, and does not play a supporting role in the normal range of motion, but only plays a supporting role when the cervical spine is dislocated to the extent of severe injury. This means that joint capsule damage does not occur except in cases of severe injury [31]. The interspinous ligament and supraspinous ligament of the cervical spine are less developed compared to the thoracic spine, and instead, the nuchal ligament, which is mixed with the ligaments at the back, exists. The nuchal ligament is very important as a support against anterior displacement of the spine or flexion injury [32].

8.2.2 Basic Application and Interpretation of Imaging Devices

8.2.2.1 Plain Radiography

Plain radiography is the most basic examination in patients suspected of cervical spine injury, but there is no need to perform imaging tests on all trauma patients. The five conditions that must be met in order not to perform plain radiography in patients suspected of cervical spine injury, as proposed in the NEXUS (National X-Radiography Use Study) conducted on more than 34,000 patients, are as follows: (1) There is no tenderness in the middle of the back of the neck. (2) There is no evidence of drug intoxication. (3) They show a normal level of consciousness. (4) There are no abnormal findings on neurological examination. (5) There is no evidence of a distracting injury accompanied by pain. If all these conditions are met, cervical spine injury can be ruled out with just a physical examination. However, if even one of these conditions is not met, it is thought that a determination of the presence of cervical spine injury through plain radiography is necessary [33]. The three basic plain radiographs used in patients suspected of cervical spine injury are lateral, anteroposterior, and open-mouth views.

The lateral plain radiograph is the most basic image, and approximately 85–90% of cervical spine injuries are detected. The interpretation of lateral images is important for identifying the presence or absence of the following findings (Fig. 8.20) [4].

① Presence or absence of cervical alignment abnormalities: The anterior spinal line, posterior spinal line, and spinolaminar line, which are imaginary lines connecting the cervical vertebrae, should form a smooth lordosis curve to be considered normal (Fig. 8.20a). If these lines do not connect smoothly and form a stair-like or broken connection, cervical fractures or ligament injuries should be suspected. However, between C2 and C3, and rarely between C3 and C4, these lines can appear broken even in normal conditions (Fig. 8.20b), which is called pseudosubluxation. It is known to occur due to the immaturity of muscles and cervical bones in children, and physiological joint flexibility in adults. Pseudosubluxation disappears in extension posture on lateral images. Also, as mentioned in the content about upper cervical injuries, the atlantodens interval (ADI) is also an important test target when examining cervical alignment abnormalities. This value is the distance between the front of the odontoid process of C2 and the back of the anterior neural arch of C1, and if it exceeds 3 mm in adults and 5 mm in children, it is judged that there is instability in the C1–C2 joint.

② Presence or absence of swelling in the anterior soft tissue of the cervical spine: It is very important to observe the thickness of the anterior soft tissue of the cervical spine in lateral plain radiographs. It is a shadow formed by

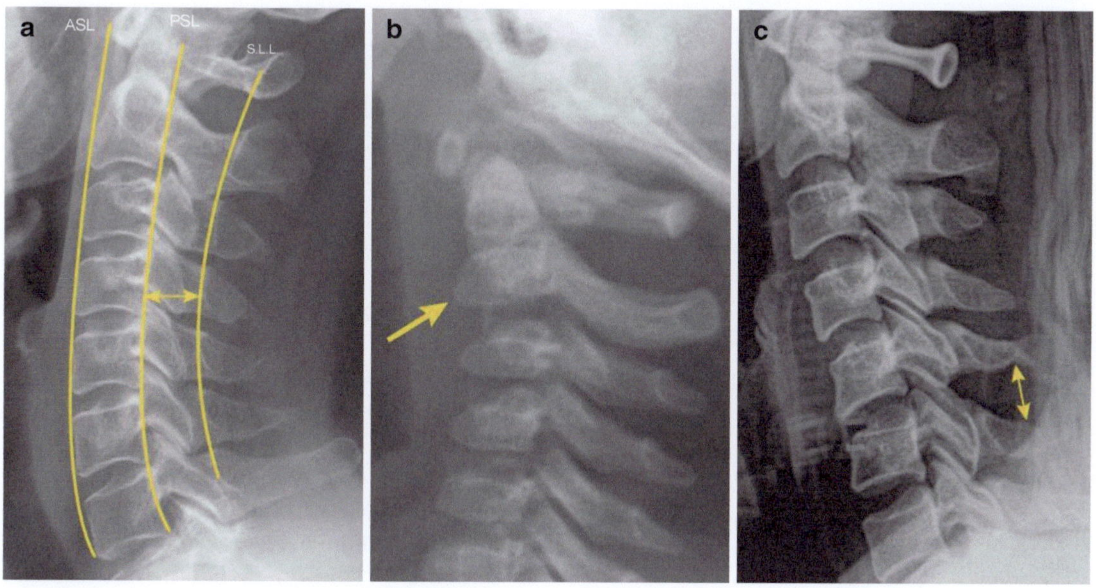

Fig. 8.20 Basics of interpreting plain radiographic lateral images of the cervical spine. (**a**) Cervical spine alignment reference lines. The anterior spinal line (ASL), posterior spinal line (PSL), and spinolaminar line (SLL) should be smoothly connected as shown in the figure, and if they are stepped or broken, fractures or ligament injuries should be suspected. The distance (bidirectional arrow) between the PSL and SLL should be measured as 13 mm or more to exclude central canal stenosis in plain radiographic images. (**b**) Pseudosubluxation. The C2 vertebra (arrow) appears to be anteriorly displaced from the C3 vertebra. However, this can be a normal finding in children or adults with flexible joints. (**c**) Increase in the width between the spinous processes. If the width between the spinous processes increases sharply compared to the nearby level, ligament damage should be suspected

the posterior wall of the pharynx and the esophagus, and if this thickness exceeds 7 mm at the C2 level, 5 mm at the C3 and C4 levels, 22 mm in adults, and 14 mm in children at the C6 level, it is judged as abnormal (Fig. 8.21) [4]. In patients with cervical injuries, these values increase due to hematomas caused by ligament or other soft tissue injuries (Fig. 8.3a).

③ Presence or absence of fractures or abnormal shadows in the cervical spine itself.

④ Increase in the width between the spinous processes: If the width between the spinous processes differs sharply compared to the adjacent level, fractures or ligament injuries should be suspected (Fig. 8.20c).

⑤ Presence or absence of angulation: If the angle between the vertebrae is more than 11°, fractures or ligament injuries should be suspected.

⑥ Presence or absence of abnormalities in the width of the central canal: The width of the central canal, i.e., the width between the posterior spinal line and the spinolaminar line should be at least 13 mm to be considered normal (Fig. 8.20a), and if it is smaller than this, it means that spinal cord compression has occurred or is imminent.

⑦ Presence or absence of abnormalities in the cervical-posterior cranial fossa: The basion-dens interval (BDI) is the most useful measurement (Fig. 8.4). The BDI should not exceed 10 mm in those over 13 years old, and 12 mm in those under 13 years old to be considered normal.

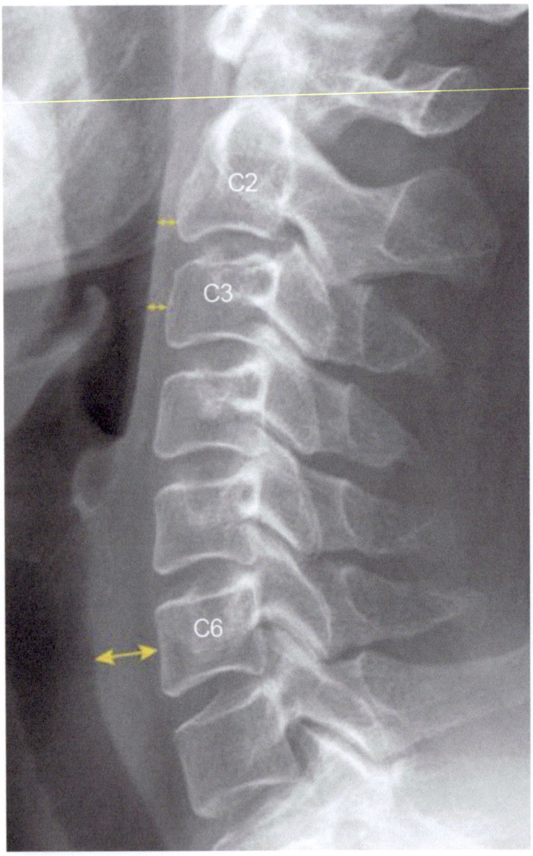

Fig. 8.21 Normal thickness of the anterior soft tissue of the cervical spine
In patients with cervical spine injuries, if the thickness of the soft tissue shadow between the cervical vertebrae and the airway and pharynx (bidirectional arrow at each level in the image) exceeds 7 mm at the C2 level, 5 mm at the C3/C4 level, and 22 mm in adults and 14 mm in children at the C6 level, ligament damage and hematoma should be considered

Lateral images can also be used to determine instability when flexing and extending the cervical spine. Such flexion-extension images can be performed in patients suspected of ligament injury where there is a very small alignment abnormality and no clear evidence of fracture or instability [34, 35]. The swimmer's view is when the cervical-thoracic junction is not clearly visible in lateral images, this method involves obtaining a lateral image by penetrating radiation through the elbow joint with the arm raised. In trauma patients, it is often impossible or unbearable to assume such a posture, so it is thought that using CT is a more rational method for this purpose.

Although anterior-posterior images provide less information than lateral images, they can always confirm the lower cervical spine, which is difficult to confirm in lateral images, and have diagnostic value in knowing whether the spinous process is located in the center of the cervical spine, indicating cervical rotation damage [4].

The open-mouth view is used to assess damage to the upper cervical spine.

8.2.2.2 Use of CT and MRI

In trauma patients, it may be difficult to obtain a proper posture for simple radiographic images due to reasons such as difficulty in obtaining patient cooperation or the patient's neck being fixed. Therefore, there are many cases where poor quality images that cannot rule out cervical injury are obtained. In lateral images, it has been reported that cervical fractures or dislocations can be overlooked up to 15%, and even after evaluating all lateral, anterior-posterior, and open-mouth views, it is known that 5–8% of fractures may not be diagnosed [4]. Therefore, in patients with high risk of cervical fracture (accidents caused by high energy, neurologic deficit, fractures of the head or pelvis, etc.), it is recommended to obtain CT images to rule out cervical injury [36]. Currently, MDCT (multidetector row CT) is being used in most institutions, and with its multiplanar capability, it is easy to obtain sagittal and coronal reformation images, so there is no doubt about the usefulness of CT in evaluating cervical injury patients. Even in previous studies before MDCT became mainstream, it has already been reported that CT is superior to simple radiographic images not only in diagnostic power but also in cost-effectiveness in patients with severe multiple injuries [37, 38].

In high-risk patients, it is often necessary to obtain CT images of the head, and considering the advantage of reducing the time spent on separate simple radiographic images by obtaining CT images of the neck at the same time, there is no need to hesitate to use MDCT. MDCT can obtain CT images in a short time compared to previous conventional CT. In addition, with MDCT, thin-section tomography is possible, allowing for isotropic voxel images. As a result, sagittal and coronal multiplanar reformation (MPR) images of almost the same quality as axial images can be obtained at the same time. The trend is increasing where CT images are used together with or instead of simple radiographic images in the evaluation of cervical fractures. Especially in the diagnosis of odontoid process fractures and vertebral endplate fractures, such coronal, sagittal MPR images are known to be essential (refer to Fig. 8.14) [39].

There is still debate about whether the use of MRI is absolutely necessary in patients with cervical trauma. There is a recent meta-analysis study reported that unless acute instability cervical injury is visible in MDCT examination, additional MRI examination is not necessary [40]. However, it is clear that MRI is superior to CT and simple radiographic images in evaluating soft tissue lesions. That is, MRI is the best means to confirm spinal cord injury, ligament injury, intervertebral disc injury, hematoma, etc. that accompany trauma patients. Many studies are being conducted to detect swelling of the vertebral body using dual-energy CT, which may replace MRI, but MRI is still an irreplaceable imaging device for the purpose of more sensitively understanding bone damage through swelling of the vertebral body. The indications for MRI in patients suspected of cervical injury can be summarized as follows [41–43].

① When more proximal nerve damage is suspected than the nerve damage predicted in simple radiographic images
② When instability is suspected or neurological symptoms worsen
③ When there are signs of suspicion of radiculopathy, myelopathy, and spinal cord injury
④ When simple radiographic images are normal but ligament injury is suspected or there are neurological symptoms
⑤ When displacement or rotation of the cervical spine that suggests soft tissue injury is suspected in simple radiographic images

Generally, to evaluate spinal injury with MRI, two pulse sequences of sagittal T1-enhanced image and T2-enhanced image are basic. In addition, it is good to include a pulse sequence (fluid-sensitive sequence) that clearly shows swelling in the imaging protocol to increase the sensitivity of ligament injury, intervertebral disc injury, and fracture, which is the biggest advantage of MRI. These pulse sequences include fat-suppressed spin-echo T2-enhanced images and short inversion recovery (hereinafter referred to as STIR) images (Fig. 8.22). These pulse sequences are also useful for evaluating spinal cord injury [44, 45]. Ligament injury in MRI is diagnosed by discontinuity of the ligament, hematoma around the injury site, and swelling of the soft tissue around the ligament [46]. There is still controversy over the accuracy of MRI in determining the injury of the posterior ligament complex of the cervical spine, and it has been reported to have high sensitivity but low specificity and positive predictive value. Therefore, the injury of the ligament in MRI should be judged considering the mechanism and degree of injury and simple radiographic findings, not just MRI findings [47]. Intervertebral disc injury caused by trauma is known to be more common in the cervical and thoracic spine than in the lumbar spine. Intervertebral disc injury shows increased signal intensity in T2-enhanced images, decreased or increased disc space, etc. The findings of disc herniation caused by trauma are known to show similar findings to disc herniation unrelated to trauma [46, 48, 49]. Spinal cord injury appears in three forms of swelling, bleeding, and swelling-bleeding in MRI, and the basic MRI images are T1 and T2. In addition to the spin-echo highlight video (Fig. 8.23), T2 highlights gradient echo images which play an

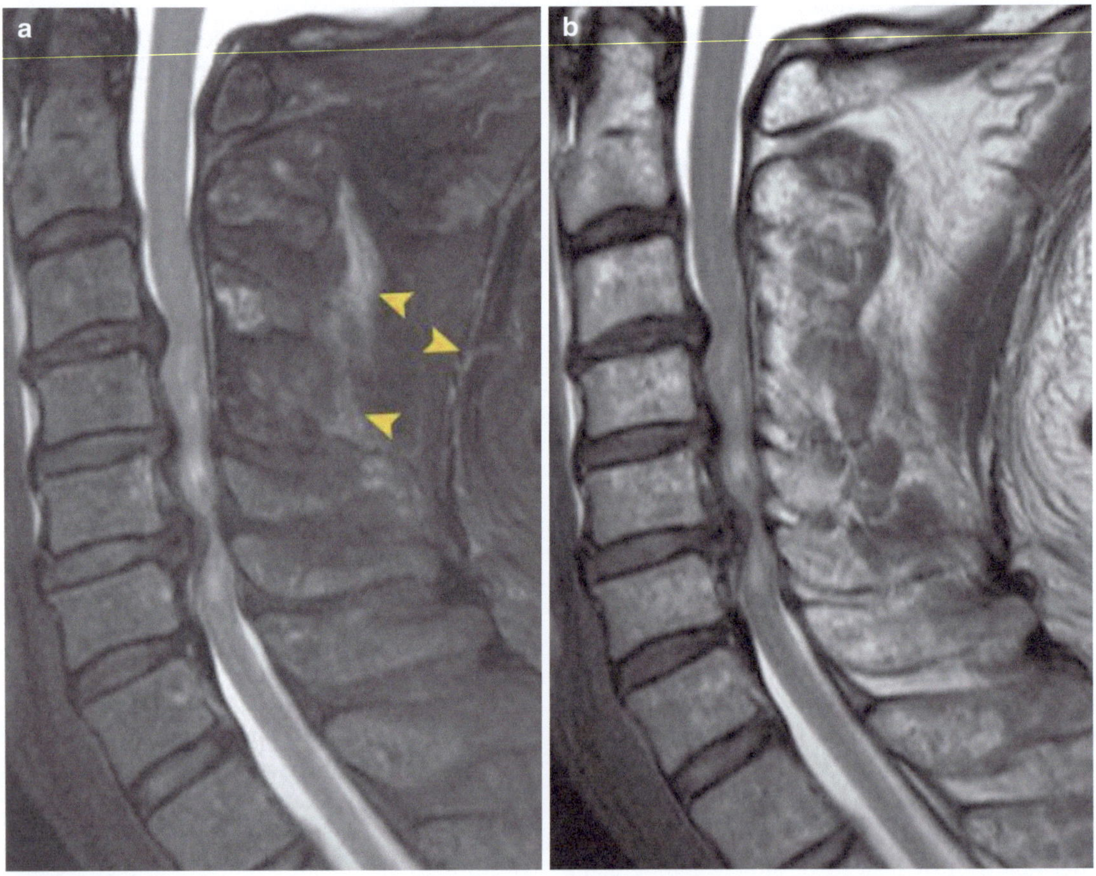

Fig. 8.22 Sensitivity of ligament damage in fat-suppressed images in patients with cervical spine injuries When comparing fat-suppressed T2-weighted images (**a**) and non-fat-suppressed T2-weighted images (**b**), the fat-suppressed images show ligament damage more sensitively (arrowhead)

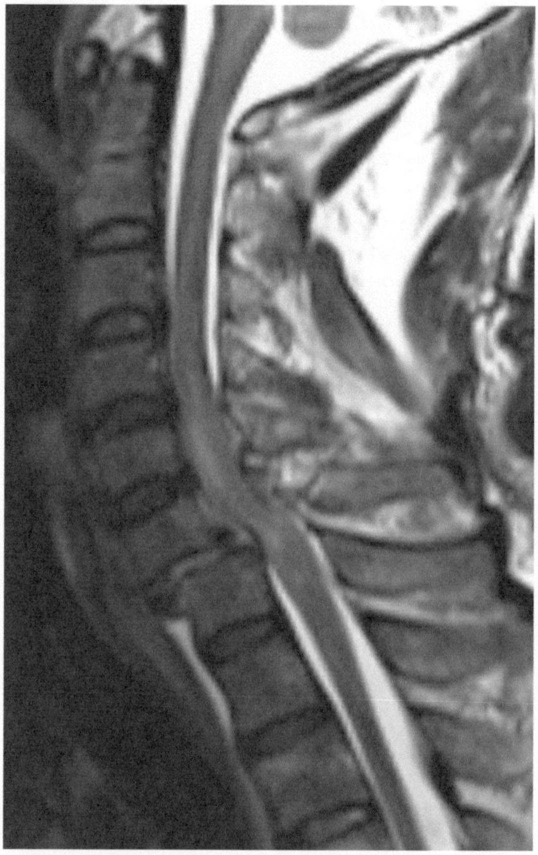

Fig. 8.23 MRI findings of spinal cord injury caused by cervical spine injury
On the T2-weighted sagittal image, swelling of the spinal cord is seen across four cervical levels

important role in the detection of hemorrhage. It is known that the prognosis is poor when there is a hemorrhage, as the likelihood of functional recovery is low [50, 51]. Furthermore, when the spinal cord is compressed by cervical vertebrae, intervertebral discs, hematoma, etc., rapid decompression through surgery is necessary, and MRI plays an important role in its detection [52]. It should also be considered that even without clear fractures or dislocations, spinal cord injuries can occur in children with relatively heavy heads and flexible musculoskeletal movements, or in adults with spinal stenosis due to degenerative changes [53].

8.2.3 Classification and Imaging Findings of Lower Cervical Injuries

The most commonly used classification for lower cervical injuries is based on the mechanism of injury. Understanding the mechanism of injury allows us to infer which structures may have been damaged in sequence and to determine treatment policies based on this. However, predicting the mechanism of injury can sometimes be very difficult. Injuries occur due to external forces of various directions and intensities in various postures, and the strength of the cervical spine and the presence or absence of degenerative changes vary greatly from person to person [1]. Also, it should be noted that the displacement, distraction, compression, and narrowing of the central canal seen in the fractured bone fragments in the images may have been more severe at the time of injury [1, 54]. The most widely used classification currently is the classification proposed by Allen and Ferguson, which infers the mechanism of injury through imaging (hereinafter referred to as the Allen-Ferguson classification) [55]. This classification, based on simple radiographic images, has disagreements about its applicability in the current era where CT and MRI are widely used, and it is difficult to apply in cases where cervical injuries occur due to complex injury mechanisms, and its reproducibility has not been properly verified [1]. In this context, Vacarro et al. proposed a new lower cervical injury classification system called Subaxial Injury Classification (SLIC), which evaluates and scores lower cervical injuries based on (1) the fracture pattern of the vertebral body, (2) the degree of intervertebral disc-ligament injury, and (3) the degree of neurological abnormalities, so that it can be used to determine treatment policies [26]. I would like to describe these two classification methods and how to analyze the images of lower cervical injuries.

8.2.3.1 Allen-Ferguson Classification

In 1982, Allen et al. retrospectively analyzed lower cervical injury patients with clear injury mechanisms and proposed a classification system that linked their simple radiographic images and injury mechanisms. This classification system is based on simple radiographic images and determines what posture the cervical spine was in at the time of injury and what direction of external force was applied in that posture. It is proposed to classify the damage to the lower vertebrae by inference. It is based on the two column theory that divides the vertebral part in front of the posterior longitudinal ligament (PLL) into the anterior column and the vertebral part in the back into the posterior column [55]. The lower vertebrae, especially at levels from C5 to C7 where fractures or dislocations are common, have a greater range of motion in the flexion-extension direction than lateral flexion or rotation [56]. Therefore, it is reported that damage mainly occurs in flexion and extension postures, and considering that the external forces of compression and distraction will be applied in these two postures, a total of four damage mechanisms (compressive flexion, distractive flexion, compressive extension, and distractive extension) combinations are obtained. Adding the damage mechanism of lateral flexion and vertical compression in the neutral posture, it is proposed to classify the damage to the lower vertebrae into a total of six damage mechanisms as follows. The percentage figures in the brackets behind each classification are the frequencies of each classification presented in the original paper.

① Compressive flexion [CF, 36 cases (22%)]
② Distractive flexion [DF, 61 cases (37%)]
③ Compressive extension [CE, 40 cases (24%)]
④ Distractive extension [DE, 9 cases (5%)]
⑤ Lateral flexion [LF, 5 cases (3%)]
⑥ Vertical compression [VC, 14 cases (8%)]

Allen et al. reported that the most common injury mechanism was the DF type, followed by the CE and CF types in order [55]. Depending on the severity of the injury, it is divided into 2–5 stages.

The general concept of the Allen-Ferguson classification can be explained as follows. In the case of injury in the flexion posture, the compressive external force of the anterior column by the compression injury mechanism (CF) and the distraction external force of the posterior column by the distraction injury mechanism (DF) are the beginning of the injury. On the other hand, in the case of injury in the extension posture, the compressive external force of the posterior column by the compression injury mechanism (CE) and the distraction external force of the anterior column by the distraction injury mechanism (DE) are the beginning of the injury. Although this classification has some disadvantages as mentioned above, it is very useful as a framework for explaining fractures of the lower vertebrae because it allows us to infer the injury mechanism from the following characteristic imaging findings. Many clinicians are describing lower vertebral fractures according to this classification.

- The CF type is characterized by a compression fracture of the anterior vertebral body.
- The DF type is characterized by ligament damage in the posterior column and dislocation or subluxation of the facet joint, with no or minimal vertebral fractures.
- The CE type is characterized by fractures appearing in various parts of the posterior column (lamina, ismuth, spinous process).
- The DE type is characterized by a slight anterior widening of the intervertebral space without a fracture or by a small avulsion fracture on the anterior aspect of the vertebral body, which sometimes might be subtle enough to be missed on radiographic imaging.

Below, detailed imaging findings are described for each type.

The CF type is a cervical injury caused by a mechanism in which pressure is applied when the cervical spine is in flexion (Fig. 8.24). Therefore, when the anterior column is compressed, the upper endplate of the spine is pressed, lowering the height of the anterior vertebral body, and if the energy of the trauma is large, the fracture line of the upper endplate extends to the lower endplate, forming a relatively large bone fragment (commonly called a flexion tear drop fracture) in the anterior vertebral body (Fig. 8.25). In the case of damage caused by stronger energy, the liga-

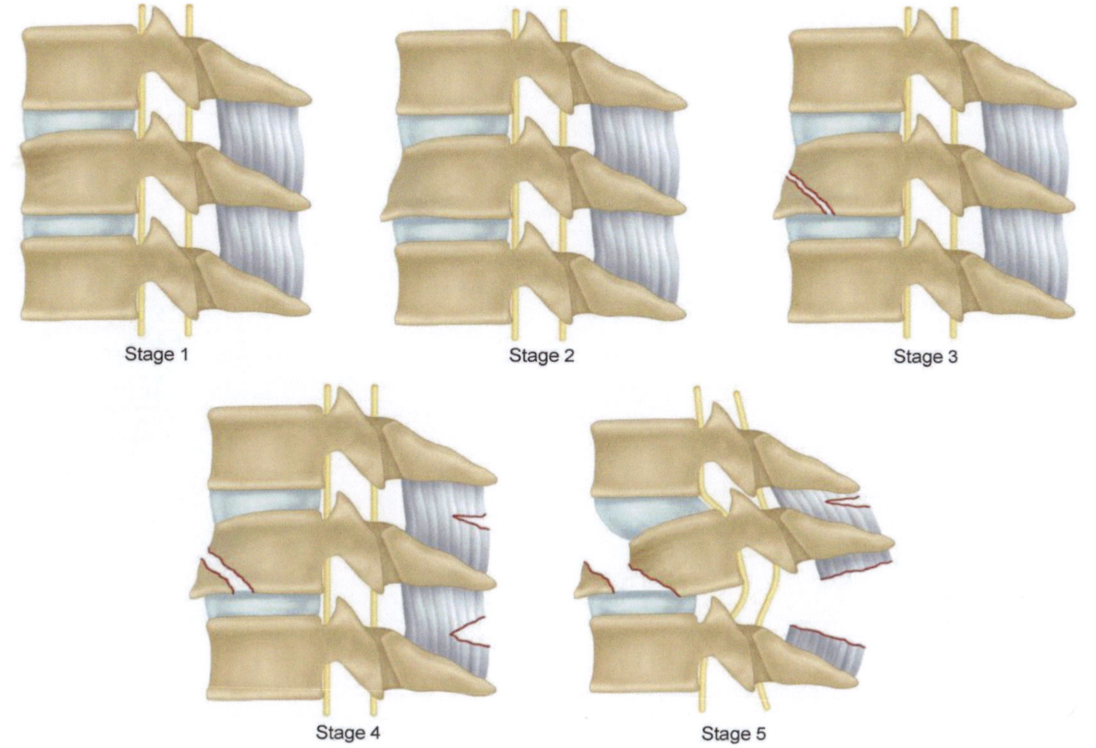

Fig. 8.24 Schematic of compressive flexion (CF) type Stage 1 refers to the shape where the front of the spinal upper endplate sinks and the margin becomes round, stage 2 is the shape where the height of the anterior part of the vertebra decreases and the anterior surface of the vertebra shows obliquity as the changes in stage 1 progress, stage 3 is the shape where the fracture starting from the anterior part of the vertebra connects to the lower endplate of the vertebra, forming a relatively large bone fragment in the anterior and lower part of the vertebra (flexion tear drop fracture), stage 4 is the shape where the fractured vertebra is displaced posteriorly, showing a small displacement of <3 mm in the posterior and lower part of the vertebra, and stage 5 refers to the shape where the fractured vertebra is displaced posteriorly, the posterior and lower part of the vertebra is displaced more than 3 mm, and the distance between the facet joint dislocation and the spinous process significantly increases

ments and nonosseous structures in the back of the cervical spine are damaged, and the damaged vertebral body is pushed back.

The DF type is a cervical injury caused by a mechanism in which distraction is applied when the cervical spine is in flexion, characterized by damage to the posterior ligaments of the cervical spine and anterior displacement of the vertebral body, resulting in dislocation of the facet joint. In contrast to the CF type, where the vertebral body at the site of injury is posteriorly displaced, the DF type is characterized by anterior displacement of the vertebral body (Fig. 8.26). Dislocation of the facet joint is the anterior displacement of the inferior articular process of the upper cervical spine over the superior articular process of the lower cervical spine, and the inability of the anteriorly displaced inferior articular process of the upper cervical spine to return due to being caught on the superior articular process of the lower cervical spine is called "facet locking." In cases where dislocation occurs in the unilateral facet joint (DF stage 2), even if the posterior ligament complex is damaged, if the facet joint on the opposite side is stable, it forms a locked vertebra, which is known to be a relatively stable injury [4], in this case, the upper cervical spine shows <50% anterior displacement compared to the lower cervical spine in simple radiographic lateral images. Also, if only the unilateral facet joint is dislocated, the cervical spine located above the injury level rotates, so the oblique image of these

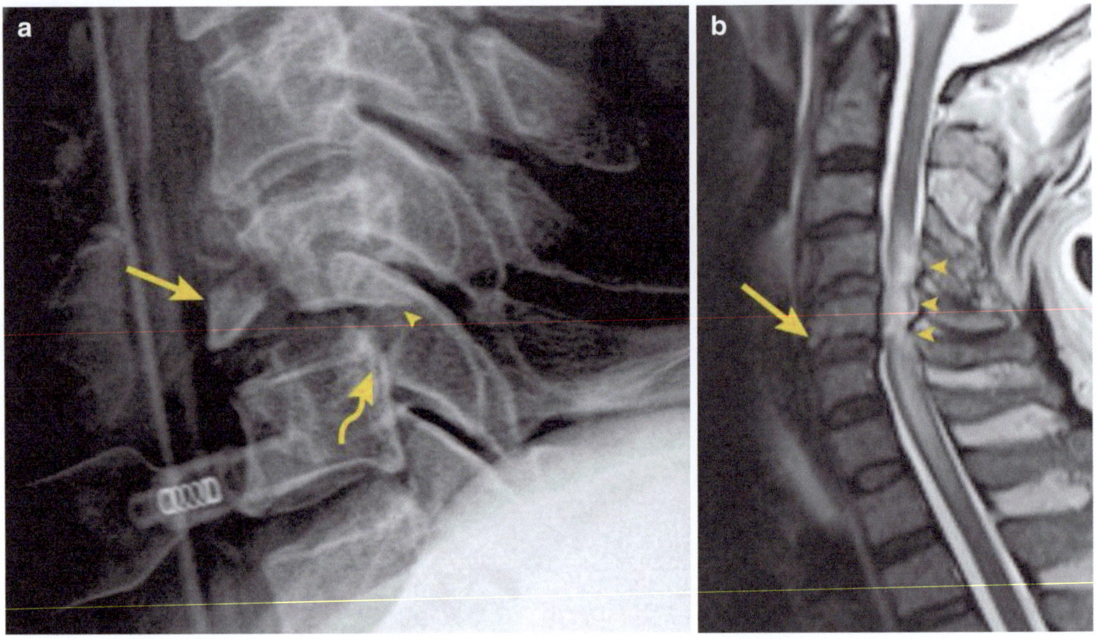

Fig. 8.25 Imaging findings of compressive flexion (CF) type. (**a**) In the simple radiographic lateral image, a relatively large bone fragment (flexion tear drop fracture, arrow) is seen in the anterior part of the vertebra, and the upper vertebra (arrowhead) is posteriorly displaced compared to the lower vertebra (curved arrow), which is a finding of CF stage 4. (**b**) In the same patient's MRI sagittal T2-weighted image, severe spinal cord injury is accompanied (arrowhead). As in the simple radiographic image, a "flexion tear drop fracture" (arrow) is seen

cervical spines is seen in the lateral image, so the articular processes of one vertebra do not overlap each other in simple radiographic lateral images, showing a bow tie appearance [55, 57]. Such facet joint dislocation and facet locking are often difficult to judge with simple radiographic images alone and are best evaluated on CT (Fig. 8.27) [58]. In cases where bilateral facet joint dislocation occurs, the upper cervical spine shows more than 50% anterior displacement compared to the lower cervical spine, and cases showing about 50% anterior displacement in simple radiographic lateral images are defined as DF stage 3, and cases where the entire upper cervical spine has moved forward to the lower cervical spine or appears to be floating unstably are defined as DF stage 4 [55]. Bilateral facet joint dislocation is a very unstable fracture, and in many cases, ALL, PLL, interspinous ligament, supraspinous ligament, intervertebral disc, etc. are all damaged at the injury level, so if it is suspected clinically or if bilateral facet joint dislocation is suspected in simple radiographic/CT images, it is recommended to perform MRI (Fig. 8.28) [4, 59].

The CE type refers to a case where the main fractures are fractures of the lamina, pedicle, articular process, etc., caused by a mechanism in which pressure is applied when the cervical spine is in extension. The CE type is divided into five stages (Fig. 8.29), and among them, stage 1 is in the case of unilateral lamina, pedicle, articular process fractures, etc., it is stage 2 characterized by lamina fractures at multiple levels. Stage 3 involves bilateral lamina, pedicle, articular process fractures, but no cervical displacement, and stage 4 involves partial anterior displacement of the spine. Stage 5 is a progression of stage 4, where the entire width of the vertebral body is anteriorly displaced on lateral plain radiographs. CE type injuries often make it difficult to fully understand the presence and shape of fractures with plain radiographs alone. Often, CT images must be obtained, and sometimes MRI must be performed to evaluate damage to the facet joint and ligaments [60, 61].

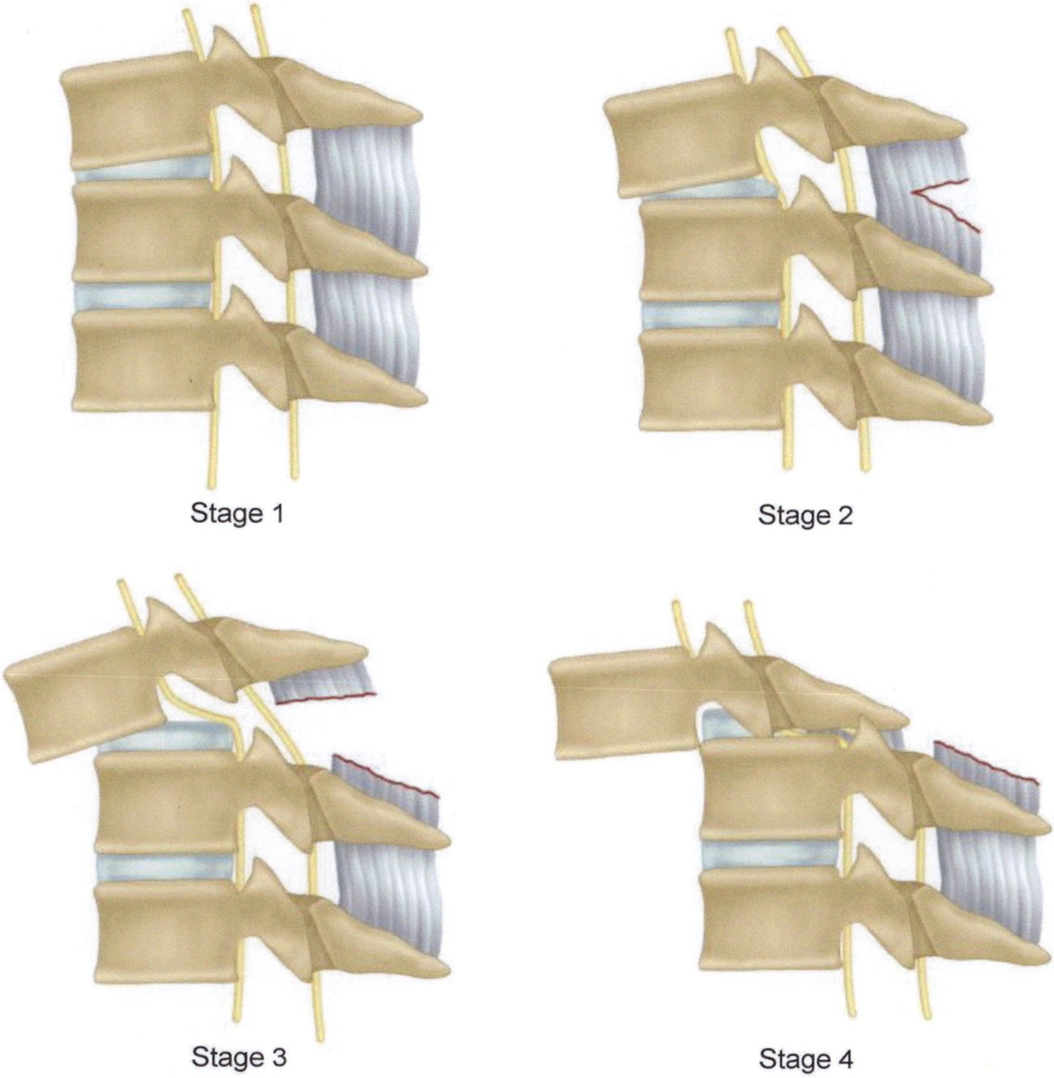

Fig. 8.26 Schematic of distractive flexion (DF) type Stage 1 shows the shape of facet joint subluxation as the distance between the spinous processes increases, stage 2 shows <50% displacement of the upper vertebra due to unilateral facet joint dislocation, stage 3 shows about 50% displacement of the upper vertebra and facet locking due to bilateral facet joint dislocation, and stage 4 refers to cases where the entire upper vertebra is anteriorly displaced compared to the lower vertebra, showing the shape of a "floating vertebra"

DE type is a fracture form that occurs when the cervical spine is extended and distraction is applied, characterized by damage to the ALL or avulsion fracture of the vertebral body by the ALL or intervertebral disc annulus fibrosus (Fig. 8.30) [55]. That is, it is characterized by an "extension tear drop fracture" that shows a different form from the "flexion tear drop fracture" seen in the aforementioned CF type. Flexion tear drop fracture and extension tear drop fracture commonly appear as triangular bone fragments in the lower anterior of the vertebral body on lateral radiographs, but they have important differences and should be distinguished from each other. Flexion tear drop fracture occurs due to severe unstable damage of CF stage 3 or higher and forms a relatively large bone fragment (Fig. 8.25), whereas extension tear drop fracture

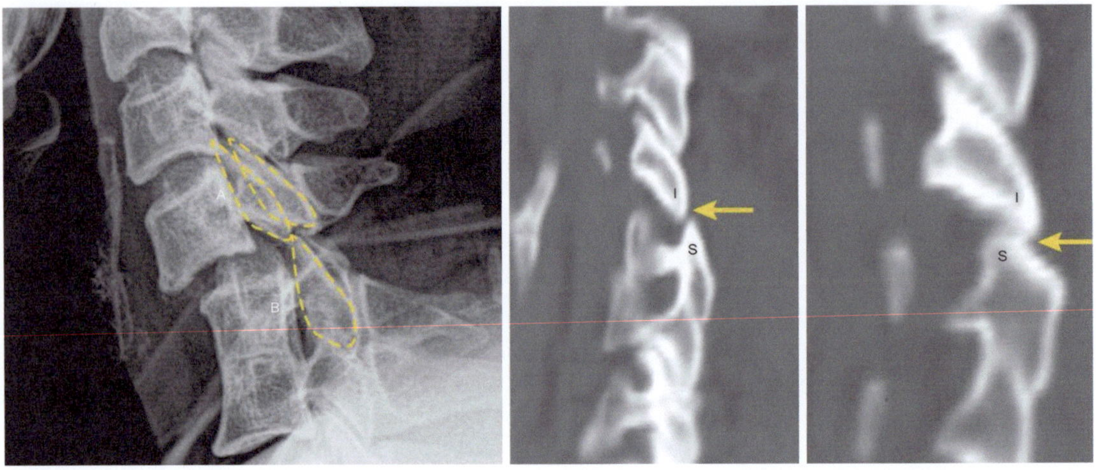

Fig. 8.27 Imaging findings of distractive flexion (DF) type stage 2 (unilateral facet joint dislocation). (**a**) Simple radiographic lateral image of unilateral facet joint dislocation. The cervical bodies located above the dislocated level rotate due to unilateral facet dislocation. Therefore, on the lateral image, both articular processes do not completely overlap, showing a bow tie appearance (refer to A dotted line). Below the dislocation level, both articular processes overlap normally and appear as one (refer to B dotted line). The upper vertebra shows <50% anterior displacement. (**b**) Sagittal reformat CT image of the dislocated facet joint. The inferior articular process (I) of the upper vertebra is dislocated anteriorly to the superior articular process (S) of the lower vertebra (arrow). (**c**) Sagittal reformat CT image of the non-dislocated contralateral side facet joint. Reformatted CT image. Although subluxation has occurred, there is no dislocation, and the normal anterior-posterior arrangement of the articular process in the facet joint is maintained (arrow)

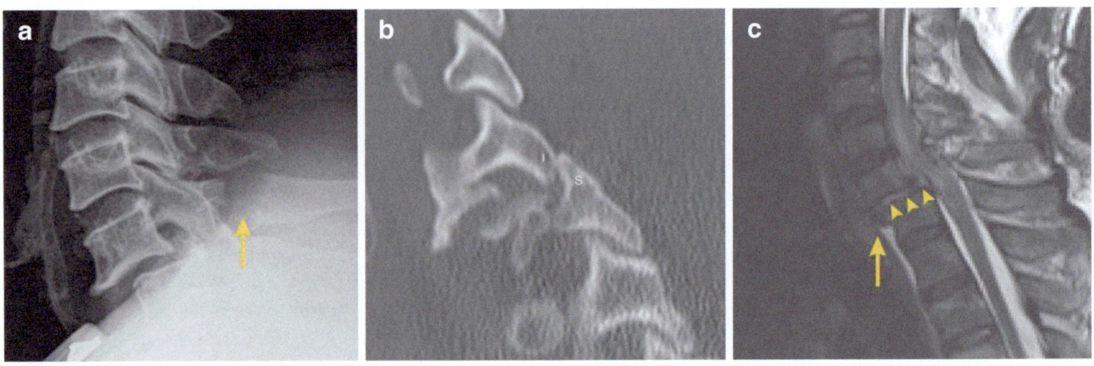

Fig. 8.28 Imaging findings of distractive flexion (DF) type stage 4

(**a**) Simple radiographic lateral image of bilateral facet joint dislocation. The upper vertebra shows about 50% anterior displacement, along with facet joint dislocation and fracture of the spinous process (arrow). (**b**) Sagittal reformat CT image of the dislocated facet joint of the same patient. Both sides show facet locking findings where the superior articular process (S) of the lower vertebra is directly connected to the anterior of the inferior articular process (I) of the upper vertebra. (**c**) Severe disc damage (arrowhead) and complete damage to the anterior longitudinal ligament (arrow) are seen in the sagittal T2-weighted MRI of the same patient, and severe damage to the spinal cord is seen. Although it may be considered as stage 3 damage in the lateral radiographic image, it is judged as the damage form of "floating vertebra" damaged from ALL to nuchal ligament across all layers in MRI, so the patient's damage was classified as stage 4

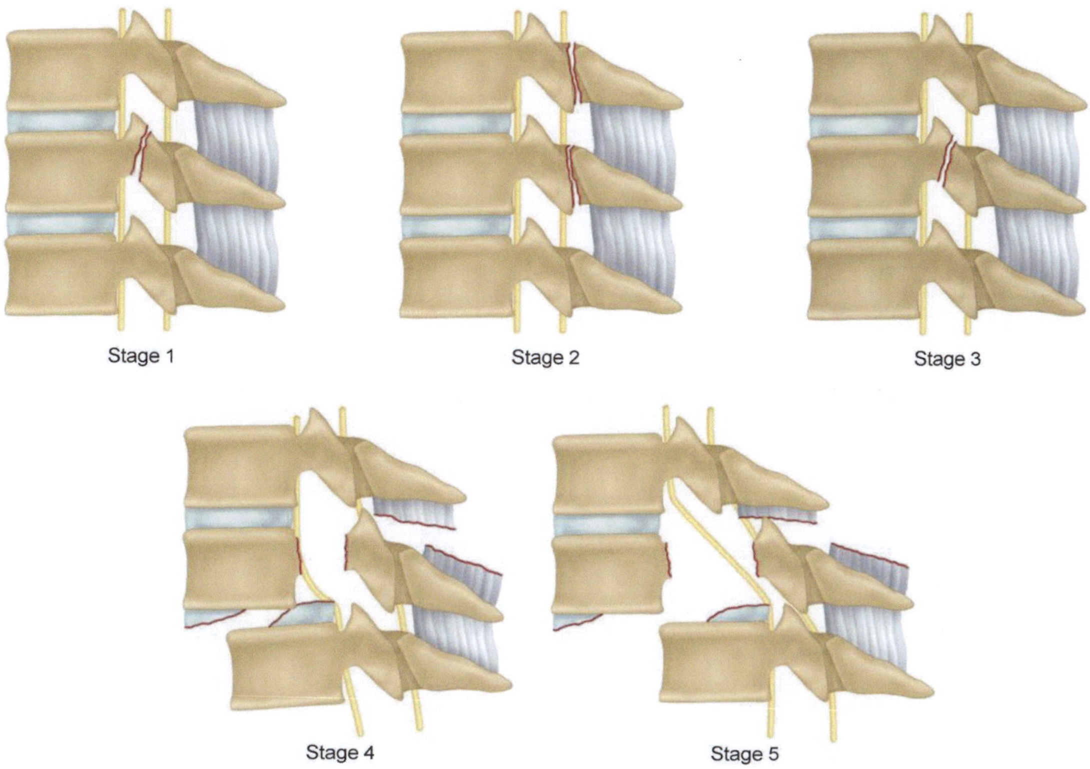

Fig. 8.29 Schematic of compressive extension (CE) type Stage 1 is when there are fractures of the articular process, pedicle, lamina, etc. on one side, stage 2 is when there are lamina fractures at multiple levels, stage 3 is when there are fractures of both lamina, pedicle, articular process, but no displacement of the vertebra, stage 4 is when there is partial anterior displacement of the spine, stage 5 is when stage 4 has progressed and the entire width of the vertebral body is anteriorly displaced in the lateral simple radiographic image. In Allen's study, stages 3 and 4 were presented as theoretical stages to logically connect stages 2 and 5, and actual patient cases were not presented

appears as a relatively small bone fragment as an avulsion fracture, and can be seen even at a low stage, so it does not necessarily mean unstable damage (Fig. 8.31) [4, 55].

LF type is the rarest form of injury in the Allen-Ferguson classification and is referred to when asymmetric compression on the cervical spine is seen in anteroposterior images (Fig. 8.32).

VC type, unlike CF type, refers to cases where the collapse of the vertebral body occurs not in the front of the cervical body but in the center, and is classified into three stages (Fig. 8.33). Stage 1 and stage 2 are described by Allen et al. in their study as having no ligament damage. Stage 3 is a concept similar to the burst fracture that will be described in detail in the thoracic spine fracture later, where the posterior displacement of the bone fragment occurs and the central canal narrows even without abnormal cervical alignment due to the posteriorly displaced bone fragment, so it is classified as an unstable fracture (Fig. 8.34).

8.2.3.2 Subaxial Injury Classification (SLIC)

Although various classification systems have been proposed, no single classification system has received unilateral support, and the Allen-Ferguson classification described above is a classification system used by relatively many clinicians. However, these previous classifications, including the Allen-Ferguson classification, have the disadvantage of not considering nerve damage, which acts as an important factor in prognosis prediction and treatment policy [26].

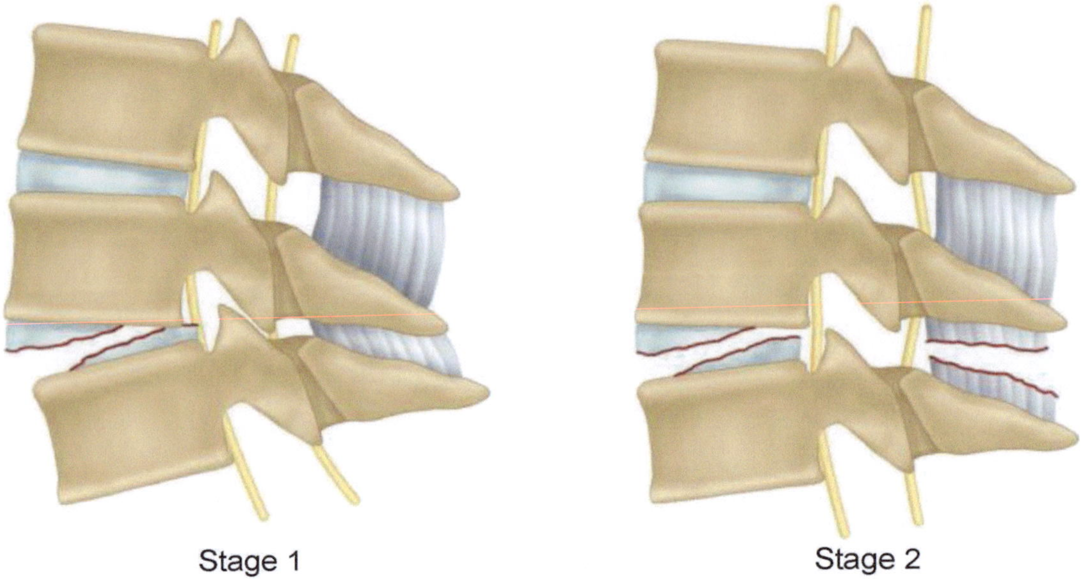

Fig. 8.30 Schematic of distraction-extension (DE) type Stage 1 involves damage to the anterior longitudinal ligament (ALL) or avulsion fracture of the vertebra by this ligament, stage 2 involves damage to the posterior ligament along with ALL. Refers to cases where the spine is posteriorly displaced at the damage level

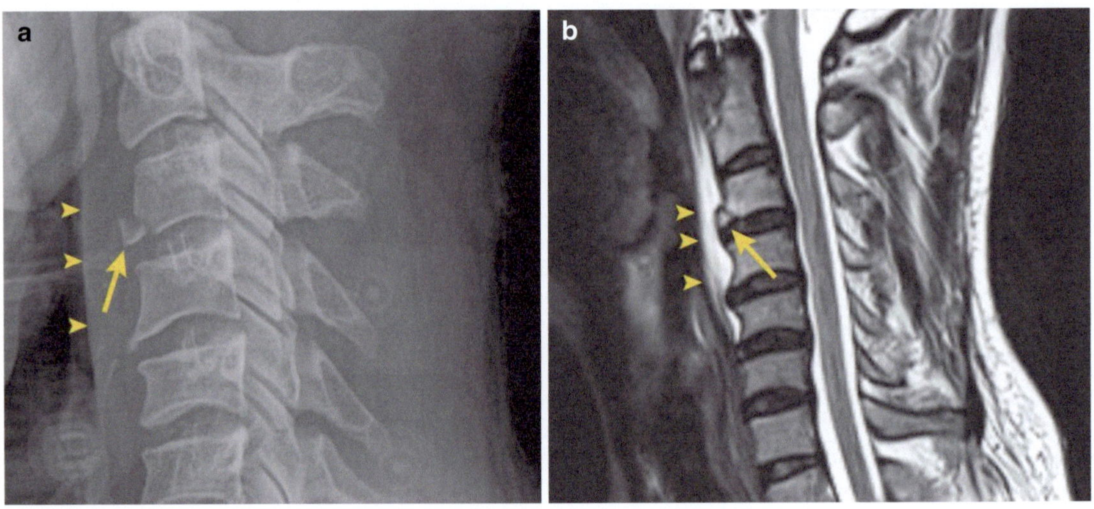

Fig. 8.31 Imaging findings of distractive extension (DE) type
(**a**) A relatively small bone fragment ("extension tear drop fracture," arrow) is seen in the anterior of the vertebral body in the simple radiographic lateral image. Note the thickened soft tissue shadow in the anterior of the vertebral body (arrowhead). (**b**) In the sagittal T2-weighted MRI of the same patient, there is severe swelling in the anterior of the spine (arrowhead), which is a finding of hematoma due to avulsion fracture of the vertebral body (arrow). There is no damage to the spinal cord, and it was classified as stage 1 DE damage

To overcome the shortcomings of the previous classification system, in 2007, a group of researchers called the "Spine Trauma Study Group (STSG)" proposed the ThoracoLumbar Injury Classification and Severity score (TLICS) devised in 2005 for thoracic spine injury classification [62]. By expanding the classification of lower cervical spine injuries, a new lower cervical spine injury classification system called Subaxial Injury Classification (SLIC) was pro-

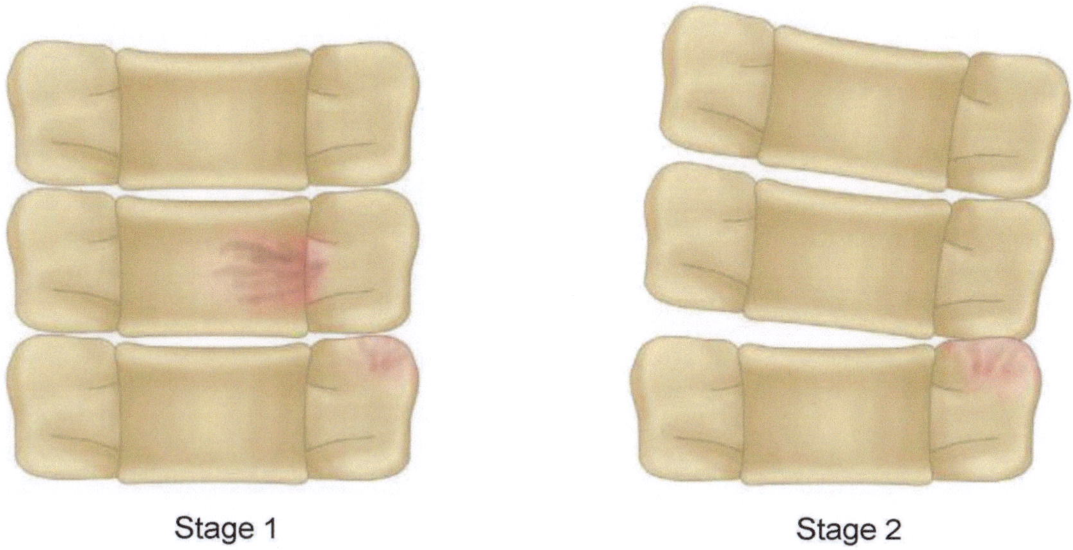

Fig. 8.32 Schematic of lateral flexion (LF) type
Stage 1 refers to an asymmetric unilateral cervical body and vertebral neural arch compression fracture, and stage 2 refers to cases where the fractured part of the spinal arch where the compression fracture occurred is displaced or the space between the opposite side vertebral bodies is widened

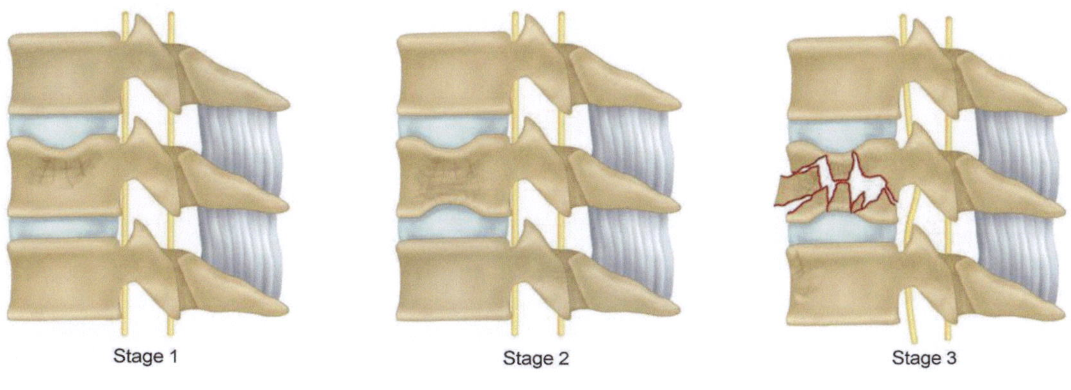

Fig. 8.33 Schematic of vertical compression (VC) type
A damage mechanism in which the center of the endplate collapses, stage 1 refers to cases where only one of the upper and lower endplates has collapsed, stage 2 refers to cases where both upper and lower endplates have collapsed, and stage 3 refers to cases where bone fragments from burst fractures are displaced into the central canal

posed [26]. The SLIC system similarly used the three variables used in the TLICS system, which was devised earlier in time [26, 62]. These three variables are injury morphology, the presence of disc-ligamentous complex (DLC) injury, and neurological status, and as shown in Table 8.1, scores are calculated for each variable and the total score is used as a basis for determining treatment policy. Non-surgical treatment is recommended when the total score is 1–3 points, and surgical treatment is recommended when it is 5 points or more. These three variables are described in more detail below.

First, the injury morphology is broadly divided into compression injury (compression, 1 point), distraction injury (distraction, 3 points), and rotation injury (rotation, 4 points). Compression injury includes all injuries caused

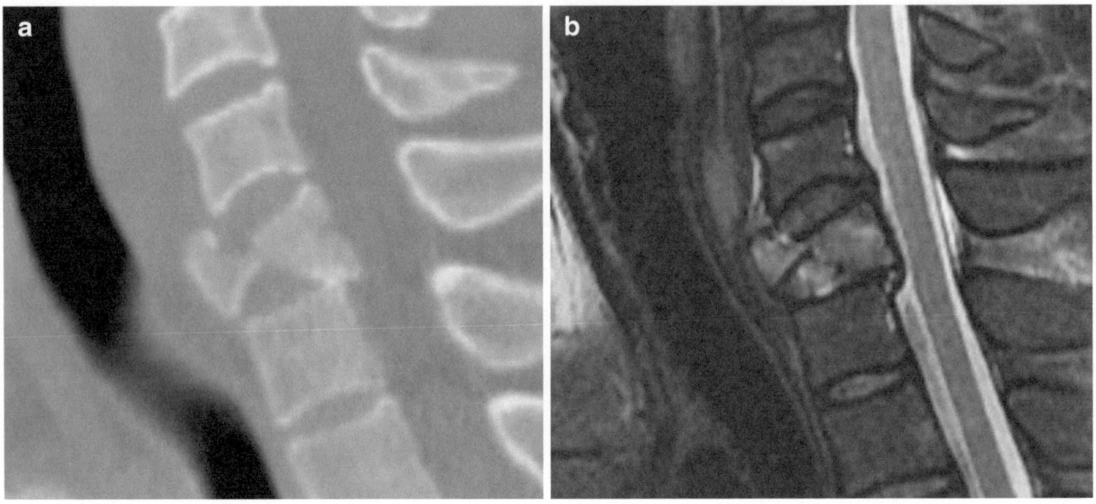

Fig. 8.34 Imaging findings of vertical compression (VC) type. (**a**) In the sagittal reformat CT image, a burst fracture is seen where the center of the vertebral body has collapsed and the vertebral body is displaced anteriorly and posteriorly (VC stage 3). (**b**) In the same patient's MRI sagittal fat-suppressed T2-weighted image, the anteriorly and posteriorly displaced vertebral body is visible, there is swelling in the vertebral body, the central canal is slightly narrowed, but there is no damage to the spinal cord

Table 8.1 Subaxial Injury Classification (SLIC)

Evaluation items	Score
Injury morphology	
No abnormality	0
Compression injury	1
Burst fracture	+1(=2)
Distraction injury (facet perch, hyperextension)	3
Rotation injury (facet dislocation, unstable tear drop/ advanced flexion compression injury)	4
Disco-ligamentous complex injury	
Intact	0
Indeterminate (isolated interspinous widening, MRI signal change only)	1
Disrupted (widening of disc space, facet perch or dislocation)	2
Neurological status	
Intact	0
Root injury	1
Complete cord injury	2
Incomplete cord injury	3
Continuous cord compression in setting of neuro deficit	+1

Note: The score is the sum of the scores for injury type, DLC injury, and neurological status. If this sum is 3 or less, non-surgical treatment is recommended, if it is 5 or more, surgical treatment is recommended, and if it is 4, the patient is advised to choose between surgical and non-surgical treatment by compression, including the lower stage forms of CF, LF, and VC in the Allen-Ferguson classification. Regardless of the anterior column and posterior column of the cervical spine, fractures caused by compression are described as included in compression injuries only when there is no displacement of the fracture fragment. Two notable points are that in the case of a burst fracture, i.e., stage 3 of VC, 1 point is added to calculate 2 points, and even in the case of a compression injury without displacement of the injured cervical body, there may be a DLC injury. Distraction injury was defined as a case where separation occurs between anatomical structures in the craniocaudal direction, the vertical axis of the body. During flexion injury, the support structures of the facet joint are damaged, and during extension injury, the ALL and intervertebral discs are damaged, and cases with almost no cervical displacement in the horizontal direction (horizontal displacement) were described as distraction injury forms. Rotation injury is a case where the injured cervical spine is displaced in the horizontal direction, and the DE type and high stage form of CF in the Allen-Ferguson classification belong here [26].

Second, the DLC is defined from front to back as ALL, intervertebral disc, PLL, facet joint capsule, ligamentum flavum, interspinous ligament, and supraspinous ligament. Because the healing of soft tissues such as ligaments is relatively late compared to bones and it is difficult to predict the recovery period, determining the presence or absence of DLC injury is very important for the prognosis of the patient and the decision of the patient's treatment policy. MRI is useful for directly diagnosing DLC injury, but the criteria for indirectly determining DLC injury are as follows.

① If the facet joint has <50% contact surface or shows a separation (diastasis) of 2 mm or more
② If the anterior disc space is abnormally widened
③ If the facet joint is separated on the lateral flexion image or the injured cervical segmentation shows an angulation of 11° or more

DLC injury can be directly diagnosed through MRI, and ligament injury can be confirmed through discontinuity of the ligament or swelling of the surrounding soft tissue and disc injury can be confirmed by checking high signal intensity in the intervertebral disc on T2-weighted images [26]. If there is a DLC injury, when in doubt or unclear, assign 1 point, and when clear, assign 2 points (Table 8.1).

Thirdly, the neurological status is evaluated based on clinical judgment, not imaging, as follows: If only nerve root damage is suspected, assign 1 point. In case of complete spinal cord injury, assign 2 points, and in case of partial spinal cord injury, assign 3 points (Table 8.1). The reason for assigning a lower score to complete spinal cord injury (2 points) than to partial injury (3 points) is because the SLIC system is designed to perform surgical treatment in case of higher score injuries. In other words, a higher score is given in case of partial injury than complete injury to induce surgical treatment. Although the neurological status depends on clinical judgment, spinal cord compression associated with neurological symptoms can only be determined by imaging, and MRI is known as a reliable test for this purpose [63]. The SLIC system reflects this by adding 1 point to the total score if neurological symptoms are associated with spinal cord compression findings on MRI (Fig. 8.35, Table 8.1) [26].

8.3 Thoracolumbar

The most commonly injured part of the thoracolumbar is the thoracolumbar junction (T10–L2). The relative frequency of thoracolumbar injuries by site is known to be 16% in the T1–T10 area, 52% in the T11–L1 area, and 32% in the L2–L5 area [64]. Thoracolumbar injuries are known to cause concurrent injuries in 50% of cases, including the thoracic cavity (20%), abdominal cavity (10%), limbs and pelvic bones (20%), so care should be taken in evaluating these areas and interpreting the images [64]. The imaging findings of thoracolumbar injuries are described with a focus on the explanation of the classification

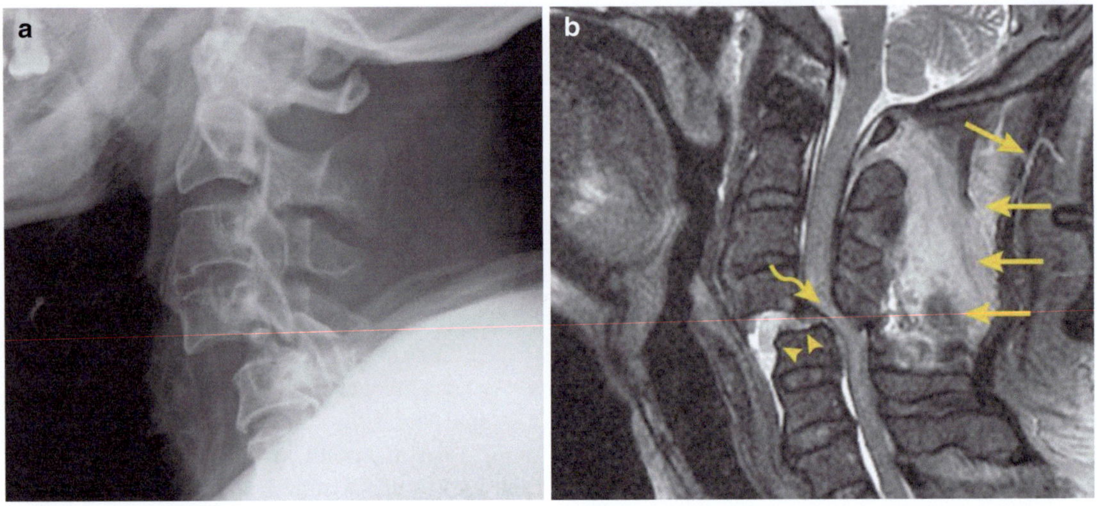

Fig. 8.35 Example of applying the subaxial injury classification (SLIC)
A 54-year-old traffic accident patient was admitted with complete paralysis and loss of sensation below the C6 level. On the simple radiographic lateral image (**a**), it showed findings of stage 4 distraction-flexion (DF) injury according to the Allen-Ferguson classification, and on the sagittal fat-suppressed T2-weighted MRI (**b**) performed at the time of admission, it showed complete damage to the disc (arrowhead) and the intervertebral disc-ligament complex (DLC) (arrow). The spinal cord is compressed within the central canal (curved arrow). According to SLIC, the score is a total of 9 points, including 4 points for rotational injury, 2 points for DLC injury, 2 points for complete spinal cord injury, and 11 points for confirming the association between spinal cord compression and neurological symptoms in the image, and it is judged that surgical treatment is required because it is 5 points or more

system by injury mechanism, as with the content for the lower cervical spine.

8.3.1 Anatomy and Biomechanics

The thoracic vertebrae are firmly fixed by the upper nine ribs, and the facet joint's articular surface is in the coronal direction, so there is less flexion-extension movement than in the cervical or lumbar spine, and lateral flexion movement is larger than in the lumbar spine but smaller than in the cervical spine [56]. Therefore, it is relatively strong against trauma. The mid-thoracic spine has a narrow central canal and less vascular distribution to the spinal cord, so if a fracture or dislocation occurs in the thoracic spine, the possibility of neurological damage is high, with frequencies reported up to 50% [65]. The axial rotation of the thoracic spine is larger than that of the lumbar spine because, as mentioned above, the direction of the facet joint's articular surface is coronal in the thoracic spine, whereas it is closer to sagittal in the lumbar spine, which restricts the rotation movement of the lumbar spine more [56]. However, the lower thoracic vertebrae, i.e., those below T10, have a facet joint direction that transitions closer to the lumbar spine, so this area has less rotational movement than the upper and middle thoracic vertebrae (Fig. 8.36) [56]. This is because the thoracic spine area has less rotation than the thoracolumbar junction or lumbar spine due to it serves as the basis for describing the characteristics of more damage occurring.

The thoracolumbar junction is the most vulnerable part of the spine to trauma than any other level. About 50% of all spinal fractures and 40% of all spinal cord injuries occur at the T11–L2 site. This is because the movement restriction by the ribs is smaller than the upper thoracic spine, the movement in the flexion-extension direction is large, the curvature of the spine transitions from the thoracic kyphotic curve to the lumbar

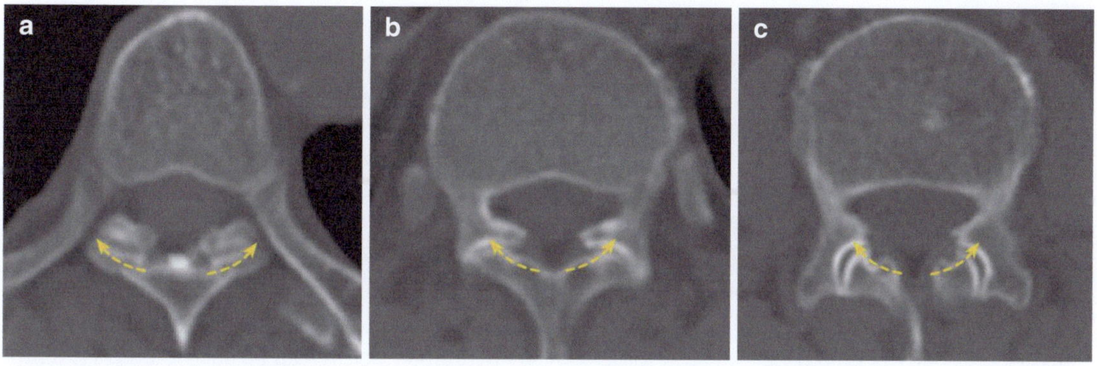

Fig. 8.36 The effect of the directionality of the facet joint of the upper thoracic, lower thoracic, and lumbar spine on spinal rotation
As seen in the axial CT images of the T5–T6 (**a**), T11–T12 (**b**), L2–L3 (**c**) facet joints, the direction of the facet joint surface is closer to coronal in the thoracic spine, and as it goes down through the lower thoracic to the lumbar spine, it becomes closer to sagittal. Therefore, the rotation of the spine (curved arrows) is relatively less restricted in the thoracic spine, but becomes more restricted as it goes down to the lumbar spine

lordotic curve, and the shape and size of the intervertebral disc changes, etc. This is a large area of biomechanical feature transition [66].

The lower lumbar spine has a lordotic curve, is structurally stronger, and the muscles around the spine are well developed, so it has the characteristic of being stronger against compression than the thoracic spine. When a fracture occurs due to compression, it is known that the posterior vertebral body is compressed by the lordotic curve, so the anterior vertebral body collapses more often in the form of an anterior wedging compression fracture than a burst fracture [64].

The injury mechanisms of the thoracolumbar region can usually be summarized into the following seven categories [66].

1. Axial compression: Appears in the form of an anterior wedging compression fracture or burst fracture.
2. Flexion: Compression in the front of the spine, distraction in the back, mainly in the form of an anterior wedging compression fracture of the vertebral body. In severe cases of compression fracture, it appears in the form of ligament damage or avulsion fracture of the bone connected to the ligament in the posterior spine.
3. Lateral compression: Similar to axial compression, trauma is biased to one side, appearing in the form of a compression fracture.
4. Flexion-rotation: When rotation of the spine accompanies flexion. As when flexion occurs, a compression fracture of the anterior vertebral body appears, and if the facet joint capsule and ligaments in the posterior spine are damaged by rotation, it causes unstable fractures.
5. Flexion-distraction: A mechanism related to chance fracture [67], where the center of spinal flexion is located anterior to the spine, causing the entire spine to be affected by the distraction mechanism. The ligaments or bones in the posterior spine are damaged and spread apart, and there are no or almost no compression fractures in the anterior spine.
6. Shear: When a force is applied in the anterior-posterior or left-right transverse direction based on the long axis of the vertebral column. It shows an unstable fracture form accompanied by severe ligament damage.
7. Extension: It usually occurs when the head or upper body part is pushed back. Distraction appears in the anterior structures of the spine, and compression mechanism in the posterior structures. It usually shows a stable fracture, but in the case of a strong injury mechanism caused by a heavy object falling on the patient's back, it can also show an unstable fracture form by causing complete damage to the anterior ligament structure.

8.3.2 Application and Basic Interpretation of Imaging Devices

8.3.2.1 Simple X-Ray Image

Anteroposterior and lateral images are the basic images for evaluating thoracolumbar injuries. Fractures are determined by findings such as cortical bone buckling, cortical bone discontinuity, and a decrease in the height of the anterior or central vertebral body (Fig. 8.37).

In the lateral image, if the anterior height of the thoracolumbar vertebrae is more than 2 mm smaller than the posterior height, a compression fracture should be suspected. However, caution is needed because the T12 and L1 vertebral bodies can show a significant difference in anterior height even in normal conditions [64]. In the lateral image, attention should also be paid to the increase in the width between the spinous processes, disc space, and facet joint. Not only the anterior but also the posterior cortical bone of the vertebral body should be evaluated carefully, and if the posterior cortical bone is lost, a posterior displacement of the bone fragment due to a burst fracture should be suspected [68].

In the anteroposterior plain radiograph, as in the lateral image, the discontinuity of the cortical bone and changes in the height of the vertebral body should be evaluated, and the width between the pedicles should be carefully evaluated. The width between the pedicles is known to gradually increase as you go down from the T6 level. If the width between the pedicles shows a difference of 2–3 mm or more from both the thoracic level above and below, a burst fracture accompanied by a lamina fracture can be suspected (Fig. 8.38), but not all burst fractures accompanied by a lamina fracture show an increase in the width between the pedicles [69–71].

8.3.2.2 CT

With the introduction of MDCT, the use of CT has expanded as isotropic voxel images and coronal and sagittal reformat images can be easily obtained. In patients with blunt trauma to the chest and abdomen, CT is performed to confirm internal organ damage, and it is important to note that there is no need to perform a separate spinal CT to evaluate spinal injuries in these patients. It is sufficient to reconstruct the image centered on the spine using the raw data of the

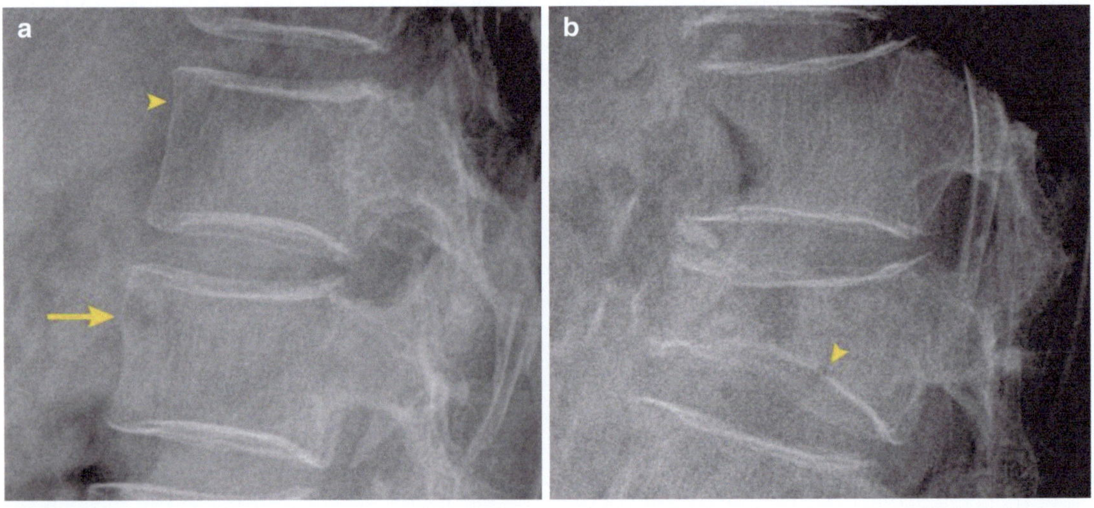

Fig. 8.37 Important findings of thoracolumbar fractures in simple radiographic lateral images. (**a**) Buckling of the cortical bone (arrow). Compare with the flatness of the normal cortical bone of the adjacent vertebra at the corresponding site (arrowhead). As in this case, it may only appear as a buckling of the cortical bone without a decrease in vertebral body height, so caution is required. (**b**) Fracture of the endplate cortical bone (arrowhead) and decrease in anterior height of the vertebral body

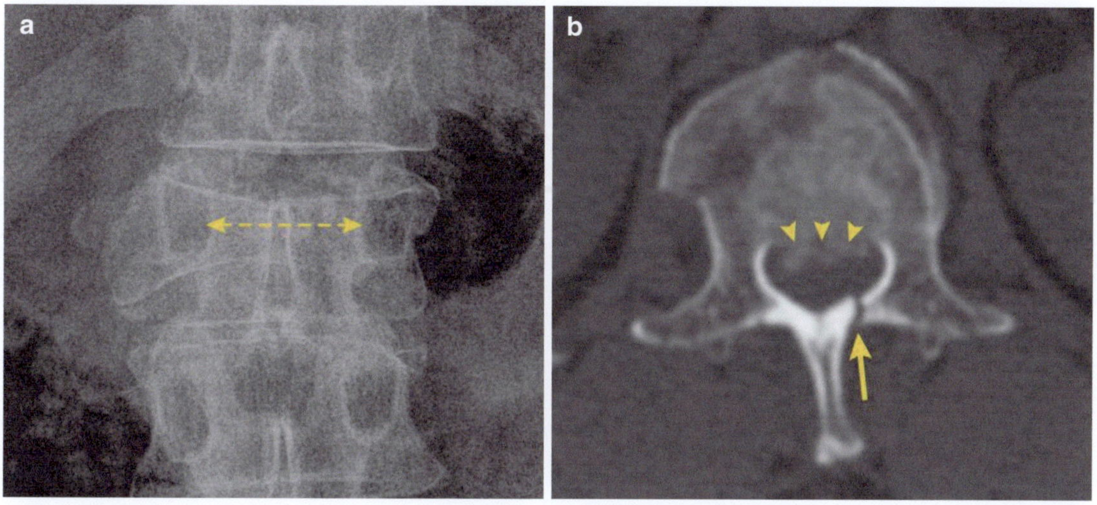

Fig. 8.38 The meaning of interpedicular distance in simple radiographic anteroposterior images
In the anteroposterior image (**a**), if the space between the pedicles is wider compared to the adjacent vertebral body (bidirectional arrows), it signifies a burst fracture accompanied by a lamina fracture. In the axial CT image (**b**) obtained at the same patient's fracture level, a burst fracture accompanied by a posteriorly displaced bone fragment (arrowhead) and lamina fracture (arrow) can be confirmed

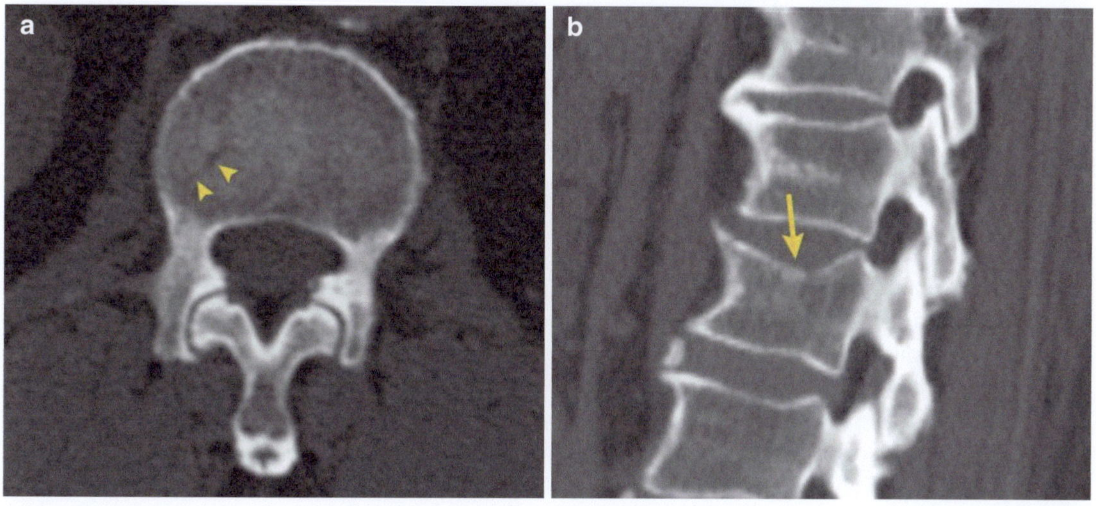

Fig. 8.39 Examples of fractures that are easy to miss in axial CT images
The compression fracture of the upper endplate, which is clearly visible in the sagittal reformat CT image (**b**), may only appear as a fracture line (arrowhead) that is easy to miss in the axial CT image (**a**)

chest and abdominal CT images [72]. What should be noted when evaluating CT images is that many fractures cannot be found with axial (axial) images alone, so sagittal and coronal images must be referred to for interpretation (Fig. 8.39) [64].

8.3.2.3 MRI

Compared to other imaging methods, the most important advantage of MRI is that it has very high soft tissue contrast. Therefore, MRI is superior as an imaging method that directly shows ligament injuries, intervertebral disc injuries, epidural bleeding, spinal cord injuries, etc. Another advantage of

MRI is that it can more sensitively detect fractures. This is because it is a test with high sensitivity to bone marrow edema and bleeding caused by minor fractures. The area with a fracture shows low signal intensity on T1-weighted images and high signal intensity on fluid-sensitive sequences, i.e., fat-suppressed spin-echo T2-weighted images or short tau inversion recovery (STIR) images. However, MRI takes longer to acquire images compared to other imaging methods. Also, pacemakers and life-sustaining and related device have the disadvantage that it cannot be applied to patients carrying medical devices in their bodies that may malfunction, generate heat, or have concerns about potential in the magnetic field [64].

8.3.3 Injury Classification and Imaging Findings

To communicate with fellow clinicians about thoracolumbar injuries, it is sufficient to understand the classification system used in the institution where you work and become familiar with that system. However, the mainstream classification systems provide important foundations for understanding thoracolumbar injury images, so the more you understand these systems, the deeper your understanding of the images. In this chapter, we explain based on the Denis classification [73], which is widely used by many clinicians today despite being an old classification, and apply the McAfee classification [74] to parts that are difficult to explain with the Denis classification alone. We also introduced the Magerl/AO classification, ThoracoLumbar Injury Classification and Severity score (TLICS) for reference.

8.3.3.1 Denis Classification and McAfee Classification

To understand the imaging findings of various injury types occurring in the thoracolumbar region, it is necessary to understand the basis of the Denis and McAfee classifications and their background. In the 1960s, Holdsworth first applied the two column theory, which divides the spine into the anterior column and the posterior column, to the interpretation of thoracolumbar injuries [75]. He also defined the mechanism of injury as flexion, flexion-rotation, extension, vertical compression, and direct shear [76]. Holdsworth's column theory and concept of injury mechanism provided the basic framework for many current injury mechanism classifications, including Denis [73] and McAfee's [74] classifications. With the introduction of CT in the early 1980s, thoracolumbar injury classifications began to converge, with the Denis classification [73] and McAfee classification [74] being representative.

In 1983, Denis first presented the three column theory, a modification of Holdsworth's two column theory, based on 412 thoracolumbar injury patients and 53 CT images obtained from some of these patients, and proposed a systematic injury classification centered on this [73]. The core of the three column theory is the application of the middle column. That is, the spine is divided into the anterior, middle, and posterior columns, and the middle column is proposed as the most important part for spinal stability [73]. The vertebral body was divided into anterior and posterior, describing the anterior as the anterior column and the posterior as the middle column, and the posterior was described as the posterior column based on the posterior longitudinal ligament (PLL) (Fig. 8.40). In the original paper where Denis first proposed the three column theory, the vertebral body was described as being divided into the anterior column and the middle column by dividing the front 1/2 and the back 1/2, but in many subsequent papers, it was often described as dividing the front 2/3 and the back 1/3, causing confusion. However, what is important as a criterion for judging the damage to the middle column is the presence or absence of damage to the posterior wall of the vertebral body, so the definition of the boundary within the vertebral body that divides the anterior column and the middle column is not actually very important. Denis divided spinal injuries into major injuries and minor injuries. Minor injuries are isolated injuries that do not cause acute instability, such as transverse process fractures, articular process fractures, pars interarticularis

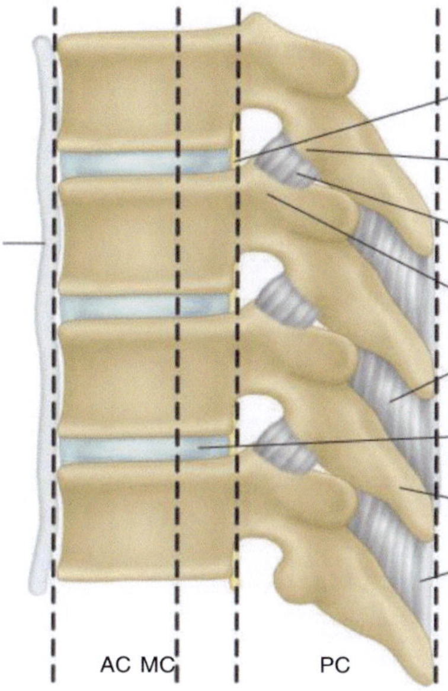

Fig. 8.40 Denis's three column theory
The anterior column (AC) includes the anterior 2/3 of the vertebral body, the anterior intervertebral disc annulus fibrosus, and the anterior longitudinal ligament. The middle column (MC) includes the posterior 1/3 of the vertebral body, the posterior intervertebral disc annulus fibrosus, and the posterior longitudinal ligament. The posterior column (PC) includes osseous structures such as the pedicle, articular process, facet joint, lamina, spinous process, and the posterior ligament complex including the facet joint capsule, ligamentum flavum, interspinous ligament, and supraspinous ligament

Table 8.2 Denis thoracolumbar injury classification and three column injury mechanism [73]

	Main injury mechanism		
Fracture type	Anterior column	Middle column	Posterior column
Compression fracture	Compression	None	None/distraction[a]
Burst fracture	Compression	Compression	None
Seat-belt type	None/Compression[b]	Distraction	Distraction
Fracture-dislocation	Compression/rotation/shear	Distraction/rotation/shear	Distraction/rotation/shear

[a]In the case of a compression fracture, a distraction mechanism occurs in the posterior column when severe energy damage has occurred
[b]Even if a compression mechanism acts on the anterior column in a seat-belt type fracture, the collapse of the anterior vertebral body does not exceed 10–20%

fractures, and spinous process fractures are included here. Major injuries are divided into four types: compression, burst, seat-belt type, and fracture-dislocation, depending on the mechanism of injury and the associated fracture pattern. It was explained that the mechanism acting on each column varies by type, resulting in different fracture patterns (Table 8.2) [73]. Each type is classified into 3–5 subtypes, with a total of 16 subtypes: 4 for compression, 5 for burst, 4 for seat-belt type, and 3 for fracture-dislocation.

A compression fracture is described as a fracture in which the anterior column is compressed and the middle column acts as a hinge, causing the anterior vertebral body to collapse (Fig. 8.41a, b). It is described that if the collapse of the anterior vertebral body is severe, distraction can be applied to the posterior column, which is important for evaluating and understanding the images of spinal fractures. That is, even if the fracture pattern is a compression fracture with anterior collapse, damage can be inflicted on the bone or

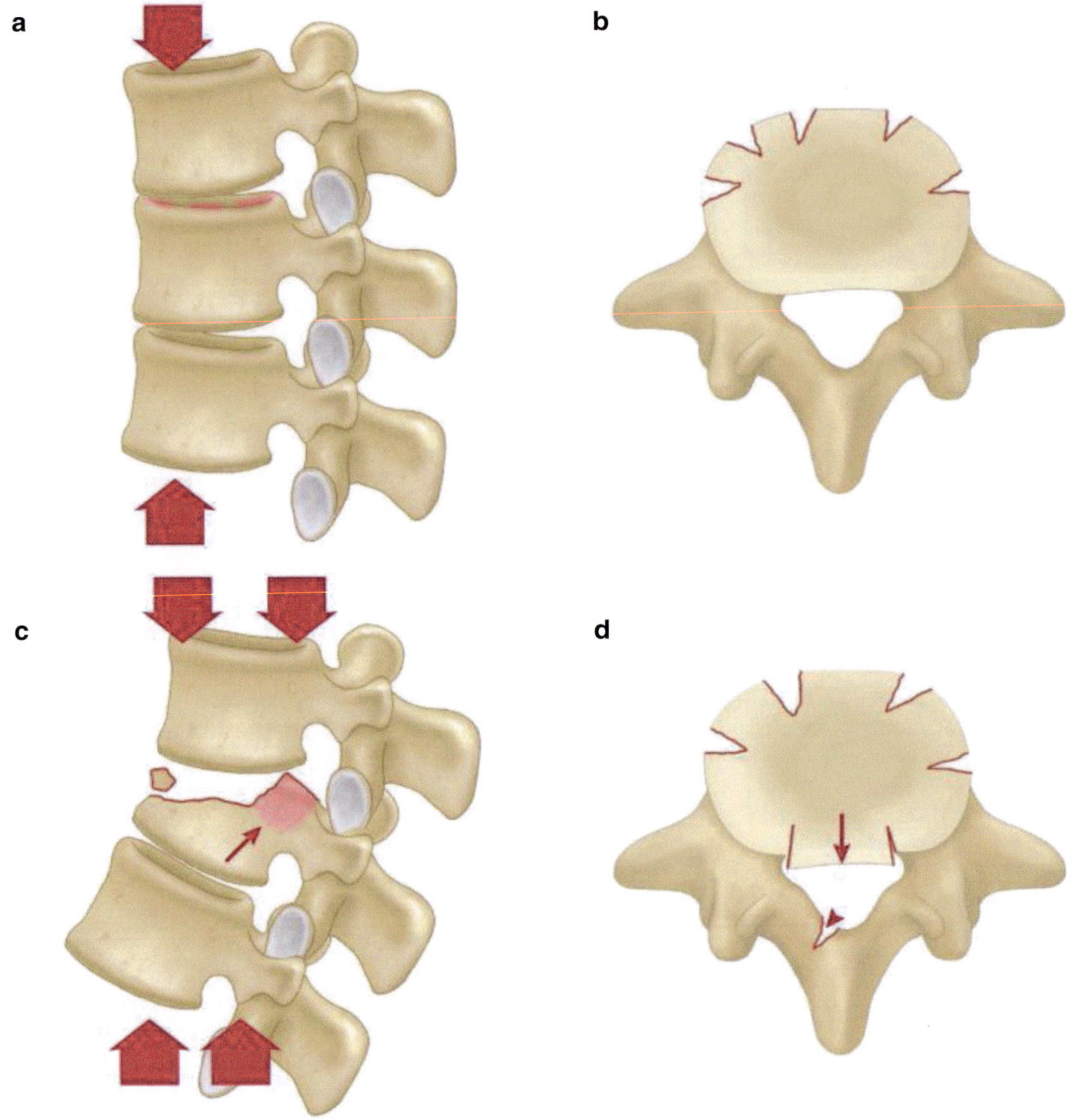

Fig. 8.41 Basic schematic of Denis classification compression type and burst type. (**a**, **b**) Compression type only applies pressure to the anterior column, causing fractures only in the front of the spine. (**c**, **d**)Burst type applies pressure to both the anterior column and middle column, causing fractures in both areas. It is characterized by bone fragments displaced to the central canal (arrows in **c**, **d**) and fractures of the lamina (arrowhead in **d**)

supraspinous ligament, interspinous ligament, ligamentum flavum, and other posterior ligament complex (PLC). In Denis's original paper in 1984, this severe compression fracture and the damage to the PLC occurring in seat-belt injuries are described as factors of "mechanical instability" to be mentioned later [73].

A burst fracture is a type in which the anterior and middle columns of the spine are compressed, causing these columns to collapse. The characteristic of this type is that the middle column collapses, causing a fracture in the posterior wall of the vertebral body, and the resulting bone fragment is retropulsed (Fig. 8.41c, d).

There is much disagreement about the name "seat-belt type." Even in Denis's original paper, it is described that there is room for disagreement about being called "seat-belt type" because this type of injury can occur in accidents other than car accidents. Denis suggested that in addition to "seat-belt type," the names "chance fracture" [67] or "flexion distraction injury" could be used, but he excluded "chance fracture" because it could only explain one of the four subtypes of seat-belt type he proposed, and he excluded "flexion distraction injury" to prevent a terminology collision with the flexion-distraction subtype of fracture-dislocation mentioned below. However, the use of terms for seat-belt type thoracolumbar injuries is still confusing, and recently, terms such as "seat-belt type injury," "flexion-distraction injury," and "chance type fracture" are being used interchangeably [77, 78]. Seat-belt type is a fracture type in which the middle and posterior columns of the spine are damaged by the mechanism of distraction due to flexion. It is described that the anterior column should not be damaged in principle, but it can receive compression damage to the extent that it does not lose its function as a hinge (Table 8.2) [73]. On the other hand, if the anterior column loses its function as a hinge and spinal displacement occurs, it should be distinguished as the flexion-distraction subtype of the fracture-dislocation type that occurs by the same mechanism as mentioned above. Denis reported that seat-belt type injuries can occur at one spinal level or across two spinal levels, and classified them into four subtypes accordingly (Fig. 8.42).

Fracture-dislocation injuries involve damage to all three columns. It is an unstable type of damage. Denis classified this into three subtypes: "flexion rotation," "shear," and "flexion distraction." The flexion-rotation subtype is a mechanism proposed by Holdsworth and others [76], and it shows a form in which the anterior vertebral body collapses as the middle column, posterior column, and anterior column are damaged together when the flexion-rotation mechanism occurs. The height of the posterior vertebral body tends to be relatively maintained (Fig. 8.43). The shear subtype refers to cases where strong force acts across the longitudinal axis of the vertebral column [66]. Most of the damage occurs due to force from the posterior to the anterior direction, but it can also occur due to force from the anterior to the posterior direction (Fig. 8.44) [73]. The flexion-distraction subtype occurs by a similar mechanism to the seat-belt type damage mentioned above, but it is described as different in that the anterior column is damaged and the posterior column does not necessarily start from the posterior (Fig. 8.45). In the Denis classification, if damage is inflicted on two or more columns out of the three columns, it is defined as unstable damage, and the instability of the thoracolumbar is defined in three stages as follows [73]. The first stage is mechanical instability, which is a case that causes damage to the PLC, such as severe compression type and seat-belt type, etc. It does not cause acute spinal instability, but it can cause chronic instability, so it is described that external fixation should be done until the damage to the PLC is healed, or sometimes surgical internal fixation may be required.

The second stage is neurological instability, and burst fractures that mildly compress the central canal belong here. At the time of imaging, it does not show morphological instability, but it is that bone fragments could have been displaced and caused nerve damage at the time of trauma. It is described that there are cases where even patients with relatively mild burst fractures have complained of temporary nerve damage symptoms. The third stage is defined as mechanical and neurologic instability, and cases that show severe burst type and fracture-dislocation type findings and are accompanied by neurological symptoms belong here. In this case, there is a possibility of additional spinal displacement occurring and neurological symptoms may worsen, so it is suggested to perform decompression surgery and internal fixation through surgery. The Denis classification concept can find historical importance in finding the morphological-neurological stability concept of the spine [75].

Although the Denis classification is criticized for its low interobserver agreement [79], it is currently the most widely used classification.

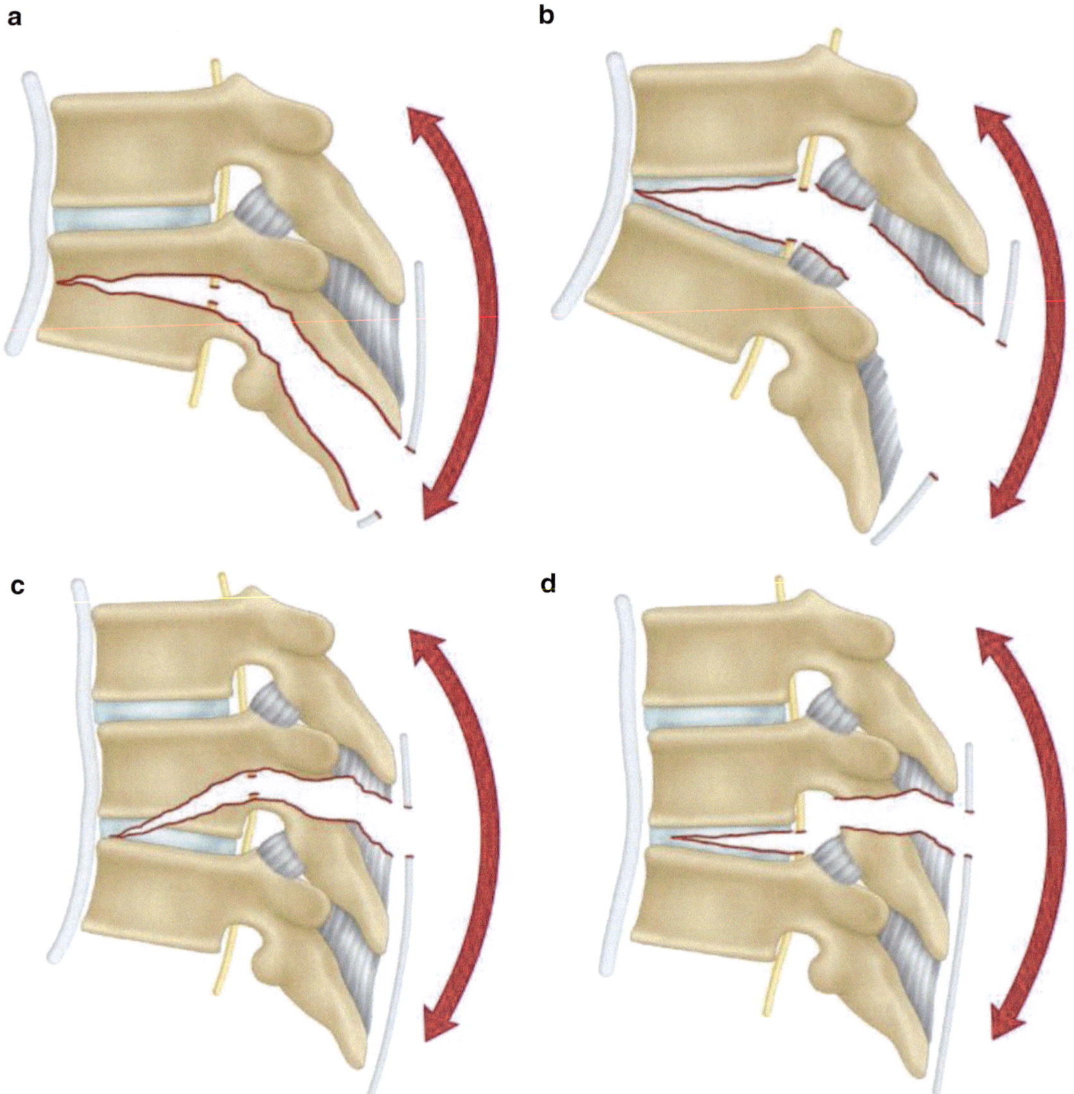

Fig. 8.42 Schematic of Denis classification seat-belt type
This is a damage caused by a distraction mechanism acting on the posterior column and middle column centered on the fulcrum located in front of the anterior longitudinal ligament. (**a**) One level type that occurs along the spine (commonly called a Chance fracture). (**b**) One level type that occurs along the ligament and disc. (**c**) Two level type that occurs along the spine in the middle column (**d**) Two level type that occurs along the disc in the middle column

However, in addition to the low agreement, it has several limitations. First, it is difficult to distinguish between morphologically stable fractures and unstable fractures. Especially in the case of burst fractures, the Denis classification describes all burst types as unstable fractures [75], but this is not actually the case [74]. Also, the core of the Denis classification theory is that the middle column is most important for the stability of the thoracolumbar, but subsequent biomechanical studies have shown that the posterior column, including the PLC, is more important for the stability of thoracolumbar fractures [80]. Moreover, the Denis classification includes 16 subtypes even when considering only major injuries, and each subtype can be further subdivided, making

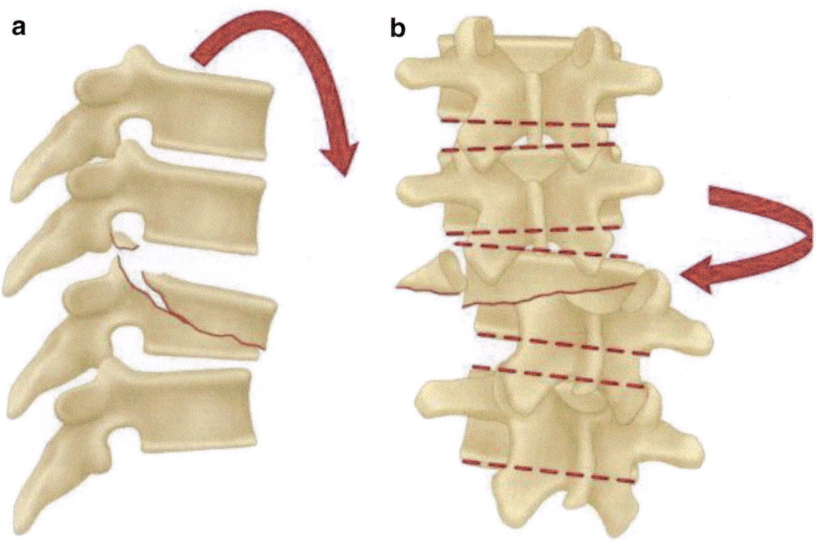

Fig. 8.43 Schematic of flexion-rotation subtype in Denis classification fracture-dislocation type
The entire spine from the anterior column to the posterior column is damaged, and while the front of the vertebral body collapses, the back of the vertebral body relatively maintains its height (**a**). Also, it is a damage where rotational force acts on the fractured level's axial plane (**b**)

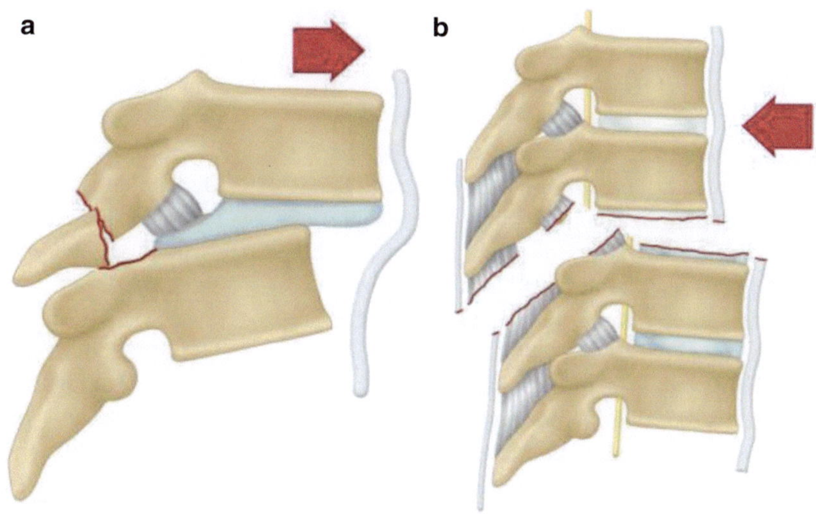

Fig. 8.44 Schematic of shear subtype in Denis classification fracture-dislocation type
Shear force refers to the case where force is applied across the longitudinal axis of the spine, and force can be applied from the back to the front of the spine (**a**) or from the front to the back (**b**)

it challenging to apply all these subtypes in actual clinical practice. On the other hand, categorizing fractures into only four main types—compression, burst, seat-belt type, and fracture-dislocation—oversimplifies the classification and fails to comprehensively describe all fracture patterns, which may lead to difficulties in communication regarding fracture morphology [75].

In 1983, McAfee et al. proposed a classification that emphasized the PLC as the main factor of injury stability. Based on the CT findings of 100 thoracolumbar injury patients, McAfee limited the injury mechanism applied to the middle column to three types: axial compression, axial distraction, and translation, and proposed a classification considering the corresponding injury forms [74, 75]. In the McAfee classification,

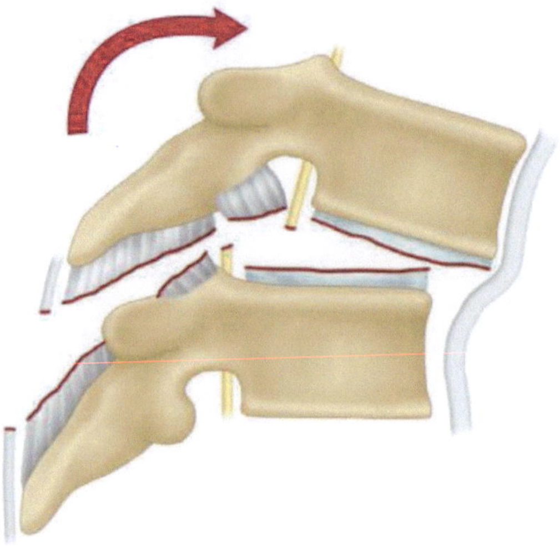

Fig. 8.45 Schematic of flexion-distraction subtype in Denis classification fracture-dislocation type
The middle column and posterior column are damaged by the distraction mechanism due to the flexion of the spine, similar to the seat-belt type, but the anterior column is also damaged, which is different from the seat-belt type where the damaged spine shows displacement

thoracolumbar injuries were divided into the following six forms [74].

1. "Anterior wedging compression fracture" is the same as the compression type in the Denis classification, a damage limited to the anterior column, and occurs due to a flexion mechanism. It was described that nerve damage is rare unless multiple spinal fractures are accompanied.
2. "Stable burst fracture" is a fracture with damage to the anterior column and middle column, which occurs due to axial compression applied to the middle column, but there is no damage to the posterior column.
3. "Unstable burst fracture" is a case where the disruption of the posterior column is accompanied by a fracture due to the compression mechanism of the anterior column and middle column. It is an unstable fracture that can be accompanied by posttraumatic kyphosis and worsening of neurological symptoms. According to McAfee's classification, the middle column is damaged by compression, so the posterior column cannot receive distraction damage [74]. However, in reality, there are cases where the form of unstable burst fracture and the form of distraction damage to the posterior column coexist [81], which will be mentioned in more detail in the description of imaging findings later.
4. "Chance-type fracture" is a case where all columns receive a distraction injury when a flexion force acts in a state where the fulcrum is in front of the ALL. It differs from the flexion-distraction injury mentioned below in that the distraction force also acts on the anterior column.
5. "Flexion-distraction injury" is a case where the fulcrum is behind the ALL, that is, within the anterior column of the vertebral body, so the anterior column receives axial compression, and the middle column and posterior column receive distraction damage. It differs from the chance-type fracture in that the anterior column receives compression damage, not distraction damage.
6. "Translational injury" is when all three columns are ruptured by shear force (shearing force), and the vertebral column is translated in the transverse direction. Compared to the Denis classification, the flexion-rotation subtype and shear subtype, excluding the flexion-distraction subtype, would fall under this category.

The McAfee classification has the advantage of clearly dividing stable fractures and unstable fractures, especially dividing burst fractures into stable and unstable, and being able to sufficiently describe the fracture form even when simplified compared to the Denis classification. However, it has the disadvantage of not having been tested for reliability and not having been prospectively validated [75].

8.3.3.2 Imaging Findings of Thoracolumbar Injury

The clinicians I have experienced often used a mix of Denis classification and some terms from McAfee classification. The content of the following radiological findings is based on the Denis classification, but it should be noted that the McAfee classification was applied to burst fractures.

(1) Compression fracture

The simple radiographic findings of a compression fracture most commonly show a wedge-shaped deformation due to a decrease in the height of the anterior vertebral body. It usually shows a decrease in height of <50%, and sometimes shows a discontinuity or buckling of the anterior cortical bone of the vertebral body, or a discontinuity of the vertebral body endplate (Fig. 8.37). In the Denis classification, a compression fracture is a "one column injury" with damage only to the anterior column, so it is a morphologically stable fracture. However, it is known that severe compression can cause damage to the PLC [73, 82], and in this case, it can be classified as unstable and may be an indication for surgery. If there is a fracture at one level, if the height of the anterior vertebral body decreases by more than 40%, or if a kyphotic angle of more than 30° is shown, there is a possibility of an unstable fracture due to damage to the PLC, and surgery may be necessary as the kyphosis may worsen [83]. Also, if there are fractures at multiple levels, unstable fractures should be suspected for similar reasons. Compression fractures can be difficult to diagnose on axial CT images when the fracture line occurs parallel to the image plane, and in this case, it can be easily diagnosed using CT reformatted in sagittal and coronal. MRI is a test with high sensitivity for edema and bleeding in the bone marrow. When evaluating MRI images of compression fracture patients, it should always be kept in mind that there may be sufficient damage to the PLC if the height of the anterior vertebral body is severely reduced as mentioned above. Also, MRI is a test that can sensitively confirm damage to ligaments or surrounding soft tissues, and it is very important to confirm the presence of PLC damage not only in burst fractures, flexion-distraction injuries, and fracture-dislocations, but also in compression fractures (Fig. 8.46).

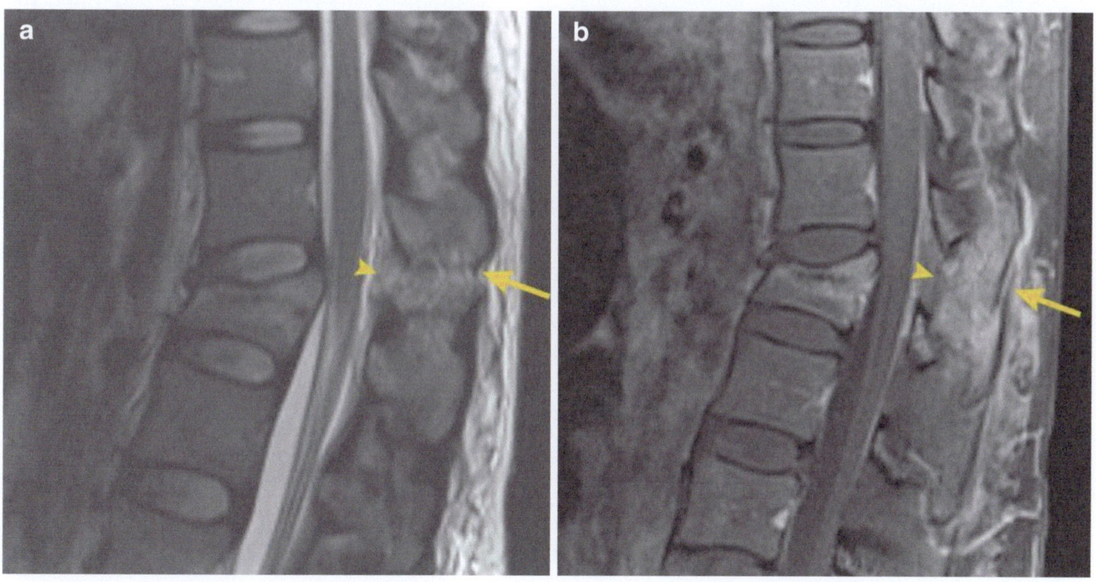

Fig. 8.46 Combination of compression fracture and posterior ligament complex damage
On T2-enhanced MRI (**a**) and contrast-enhanced fat-suppressed T1MRI using gadolinium (**b**), the posterior ligament complex is damaged from the supraspinous ligament (arrow) to the ligamentum flavum (arrowhead) due to distraction damage of the posterior column by compression fracture of the vertebral body

(2) Stable burst fracture and unstable burst fracture
Burst fractures are characterized by fractures in the posterior wall of the vertebral body due to compression applied to the middle column, and bone fragments caused by this are posteriorly displaced.

On lateral simple radiographs, a decrease in the height of the posterior vertebral body and posterior displacement of the posterior vertebral body bone fragments are seen. On anteroposterior simple radiographs, if there is an increase in the distance between the pedicles (interpedicular distance), it can be diagnosed as a burst fracture (Fig. 8.38). However, simple radiographs often fail to diagnose burst fractures or properly evaluate the degree of posterior displacement of bone fragments because they do not show the posterior of the spine well [84, 85], and CT compensates for these disadvantages.

In other words, the main role of CT in diagnosing burst fractures is to evaluate whether the fracture invades the posterior wall of the spine and the degree of narrowing of the central canal by posteriorly displaced bone fragments. However, sometimes these radiographic findings are not clear, and it is not easy to determine whether it is a burst fracture. In such cases on the apex, the posterior wall of the spine, which appears concave, can be diagnosed as a burst fracture if it shows a flattened shape (flattening) (Fig. 8.47) [86]. There are reports that there is no evidence that the degree of neurological symptoms is severe as the central canal is narrowed by the posteriorly displaced bone fragment in CT images [87–89], but this is still a subject of controversy. In one study, it was reported that the more the central canal is narrowed, the more severe the neurological damage when the neurological deficit is evaluated only in incomplete cases [90]. The reason for the different results in each study may be that these studies are very unevenly designed with different patient groups, number of patients, and various injury mechanisms, but it may also be a natural result considering that the degree of displacement of the bone fragment at the time of injury and the time of obtaining the image may be different [89]. Although there is disagreement in each study about the "correlation" between the degree of central canal invasion and the

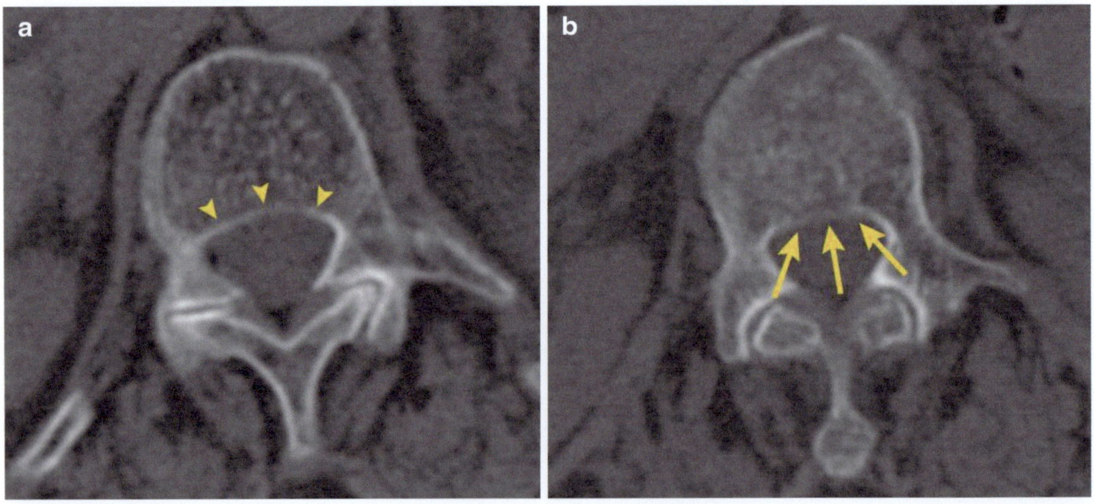

Fig. 8.47 Findings of mild-degree burst fracture in axial CT images
In a spine where a burst fracture has not occurred (**a**), the posterior part of the vertebral body shows a concave shape (arrowhead), but in a spine where a burst fracture has occurred (**b**), the vertebral body. The shape appears to flatten or slightly bulge as the boundary of the back becomes ambiguous (arrow)

degree of neurological symptoms, it is being reported consistently that the possibility of neurological symptoms is high when the central canal is invaded by the bone fragment, that is, from the perspective of the "presence or absence" of symptoms. Denis reported that the proportion of patients with neurological symptoms was high when the bone fragment invaded more than 50% of the central canal [73]. In a study involving a fairly large number of 198 patients, it was reported that the frequency of neurological damage was 12%, 41%, 78% in the thoracolumbar junction (T11–L1) and 8%, 30%, 68% in the lumbar (L2–L5) when the central canal was invaded by 25%, 50%, 75% of the bone fragment, respectively [90].

MRI directly shows the shape of the spinal cord or other neural structures being pressed by the posteriorly displaced bone fragment and is useful for sensitively determining the presence or absence of fractures at other spinal levels.

Denis classified cases with damage to two or more columns as unstable fractures, so according to this classification, burst fractures caused by compression damage to the anterior column and middle column should all be classified as unstable fractures. However, many burst fractures are actually stable fractures, and McAfee distinguished between stable burst fractures and unstable burst fractures, with the criterion for unstable burst fractures being the severance of the posterior column [74]. However, currently, the instability of burst fractures is not determined solely by the severance of the posterior column, and if a decrease in vertebral body height of more than 50%, an invasion of the central canal of more than 40% by the posteriorly displaced spinal bone fragment, and a kyphotic angle displacement of 25° or more at the injury level are confirmed in the image, it is judged as unstable (Fig. 8.48). Regardless of the imaging findings, if neurological damage progresses clinically, it is considered an unstable burst fracture and surgical treatment is considered [83].

(3) Seat-belt type injury

This type of injury is probably the most confusing in terms of the classification and naming of thoracolumbar injuries. Even now, many documents describe the seat-belt type injury mechanism using different names, and "seat-belt type injury," [73] "flexion-distraction injury," [77] and "chance-type fracture" [78] all mean the same injury mechanism and shape. It is believed that there will be no problem if understood. Here, I will use the term "seat-belt type" faithfully to Denis's original work.

This damage refers to a case where the fulcrum of the lever is in front of the vertebral body, i.e., the ALL, and when flexion force is applied to the vertebral column, the spine at the level where the fulcrum is located is separated transversely from the back, creating a fracture line on the cross-section and showing a wide-open shape of the back of the spine around it (Fig. 8.49). At this time, it can be classified as a seat-belt type injury if the ALL is not damaged, and if the ALL is damaged and the upper spine is anteriorly displaced, it is classified as a fracture-dislocation type to be mentioned later, and it corresponds to the "flexion-distraction subtype." [73] Seat-belt type injuries occur almost entirely at the T12–L2 level, and they can also show injuries at nearby or distant levels, and these injuries can be easily found using MRI [77, 78]. The transverse fracture line caused by seat-belt type injury appears along the spine, along the ligaments and intervertebral discs, and across the spine and ligaments (Fig. 8.42) [73].

Seat-belt type injuries show fractures in the middle column and posterior column while maintaining the height of the anterior vertebral body in simple radiographic images, and changes in the posterior column alone or both the posterior column and middle column are spread by distraction injuries. In anteroposterior radiographic images, the "empty vertebral body sign," which is characterized by a decrease in the shadow inside the vertebral body due to angulation of the

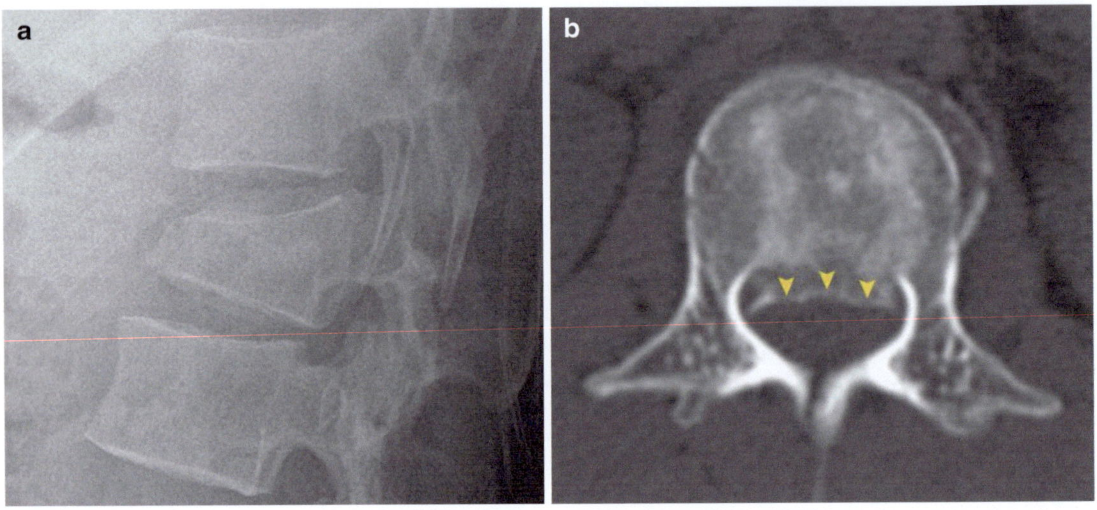

Fig. 8.48 If more than 50% of the vertebral body height is reduced and a kyphotic angle of more than 25 degrees is shown in the simple radiographic lateral image (a), and in CT (b), if the posteriorly displaced bone fragment (arrowhead) invades more than 40% of the central canal, it is considered unstable and surgical treatment is considered

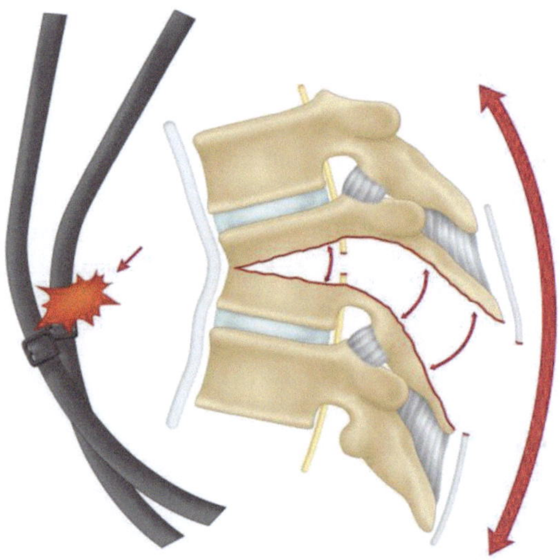

Fig. 8.49 Mechanism of seat-belt type injury
When the fulcrum point (middle arrow of the belt) is located in front of the anterior longitudinal ligament due to seat belts, etc., and flexion force is applied to the vertebral column, a distraction mechanism works from the posterior column and middle column of the spine, causing a cross-sectional separation injury

upper vertebral body based on the fracture or injury site, is characteristic (Fig. 8.50) [78]. Other findings suggesting seat-belt type injuries in anteroposterior images include transverse fracture lines along the pedicle, increased distance between ribs, transverse fracture lines of the transverse process, lamina, and articular process. In lateral images, transverse fractures of the pedicle, vertebral body, and spinous process and spread fracture sites are shown, and if the posterior ligament complex is damaged, the space between the spinous processes widens and the intervertebral neural foramen widens or facet joint subluxation or dislocation is observed. When the PLC is damaged, the disc space can also spread [78, 91].

In cases where seat-belt type injuries invade the lumbar spine, more than 40% of the time they are accompanied by abdominal injuries [78], so many patients undergo abdominal CT. In this case, it is known that fractures are easily overlooked with axial CT images alone [91]. However, seat-belt type injuries can be diagnosed with findings such as the "dissolving pedicle sign" and "naked-facet sign" even in axial CT images. The "Dissolving pedicle sign" (Fig. 8.51) refers to the disappearance of the pedicle at the level where there is a transverse fracture, and the "naked-facet sign" refers to the case where the inferior articular process of the

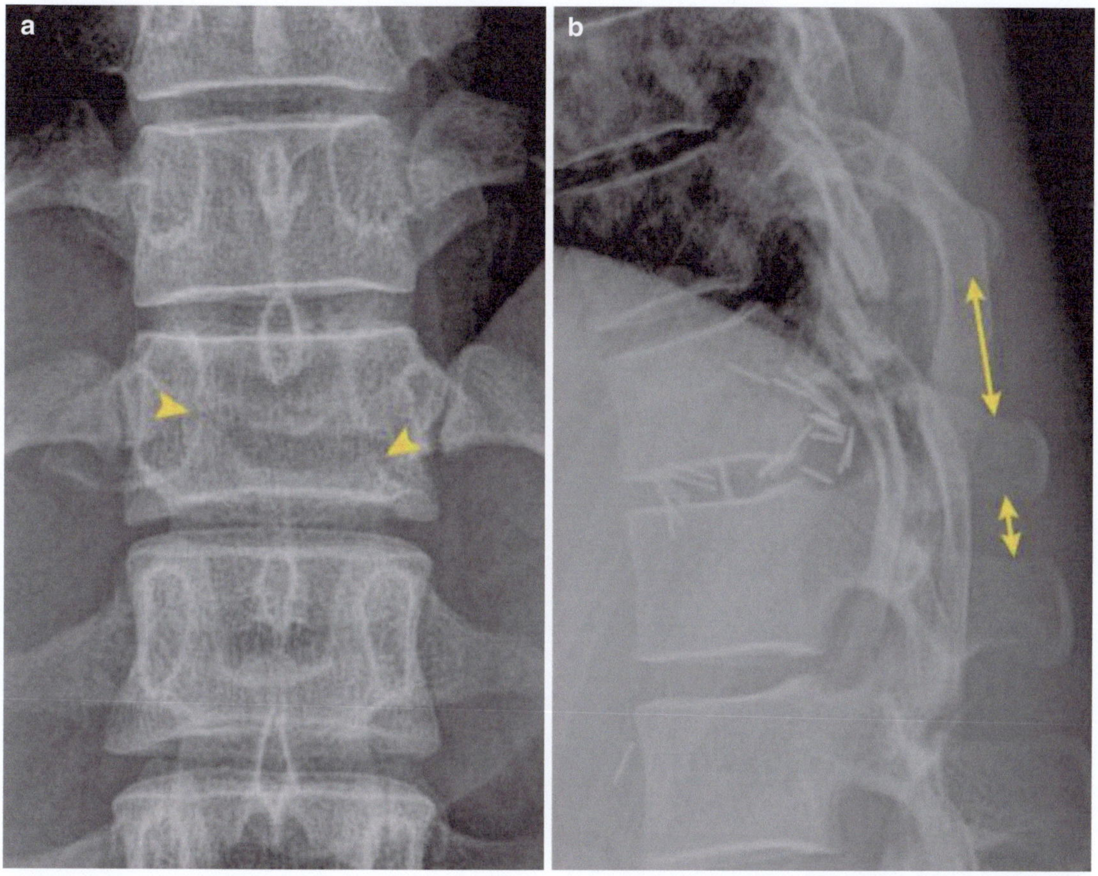

Fig. 8.50 Simple radiographic findings of seat-belt type injury. (**a**) "Empty vertebra sign" in the simple radiographic anteroposterior image. The fracture of the inner wall cortical bone of the pedicle is also shown (arrowhead). (**b**) Simple radiographic lateral image. The distance between the spinous processes is significantly larger at the injury level (long bidirectional arrow) compared to the normal level (short bidirectional arrow). This is a finding suggesting damage to the posterior ligament complex. The high-density foreign bodies on the line are clips related to previous abdominal surgery

upper spine, which should be seen behind the superior articular process of the lower spine at the corresponding facet joint level, is not seen when the facet joint dislocation occurs due to distraction injury [78]. However, since these findings do not appear in all patients, it is necessary to obtain sagittal/coronal reformat images as much as possible and directly confirm the transverse fracture/facet joint dislocation to make a diagnosis (Fig. 8.51).

MRI is used to confirm PLC damage and the presence of fractures at other levels (Fig. 8.52) [77, 78]. The accuracy of MRI in diagnosing PLC damage has been reported to vary widely. A study in 2000 that evaluated the diagnostic accuracy of MRI for PLC damage through fat-suppressed T2-weighted images in 34 patients reported high accuracy for damage to the supraspinous ligament, interspinous ligament, and ligamentum flavum [92]. However, a prospective evaluation of the diagnostic power of fat-suppressed T2-weighted images for PLC damage performed by Vaccaro et al. in 2009 showed lower accuracy than previously published papers, especially with low specificity (between 53–65%), and it was argued in this

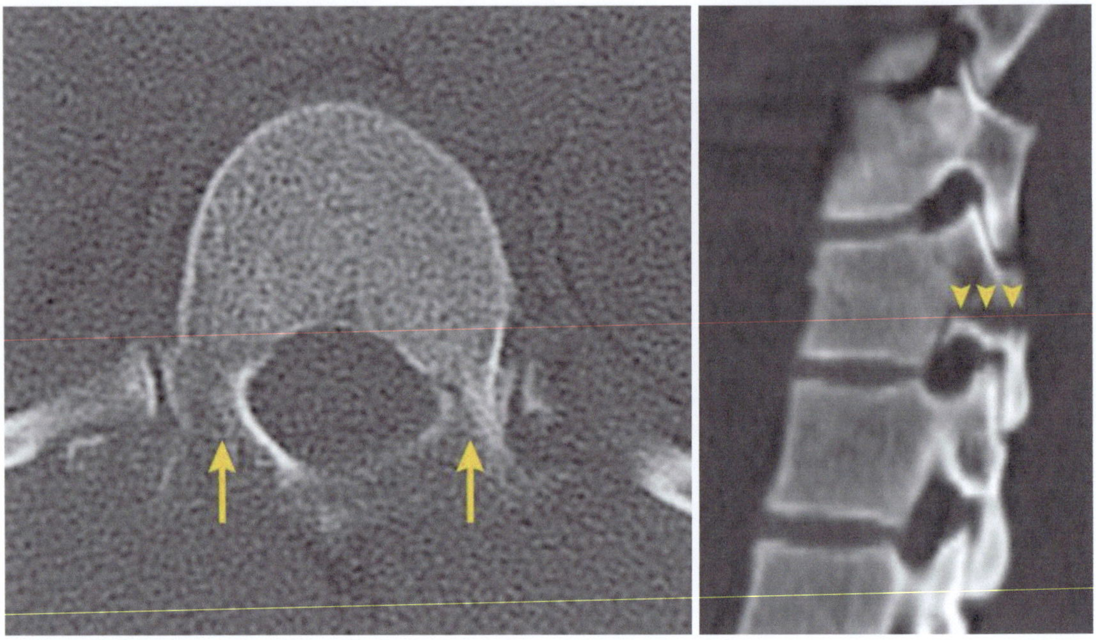

Fig. 8.51 CT findings of seat-belt type injury. (**a**) In the axial CT image, if the image is obtained at the level where there is a cross-sectional fracture of the pedicle, the "dissolving pedicle sign" appears where part or all of the pedicle is not visible (arrow). (**b**) Cross-sectional fracture of the pedicle is seen in the sagittal reformat CT image of the same spine (arrowhead)

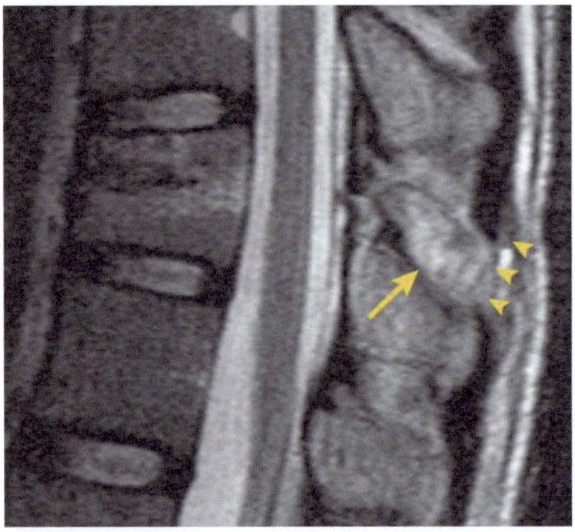

Fig. 8.52 MRI findings of posterior ligament complex injury in seat-belt type injury
In the T2-enhanced image, the supraspinous ligament (arrowhead) and interspinous ligament (arrow) are damaged due to the distraction injury of the posterior column. The relatively almost unchanged height of the anterior vertebral body is one of the characteristics of seat-belt type injury

study that it is difficult to determine treatment policy solely by MRI [93].

Although there are such disagreements about the diagnostic accuracy of MRI for PLC damage, MRI is still considered an important means in diagnosing PLC damage and its use is increasing [93]. Accordingly, in clinical practice, we often encounter cases where PLC damage or transverse fractures of the posterior column, which appear to be due to distraction mechanisms on MRI, are also confirmed in burst fractures and compression fractures [92]. The concept of distraction mechanism in the posterior column accompanying severe compression fracture, as discussed above, was also mentioned in Denis's original paper, but the distraction mechanism damage in the posterior column in burst fracture is contrary to the basic concept in Denis classification. However, there have already been reports that there are fracture types where distraction mechanism damage and burst fracture coexist [81, 94], and recently, the inability to explain the coexistence of these two is being presented as a weakness of Denis classification [66]. Recently, two mechanisms have been proposed for the cause of the coexistence of seat-belt type damage and burst fracture [77, 78], Bernstein said that due to strong energy, the fulcrum of seat-belt type damage is in front of ALL and moves to the middle column, causing pressure on the middle column and resulting in burst fracture [78], Groves et al. suggested a mechanism in which the anterior column and middle column of the spine, which had been spread up and down by severe seat-belt type damage, collide strongly as they return to their original position (recoil), resulting in secondary burst fracture [77]. It is difficult to prove which mechanism is correct, but it is starting to be accepted that seat-belt type damage and burst fracture can appear together at one level, and in this case, the preceding mechanism is seat-belt type damage (Fig. 8.53). This is an important concept because when seat-belt type damage occurs in the lumbar spine, it is often accompanied by more abdominal damage than pure burst fracture [77].

Seat-belt type damage is classified as unstable fracture, but the frequency of neurological damage is relatively low. In the thoracic region, a neurological damage frequency of 30–40% has been reported [77, 95, 96]. In the lumbar region, a smaller neurological damage frequency has been reported [78]. Surgical fixation can be considered to prevent progressive kyphotic deformity, and the criteria are 15° or more of kyphosis on imaging, or pure PLC ligament damage without accompanying fractures of the posterior column and avulsion fractures. It is recommended that surgical treatment be performed regardless of imaging findings in cases accompanied by neurological symptoms [83].

(4) Fracture-dislocation

Denis divided this injury into three mechanisms: flexion-rotation, shear, and flexion-distraction [73]. It is characterized by damage to all three columns, and the upper vertebrae at the injury level are anteriorly, posteriorly, or laterally displaced relative to the lower vertebrae [97]. Rotation of the vertebral body can also occur. Anterior displacement of the vertebral body is much more common, lateral displacement is relatively rare, and posterior displacement is rare [97].

The most common places for fracture-dislocation to occur are at the T4–T5 and T5–T6 levels in the upper thoracic spine and in the thoracolumbar transition area in the lumbar spine. Fracture-dislocation is very likely to be accompanied by neurological damage. Almost all fracture-dislocations occurring from T1 to T8 level are known to be accompanied by neurological damage, and fracture-dislocations occurring in the thoracolumbar transition area are known to be accompanied by neurological damage in 60–70% of cases [97].

On simple radiographs, the displacement of the vertebral body located above the injury level can be confirmed. The vertebral body located below the injury level shows various degrees of compression fracture and a characteristic triangular bone fragment on the anterior upper endplate ("ripped can top appearance," Fig. 8.54). Since the PLC is completely damaged from the posterior supraspinous ligament to the anterior facet joint, various degrees of dislocation occur in the facet joint. In cases where rotation or shear force is involved, fractures of the ribs or transverse processes of the spine may occur, and the alignment of the vertebral column may be displaced laterally ("windswept appearance," Fig. 8.54).

In cases of fracture-dislocation in the thoracolumbar spine, there are many accompanying thoracic or abdominal injuries, so CT is performed in most cases. On axial CT images, the so-called double vertebrae sign

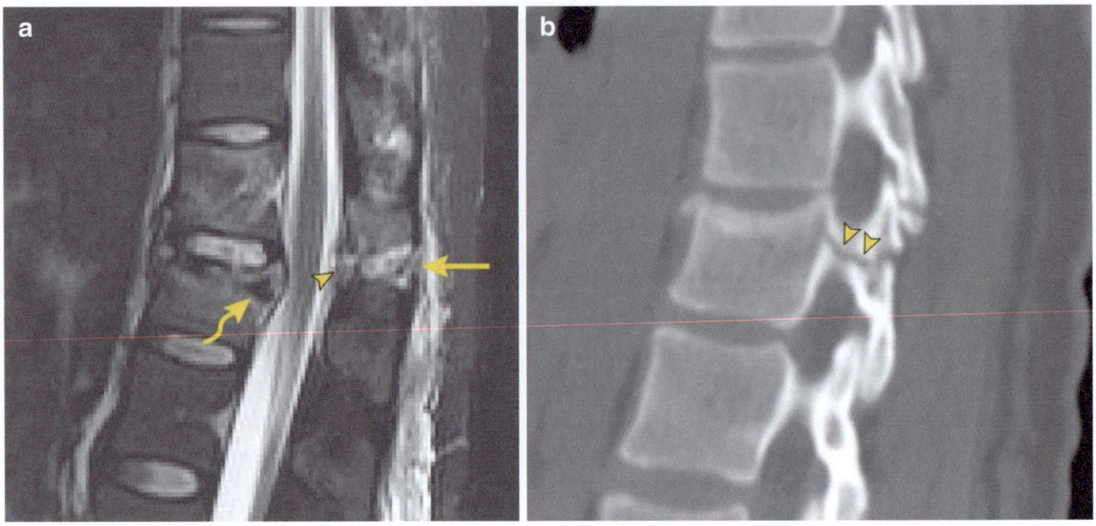

Fig. 8.53 Co-occurrence of seat-belt type injury and burst fracture
In the fat-suppressed T2-enhanced sagittal image (**a**) of the thoracolumbar junction, the cross-sectional fracture of the spinous process (arrow) suggests damage to the posterior column and posterior ligament complex, accompanied by rupture of the ligamentum flavum (arrowhead). It is accompanied by the form of a burst fracture where the back of the vertebral body is posteriorly displaced (curved arrow). In the sagittal reformat CT image (b) of the same patient, a cross-sectional fracture line of the pedicle suggesting a seat-belt type injury is seen (arrowhead)

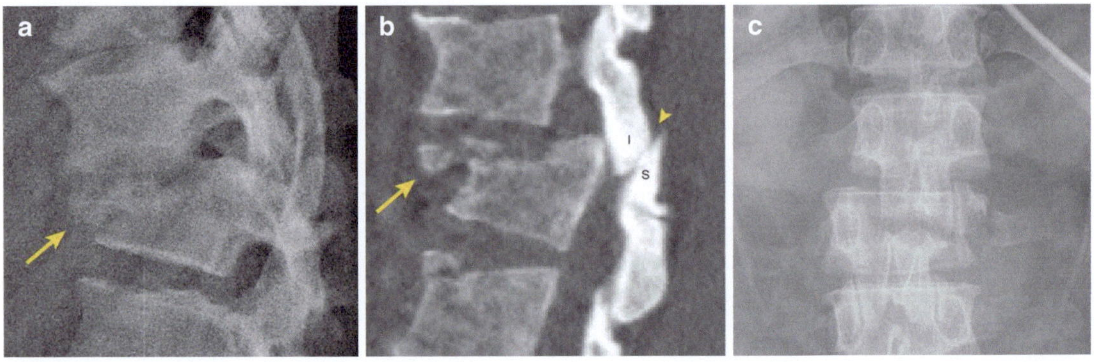

Fig. 8.54 Simple radiographic findings of thoracolumbar fracture-dislocation. (**a**, **b**) Fracture-dislocation findings at the T12–L1 level. In the simple radiographic lateral image (**a**), the T12 vertebral body is anteriorly displaced. The L1 vertebral body has a severe compression fracture, and a small triangular bone fragment from the L1 vertebral body maintains alignment with the T12 vertebral body, maintaining alignment, showing a typical "ripped can top appearance." The "ripped can top appearance" seen in simple radiographs is clearly visible in the sagittal reformat CT (**b**) of the same patient. Accompanied facet locking is seen (arrowhead). S: superior articular process of the lower vertebra, I: inferior articular process of the upper vertebra. (**c**) Thoracic lumbar fracture-dislocation findings due to lateral shear force. It shows a typical "windswept appearance"

can be seen where two vertebrae are seen in one axial image as the upper vertebrae are displaced and fall to the lower level, and when the facet joint is completely dislocated, the "naked facet sign" where the inferior articular process of the upper vertebrae, which should be seen behind the superior articular process of the lower vertebrae at the facet joint level, is not seen, or the "reverse hamburger sign," a finding of facet

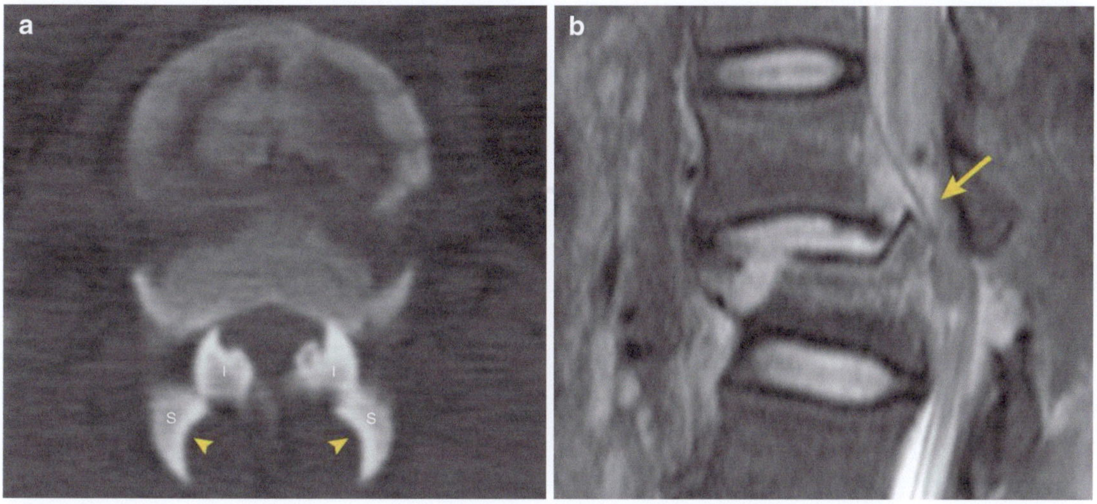

Fig. 8.55 CT and MRI imaging findings of thoracic lumbar fracture-dislocation
(**a**) Axial CT imaging findings of facet joint dislocation and facet joint locking in the thoracic lumbar transition. The inferior articular process (I) of the upper vertebra is not seen behind the superior articular process (S) of the lower vertebra ("naked facet sign," arrowhead) and is anteriorly displaced (facet locking). (**b**) Sagittal fat-suppressed T2-weighted MRI findings of a flexion-rotation subtype case. The anterior longitudinal ligament, intervertebral disc, posterior longitudinal ligament, and posterior ligament complex including the facet joint are all completely damaged. The conus medullaris is also damaged (arrow)

locking where the inferior articular process of the upper vertebrae is seen in front of the superior articular process of the lower vertebrae, can be seen. However, these axial image findings can be more easily evaluated on sagittal or coronal reformat images (Fig. 8.55) [97].

MRI is an important imaging tool for determining the cause and degree of neurological damage and is used to evaluate spinal cord injury, surrounding hematoma at the injury site, intervertebral disc injury, and degree of herniation (Fig. 8.55).

8.3.3.3 Other Classifications of Thoracolumbar Injuries

(1) AO classification

In the early 1990s, the AO (Arbeitsgemeinschaft fur Osteosynthesegragen) group, a group of researchers studying the diagnosis and treatment of fractures, proposed various spinal classifications. After reviewing the damage classification methods, a new classification method was devised that could comprehensively describe all types of spinal injuries and was proposed through a research paper by Magerl et al. in 1994 [98]. At that time, the AO classification was described based on the Magerl classification, and the damage mechanism applied to the spine was divided into three categories: compression, distraction, and rotation. Each type of damage caused by these mechanisms was classified into types A, B, and C, establishing a classification system. Each type is further subdivided according to the type and severity of the fracture, and according to Magerl's original paper, it is classified into more than 50 types [98]. This classification has the advantage of being able to explain all types of fractures because it comprehensively covers the shape of the fractures, and it has the advantage of logically hierarchizing thoracolumbar injuries. However, it was overly complicated to the point where the table had to be looked up one by one, and there was no consideration for clinical information, making it difficult to apply directly to the clinic and the usefulness verification was not well performed [99].

To overcome these disadvantages, a new AO classification was proposed in 2013. Based on the ThoracoLumbar Injury Classification and Severity Score (TLICS) described below, the morphology part of the existing AO classification was classified more simply, and new factors (modifiers) that affect neurological signs and stability were added to strengthen clinical elements, thereby revising it into a classification system that can be used for treatment policy decisions. Like the existing AO classification, it is comprehensive but simpler than before (Fig. 8.56) [100]. Following the revised AO classification, for example, if there is a clear displacement of the vertebral column at the T8–9 level, a burst fracture is seen in the T9 vertebra, and the patient has incomplete spinal cord injury and ankylosing spondylitis as a basic disease, the primary injury is described as T8–9: C, and the secondary injury, neurologic status, modifier is put in parentheses as (T9: A3; N3; M2). In summary, the patient's injury can be described as T8–9: C (T9: A3; N3; M2) according to the AO classification.

(2) Thoracolumbar Injury Classification and Severity Score

The Denis and McAfee classifications have the disadvantage of not being able to explain all fracture types, and the AO classification has the disadvantage of being overly complicated. To overcome this, the "Spine Trauma Study Group (STSG)," led by Vaccaro et al., proposed a new classification for thoracolumbar injuries called "Thoracolumbar Injury Severity Score (TLISS)" in 2005 [101]. The STSG is a research group that proposed the Subaxial Injury Classification (SLIC) as a classification method for lower cervical injuries, and the TLISS classification is an algorithm proposed about two years before the SLIC was proposed, and is a classification method that is currently receiving attention. The TLISS classification allows for treatment policy

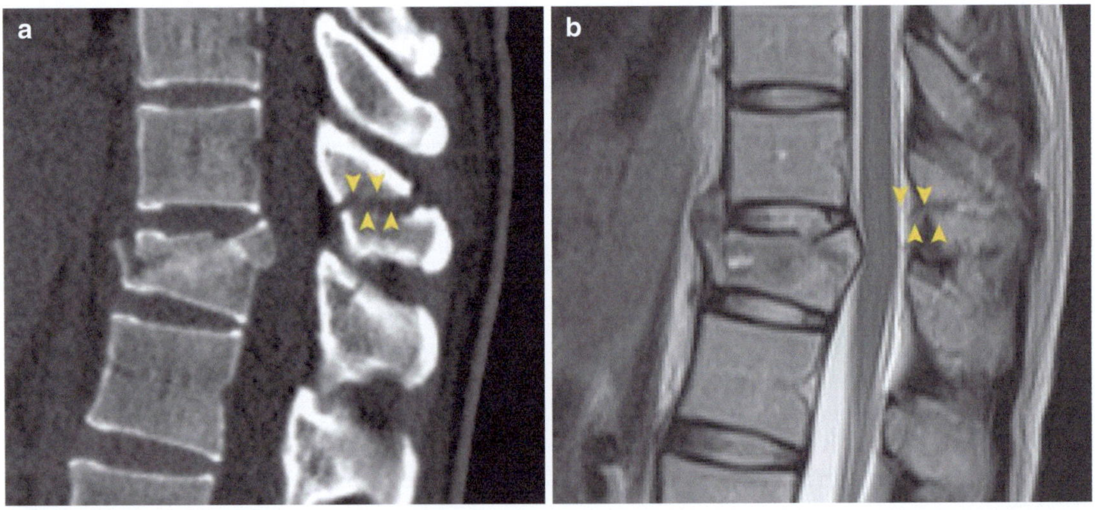

Fig. 8.56 Example of applying the Thoracolumbar Injury Classification and Severity Score (TLICS)
A 34-year-old traffic accident patient was admitted without neurological symptoms. The sagittal reformat CT image (**a**) shows a burst fracture form due to compression mechanism, and a transverse fracture line that appears to be due to distraction damage is seen on the spinous process one level above (arrowhead). The sagittal T2-weighted image (**b**) performed at the time of admission shows no spinal cord injury, and the damage to the posterior ligament complex (posterior ligament complex, PLC) associated with the transverse fracture of the spinous process (arrowhead) is clear. When calculating the score according to TLICS, the highest score is 4 points for morphology score, including compression mechanism (1 point), burst fracture form (1 point), distraction mechanism (4 points), clear PLC damage (3 points), and normal neurological status (0 points), for a total of 7 points. Since it is 5 points or more, it can be judged that surgical treatment is required

decisions through scoring of three variables when evaluating thoracolumbar injuries, the three variables being (1) suspected injury mechanism through imaging, (2) presence or absence of PLC damage, and (3) the patient's neurological damage status were defined [100]. However, the first variable, the injury mechanism, had the disadvantage that some subjectivity could be involved in the process of inferring the mechanism through the shape of the fracture [102, 103]. To overcome this, the classification was changed to a classification that scores the "shape of the fracture" rather than the "mechanism of injury," and this was announced by Vaccaro et al. in 2015 under the name "Thoracolumbar Injury Classification and Severity Score (TLICS)." Here, the first of the three variables above was changed from "injury mechanism" to "injury morphology" [62]. In addition, in the TLISS classification, if multiple injury mechanisms are suspected in one spine, the scores of these are all added up, but in TLICS, it was changed to score only the injury shape caused by the most severe injury mechanism. For example, if a spine showing the shape of a burst fracture (2 points) shows a shape caused by a distraction mechanism (distraction) (4 points), in the TLISS classification, 6 points are given focusing on the mechanism, but in TLICS, only 4 points are given focusing on the shape of the distraction mechanism.(Table 8.3) [104]. In the TLICS classification, the provision to add 1 point to lateral compression was also deleted unlike the TLISS classification. Subsequent studies comparing the usefulness and reliability of the TLISS and TLICS classification systems reported that both classifications showed relatively high interobserver agreement. Here, it is described according to the TLICS classification [66, 103, 105].

In the TLICS classification (Table 8.4), as mentioned above, the injury mechanism based on the injury shape, neurologic status, and the presence or absence of PLC injury are scored as in Table 8.3, and if the sum of the scores is 3 points or less, non-surgical treatment is recommended, and if it is 5 points or more, surgical treatment is recommended. If it is 4 points, it is recommended that the clinician decides according to the situations (Fig. 8.56).

First, in the injury mechanism, the three mechanisms of compression, rotational/translational, and distraction applied in the AO classification were applied. Here, 1 point was assigned to compression, 3 points to rotational/translational, and 4 points to distraction, and 1 point was added if there was a burst fracture. If there are injuries at multiple levels, the most severe level of injury is used as the basis for scoring, and if multiple mechanisms of injury are suspected at the level decided to be scored, the highest score among them is used as the basis for scoring.

The neurological injury status is judged clinically, and it is divided into four categories based on severity and recovery potential. Two points were given for nerve root injury, 2 points for complete injury of the spinal cord or conus medullaris, and 3 points were given for incomplete injury of the spinal cord or conus medullaris or cauda equina injury.

The damage to the PLC is comprehensively evaluated using physical examination, plain radiography, CT, MRI, etc. It is judged as follows: if there is no damage, 0 points are given, if the damage is uncertain, 2 points are given, and if the damage is certain, 3 points are given.

This classification has the advantage of being directly linked to treatment and prognosis, and as mentioned above, it was used as the basis for the revised AO classification.

Table 8.3 AO classification

Evaluation item	Description
Morphology (fracture shape)	
Type A. Compression injuries. Anterior structure damage due to compression	
A0. Minor, nonstructural fractures	Fractures do not weaken the structural integrity of the spinal column (such as transverse process, spinous process fractures, etc.)
A1. Wedge-compression	Only one of the upper and lower endplates is fractured. No involvement of the vertebral body posterior wall
A2. Split	Both the upper and lower endplates are fractured. No involvement of the vertebral body posterior wall
A3. Incomplete burst	Involvement of the vertebral body posterior wall. Only one of the upper and lower endplates is fractured. There is usually a vertical fracture of the lamina, but it does not involve the failure of the tension band
A4. Complete burst	Involvement of the vertebral body posterior wall. Both the upper and lower endplates are fractured. There is usually a vertical fracture of the lamina, but it does not involve the failure of the tension band
Type B. Failure of the posterior or anterior tension band	
B1. Transosseous tension band disruption/chance fracture	Limited to one segmentation
	Pure osseous failure of the posterior tension band. Classic chance fracture
B2. Posterior tension band disruption (bone and/or ligament)	Accompanied by Type A fracture. Type A fracture should be described separately
B3. Hyperextension	Causes a hyperextension posture due to damage through the disc or vertebral body.
	Commonly occurs in diseases that cause ankylosis
	The anterior structure, especially the ALL, is damaged, but there is a posterior hinge to prevent displacement
Type C. Failure of all elements leading to dislocation or displacement	
C. Displacement or dislocation	No subtypes If necessary, it can be described along with the subtype of Type A as a secondary injury
Neurologic injury (at the time of admission)	
N0	No neurological symptoms
N1	Temporary neurological damage, not present at the time of admission
N2	Radicular symptoms
N3	Incomplete spinal cord injury or cauda equina injury
N4	Complete spinal cord injury or cauda equina injury
NX	Unknown due to sedation or cranial injury
Modifiers	
M1	Refers to cases where ligament injury is uncertain in imaging (regardless of the presence of MRI). In cases of stable fractures from the osseous structure perspective, ligament insufficiency can help consider surgery
M2	Comorbidities that the injured patient has (e.g., ankylosing spondylitis, burns on the skin covering the injured spinal level)

Table 8.4 Thoracolumbar Injury Classification and Severity Score (TLICS)

Evaluation items	Score
Injury morphology[a]	
Compression	1
Burst fracture	+1(=2)
Rotational/translational	3
Distraction	4
Posterior Ligament Complex (PLC) injury	
Intact	0
Suspected/indeterminate	2
Injured	3
Neurologic status	
Root injury	2
Complete cord/conus medullaris injury	2
Incomplete cord/conus medullaris injury	3
Cauda equina involvement	3

[a]When scoring the injury morphology, if there are injuries at multiple levels, the most severe the level with damage is used as the standard, and if multiple types of damage are suspected at one level, the highest score is used as the standard. For example, if compression (1 point) and distraction (4 points) are suspected, and the burst (1 point) form appears at the level with the most severe damage, the score for the type of damage is 4 points corresponding to distraction. Non-surgical treatment is recommended if the score is 3 points or less, surgical treatment is recommended if the score is 5 points or more, and if the score is 4 points, the patient is advised to choose between surgical and non-surgical treatment

Bibliography

1. France JC, Gocke RT. Injuries of the cervicocranium. In: Browner BD, Jupiter JB, Levine AM, Trafton PG, Krettek C, editors. Skeletal trauma. 4th ed. Philadelphia: Saunders Elsevier; 2009. p. 813–62.
2. Garrett M, Consiglieri G, Kakarla UK, Chang SW, Dickman CA. Occipitoatlantal dislocation. Neurosurgery. 2010;66:48–55.
3. Traynelis VC, Marano GD, Dunker RO, Kaufman HH. Traumatic atlanto-occipital dislocation. Case report. J Neurosurg. 1986;65:863–70.
4. Ozsarlak O. Cervical trauma. In: Van Goethem JWM, Den Hauwe LV, Parizel PM, editors. Spinal imaging. 1st ed. Heidelberg: Springer; 2007. p. 279–324.
5. Wholey MH, Bruwer AJ, Baker HL Jr. The lateral roentgenogram of the neck; with comments on the Atlanto-odontoid-Basion relationship. Radiology. 1958;71:350–6.
6. Harris JH Jr, Carson GC, Wagner LK. Radiologic diagnosis of traumatic occipitovertebral dissociation: 1. Normal occipitovertebral relationships on lateral radiographs of supine subjects. AJR Am J Roentgenol. 1994;162:881–6.
7. Hadley MN, Walters BC, Grabb PA, Oyesiku NM, Przybylski GJ, Resnick DK, et al. Guidelines for the management of acute cervical spine and spinal cord injuries. Clin Neurosurg. 2002;49:407–98.
8. Pang D, Nemzek WR, Zovickian J. Atlanto-occipital dislocation—part 2: The clinical use of (occipital) condyle-C1 interval, comparison with other diagnostic methods, and the manifestation, management, and outcome of atlanto-occipital dislocation in children. Neurosurgery. 2007;61:995–1015. discussion 1015
9. Pang D, Nemzek WR, Zovickian J. Atlanto-occipital dislocation: part 1—normal occipital condyle-C1 interval in 89 children. Neurosurgery. 2007;61:514–21. discussion 521
10. Kakarla UK, Chang SW, Theodore N, Sonntag VK. Atlas fractures. Neurosurgery. 2010;66:60–7.
11. Jefferson G. Fractures of the atlas vertebra: report of four cases and a review of those previously recorded. Br J Surg. 1920;7:407–22.
12. Gehweiler J, Duff D, Salutario M, Miller M, Clark M. Fractures of the atlas vertebra. Skeletal Radiol. 1976;23:97–102.
13. Spence KF Jr, Decker S, Sell KW. Bursting atlantal fracture associated with rupture of the transverse ligament. J Bone Joint Surg Am. 1970;52:543–9.
14. Dickman CA, Greene KA, Sonntag VK. Injuries involving the transverse atlantal ligament: classification and treatment guidelines based upon experience with 39 injuries. Neurosurgery. 1996;38:44–50.
15. Pang D. Atlantoaxial rotatory fixation. Neurosurgery. 2010;66:161–83.
16. Wortzman G, Dewar FP. Rotary fixation of the atlantoaxial joint: rotational atlantoaxial subluxation. Radiology. 1968;90:479–87.
17. Jones RN. Rotatory dislocation of both atlanto-axial joints. J Bone Joint Surg Br. 1984;66:6–7.
18. Pryputniewicz DM, Hadley MN. Axis fractures. Neurosurgery. 2010;66:68–82.

19. Greene KA, Dickman CA, Marciano FF, Drabier JB, Hadley MN, Sonntag VK. Acute axis fractures. Analysis of management and outcome in 340 consecutive cases. Spine (Phila Pa 1976). 1997;22:1843–52.
20. Anderson LD, D'Alonzo RT. Fractures of the odontoid process of the axis. J Bone Joint Surg Am. 1974;56:1663–74.
21. Grauer JN, Shafi B, Hilibrand AS, Harrop JS, Kwon BK, Beiner JM, et al. Proposal of a modified, treatment-oriented classification of odontoid fractures. Spine J. 2005;5:123–9.
22. Arvin B, Fournier-Gosselin MP, Fehlings MG. Os odontoideum: etiology and surgical management. Neurosurgery. 2010;66:22–31.
23. Fielding JW, Hensinger RN, Hawkins RJ. Os Odontoideum. J Bone Joint Surg Am. 1980;62:376–83.
24. Levine AM, Edwards CC. The management of traumatic spondylolisthesis of the axis. J Bone Joint Surg Am. 1985;67:217–26.
25. Burke JT, Harris JH Jr. Acute injuries of the axis vertebra. Skeletal Radiol. 1989;18:335–46.
26. Vaccaro AR, Hulbert RJ, Patel AA, Fisher C, Dvorak M, Lehman RA Jr, et al. The subaxial cervical spine injury classification system: a novel approach to recognize the importance of morphology, neurology, and integrity of the disco-ligamentous complex. Spine (Phila Pa 1976). 2007;32:2365–74.
27. Goldberg W, Mueller C, Panacek E, Tigges S, Hoffman JR, Mower WR. Distribution and patterns of blunt traumatic cervical spine injury. Ann Emerg Med. 2001;38:17–21.
28. Mercer S, Bogduk N. The ligaments and annulus fibrosus of human adult cervical intervertebral discs. Spine (Phila Pa 1976). 1999;24:619–26. discussion 627–618
29. Shea M, Wittenberg RH, Edwards WT, White AA 3rd, Hayes WC. In vitro hyperextension injuries in the human cadaveric cervical spine. J Orthop Res. 1992;10:911–6.
30. Przybylski GJ, Carlin GJ, Patel PR, Woo SL. Human anterior and posterior cervical longitudinal ligaments possess similar tensile properties. J Orthop Res. 1996;14:1005–8.
31. Onan OA, Heggeness MH, Hipp JA. A motion analysis of the cervical facet joint. Spine(Phila Pa 1976). 1998;23:430–9.
32. Kwon BK, Anderson PA. Injuries of the lower cervical spine. In: Browner BD, Jupiter JB, Levine AM, Trafton PG, Krettek C, editors. Skeletal trauma. 4th ed. Philadelphia: Saunders Elsevier; 2009. p. 863–914.
33. Hoffman JR, Mower WR, Wolfson AB, Todd KH, Zucker MI. Validity of a set of clinical criteria to rule out injury to the cervical spine in patients with blunt trauma. National Emergency X-Radiography Utilization Study Group. N Engl J Med. 2000;343:94–9.
34. Dwek JR, Chung CB. Radiography of cervical spine injury in children: are flexion-extension radiographs useful for acute trauma? AJR Am J Roentgenol. 2000;174:1617–9.
35. Fazl M, LaFebvre J, Willinsky RA, Gertzbein S. Posttraumatic ligamentous disruption of the cervical spine, an easily overlooked diagnosis: presentation of three cases. Neurosurgery. 1990;26:674–8.
36. Nunez DB Jr, Quencer RM. The role of helical CT in the assessment of cervical spine injuries. AJR Am J Roentgenol. 1998;171:951–7.
37. Blackmore CC, Ramsey SD, Mann FA, Deyo RA. Cervical spine screening with CT in trauma patients: a cost-effectiveness analysis. Radiology. 1999;212:117–25.
38. Hanson JA, Blackmore CC, Mann FA, Wilson AJ. Cervical spine injury: a clinical decision rule to identify high-risk patients for helical CT screening. AJR Am J Roentgenol. 2000;174:713–7.
39. Van Goethem JW, Ozsarlak O, Parizel PM. Cervical spine fractures and soft tissue injuries. JBR-BTR. 2003;86:230–4.
40. Panczykowski DM, Tomycz ND, Okonkwo DO. Comparative effectiveness of using computed tomography alone to exclude cervical spine injuries in obtunded or intubated patients: meta-analysis of 14,327 patients with blunt trauma. J Neurosurg. 2011;
41. Brohi K, Wilson-Macdonald J. Evaluation of unstable cervical spine injury: a 6-year experience. J Trauma. 2000;49:76–80.
42. Geck MJ, Yoo S, Wang JC. Assessment of cervical ligamentous injury in trauma patients using MRI. J Spinal Disord. 2001;14:371–7.
43. Van Goethem JW, Maes M, Ozsarlak O, van den Hauwe L, Parizel PM. Imaging in spinal trauma. Eur Radiol. 2005;15:582–90.
44. Benedetti PF, Fahr LM, Kuhns LR, Hayman LA. MR imaging findings in spinal ligamentous injury. AJR Am J Roentgenol. 2000;175:661–5.
45. Gunzburg R, Szpalski M, Van Goethem J. Initial assessment of whiplash patients. Pain Res Manag. 2003;8:24–7.
46. Looby S, Flanders A. Spine trauma. Radiol Clin North Am. 2011;49:129–63.
47. Rihn JA, Fisher C, Harrop J, Morrison W, Yang N, Vaccaro AR. Assessment of the posterior ligamentous complex following acute cervical spine trauma. J Bone Joint Surg Am. 2010;92:583–9.
48. Flanders AE, Schaefer DM, Doan HT, Mishkin MM, Gonzalez CF, Northrup BE. Acute cervical spine trauma: correlation of MR imaging findings with degree of neurologic deficit. Radiology. 1990;177:25–33.
49. Katzberg RW, Benedetti PF, Drake CM, Ivanovic M, Levine RA, Beatty CS, et al. Acute cervical spine injuries: prospective MR imaging assessment at a level 1 trauma center. Radiology. 1999;213:203–12.
50. Kulkarni MV, Bondurant FJ, Rose SL, Narayana PA. 1.5 tesla magnetic resonance imaging of acute spinal trauma. Radiographics. 1988;8:1059–82.
51. Miyanji F, Furlan JC, Aarabi B, Arnold PM, Fehlings MG. Acute cervical traumatic spinal cord injury:

MR imaging findings correlated with neurologic outcome—prospective study with 100 consecutive patients. Radiology. 2007;243:820–7.
52. Quencer RM, Nunez D, Green BA. Controversies in imaging acute cervical spine trauma. AJNR Am J Neuroradiol. 1997;18:1866–8.
53. Richards PJ. Cervical spine clearance: a review. Injury. 2005;36:248–69. discussion 270
54. Chang DG, Tencer AF, Ching RP, Treece B, Senft D, Anderson PA. Geometric changes in the cervical spinal canal during impact. Spine (Phila Pa 1976). 1994;19:973–80.
55. Allen BL Jr, Ferguson RL, Lehmann TR, O'Brien RP. A mechanistic classification of closed, indirect fractures and dislocations of the lower cervical spine. Spine (Phila Pa 1976). 1982;7:1–27.
56. White AA 3rd, Panjabi MM. The basic kinematics of the human spine. A review of past and current knowledge. Spine (Phila Pa 1976). 1978;3:12–20.
57. Young JW, Resnik CS, DeCandido P, Mirvis SE. The laminar space in the diagnosis of rotational flexion injuries of the cervical spine. AJR Am J Roentgenol. 1989;152:103–7.
58. Shapiro S, Snyder W, Kaufman K, Abel T. Outcome of 51 cases of unilateral locked cervical facets: interspinous braided cable for lateral mass plate fusion compared with interspinous wire and facet wiring with iliac crest. J Neurosurg. 1999;91:19–24.
59. Vaccaro AR, Madigan L, Schweitzer ME, Flanders AE, Hilibrand AS, Albert TJ. Magnetic resonance imaging analysis of soft tissue disruption after flexion-distraction injuries of the subaxial cervical spine. Spine (Phila Pa 1976). 2001;26:1866–72.
60. Argenson C, Lovet J, Sanouiller JL, de Peretti F. Traumatic rotatory displacement of the lower cervical spine. Spine (Phila Pa 1976). 1988;13:767–73.
61. Halliday AL, Henderson BR, Hart BL, Benzel EC. The management of unilateral lateral mass/facet fractures of the subaxial cervical spine: the use of magnetic resonance imaging to predict instability. Spine (Phila Pa 1976). 1997;22:2614–21.
62. Vaccaro AR, Lehman RA Jr, Hurlbert RJ, Anderson PA, Harris M, Hedlund R, et al. A new classification of thoracolumbar injuries: the importance of injury morphology, the integrity of the posterior ligamentous complex, and neurologic status. Spine (Phila Pa 1976). 2005;30:2325–33.
63. Furlan JC, Fehlings MG, Massicotte EM, Aarabi B, Vaccaro AR, Bono CM, et al. A quantitative and reproducible method to assess cord compression and canal stenosis after cervical spine trauma: a study of interrater and intrarater reliability. Spine (Phila Pa 1976). 2007;32:2083–91.
64. Bhatia RG, Bower BC. Thoracolumbar spine trauma. In: Van Goethem JWM, Den Hauwe LV, Parizel PM, editors. Spinal imaging. 1st ed. Heidelberg: Springer; 2007. p. 325–57.
65. Hanley EN Jr, Eskay ML. Thoracic spine fractures. Orthopedics. 1989;12:689–96.
66. Lee YP, Templin C, Eismont F, Garfin SR. Thoracic and upper lumbar spine injuries. In: Browner BD, Jupiter JB, Levine AM, Trafton PG, Krettek C, editors. Skeletal trauma. 4th ed. Philadelphia: Saunders Elsevier; 2009. p. 915–77.
67. Chance CQ. Note on a type of flexion fracture of the spine. Br. J Radiol. 1948;21:452.
68. Daffner RH, Deeb ZL, Goldberg AL, Kandabarow A, Rothfus WE. The radiologic assessment of post-traumatic vertebral stability. Skeletal Radiol. 1990;19:103–8.
69. Atlas SW, Regenbogen V, Rogers LF, Kim KS. The radiographic characterization of burst fractures of the spine. AJR Am J Roentgenol. 1986;147:575–82.
70. Martijn A, Veldhuis EF. The diagnostic value of interpediculate distance assessment on plain films in thoracic and lumbar spine injuries. J Trauma. 1991;31:1393–5.
71. Ballock RT, Mackersie R, Abitbol JJ, Cervilla V, Resnick D, Garfin SR. Can burst fractures be predicted from plain radiographs? J Bone Joint Surg Br. 1992;74:147–50.
72. Roos JE, Hilfiker P, Platz A, Desbiolles L, Boehm T, Marincek B, et al. MDCT in emergency radiology: is a standardized chest or abdominal protocol sufficient for evaluation of thoracic and lumbar spine trauma? AJR Am J Roentgenol. 2004;183:959–68.
73. Denis F. The three column spine and its significance in the classification of acute thoracolumbar spinal injuries. Spine (Phila Pa 1976). 1983;8:817–31.
74. McAfee PC, Yuan HA, Fredrickson BE, Lubicky JP. The value of computed tomography in thoracolumbar fractures. An analysis of one hundred consecutive cases and a new classification. J Bone Joint Surg Am. 1983;65:461–73.
75. Sethi MK, Schoenfeld AJ, Bono CM, Harris MB. The evolution of thoracolumbar injury classification systems. Spine J. 2009;9:780–8.
76. Holdsworth F. Fractures, dislocations, and fracture-dislocations of the spine. J Bone Joint Surg Am. 1970;52:1534–51.
77. Groves CJ, Cassar-Pullicino VN, Tins BJ, Tyrrell PN, McCall IW. Chance-type flexion-distraction injuries in the thoracolumbar spine: MR imaging characteristics. Radiology. 2005;236:601–8.
78. Bernstein MP, Mirvis SE, Shanmuganathan K. Chance-type fractures of the thoracolumbar spine: imaging analysis in 53 patients. AJR Am J Roentgenol. 2006;187:859–68.
79. Wood KB, Khanna G, Vaccaro AR, Arnold PM, Harris MB, Mehbod AA. Assessment of two thoracolumbar fracture classification systems as used by multiple surgeons. J Bone Joint Surg Am. 2005;87:1423–9.
80. James KS, Wenger KH, Schlegel JD, Dunn HK. Biomechanical evaluation of the stability of thoracolumbar burst fractures. Spine (Phila Pa 1976). 1994;19:1731–40.
81. Gertzbein SD, Court-Brown CM. Flexion-distraction injuries of the lumbar spine. Mechanisms of injury and classification. Clin Orthop Relat Res. 1988;227:52–60.

82. Ferguson RL, Allen BL Jr. A mechanistic classification of thoracolumbar spine fractures. Clin Orthop Relat Res. 1984;77:88.
83. Mikles MR, Stchur RP, Graziano GP. Posterior instrumentation for thoracolumbar fractures. J Am Acad Orthop Surg. 2004;12:424–35.
84. Barker L, Anderson J, Chesnut R, Nesbit G, Tjauw T, Hart R. Reliability and reproducibility of dens fracture classification with use of plain radiography and reformatted computer-aided tomography. J Bone Joint Surg Am. 2006;88:106–12.
85. Brant-Zawadzki M, Jeffrey RB Jr, Minagi H, Pitts LH. High resolution CT of thoracolumbar fractures. AJR Am J Roentgenol. 1982;138:699–704.
86. Wilson BP, Finlay D. Computerized tomography of injury to the thoracolumbar spine. Injury. 1987;18:185–9.
87. Kilcoyne RF, Mack LA, King HA, Ratcliffe SS, Loop JW. Thoracolumbar spine injuries associated with vertical plunges: reappraisal with computed tomography. Radiology. 1983;146:137–40.
88. Lindahl S, Willen J, Nordwall A, Irstam L. The crush-cleavage fracture. A "new" thoracolumbar unstable fracture. Spine (Phila Pa 1976). 1983;8:559–69.
89. Shuman WP, Rogers JV, Sickler ME, Hanson JA, Crutcher JP, King HA, et al. Thoracolumbar burst fractures: CT dimensions of the spinal canal relative to postsurgical improvement. AJR Am J Roentgenol. 1985;145:337–41.
90. Meves R, Avanzi O. Correlation between neurological deficit and spinal canal compromise in 198 patients with thoracolumbar and lumbar fractures. Spine (Phila Pa 1976). 2005;30:787–91.
91. Pathria MN. Physical injury: spine. In: Resnick D, editor. Diagnosis of bone and joint disorders. 4th ed. Philadelphia: Saunders; 2002. p. 2934–3015.
92. Lee HM, Kim HS, Kim DJ, Suk KS, Park JO, Kim NH. Reliability of magnetic resonance imaging in detecting posterior ligament complex injury in thoracolumbar spinal fractures. Spine (Phila Pa 1976). 2000;25:2079–84.
93. Vaccaro AR, Rihn JA, Saravanja D, Anderson DG, Hilibrand AS, Albert TJ, et al. Injury of the posterior ligamentous complex of the thoracolumbar spine: a prospective evaluation of the diagnostic accuracy of magnetic resonance imaging. Spine (Phila Pa 1976). 2009;34:E841–7.
94. Gumley G, Taylor TK, Ryan MD. Distraction fractures of the lumbar spine. J Bone Joint Surg Br. 1982;64:520–5.
95. Anderson PA, Henley MB, Rivara FP, Maier RV. Flexion distraction and chance injuries to the thoracolumbar spine. J Orthop Trauma. 1991;5:153–60.
96. Frankel HL, Rozycki GS, Ochsner MG, Harviel JD, Champion HR. Indications for obtaining surveillance thoracic and lumbar spine radiographs. J Trauma. 1994;37:673–6.
97. Daffner RH. The thoracic and lumbar spine. In: Rogers LF, editor. Radiology of Skeletal Trauma. 3rd ed. Philadelphia: Churchill Livingstone; 2002. p. 453–540.
98. Magerl F, Aebi M, Gertzbein SD, Harms J, Nazarian S. A comprehensive classification of thoracic and lumbar injuries. Eur Spine J. 1994;3:184–201.
99. Aebi M. Classification of thoracolumbar fractures and dislocations. Eur Spine J. 2010;19(Suppl. 1):S2–7.
100. Vaccaro AR, Oner C, Kepler CK, Dvorak M, Schnake K, Bellabarba C, et al. AO Spine thoracolumbar spine injury classification system: fracture description, neurological status, and key modifiers. Spine. 2013;38:2028–37.
101. Vaccaro AR, Zeiller SC, Hulbert RJ, Anderson PA, Harris M, Hedlund R, et al. The thoracolumbar injury severity score: a proposed treatment algorithm. J Spinal Disord Tech. 2005;18:209–15.
102. Schweitzer KM Jr, Vaccaro AR, Lee JY, Grauer JN. Confusion regarding mechanisms of injury in the setting of thoracolumbar spinal trauma: a survey of The Spine Trauma Study Group (STSG). J Spinal Disord Tech. 2006;19:528–30.
103. Whang PG, Vaccaro AR, Poelstra KA, Patel AA, Anderson DG, Albert TJ, et al. The influence of fracture mechanism and morphology on the reliability and validity of two novel thoracolumbar injury classification systems. Spine(Phila Pa 1976). 2007;32:791–5.
104. Vaccaro AR, Baron EM, Sanfilippo J, Jacoby S, Steuve J, Grossman E, et al. Reliability of a novel classification system for thoracolumbar injuries: the Thoracolumbar Injury Severity Score. Spine (Phila Pa 1976). 2006;31:S62–9. discussion S104
105. Patel AA, Vaccaro AR, Albert TJ, Hilibrand AS, Harrop JS, Anderson DG, et al. The adoption of a new classification system: time-dependent variation in interobserver reliability of the thoracolumbar injury severity score classification system. Spine (Phila Pa 1976). 2007;32:E105–10.

Osteoporosis

9

Jee Won Chai

Osteoporosis is the most common metabolic bone disease, which refers to a state where fractures are likely to occur due to decreased bone strength. Bone strength is related to both bone quantity and bone quality, and these two factors are important in evaluating bone strength and fracture risk. Among them, the variable mainly used to represent bone quantity is bone density, which is known to determine 60–90% of bone strength, so bone density has a close relationship with bone strength, and therefore, it can be said to be the most important factor in the diagnosis of osteoporosis. In this chapter, we will learn about the concept and importance of osteoporosis, the diagnosis of osteoporosis using DXA, and the imaging findings of osteoporosis appearing in the other imaging techniques.

9.1 Introduction

Until the twentieth century, the definition of osteoporosis was "a reduced amount of bone that is qualitatively normal," and it was thought that the decrease in bone quantity was the main cause of osteoporosis [1]. However, it was later revealed that not only bone quantity but also bone quality is important in causing osteoporotic fractures, and in 1994, the World Health Organization (WHO) Study Group defined osteoporosis as "a systemic skeletal disease characterized by low bone mass and microarchitectural deterioration of bone tissue, with a consequent increase in bone fragility and susceptibility to fracture" [2], and in 2000, the NIH Consensus Development Conference summarized it as "a skeletal disorder characterized by compromised bone strength predisposing a person to an increased risk of fracture."

According to a survey using the claim data of the National Health Insurance Corporation from January 2008 to December 2013, the prevalence of osteoporosis in the Korean population aged 50 and over was 22.4%, and the prevalence of osteopenia was 47.9%. In women, osteoporosis doubled every 10 years, and 68.5% of women over 70 were osteoporotic. Osteoporotic fractures increased by 4% each year from 2008 to 2013, and it was estimated that the estimated number of hip and vertebral fractures would increase by 1.4 times in the next 10 years [3]. According to one study, only 40% of patients can recover to the level of activity before the fracture after an osteoporotic fracture, 20% need long-term care, and mortality can increase by 8–36% within one year after a hip fracture.

As such, osteoporotic fractures not only cause serious physical and economic difficulties for patients, but also lead to significant societal losses. Therefore, it is most important to detect and treat them early to prevent fractures [5].

J. W. Chai (✉)
Department of Radiology, Seoul National University College of Medicine, Seoul, Republic of Korea

© The Author(s), under exclusive license to Springer Nature Singapore Pte Ltd. 2025

H. S. Kang, J. W. Lee (eds.), *Spinal Imaging*, https://doi.org/10.1007/978-981-95-1386-4_9

9.2 Diagnosis of Osteoporosis, Focusing on DXA

In 1994, the WHO established the diagnostic criteria for osteoporosis based on the *T*-score of bone density measured using dual-energy X-ray absorptiometry (DXA), which is still the most commonly used method for diagnosing osteoporosis. The criteria are as follows [6].

- Normal: *T*-score –1.0 or higher
- Osteopenia (Low bone mass): *T*-score between –1.0 and –2.5
- Osteoporosis: *T*-score of –2.5 or lower
- Severe osteoporosis: *T*-score –2.5 or lower, accompanied by one or more fragility fractures

Introduced in 1987, DXA has low radiation exposure, short examination time, and high precision, making it easy to diagnose and follow-up. The central DXA, which captures the central bone (spine and femur), can measure the bone density of the spine and femur where osteoporotic fractures commonly occur, and is recognized as the standard test for bone density (Fig. 9.1). DXA is highly accurate, but it must be backed by the assumption that the measurement was done correctly, and the appropriate site must be correctly selected for the interpretation of the test [7, 8]. The International Society for Clinical Densitometry (ISCD) provides standards for the interpretation of DXA based on regularly updated research results. The ISCD Official Positions updated in 2019 can be referred to as the most

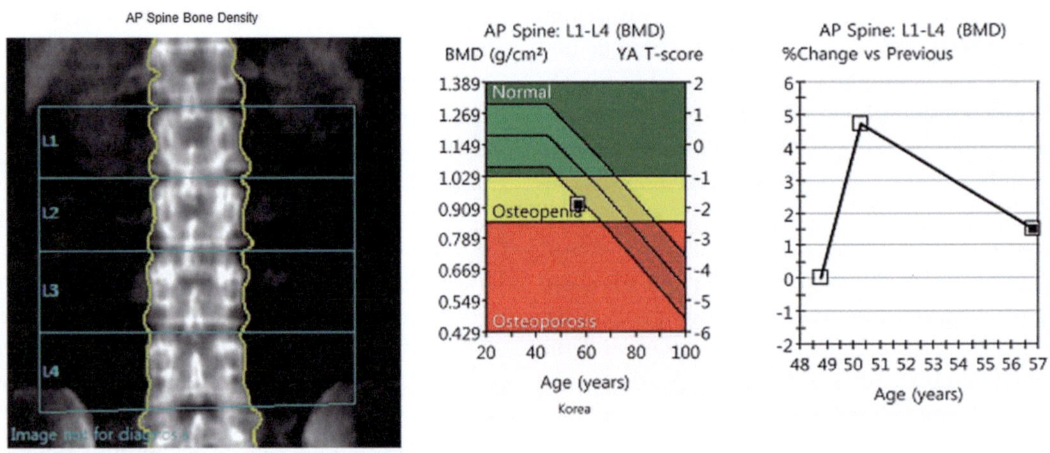

		Young-Adult		Age-Matched	
Region	BMD (g/cm²)	YA (%)	YA T-score	AM (%)	AM Z-score
L1	0.860	80	−1.7	87	−1.0
L2	0.927	82	−1.7	89	−1.0
L3	0.937	78	−2.2	83	−1.6
L4	0.950	80	−2.0	84	−1.5
L1-L2	0.895	81	−1.7	88	−1.0
L1-L3	0.911	80	−1.9	86	−1.2
L1-L4	0.921	80	−1.9	86	−1.2
L2-L3	0.933	80	−1.9	86	−1.2
L2-L4	0.938	80	−1.9	85	−1.4
L3-L4	0.943	79	−2.1	84	−1.4

Fig. 9.1 DXA results of a 57-year-old woman
From L1 to L4, the bone marrow density (BM8D) and *T*-score, which indicates the level of this bone density in the distribution of normal adult bone density, and *Z*-score, which indicates the level of this bone density in the distribution of the same age group, are presented for each combination of areas. The average bone density of this patient's L1–L4 VB is 0.921 g/cm³, and since the *T*-score is –1.9, it can be diagnosed as osteopenia (bone loss) (underline)

recent data (https://iscd.org/learn/official-positions/adult-positions/).

9.2.1 DXA Interpretation

9.2.1.1 Lumbar Spine

The lumbar spine, rich in trabecular bone, can most sensitively reflect changes in bone metabolism in postmenopausal women and responds quickly to treatment, making it suitable for follow-up examinations. During follow-up examinations, it is important to ensure that the measured level does not change compared to the previous one. To correctly measure the lumbar spine, use leg supports to reduce lordosis and include parts of T12 and L5 in the shot. L1–L4 are included in the analysis, but L5 is excluded because it is larger than other vertebral bodies, resulting in a higher measured bone density, and it is difficult to measure consistently in the case of a transitional lumbosacral vertebra. As you go from L1 to L4, the bone density generally appears higher, but if this trend reverses, there may be degenerative changes, so caution is needed. Check that the region of interest (ROI) is accurately set along the margin and endplate of the vertebral body (Fig. 9.2).

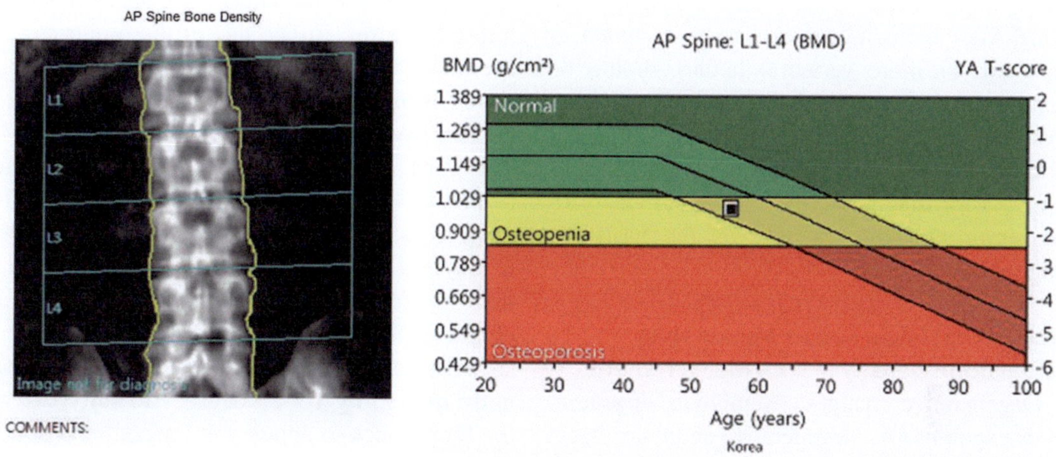

		Young-Adult		Age-Matched	
Region	BMD (g/cm^2)	YA (%)	YA T-score	AM (%)	AM Z-score
L1	0.929	87	−1.2	95	−0.4
L2	1.004	89	−1.0	97	−0.3
L3	1.013	85	−1.5	91	−0.9
L4	0.982	83	−1.7	87	−1.2
L1-L2	0.967	88	−1.1	96	−0.4
L1-L3	0.983	87	−1.3	94	−0.5
L1-L4	0.983	86	−1.4	93	−0.6
L2-L3	1.009	87	−1.3	94	−0.6
L2-L4	0.999	85	−1.4	91	−0.8
L3-L4	0.997	84	−1.6	90	−0.9

Fig. 9.2 Bone density measurement of the lumbar spine using DXA
The L1–4 level is used, and it is confirmed that the region of interest is accurately set along the margin and endplate of the vertebral body. The *T*-score calculated by the standard deviation of bone density measured from L1–4 VB is −1.4 and can be easily confirmed on the graph (This case was diagnosed as osteopenia in a 56-year-old woman)

During AP lumbar spine DXA imaging, factors such as compression fractures, aortic calcification, degenerative changes, changes due to surgery or artificial objects, and the presence of intestinal contrast agents like barium can result in higher or lower values than the actual bone density. Therefore, these areas are excluded from consideration. Degenerative changes can be difficult to discern visually, but if the *T*-score differs by more than 1 from the adjacent vertebral body, or if the upper vertebral body has a higher bone density than the lower one, it is likely unsuitable for diagnosis and is excluded (Fig. 9.3). If there are no levels to exclude in the lumbar spine, the diagnosis is based on the *T*-score or *Z*-score corresponding to L1–L4, and the diagnosis should not be made based on the lowest measured area alone. After excluding all areas to be excluded, at least two or more vertebral bodies should be included in the analysis for an appropriate diagnosis. If only one analyzable vertebral body remains, the bone density of the lumbar spine is not used for diagnosis, and the bone density of the femur or radius is used as the basis for diagnosis.

Factors That Show Higher Values Than Actual Bone Density in DXA Measurement

- Degenerative changes; osteophyte, degenerative spondylosis, degenerative endplates, facet arthrosis
- Aortic calcification
- Compression fracture
- Abdominal artificial objects such as kidney stones, barium
- Hardening bone lesions such as acromegaly, osteopetrosis, osteoblastic metastasis

Lateral spine DXA allows for the measurement of trabecular bone density, which can be used for early detection of bone loss depending on age before and after menopause. However, because the patient must be laid on their side for measurement, the reproducibility depending on the position is not good, and the precision is worse than the anterior-posterior measurement method. To improve these disadvantages, devices that can collect lateral spine DXA data in a supine position have been developed, but they are not widely used yet, and there is a lack of reference data, so they are not used for the diagnosis of osteoporosis.

9.2.1.2 Femur

It is useful for predicting the occurrence of femur fractures. Either side of the femur can be examined without any problem, and bone density is measured in areas such as the femur neck, greater trochanter, total femur, and ward area. The ward area, which is rich in trabecular bone, responds sensitively to bone metabolism, but its range is smaller than other areas, so its precision is low, and its association with fractures is lower than the femur neck, so it is not used for the diagnosis of osteoporosis. For accurate measurement of the femur, the foot should be internally rotated by 15–20 degrees to fully extend the femur neck to appear the longest, and at this time, the lesser trochanter should appear halfway. The area of interest should not include artificial objects or the ischium other than the femur, and areas with changes due to surgery or lesions on the bone to be measured should be excluded (Fig. 9.4). The presence or absence of osteoporosis is determined based on the lower

Fig. 9.3 Decision on the level to exclude
In cases of compression fractures, degenerative changes, changes due to surgery, or the presence of artificial materials, the corresponding level is excluded from the analysis. (**a**) If the L1 vertebral body is flattened due to a compression fracture and shows a *T*-score difference >1.0 compared to the adjacent L2, it should be excluded. (**b**) If the L3 and L4 vertebral bodies show a *T*-score difference >1 compared to the adjacent L2 due to facet arthrosis, they should be excluded. (**c**) The L4 vertebral body should be excluded from the analysis due to deformation caused by laminectomy. (**d**) If there are artificial materials due to surgery across L2–L4, L2, L3, L4 should be excluded from the analysis. Eventually, only the L1 vertebral body remains, but if there is only one vertebra that can be analyzed like this, the BMD value of the lumbar spine is unreliable, so it is excluded from the analysis

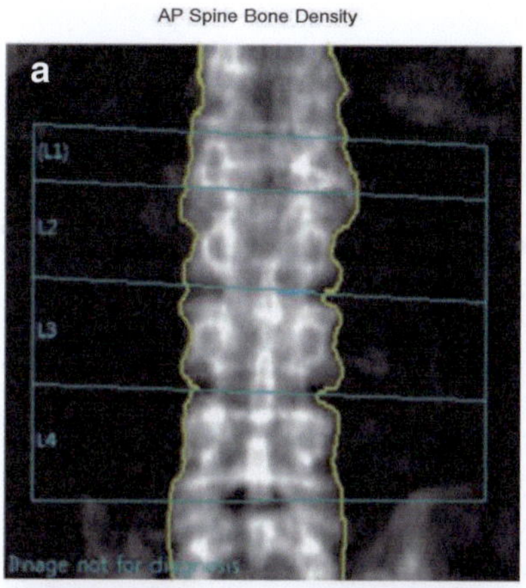

Region	BMD (g/cm²)	Young-Adult YA (%)	Young-Adult YA T-score	Age-Matched AM (%)	Age-Matched AM Z-score
L1	1.128	96	−0.4	104	0.4
L2	1.074	86	−1.5	92	−0.7
L3	1.108	88	−1.2	95	−0.5
L4	1.089	87	−1.3	94	−0.6
L2-L3	1.091	87	−1.3	94	−0.6
L2-L4	1.090	87	−1.3	94	−0.6
L4-L4	1.098	88	−1.3	94	−0.6

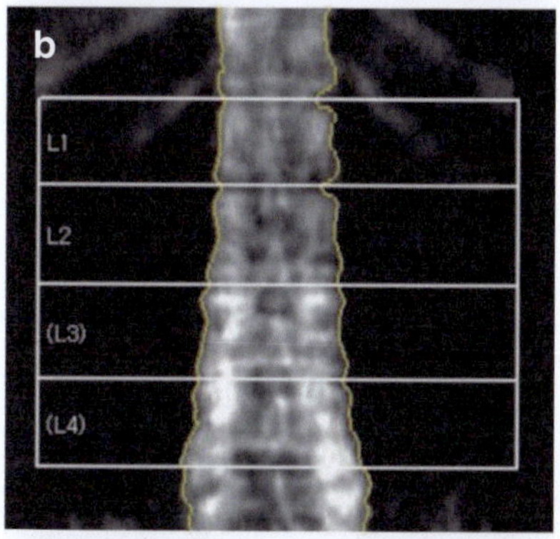

Region	BMD (g/cm²)	Young-Adult (%)	Young-Adult T-score	Age-Matched (%)	Age-Matched Z-score
L1	0.743	69	−2.7	101	0.0
L2	0.783	69	−2.9	102	0.1
L3	1.110	93	−0.7	138	2.5
L4	1.084	92	−0.8	130	2.1
L1-L2	0.765	70	−2.8	103	0.2

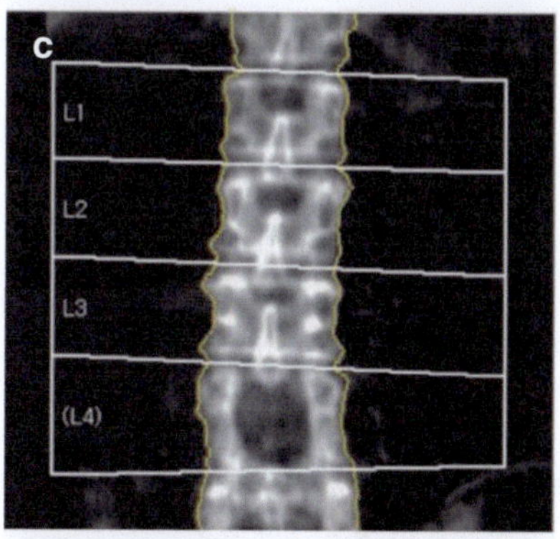

Region	BMD (g/cm²)	Young-Adult (%)	Young-Adult T-score	Age-Matched (%)	Age-Matched Z-score
L1	0.787	74	−2.4	86	−1.1
L2	0.891	79	−2.0	92	−0.7
L3	1.013	85	−1.5	96	−0.4
L4	0.789	67	−3.3	73	−2.4
L1-L2	0.842	77	−2.1	89	−0.9
L1-L3	0.903	79	−1.9	92	−0.7
L2-L3	0.953	82	−1.9	94	−0.5

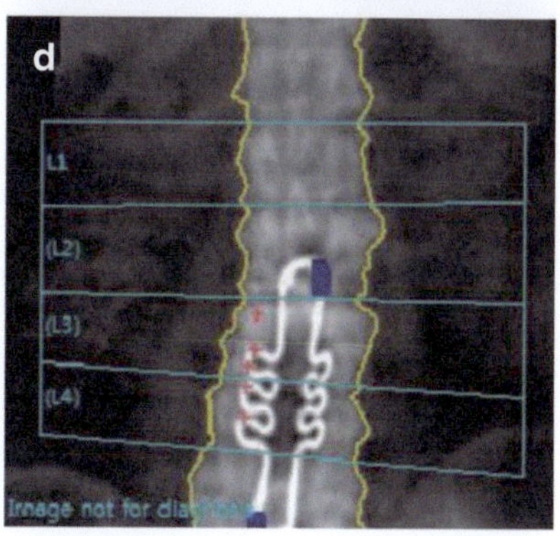

Region	BMD (g/cm²)	Young-Adult YA (%)	Young-Adult YA T-score	Age-Matched AM (%)	Age-Matched AM Z-score
L1	1.066	100	0.0	132	2.2
L2	1.269	113	1.2	150	3.5
L3	1.558	130	3.0	171	5.4
L4	1.400	118	1.8	150	3.9

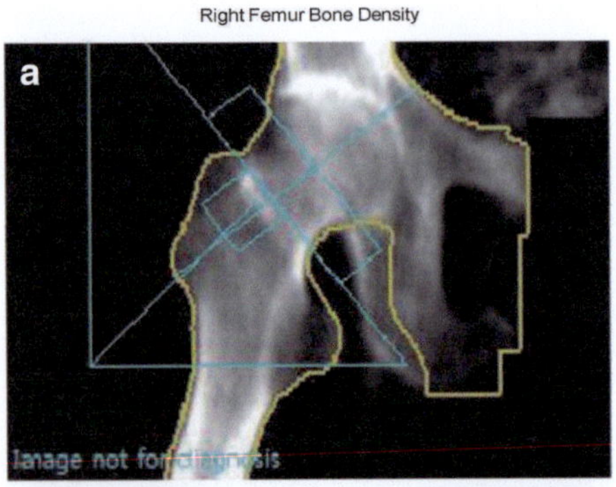

Region	BMD (g/cm²)	Young-Adult YA (%)	Young-Adult YA T-score	Age-Matched AM (%)	Age-Matched AM Z-score
Neck	0.942	100	0.0	157	2.9
Upper Neck	0.774	-	-	-	-
Lower Neck	1.107	-	-	-	-
Wards	0.880	105	0.3	214	3.3
Troch	0.634	86	−0.9	131	1.4
Shaft	0.841	-	-	-	-
Total	0.826	85	−1.2	128	1.5

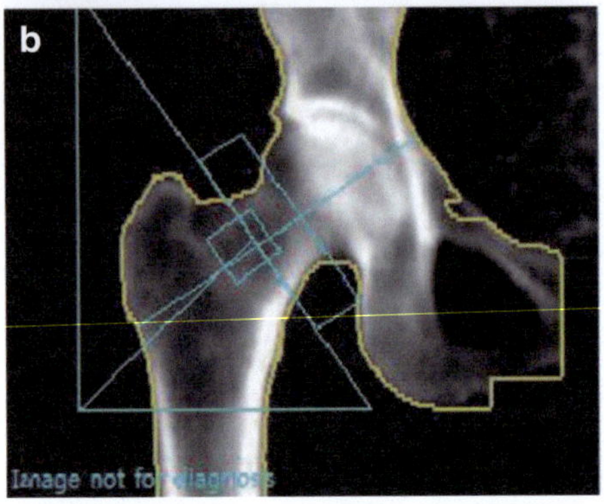

Region	BMD (g/cm²)	Young-Adult YA (%)	Young-Adult YA T-score	Age-Matched AM (%)	Age-Matched AM Z-score
Neck	0.690	73	−2.1	101	0.1
Upper Neck	0.492	-	-	-	-
Lower Neck	0.880	-	-	-	-
Wards	0.418	50	−3.0	89	−0.4
Troch	0.404	55	−3.0	70	−1.6
Shaft	0.726	-	-	-	-
Total	0.602	62	−3.1	81	−1.1

Fig. 9.4 Bone density measurement of the femur using DXA. (**a**) Inappropriate position. The Rt femur neck does not appear long, and the lesser trochanter appears large, indicating insufficient internal rotation. The ROI, which should be located on the femur neck, has risen considerably to the femur head. (**b**) Correct position. The Rt femur neck appears long, and the lesser trochanter is barely visible, indicating appropriate internal rotation. At this time, the *T*-score of the femur total is lower at −3.1, falling into the category of osteoporosis

value between the femur neck and the total femur.

9.2.1.3 Forearm

Software capable of measuring the forearm and an arm fixation device are required. Although the ISCD has defined the lumbar spine and femur as standard measurement sites, it is recommended to measure the forearm bone density in cases where it is difficult to perform or interpret bone density measurements in the spine or femur, when bone loss in the cortical bone is significant as in hyperparathyroidism, or when it is difficult to perform central bone DXA due to excessive obesity.

<Cases where the ISCD recommends forearm bone density measurement>

- When it is difficult to perform or interpret bone density measurements in the lumbar spine or femur
- When bone loss in the cortical bone is significant, as in hyperparathyroidism
- When it is difficult to perform central bone DXA due to excessive obesity

For accurate measurement of the forearm, the subject sits next to the examination table and places their arm on the table for imaging. The degree of forearm rotation must always be constant, so always use the same chair and do not adjust the height. Since the dominant arm is known to have about 3% higher bone density than the non-dominant arm, the non-dominant arm is imaged, and if there is asymmetric arthritis or a past fracture, the other side is examined. The ISCD recommends measuring the middle 33% of the radius, which is rich in cortical bone [7, 9].

9.2.2 *T*-score

The *T*-score is a value obtained by dividing the standard deviation compared to the average bone density of the same sex, young adult group. For example, a *T*-score of −1.0 means that it is 1 standard deviation lower than the average bone density of the young adult group. The *Z*-score is a value obtained by dividing the standard deviation compared to the average bone density of the same sex, similar age group. For example, a *Z*-score of −1.0 means that it is 1 standard deviation lower than the average bone density of a similar age group.

According to the WHO's diagnostic criteria, if the *T*-score is −1.0 or higher, it is normal, if it is <−1.0 and more than −2.5, it is diagnosed as osteopenia (or low bone density), and if it is −2.5 or less, it is diagnosed as osteoporosis. However, the ISCD recommends making such a diagnosis only in postmenopausal women or men over 50, and in premenopausal women or men under 50, it is judged as "below the expected range for age" if the *Z*-score is −2.0 or less, and "within the expected range for age" if the *Z*-score is higher than −2.0. In particular, in children, it is mandatory to make a judgment based on the *Z*-score.

9.3 Imaging Findings of Osteoporosis, Focusing on Other Imaging Techniques

9.3.1 Plain Radiography

The plain radiographic findings of osteoporosis include decreased bone density (osteopenia, bone deficiency), coarse trabeculation, decreased cortical thickness, changes in vertebral body shape, and insufficiency fractures [8, 10]. Compared to the vertebral bodies of healthy adults, those of osteoporosis patients show decreased bone density, appearing darker on plain radiographs. Horizontal trabeculae disappear first, emphasizing the appearance of vertical trabeculae. The remaining trabeculae are sparse, making them appear coarse on plain radiographs. Although the thickness of the cortical bone decreases, the loss of adjacent trabeculae makes it more apparent, making the vertebral body appear like an empty box on plain radiographs (Fig. 9.5). The endplates of the vertebral body may deform concavely, possibly showing the shape of a Codfish vertebra, and the anterior height of the vertebral body may decrease, showing an anterior wedging deformity.

Acute osteoporotic vertebral fractures can be diagnosed by confirming the decrease in vertebral body height along with depression or discontinuity of the endplate, bone sclerosis due to trabecular impaction, and buckling or disconti-

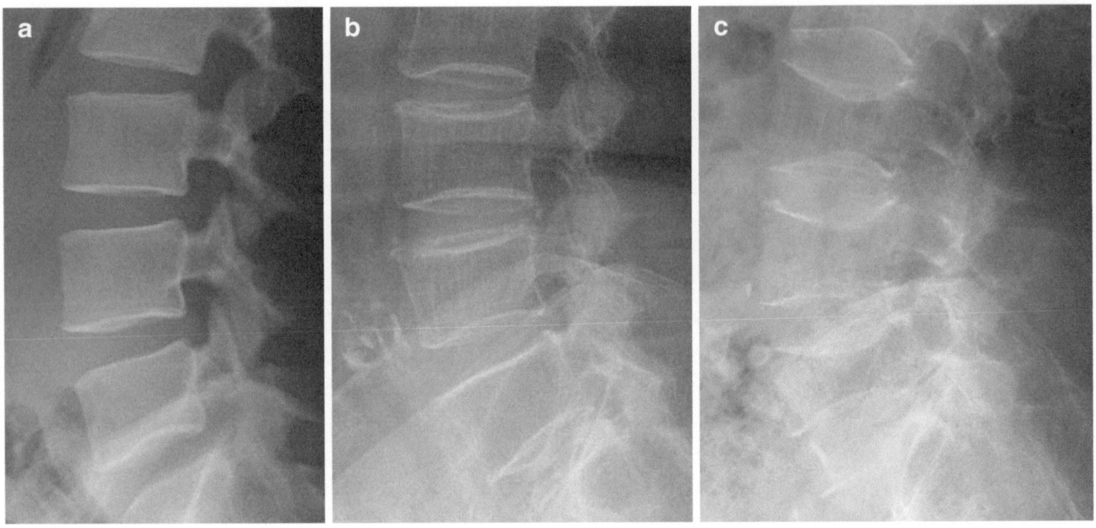

Fig. 9.5 Simple lumbar radiography of normal individuals and osteoporosis patients. (**a**) Lumbar of a normal adult. (**b**) The vertebral body of a patient with osteoporosis shows a decrease in bone shadow on simple radiography, the horizontal trabeculae disappear first, and only the vertical trabeculae are emphasized. The trabeculae are sparse and the inside looks like an empty box. (**c**) The vertebral body of an 85-year-old female patient with osteoporosis shows a concave deformation without a clear fracture on the upper and lower endplates

nuity of the anterior wall. However, in cases where these findings are not clear, and only the height of the vertebral body is reduced, or in cases of old fractures, or in the thoracic region where normal anterior wedging is present, differentiation can often be difficult. At this time, a difference of 1–3 mm between the posterior and anterior vertebral body height is normal in the thoracic region, but if the height difference is 4 mm or more, it can be diagnosed as a fracture, and in areas other than the thoracic region, a difference of 2 mm or more can also be diagnosed as a fracture [8].

The most commonly used classification in osteoporotic vertebral fractures is the semi-quantitative method proposed by Genant (Fig. 9.6) [11]. The decreased height of the anterior, middle, and posterior parts of the vertebral body is divided into wedge, biconcave, and crush shapes according to their shape, and when the height of the vertebral body is reduced by up to 20% compared to the corresponding or adjacent vertebral body, it is grade 0.5, a decrease of 20–25% is grade 1, a decrease of 25–40% is grade 2, and a decrease of more than 40% is grade 3 (Fig. 9.7).

Plain radiography has the advantage of being able to examine a wide range with minimal radiation exposure and cost, and it allows for easy comparison with previous examinations. However, it is known that a decrease in bone density of more than 30% can only be recognized as osteopenia (bone deficiency) on plain radiographs after significant bone loss has occurred, and there are limitations in evaluation when severe osteoporosis is present, or when it is necessary to rule out malignant fractures. Osteoporotic fractures are not common above the 7th thoracic vertebra, so if fractures are found above this level in elderly patients, or if severe compression fractures like vertebra plana are found, metastasis, multiple myeloma, tuberculous spondylitis, etc. should be considered.

It is necessary to confirm whether it is not due to these conditions, CT or MRI should be performed.

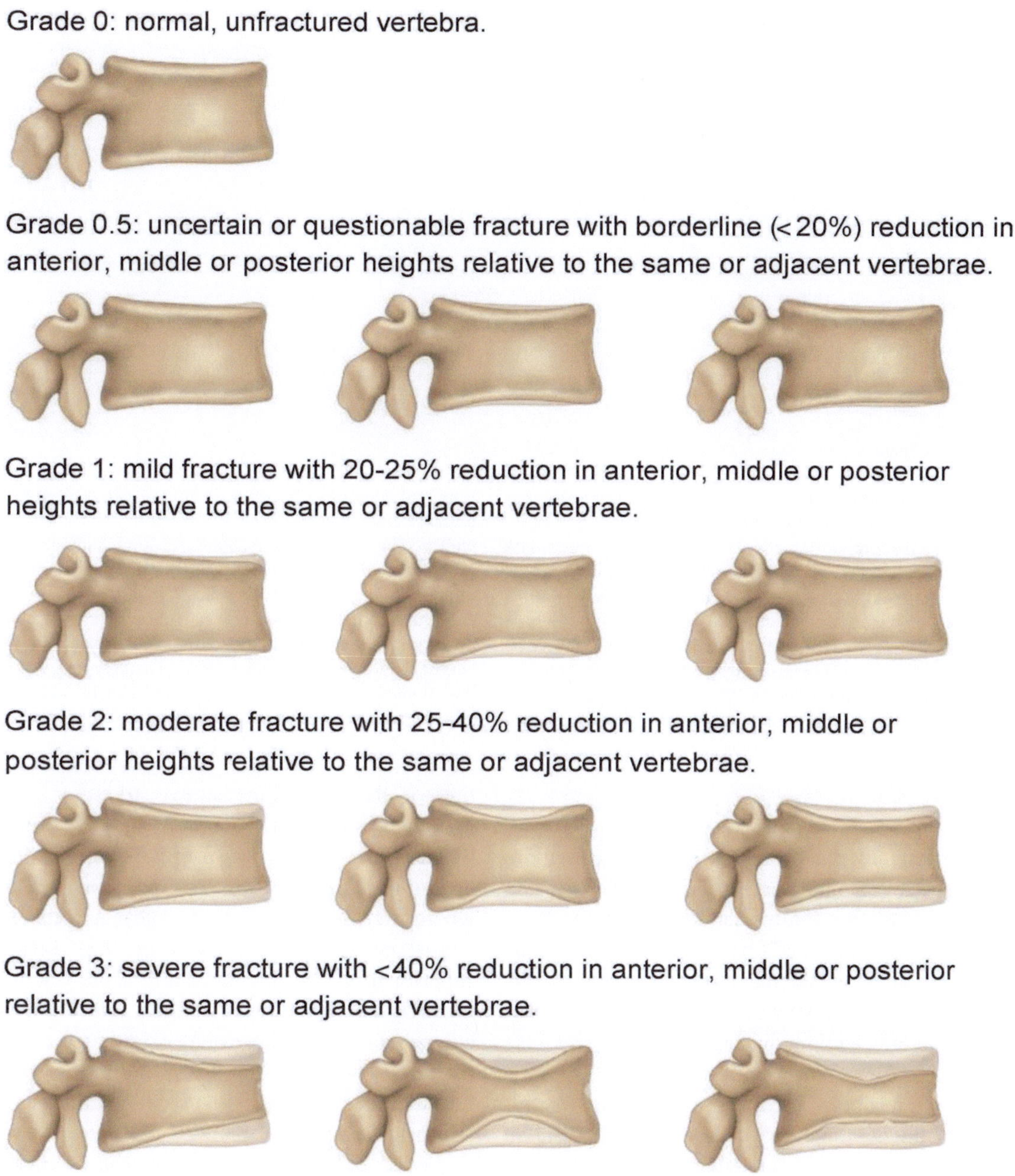

Fig. 9.6 Classification of vertebral fractures by the Genant Semiquantitative method

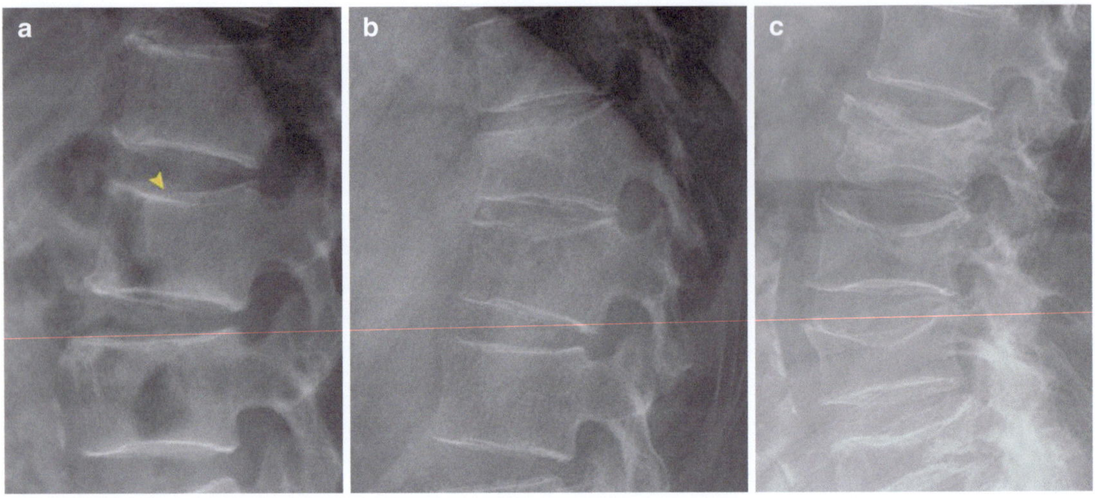

Fig. 9.7 Various forms of osteoporotic fractures. (**a**) Plain lumbar radiograph of a 77-year-old male patient. Only the discontinuity (arrowhead) of the upper endplate of the L2 vertebral body is visible, and the height difference compared to the adjacent L3 vertebral body is minimal. It can be judged as grade 0.5 according to the Genant classification. (**b**) Plain lumbar radiograph of a 74-year-old female patient. The anterior heights of the T12 and L1 vertebral bodies are reduced. Visually, the T12 vertebral body has a height reduction of more than 25%, and the L1 vertebral body has a height reduction of <25%. According to the Genant classification, T12 is grade 2, L1 is grade 1, and the shape is a wedge shape. (**c**) Plain lumbar radiograph of a 73-year-old female patient. There are fractures in the L2, L3, L4 vertebral bodies. The L2 vertebral body is a crush shape with a height reduction extending to the posterior, and it corresponds to Genant grade 3 with a height reduction of more than 40%. The L3 and L4 vertebral bodies are biconcave shapes and can be judged as Genant grades 2 and 3, respectively

9.3.2 CT

Compared to plain radiography, CT can more clearly evaluate the decrease in bone density and changes in bone marrow and can identify small fractures, the range of fracture lines, the shape of fracture lines, and edema of bone marrow and surrounding tissues. However, in severe osteoporosis, fractures without displacement, etc., even this evaluation can be difficult (Fig. 9.8). Recently, research has been attempted to increase sensitivity in finding fractures without displacement in osteoporosis patients by detecting hemorrhage in the bone marrow using dual-energy CT. It is an area where much development is expected in the future, but its utilization is still low [12].

9.3.3 MRI

MRI is considered the best imaging technique for diagnosing osteoporotic fractures. It is very helpful in understanding the direction of the fracture line or the three-dimensional structure in the diagnosis of traumatic fractures, so CT is primarily used, but MRI is more useful than CT in diagnosing initial osteoporotic compression fractures where the fracture line is not clear and there is almost no height reduction (Fig. 9.9). MRI is superior to CT in distinguishing acute fractures from chronic fractures, assessing adjacent nerve compression, and the extent of damage to surrounding soft tissues, and is also considered the best imaging technique when malignant fractures are suspected.

In the case of acute osteoporotic vertebral fractures, the fracture line appears as a low signal intensity on T1-, T2-weighted images in MRI, a fluid signal may be seen within the fracture line, and a T1 low/T2 high signal area due to edema is seen in the adjacent bone marrow. Fat-suppressed T2-weighted images are easy to observe edema of the bone marrow and soft tissues, and the use of such imaging techniques is helpful in patients suspected of acute injury (Fig. 9.10). It is known that bone marrow edema lasts for about 1–3

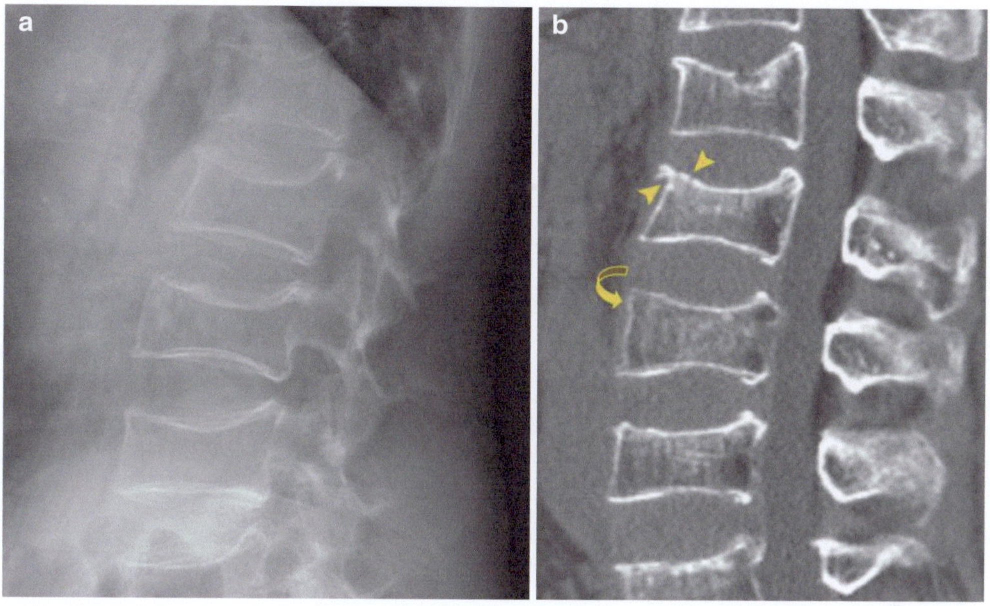

Fig. 9.8 CT imaging findings of osteoporotic vertebral fractures. (**a**) In the plain radiograph, vertebral fractures are visible at multiple levels from L1 to L4. However, it is difficult to tell whether it is an acute or chronic fracture from the plain radiograph. (**b**) In the CT sagittal reformatted scan, the L1 vertebral body has anterior wedging and a Schmorl's node formed on the upper endplate, but since the endplate is all connected and there is no bone marrow edema, it can be judged as a chronic fracture. The L2 vertebral body has discontinuity (arrowhead) on the anterior wall and upper endplate, and increased attenuation is shown by the impaction of the trabecula below the upper endplate, so it can be judged as an acute fracture. The L3 vertebral body can be judged as an acute fracture as it has a reduced height, discontinuity and buckling (bent arrow) on the anterior wall, and the connectivity of the vertical bone marrow inside appears to be broken. The L4 vertebral body has no discontinuity on the endplate or anterior wall, but increased attenuation within the bone marrow indicates an acute fracture. It is difficult to estimate the timing of the fracture in L4 vertebral body, and in such cases, taking an MRI can be helpful

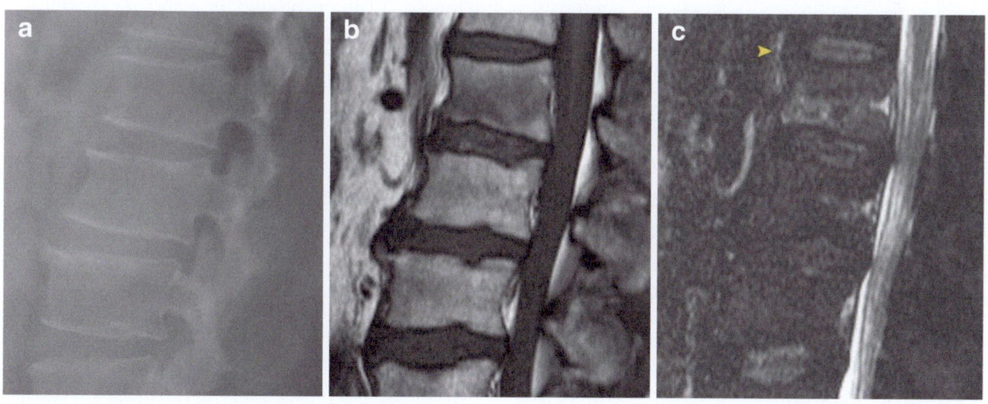

Fig. 9.9 MR imaging findings of osteoporotic vertebral fractures. (**a**) In the plain lumbar radiograph, there are several concave parts on the endplate of the L1, L2, L3 vertebral bodies, and the height of the vertebral body is slightly reduced, making it difficult to determine the presence or timing of fractures. (**b**) In the MR T1-weighted image, a horizontal fracture line is visible connected to the lower endplate of the L1 vertebral body, and the surrounding bone marrow edema allows for a diagnosis of acute fracture. There are Schmorl's nodes on the endplates of the L2 and L3 vertebral bodies, but there is no bone marrow edema, so it can be judged that there is no acute fracture. (**c**) In the MR fat-suppressed T2-weighted image, not only the bone marrow edema within the vertebral body but also the edema of the surrounding soft tissue (arrowhead) is more clearly visible than in the T1-weighted image

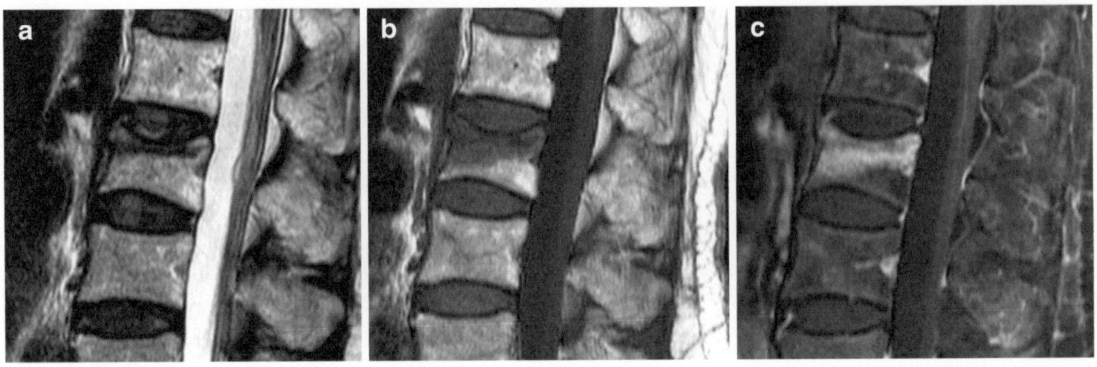

Fig. 9.10 Imaging findings of benign osteoporotic vertebral fractures. (**a**) In MR T2-weighted images, the fracture line appears as a T2 low signal intensity line parallel to the endplate. (**b**) In MR T1-weighted images, a weak low signal intensity bone marrow edema is seen around the low signal intensity fracture line. Normal bone marrow remains at the bottom of the vertebral body. (**c**) In MR T1 contrast-enhanced images, the area with bone marrow edema around the fracture line appears enhanced, but the enhancement intensity is weak, and findings such as forming a mass around are not seen

Table 9.1 Commonalities and differences between benign osteoporotic vertebral fractures and malignant vertebral fractures

	Benign osteoporotic vertebral fractures	Malignant vertebral fractures
Commonalities	Compression fractures or burst fractures of the vertebral body occurred without significant trauma	
Differences	Preservation of normal fatty bone marrow within the fractured vertebral body Weak low signal intensity on T1-weighted images Weak enhancement Linear or box-shaped non-enhancing area Retropulsion of the posterior vertebral body Space filled with fluid or air Findings of other chronic compression fractures	Signal changes throughout the entire vertebral body Strong low signal intensity on T1-weighted images Strong enhancement Small and irregularly shaped non-enhancing area Convexity of the posterior vertebral body Tumors around the spine or extradural Other metastatic findings

Reprinted from Ref. [13] with permission

months, and in chronic fractures, it usually shows similar bone marrow signal intensity to adjacent vertebrae, but low signal intensity can persist for a longer time due to Kummell's disease, etc.

Findings that should suspect malignant fractures are very low T1 signal intensity throughout the vertebral body, and the posterior of the vertebral body protrudes convexly toward the spinal canal or shows strong enhancement during contrast enhancement, and can be more suspected if it forms a tumor around the vertebral body or is accompanied by metastatic lesions in other parts (Table 9.1; Fig. 9.11) [13]. Also, in DWI images, it shows high signal intensity, and in ADC map, it shows low signal intensity, which is one of the differential points between malignant fractures and benign fractures [14–17]. However, not all of the above imaging findings are always distinguishable, so it is desirable to judge by integrating the patient's medical history, clinical symptoms, and other imaging findings, and if differentiation is difficult despite this, a biopsy may be needed.

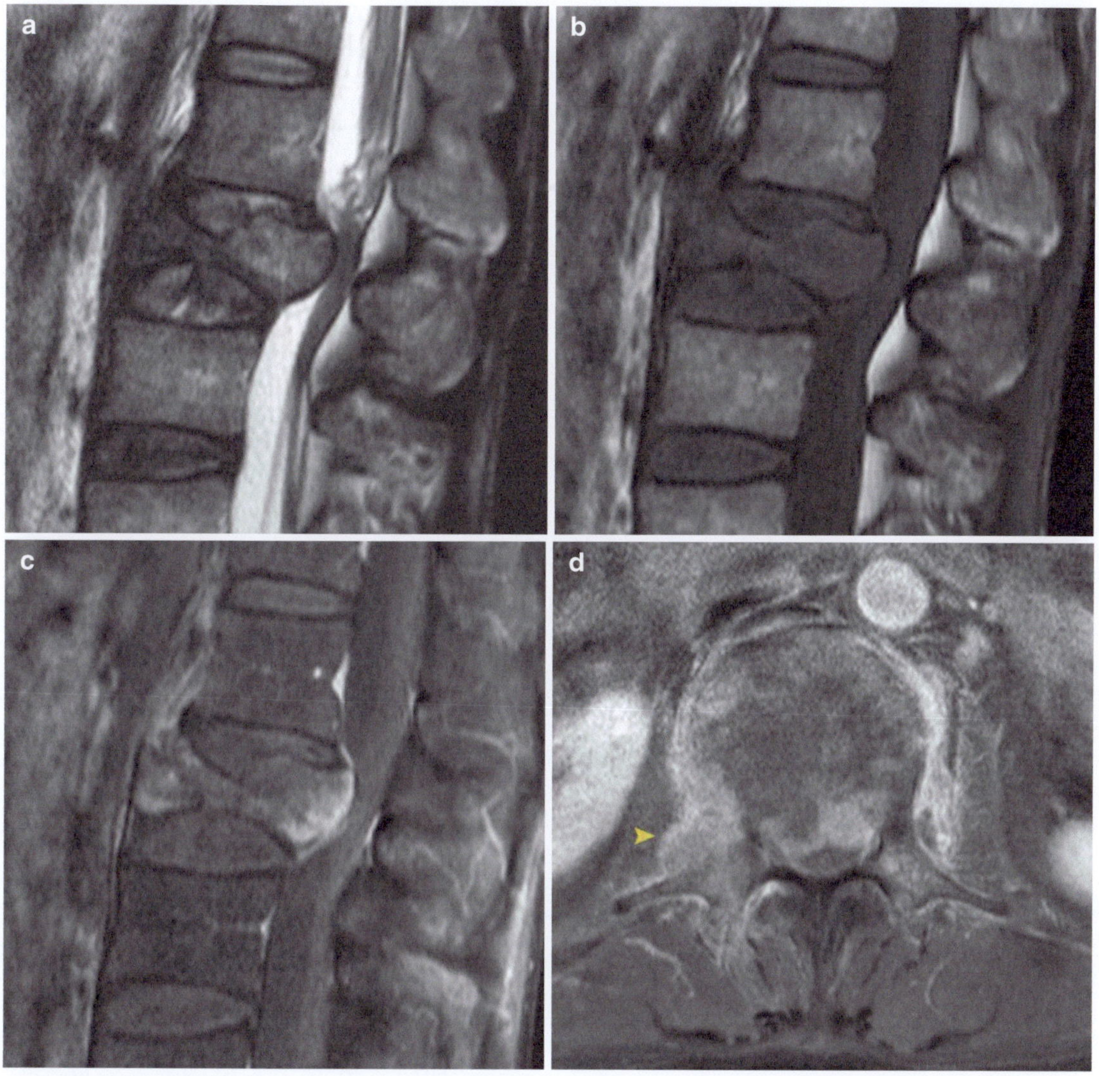

Fig. 9.11 Imaging findings of malignant vertebral fractures due to metastasis. (**a**) In MR T2-weighted images, the vertebral body is flattened with a fracture and the vertebral body's posterior part is protruding convexly toward the spinal canal, compressing the cauda equina. (**b**) In the MR T1-enhanced image, there are low signal intensity marrow changes that invade the entire vertebral body, and the fracture line is not clearly visible. (**c**) In the MR T1 contrast-enhanced image, most of the low signal intensity area that invades the entire vertebral body is enhanced, and there are irregular parts where the enhancement is less in the center. (**d**) In the MR T1 contrast-enhanced axial image, there are lesions that are enhanced not only in the vertebral body but also up to the transverse process, and a mass formation (arrowhead) spreading around the right pedicle can be seen

9.4 Conclusion

Osteoporosis is still not receiving enough attention in our country, considering its high prevalence, risk, and personal/social losses related to fractures. In order to properly diagnose and start treatment for osteoporosis, not only patients and clinicians but also radiologists must participate, one of the methods being the proper diagnosis of osteoporotic vertebral fractures. If a non-traumatic vertebral fracture is found, it can be diagnosed as osteoporosis itself, and it indicates that the current bone strength has decreased regardless of the bone density value, so it becomes an indication for drug treatment [4, 18, 19]. In patients with osteoporosis, asymptomatic vertebral fractures are relatively common, so they are often found incidentally in imaging tests (such as abdominal CT or chest CT) performed for other purposes, and these cases are often overlooked in the interpretation of imaging tests, which is increasingly becoming a problem. Also, patients with recent high grade, multiple fractures are more likely to be candidates for drug treatment, so if a vertebral fracture is found in an imaging test, it would be helpful to determine the appropriate treatment plan by accurately interpreting the location, number, degree, and if possible, whether it occurred recently [18, 20]. In addition, it can be said that it is an important role of a radiologist to ensure that patients with malignant tumors that are first discovered as spinal metastases can be properly diagnosed and treated by recognizing the imaging findings of malignant fractures and interpreting them.

Bibliography

1. Glaser DL, Kaplan FS. Osteoporosis. Definition and clinical presentation. Spine (Phila Pa 1976). 1997;22:12S–6S.
2. WA P. Consensus development conference: diagnosis, prophylaxis, and treatment of osteoporosis. Am J Med. 1993;94:646–50.
3. Korean Society for Bone and Mineral Research. Osteoporosis and osteoporotic fracture fact sheet; 2014.
4. Cosman F, de Beur SJ, LeBoff MS, Lewiecki EM, Tanner B, et al. Clinician's guide to prevention and treatment of osteoporosis. Osteoporos Int. 2014;25:2359–81.
5. Jeremiah MP, Unwin BK, Greenawald MH, Casiano VE. Diagnosis and management of osteoporosis. Am Fam Physician. 2015;92:261–8.
6. Kanis JA. Assessment of fracture risk and its application to screening for postmenopausal osteoporosis: synopsis of a WHO report. WHO Study Group. Osteoporos Int. 1994;4:368–81.
7. Korean Society of Osteoporosis. Bone density measurement guide, 2nd ed. Cheongun; 2018
8. Korean Society for Bone and Mineral Research. Osteoporosis. 5th ed. Gunja Publishing Company; 2016.
9. Shepherd JA, Schousboe JT, Broy SB, Engelke K, Leslie WD. Executive summary of the 2015 ISCD position development conference on advanced measures from DXA and QCT: fracture prediction beyond BMD. J Clin Densitom. 2015;18:274–86.
10. Kang H-s, Hong S-h, Kang C-h. Musculoskeletal radiology. Beommun Education; 2013.
11. Genant HK, Wu CY, van Kuijk C, Nevitt MC. Vertebral fracture assessment using a semiquantitative technique. J Bone Miner Res. 1993;8:1137–48.
12. Kaup M, Wichmann JL, Scholtz JE, Beeres M, Kromen W, et al. Dual-energy CT-based display of bone marrow edema in osteoporotic vertebral compression fractures: impact on diagnostic accuracy of radiologists with varying levels of experience in correlation to MR imaging. Radiology. 2016;280:510–9.
13. Kang H-s, Lee J-w, Kwon J-w. Radiology illustrated spine. Sejong Medical; 2017.
14. Wonglaksanapimon S, Chawalparit O, Khumpunnip S, Tritrakarn SO, Chiewvit P, Charnchaowanish P. Vertebral body compression fracture: discriminating benign from malignant causes by diffusion-weighted MR imaging and apparent diffusion coefficient value. J Med Assoc Thai. 2012;95:81–7.
15. Mubarak F, Akhtar W. Acute vertebral compression fracture: differentiation of malignant and benign causes by diffusion weighted magnetic resonance imaging. J Pak Med Assoc. 2011;61:555–8.
16. Park SW, Lee JH, Ehara S, Park YB, Sung SO, et al. Single shot fast spin echo diffusion-weighted MR imaging of the spine; is it useful in differentiating malignant metastatic tumor infiltration from benign fracture edema? Clin Imaging. 2004;28:102–8.
17. Spuentrup E, Buecker A, Adam G, van Vaals JJ, Guenther RW. Diffusion-weighted MR imaging for differentiation of benign fracture edema and tumor infiltration of the vertebral body. AJR Am J Roentgenol. 2001;176:351–8.
18. Kendler DL, Bauer DC, Davison KS, Dian L, Hanley DA, et al. Vertebral fractures: clinical importance and management. Am J Med. 2016;129(221):e1–10.
19. Chou SH, LeBoff MS. Vertebral imaging in the diagnosis of osteoporosis: a clinician's perspective. Curr Osteoporos Rep. 2017;15:509–20.
20. Broy SB. The vertebral fracture cascade: etiology and clinical implications. J Clin Densitom. 2016;19:29–34.

Bone Marrow Disease

10

Jung Mee Park

Plain radiography or CT can only detect abnormalities when there is destruction in the trabecular bone or cortical bone. Technetium-99m methylene diphosphonate (Tc-MDP) bone scintigraphy is an imaging diagnostic method that indirectly evaluates the state of the bone marrow, but it cannot accurately describe it anatomically, and it has the disadvantage of low specificity. Also, lesions that do not cause an osteoblastic reaction are difficult to detect on bone scintigraphy. 18F-fluorodeoxyglucose positron emission tomography (FDG-PET) imaging is a useful imaging diagnostic method for evaluating primary lesions, lymph node invasion, and metastatic cancer through abnormalities in the metabolic function of the bone marrow.

Magnetic resonance imaging is a diagnostic imaging method that can directly depict lesions invading the bone marrow, and because it has high soft tissue contrast and no ionizing radiation, it is a preferred imaging diagnostic method that can non-invasively evaluate many parts of the bone marrow. Although its histological diagnostic specificity is lower than that of bone marrow aspiration or biopsy, if interpreted in conjunction with the patient's clinical symptoms and blood picture, it can provide useful information for diagnosing bone marrow lesions, understanding various findings according to the patient's condition, and interpreting responses to treatment [1–8].

J. M. Park (✉)
Department of Radiology, College of Medicine,
The Catholic University of Korea, Seoul,
Republic of Korea
e-mail: jmpark@catholic.ac.kr

10.1 Anatomy and Physiology of Normal Bone Marrow

Bone marrow, the fourth largest organ after bones, muscles, fat, and skin, is responsible for the hematopoietic function of producing and regulating red blood cells, white blood cells, and platelets, and is composed of hematopoietic bone marrow, fatty bone marrow, and stromal bone. The bone marrow is supplied with blood from the nutrient artery, each bone has one or more nutrient arteries that penetrate the vertebral bone cortex and enter the bone marrow cavity to form a sinusoidal network, providing nutrients to hematopoietic cells and stromal cells, and then these sinusoidal veins penetrate the bone marrow and cortex.

It is drained out through numerous small veins to the Batson's venous plexus [9–11].

While adipose bone marrow has fewer capillaries and veins, the vascular network of hematopoietic bone marrow is abundant and branches out a lot, so malignant tumors or infections and other bone marrow diseases mainly invade the hematopoietic bone marrow [1–3].

The adipocytes of the bone marrow account for about 75% of the weight of adult bone marrow and are smaller than the adipocytes in other

© The Author(s), under exclusive license to Springer Nature Singapore Pte Ltd. 2025

H. S. Kang, J. W. Lee (eds.), *Spinal Imaging*, https://doi.org/10.1007/978-981-95-1386-4_10

parts of the body. It is not clear what role adipocytes play in hematopoiesis, but when the production of hematopoietic cells is reduced, their size or number increases, and during periods of active hematopoiesis, cell size decreases. After cancer treatment or radiation therapy, the increased adipocytes seem to stimulate hematopoiesis, suggesting that the adipocytes of the bone marrow supply nutrients to the blood cells and act as growth factors [12, 13].

In adult bone marrow, 60% of hematopoietic bone marrow is composed of hematopoietic cells, and 95% of adipose bone marrow is composed of adipocytes. The chemical composition is also different; hematopoietic bone marrow is composed of 40% water, 40% fat, and 20% protein, while adipose bone marrow is 80% fat (Table 10.1).

Table 10.1 Vertebral bone marrow composition

	Red marrow	Yellow marrow
Cellular component		
Hematopoietic cells	60%	5%
Fat cells	40%	95%
Chemical composition		
Fat	40~60%	80%
Water	30~40%	15%
Protein	10~20%	5%

Therefore, the proportion of adipocytes in the total bone marrow is about 75%. In magnetic resonance imaging, the signal intensity of the bone marrow is determined by these fats, water, and protein, and the main component determining this is fat, and even if there is only 20% fat, the signal intensity of the bone marrow shows the signal intensity of fat [14].

Adipose bone marrow and hematopoietic bone marrow are in a dynamic regulatory relationship, regulated by two mechanisms: conversion from hematopoietic bone marrow to adipose bone marrow and the opposite phenomenon, reconversion from adipose bone marrow to hematopoietic bone marrow. Immediately after birth, most of the bone marrow is hematopoietic bone marrow, and the conversion to adipose bone marrow, which begins immediately after birth, ends around the age of 25, starting from the extremities of the limbs and progressing to the central bones in the expected order [15, 16]. In the limb bones, it starts from the diaphysis and progresses to the metaphysis, and in the spine, it starts from the subcortical and subendplate and progresses to the center of the vertebral body, eventually leaving hematopoietic bone marrow in the spine, pelvis, sternum, skull, ribs, and the metaphysis of the humerus or femur (Fig. 10.1).

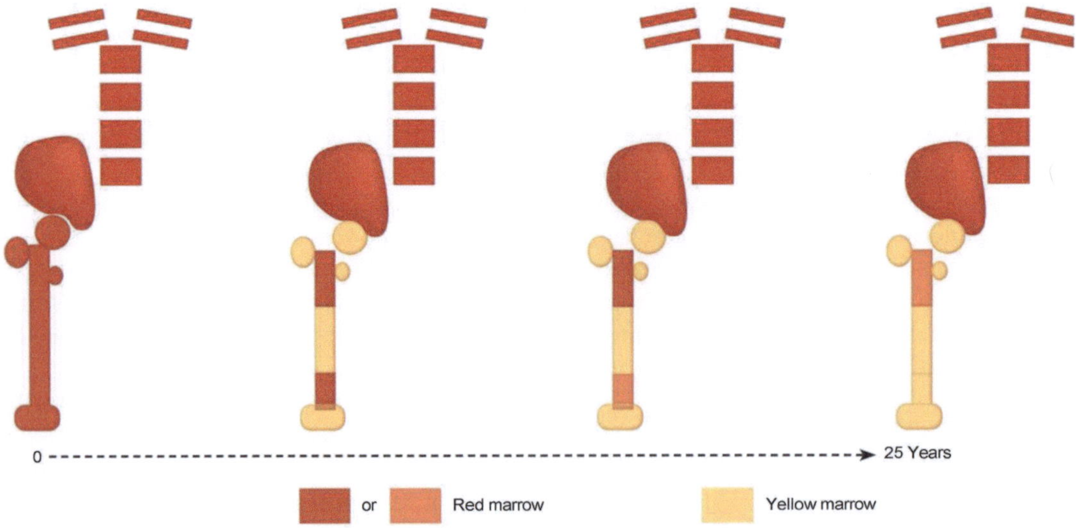

Fig. 10.1 Physiologic conversion of normal bone marrow

Factors regulating conversion include body temperature, blood flow, oxygen partial pressure, and mechanical stress. When body temperature drops, perfusion decreases, or mechanical stress increases, conversion occurs rapidly [2, 17]. On the other hand, as one ages and osteoporosis occurs, the amount of trabecular bone decreases and the amount of adipose bone marrow increases accordingly [15].

When the body's hematopoietic demand increases, reconversion occurs, and this process is different from conversion. In the opposite direction, that is, reversion first occurs from the trunk bone, and the bone marrow proliferates in the limb bone, and also reversion occurs from the proximal part to the distal part within a single bone. The range of these reversions is determined by the degree or duration of the required stimulus [18–20].

10.2 Magnetic Resonance Imaging Findings and Techniques (Fig. 10.2)

Magnetic resonance imaging findings vary depending on the imaging technique, so an imaging technique that can easily find lesions depending on the distribution of fat and water and the use of contrast agents should be used. Generally, since the lesion is mainly in the bone marrow, magnetic resonance images should be obtained focusing on the thoracic spine, pelvis, and proximal femur.

10.2.1 Spin Echo Sequence

In the most basic spin echo technique, T1-weighted images, the bone marrow of a normal adult appears as a homogeneous high signal intensity, which is lower than the signal intensity of pure fat but higher than the signal intensity of muscle. At this time, if a lesion with increased water content, that is, a lesion with high cellularity, is locally invaded, it shows low signal intensity and the lesion can be easily found [2–4, 23]. However, if the bone marrow is uniformly invaded overall, it may be difficult to find the lesion, but even then, if the signal intensity of the bone marrow appears lower than the muscle or intervertebral disc, this bone marrow is always abnormal (Fig. 10.3). If hematopoietic bone marrow is deposited locally, it may be difficult to distinguish from the lesion, but usually it shows a bull's eye sign that includes high signal intensity of fatty bone marrow with bilateral, indistinct boundaries, and the center, and increased peripheral hematopoietic demand such as obesity, smoking, and marathon running can be the cause [24–26].

The hematopoietic bone marrow of children has less fat and higher cellularity compared to adults, so the contrast of the lesion in T1-weighted images is low, so T2-weighted images, fat-saturated T2-weighted images, and STIR images are useful for confirming the lesion [27–29].

In T2-weighted images, fat is somewhat low signal intensity and water is high signal intensity, so the contrast is reversed, and because the contrast between fatty bone marrow and hematopoietic bone marrow is low, the usefulness in diagnosing bone marrow lesions is lower than T1-weighted images. Also, in fast spin echo T2-weighted images, the signal intensity of bone marrow and subcutaneous fat increases compared to the conventional spin echo method, so the sensitivity of the lesion decreases. Therefore, when examining the bone marrow, fat-suppressed fast spin echo T2-weighted images should be obtained to increase the contrast of the lesion. In fat-suppressed fast spin echo T2-weighted images, bone marrow lesions show similar sensitivity to STIR images, images can be obtained in a shorter time, and tissue specificity can also be increased [23, 30].

10.2.2 Fat Suppression Sequence

T1-weighted image, STIR images or fat-saturated fast spin echo T2-weighted image, which suppresses fat signals, is often used in bone marrow imaging. STIR images select an inversion time where fat can appear black. The signal intensity of fat is suppressed, and the signal intensity of nor-

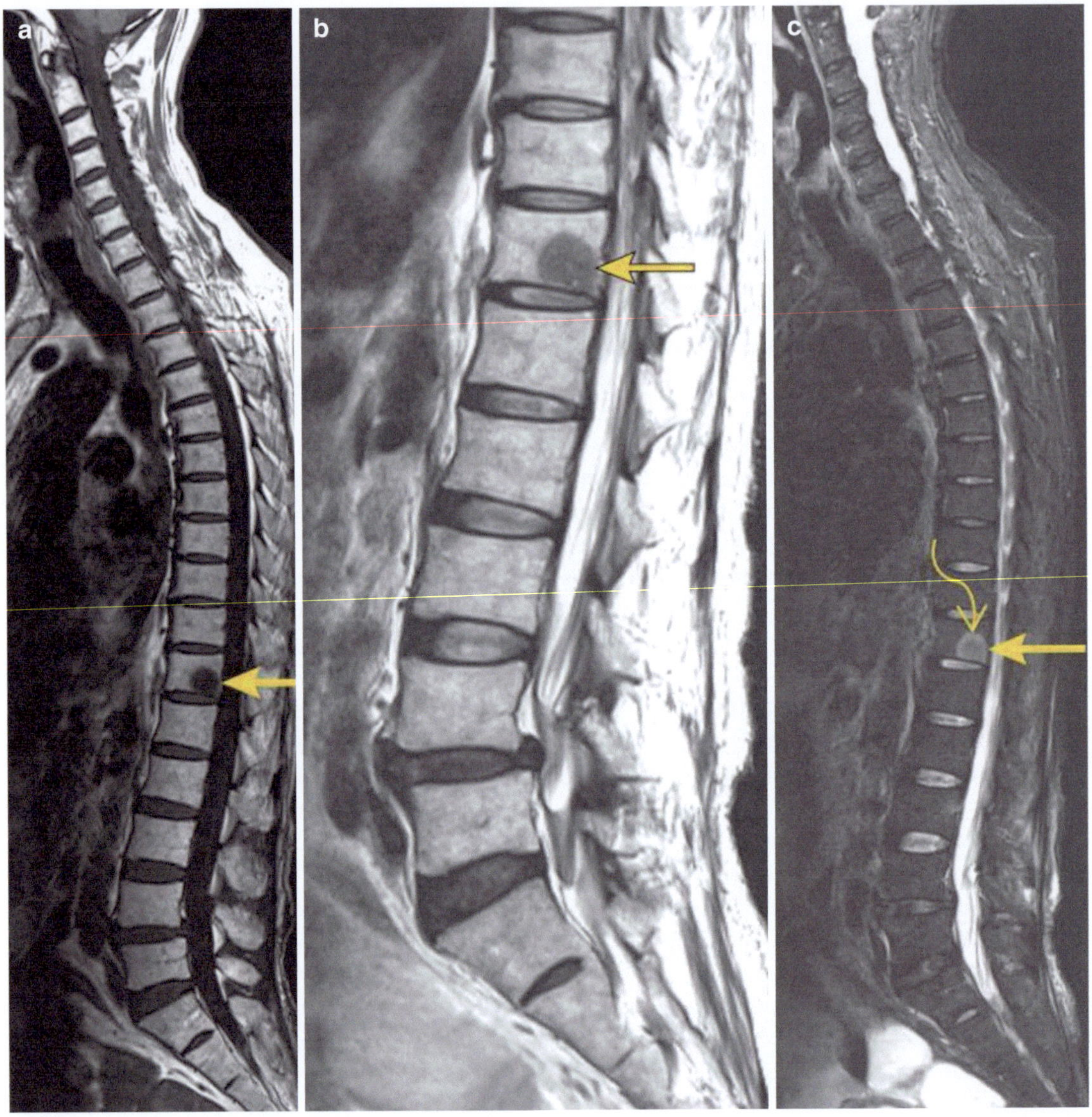

Fig. 10.2 Various magnetic resonance imaging techniques: T12 bone metastasis of pancreatic cancer (arrow). It shows low signal intensity on T1-weighted image (**a**), isointensity on fast spin echo T2-weighted image (**b**), high signal intensity and halo sign (curved arrow) on fat-saturated fast spin echo T2 image (**c**), signal increase on out-of-phase gradient echo image (**d**), high signal intensity on diffusion-weighted image (**e**), and shows diffusion restriction with a low value on ADC map (**f**)

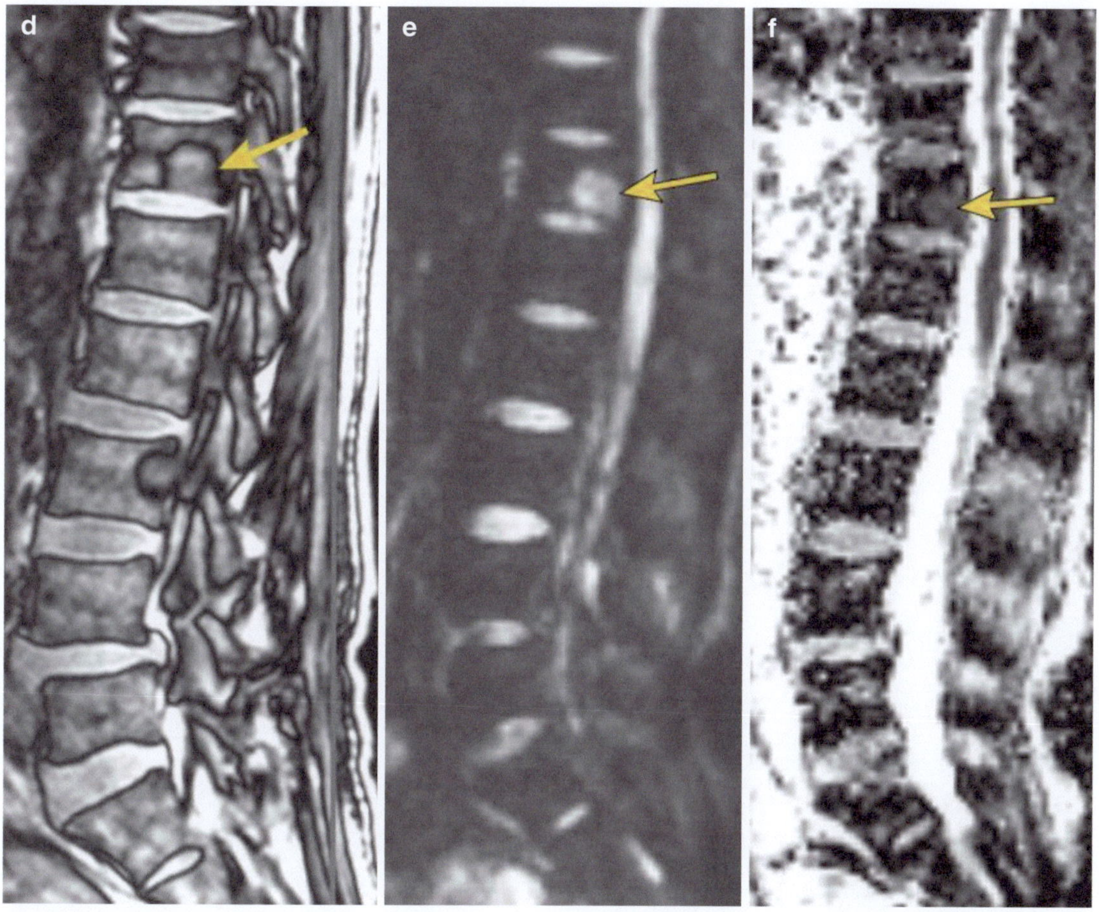

Fig. 10.2 (continued)

mal hematopoietic bone marrow is slightly increased. Bone marrow lesions appear as low signal intensity on T1-weighted MR images and high signal intensity on T2-weighted MR images. The contrast of the lesion is enhanced [30, 31].

Although the signal-to-noise ratio of STIR images falls, it is less affected by motion artifacts. Compared to fast spin echo T2-weighted image, lesions are more clearly visible, but the number of images acquired per hour is small. On the other hand, fat-saturated fast spin echo T2-weighted image, there is a disadvantage that the image becomes uneven when the field of view (FOV) is large, and STIR images are advantageous when examining the bone marrow of the body or a wide area. Both STIR images and fat-saturated T2-enhanced images have a low signal-to-noise ratio, so the bone marrow looks a bit hazy [30]. Most bone marrow lesions show higher signal intensity than surrounding normal bone marrow in fat-suppressed images.

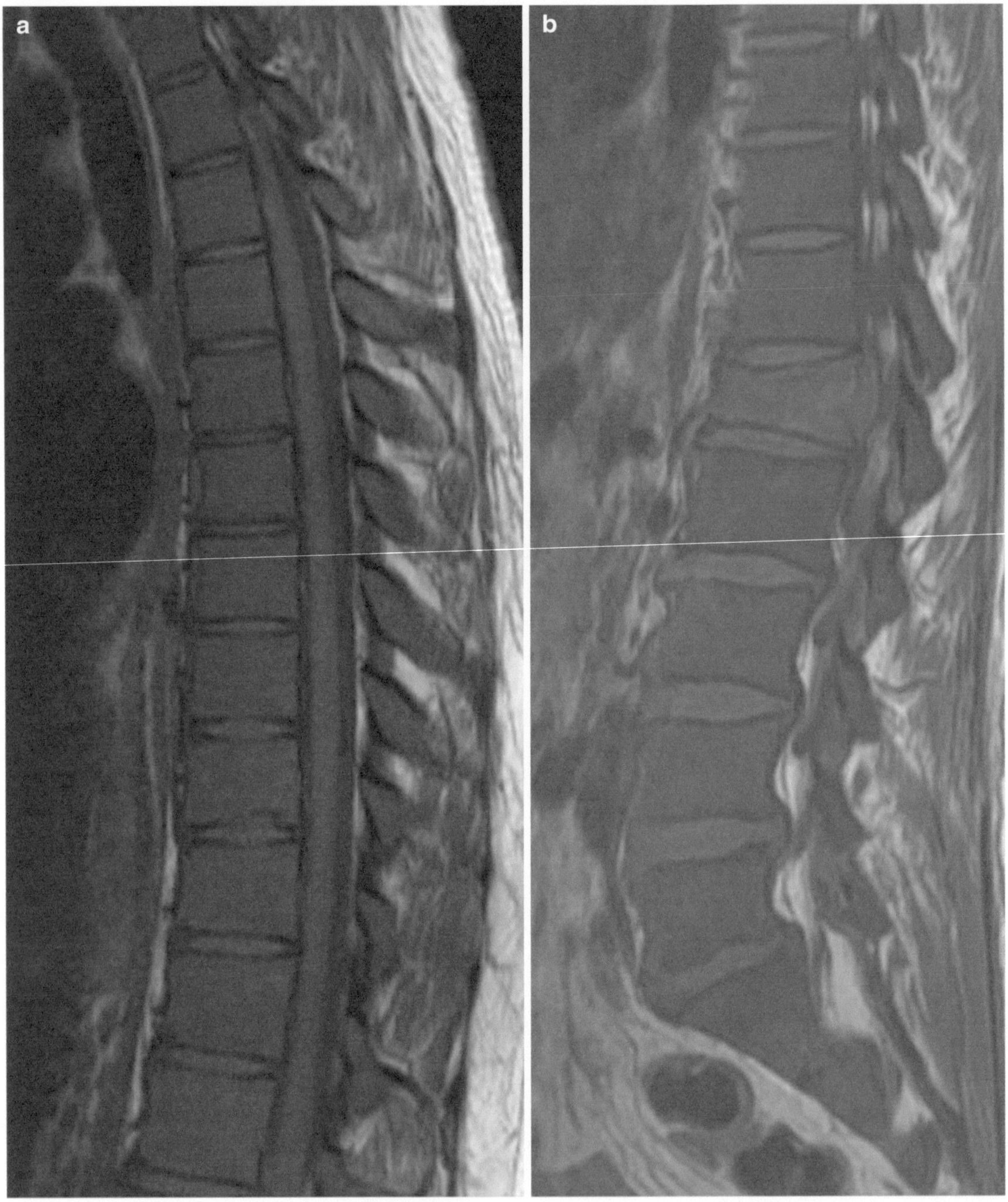

Fig. 10.3 If the signal intensity of the vertebral body on T1-weighted image is lower than that of adjacent muscles or discs, it is always abnormal [(**a**) 16-year-old male, (**b**) 63-year-old male]

10.2.3 Chemical Shift Image

Chemical shift imaging utilizes the difference in spin speed between water and fat protons, which is 3.5 ppm, or resonance frequency difference of 75~150 Hz at 1.5 T device. It is obtained by separating the signals of water and fat and obtaining images, and in the out-of-phase gradient echo images, normal hematopoietic bone marrow shows a lower signal intensity compared to fat bone marrow as the signals of water and fat cancel each other out. Relatively water-rich, i.e., lesions with bone destruction or areas with a lot of fat bone marrow are seen in the out-of-phase gradient echo images with higher signal intensity than surrounding hematopoietic bone marrow (Fig. 10.4) [30–34]. However, in the case of metastatic cancer containing fat, the signal intensity does not decrease, leading to false negatives, fibrosis, or osteosclerotic metastatic cancer, and hematoma cases may increase signal intensity, leading to false positives [35].

10.2.4 Contrast Agent

When Gadolinium-chelates contrast agent is injected, normal bone marrow increases signal intensity by less than about 15%. However, such changes are not clearly distinguished in T1-enhanced images [36, 37]. On the other hand, if there is malignant infiltration, it shows a clear contrast enhancement. In fat-saturated contrast-enhanced T1-enhanced images, even minor signal changes can be found, showing a similar level of lesion detection rate as in fat-saturated T2-enhanced images. On the other hand, if contrast-enhanced images are obtained using the out of phase gradient echo technique, the contrast between normal bone marrow and bone marrow with lesions increases, which can be useful. However, since most of the bone marrow in children is hematopoietic bone marrow, contrast enhancement imaging does not significantly aid in detection for minor bone marrow lesions [38].

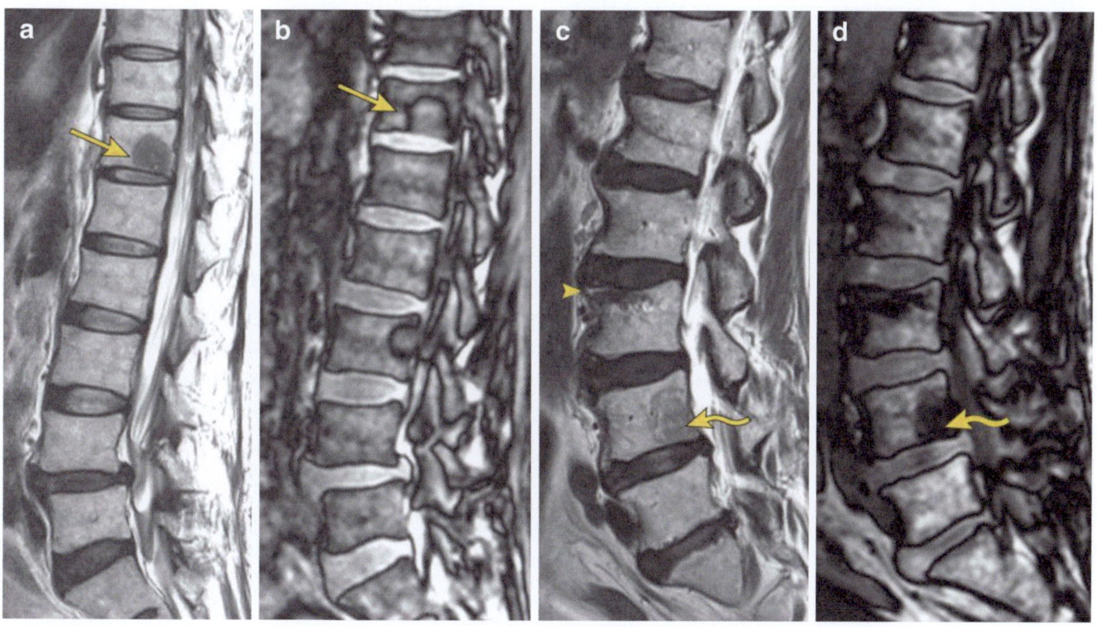

Fig. 10.4 Out-of-phase gradient echo imaging. In the T2-weighted image (**a**) of a 71-year-old male patient with pancreatic cancer, there is a round low signal intensity mass (arrow) at T12, which is a metastatic cancer with increased signal intensity in the out-of-phase gradient (**b**) image. In the T1-weighted image (**c**) of an 85-year-old female patient with an L3 compression fracture (arrowhead), the low signal intensity (curved arrow) seen at L4 is a benign lesion, a hemangioma, which appears to have decreased signal intensity in the out-of-phase image (**d**)

Ultrasmall superparamagnetic iron dioxide (USPIO), a contrast agent specifically absorbed in normal bone marrow, can significantly reduce the relaxation time of normal bone marrow due to its very small particle size, which allows it to enter the space of blood vessels in the bone marrow. On the other hand, in cases of malignant infiltration, there is no phagocytic ability, so the signal intensity does not change. Therefore, clinical trials using USPIO as a contrast agent for bone marrow in patients with blood diseases are being attempted [39, 40].

10.2.5 Diffusion-Weighted Imaging

Diffusion-weighted imaging maximizes the phenomenon of signal intensity reduction due to the diffusion phenomenon caused by the irregular Brownian motion of water molecules in the human body. The apparent diffusion coefficient (ADC) value reflects the cellularity and the state of the cell membrane. If the ADC value of the lesion is low, it suggests a malignant tumor with high cellularity, whereas a high ADC value indicates necrosis, which can be used to determine the treatment effect of malignant bone marrow lesions (Fig. 10.5). In the case of malignant compression fractures of the vertebral body, the diffusion of water molecules is limited due to tumor cell infiltration, so high signal intensity is shown in diffusion-weighted imaging, while benign compression fractures show low signal intensity [41, 42].

Hematopoietic bone marrow does not diffuse well, so diffusion-weighted imaging should be carefully interpreted in children with a lot of hematopoietic bone marrow, and there are reports that ADC values overlap a lot between benign and malignant lesions [43, 44].

10.2.6 Whole-Body Magnetic Resonance Imaging

With the advancement of technology that can obtain whole-body images in a short time and the use of techniques such as testing without stopping breathing in children, the use of whole-body magnetic resonance imaging is increasing. Fat-saturated T2-weighted imaging and diffusion-weighted imaging are primarily used [45–48]. It is very useful for initial staging and follow-up examinations of tumors because it can sensitively diagnose metastatic tumors to bones and extraosseous tissues. Whole-body magnetic resonance imaging shows similar results to PET-CT in the diagnosis of malignant bone marrow lesions [49]. However, its use is limited because there is no standardized protocol yet and the image acquisition time is long.

10.2.7 Quantitative Technique

Spectroscopy is a method of quantifying the amount of fat by examining the chemical components of the bone marrow. It has been reported how the fat of the bone marrow changes according to age and gender, but it is not widely used clinically [50, 51].

In cases where blood cancer has invaded the bone marrow in a chronic manner, measuring fat quantitatively rather than analyzing signal intensity can yield more objective results, and can increase sensitivity in evaluating bone marrow infiltration and response to treatment [26, 27]. However, when there is little cancer infiltration in the bone marrow, T1 relaxation time or the measurement of water/fat ratio was not helpful.

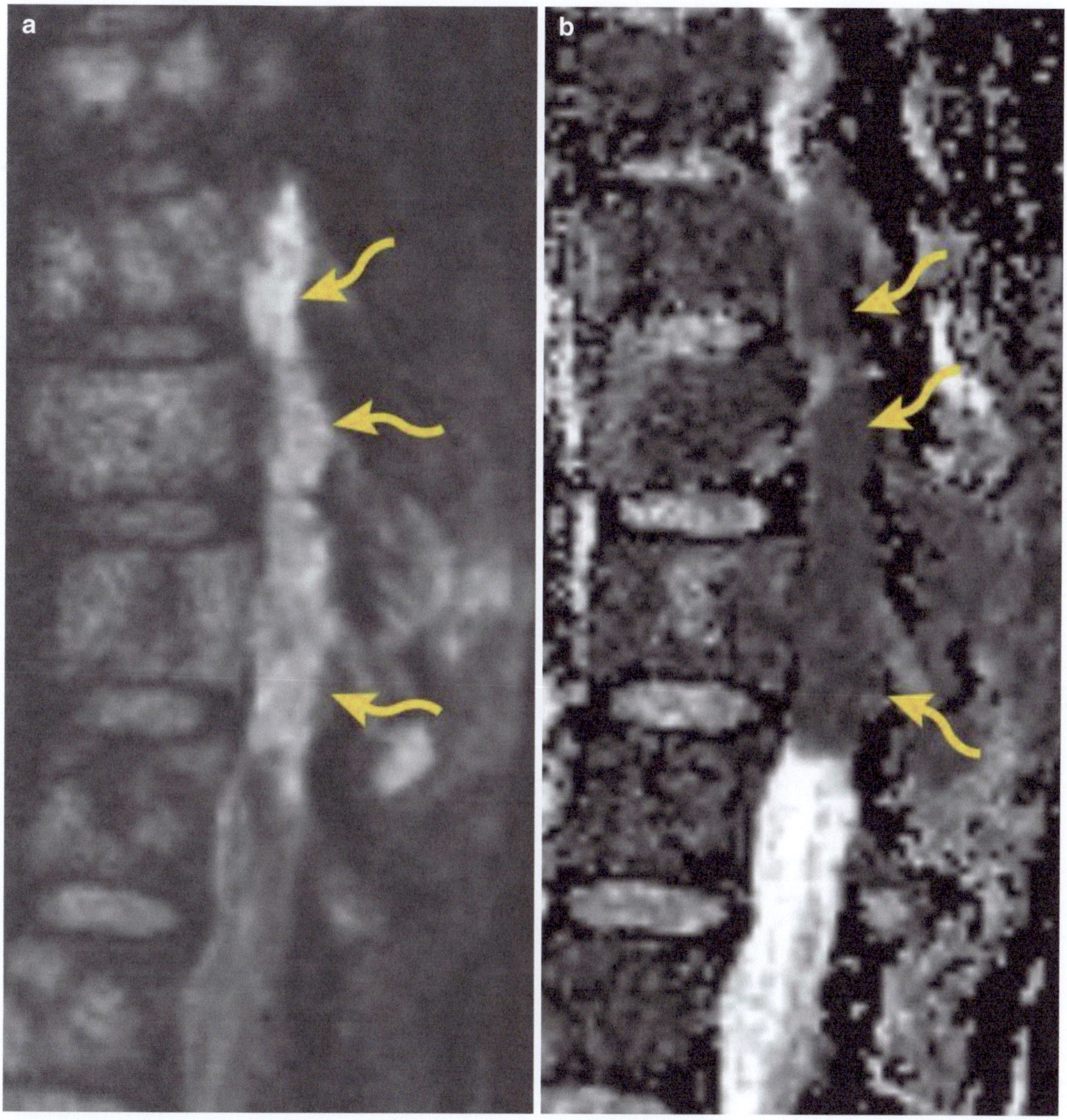

Fig. 10.5 Diffusion-weighted image and ADC map of a 56-year-old lymphoma patient. In the diffusion-weighted image (**a**), there is a high signal intensity in the midthoracic spine and spinous process, and a posterior epidural mass (curved arrow). In the ADC map (**b**), it shows low signal intensity, and its value is about 0.6 31,023 mm^2/s, indicating a malignant tumor with high cellularity

10.3 Magnetic Resonance Imaging Findings of Normal Bone Marrow

The bone marrow of the spine is a mixture of hematopoietic and fatty marrow, which is supported by trabeculae. Trabeculae appear as low signal intensity lines in all images, and their impact on the signal intensity of spinal magnetic resonance imaging is minimal. The signal intensity of spinal magnetic resonance imaging is determined by the relative ratio of fat and water [2, 3, 19–23, 53].

In T1-weighted images, the spinal marrow of adults shows a high signal intensity similar to subcutaneous fat. However, immediately after birth, most of the marrow is water-rich hematopoietic marrow, so the vertebral body shows a low signal intensity compared to adjacent discs or muscles in T1-weighted images. As age increases, fat gradually increases, mainly depositing under the endplate and toward the front of the vertebral body, showing heterogeneous signal intensity (Fig. 10.6). In particular, lumbar T1-weighted images show areas of high signal intensity of various degrees and shapes with age increase, such as appearing linearly along the basivertebral vein, appearing as a belt or triangular shape at the edge of the vertebral body, scattered small areas showing high signal intensity, and several relatively large areas with clear boundaries. It was reported that the younger the age group, the more often it appears linearly along the basivertebral vein [15]. In adults under 40, hematopoietic marrow is distributed minimally and a small amount of fatty marrow is distributed around the basivertebral vein, but after 40, it is gradually replaced by fatty marrow. However, even at the age of 70, about 50% of the hematopoietic marrow remains in the spine [15, 55].

The ratio of hematopoietic marrow to fatty marrow varies greatly depending on age, patient's condition, and individual (Fig. 10.7). In the case

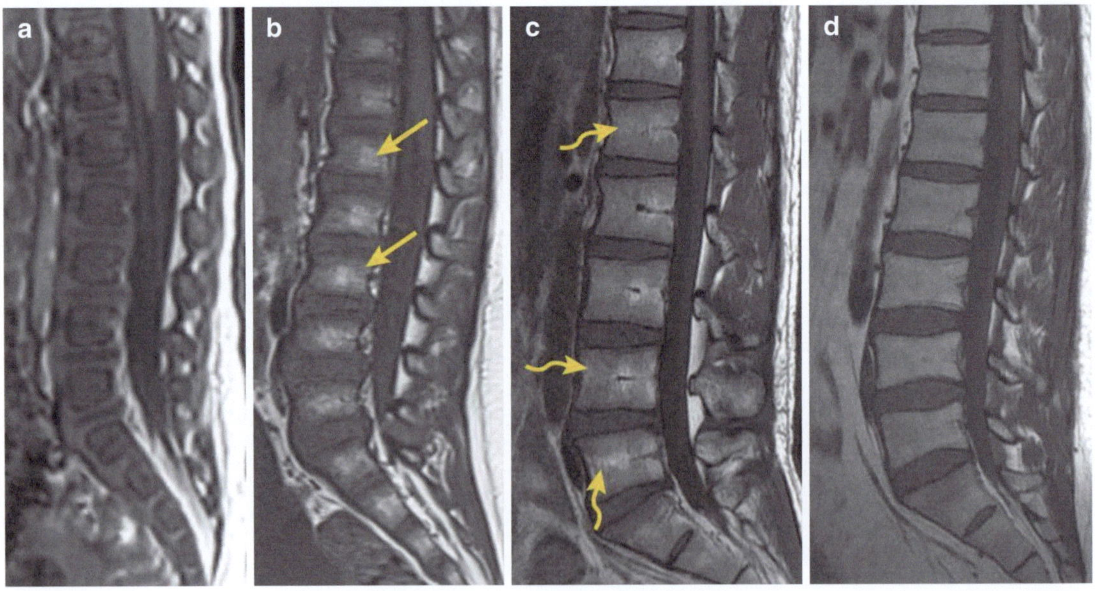

Fig. 10.6 Signal intensity of vertebral body marrow in T1-weighted images according to age. (**a**) The marrow of the vertebral body of a 6-month-old girl is mostly hematopoietic marrow, showing lower signal intensity than the intervertebral disc. (**b**) In a 5-year-old girl, conversion to fatty marrow, which shows higher signal intensity than the intervertebral disc, is occurring around the basivertebral vein (arrow). (**c**) In a 25-year-old man, high signal intensity due to fat is mainly seen in the anterior part of the vertebral body (curved arrow) and around the basivertebral vein, and (**d**) The marrow of the vertebral body of a 40-year-old man shows homogeneous high signal intensity

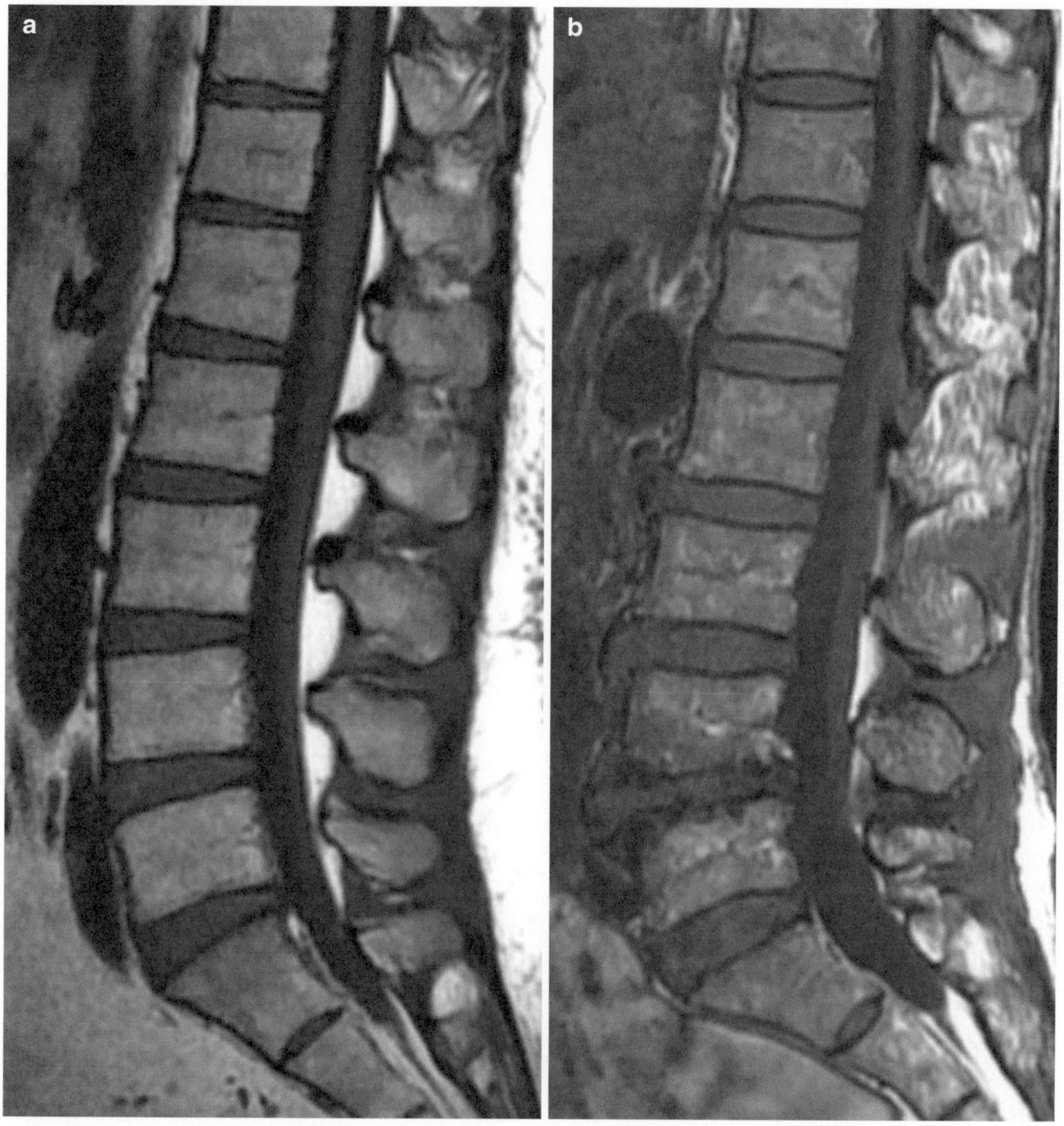

Fig. 10.7 The signal intensity of the marrow varies depending on the individual and age, so the signal intensity of the lumbar spine of a 40-year-old man (**a**) shows homogeneous high signal intensity in the T1-weighted image, but even in an 80-year-old woman (**b**), it includes heterogeneous low signal intensity (red marrow hyperplasia)

of young adult women, there is a lot of hematopoietic marrow and fat gradually increases after 60, while in men, the proportion of fat increases after 25 [23, 54]. In the elderly, malnourished, or osteoporotic, the spinal marrow can be completely replaced by fat [56]. In adults, the signal intensity of the vertebral body in T1-weighted images is higher than that of the intervertebral disc, and if the signal intensity is lower than that of the disc or muscle, it can be considered to have a bone marrow disease.

Since there is a considerable amount of fat in the hematopoietic marrow, the marrow conversion seen in T1-weighted images appears faster than histological marrow conversion.

In T2-weighted images, fatty marrow also shows a signal intensity similar to subcutaneous fat, so fat-suppressed images are needed to diagnose bone marrow lesions. In fat-saturated T2-weighted images or STIR images, hematopoietic marrow shows a slightly higher It shows a moderate signal intensity, contrasting with fatty marrow, and is useful for detecting lesions with many cells or water [23].

10.4 Bone Marrow Disease

Vogler and Murphy, among others, classified bone marrow diseases in magnetic resonance imaging as reconversion, myeloid depletion, ischemia, infiltration, and edema of the bone marrow, which helps to understand the signal intensity of the bone marrow and the diseases that invade the bone marrow [2]. Vande Berg et al. [20] classified bone marrow lesions based on how the balance between fatty marrow and non-fatty marrow components breaks down in T1-enhanced images, based on the fact that fat determines the signal intensity of the bone marrow in magnetic resonance imaging. They classified an increase in fat and an increase in signal intensity in T1-enhanced images as depletion of hematopoietic marrow, a partial loss of fat and a moderate decrease in signal intensity as bone marrow infiltration, a complete loss of fat and a lower, more homogeneous signal intensity as bone marrow replacement, and a very low signal intensity like cortical bone as bone marrow signal void. They also divided these into focal, regional, or diffuse distribution patterns.

10.4.1 Reconversion

Reconversion occurs when the demand for hematopoiesis increases and the existing hematopoietic marrow cannot handle it, causing the fatty marrow to be reconverted to hematopoietic marrow or hematopoietic hyperplasia. This process occurs in the opposite direction to the conversion where normal hematopoietic marrow is replaced by fatty marrow [57].

It starts from the axial bone and progresses to the proximal limb bone, and from the proximal to the distal part in the limb bone. Therefore, if there is reconversion in the limb bone, it can be predicted that more severe reconversion has occurred in the axial bone. Pathologically, capillaries proliferate in the subendosteal marrow of the fatty marrow, a sinusoid network is formed, and blood supply increases.

Causes of reconversion (Fig. 10.8) and hematopoietic marrow hyperplasia include diseases that replace the bone marrow, such as chronic anemia and metastatic cancer, bone marrow proliferative diseases such as myeloma and leukemia, and congenital heart disease. Reconversion is also promoted when hematopoietic growth factors are injected in conjunction with chemotherapy or bone marrow transplantation [58]. Long-term smoking causing tissue hypoxia (Fig. 10.9), chronic anemia due to hemolysis in marathoners, and anemia due to folate deficiency during pregnancy can also cause bone marrow reconversion [59, 60].

The extent of these reconversions is determined by the degree or duration of the required stimulus. For example, in the case of sickle cell anemia, the amount of bone marrow that can regenerate has already significantly decreased due to osteonecrosis, so the distribution and degree of reconversion are affected [61]. In a similar way, when there are bone metastases or bone marrow proliferative diseases, the proximal bone marrow is invaded by these lesions, so more distal bone marrow reconversion occurs. Typically, malignant diseases primarily invade the hematopoietic bone marrow of the axial skeleton, so if proliferation of hematopoietic bone marrow is seen in the limb bones of a patient with a tumor, it can be inferred that the tumor has already extensively invaded the axial skeleton. However, extensive reconversion of limb bones is not a common phenomenon, so caution is needed when diagnosing reconversion based on MR images. Currently, there are no specific MR sig-

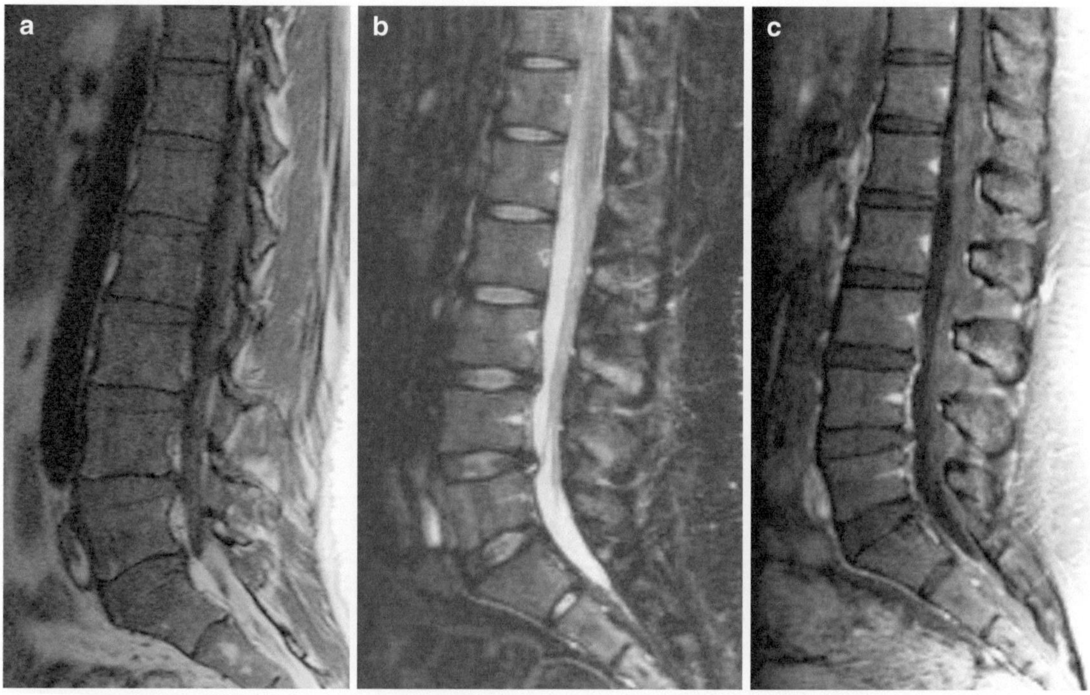

Fig. 10.8 Diffuse red marrow reconversion. The marrow signal intensity of a 26-year-old female patient with thrombocytopenia appears darker than the intervertebral disc in the T1-weighted image (**a**) and shows a slight increase in signal intensity in the STIR (**b**) and fat-saturated contrast-enhanced T1-weighted image (**c**), indicating reconversion to hematopoietic marrow

nal intensity characteristics to distinguish proliferated, i.e., reconversion, bone marrow from other bone marrow invasion diseases, so bone marrow biopsy is necessary for confirmation.

The signal intensity of proliferated bone marrow varies depending on the degree of proliferation, i.e., cellularity, which is determined by the degree of cellularity, the water content in the hematopoietic bone marrow, and the selected imaging parameters. If there is extensive bone marrow proliferation, the signal intensity on T1-weighted images appears similar to or slightly lower than muscle, higher than adipose bone marrow on T2-weighted images, and has moderate signal intensity similar to muscle on STIR images.

In the case of reconversion or hematopoietic bone marrow proliferation, the shape or distribution of signal intensity on magnetic resonance images is non-specific. However, bone marrow that has regenerated more extensively and unevenly than normal bone marrow is distributed in a very inappropriate location for the patient's age. In children, if there is a disease that can cause proliferation of hematopoietic bone marrow, the conversion of normal bone marrow is delayed. Therefore, it can be very difficult to distinguish between variations in the distribution of normal hematopoietic bone marrow and proliferation of hematopoietic bone marrow, and metastatic cancer, myeloma, leukemia, lymphoma, and other lesions may have similar distribution and signal intensity to proliferated normal hematopoietic bone marrow, making it difficult to distinguish them.

10.4.2 Bone Marrow Depletion (Myeloid Depletion)

This refers to the destruction or disappearance of all bone marrow cells other than fat, which occurs when conversion occurs early or is abnormally accelerated, depleting the hematopoietic cells in

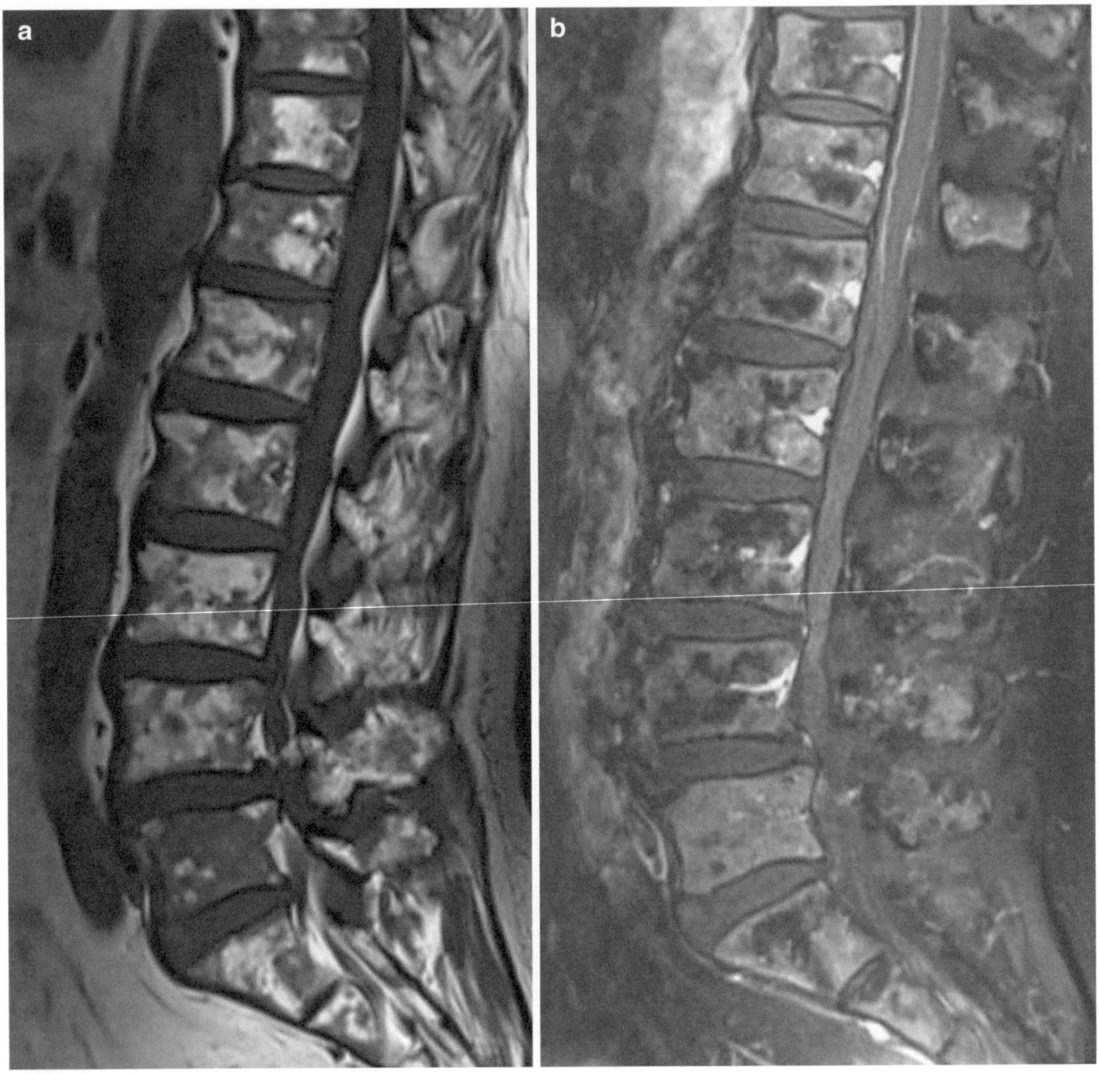

Fig. 10.9 Focal red marrow reconversion. This is an 85-year-old heavy smoker. Hematopoietic marrow is locally and unevenly deposited, so the signal intensity of the marrow appears as low signal intensity in the T1-weighted image (**a**), and after contrast enhancement (**b**), it shows partially heterogeneous high signal intensity

the bone marrow. The spaces where these cells were are filled with adipose bone marrow, and at this time, the signal intensity of the bone marrow on magnetic resonance images shows the characteristic signal intensity of fat.

Causes include aplastic anemia, radiation therapy, and chemotherapy [25].

In the case of aplastic anemia or those who have received chemotherapy, it occurs chronically, and in the case of radiation therapy, fat is deposited in the bone marrow of the treated area.

Aplastic anemia is a blood disease in which all lines of hematopoietic cells in the bone marrow decrease and are replaced by fat, resulting in pancytopenia in peripheral blood. In about 50% of cases, bone marrow formation decreases without a specific cause, and it can also occur secondarily due to drugs, viral infections, toxins, etc. Depending

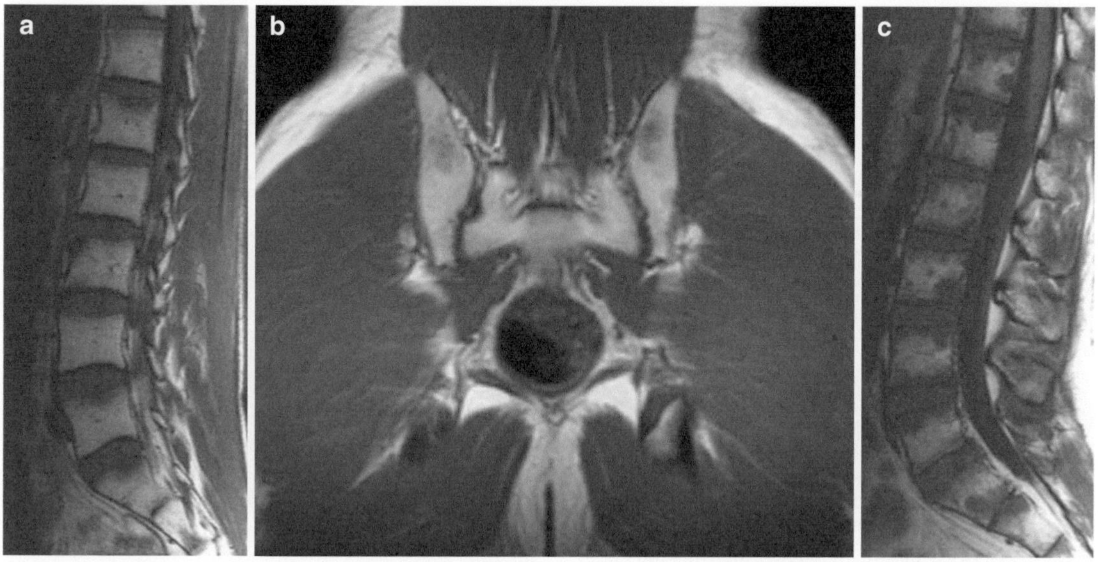

Fig. 10.10 MR of aplastic anemia (AA). (**a**, **b**) A 22-year-old male shows a significant increase in bone marrow signal intensity compared to adjacent discs on lumbar and pelvic T1-weighted images. This is severe AA with <5% bone marrow cellularity, and the signal intensity of the bone marrow has increased, indicating almost no remaining hematopoietic bone marrow. (**c**) A 25-year-old male with 30% cellularity, where low signal intensity hematopoietic bone marrow remains in places, but there is increased fatty marrow compared to his age, indicating moderate AA

on the amount of remaining hematopoietic bone marrow in the adipose bone marrow, it shows various degrees of signal intensity, but in MR T1-enhanced image (Fig. 10.10), the remaining hematopoietic marrow in the fatty marrow showing high signal intensity contains varying degrees of low signal intensity depending on the amount. When cellularity is significantly reduced, most of the marrow is replaced by fatty marrow, showing high signal intensity due to hypoplasia [25, 62].

Depending on the treatment, the low signal intensity area caused by regenerated hematopoietic marrow is deposited in the hypoplastic fatty marrow, showing quite heterogeneous signal intensity. The marrow changes resulting from aplastic anemia usually show extensive changes primarily in the axial skeleton, so changes in the spine are expected to be more severe than in the pelvis or femur.

Within the first week after radiation therapy or cancer treatment, swelling and congestion in the marrow appear as low signal intensity in T1-enhanced images and high signal intensity in STIR images, and the cellularity in the marrow decreases and the vessels are destroyed. After the acute phase, the treatment area transitions to fatty marrow, starting from about 2 weeks and rapidly transitioning the damaged marrow to fat during the first 6 weeks, and then slowly continuing for about 2 years (Figs. 10.11 and 10.12). Then, hematopoietic cells move from untreated distant areas, increasing the cellularity of the marrow and recovering hematopoietic function, usually around 6 months when regeneration becomes vigorous (Fig. 10.5). In young people, a band-shaped marrow regeneration can also be seen in MRI. However, if the radiation dose is 50 Gy or more and the vascular damage is severe, regeneration does not occur and permanent fat deposition may remain [63].

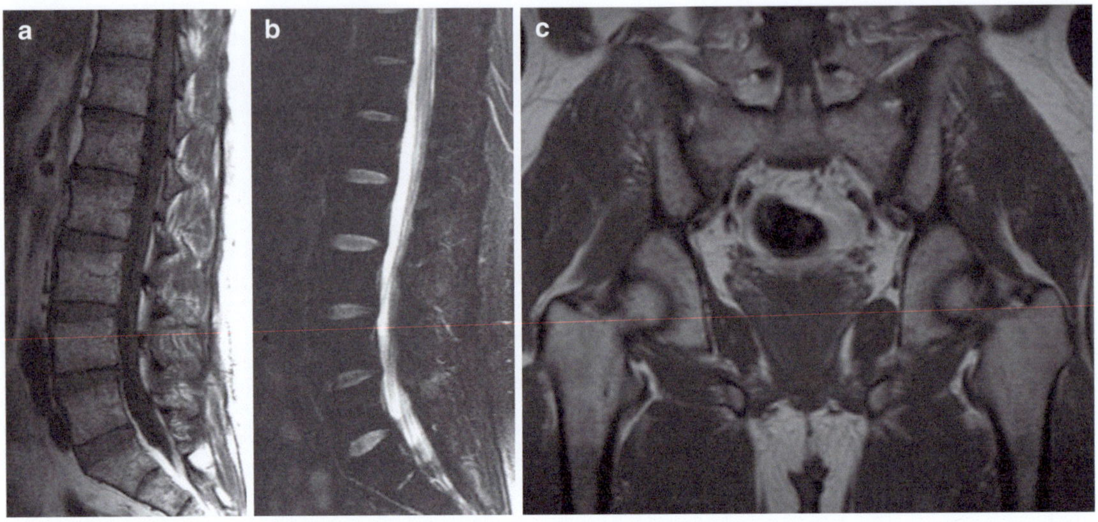

Fig. 10.11 Bone marrow depletion after chemotherapy for acute myeloid leukemia. A 46-year-old male patient, after cancer treatment, continues to suffer from pancytopenia. The results of the magnetic resonance imaging show severe bone marrow depletion with increased signal intensity in the spine on T1-weighted images (**a**), low signal intensity on STIR (**b**) images, and increased signal intensity in the pelvic bone and proximal femur on T1-weighted images (**c**)

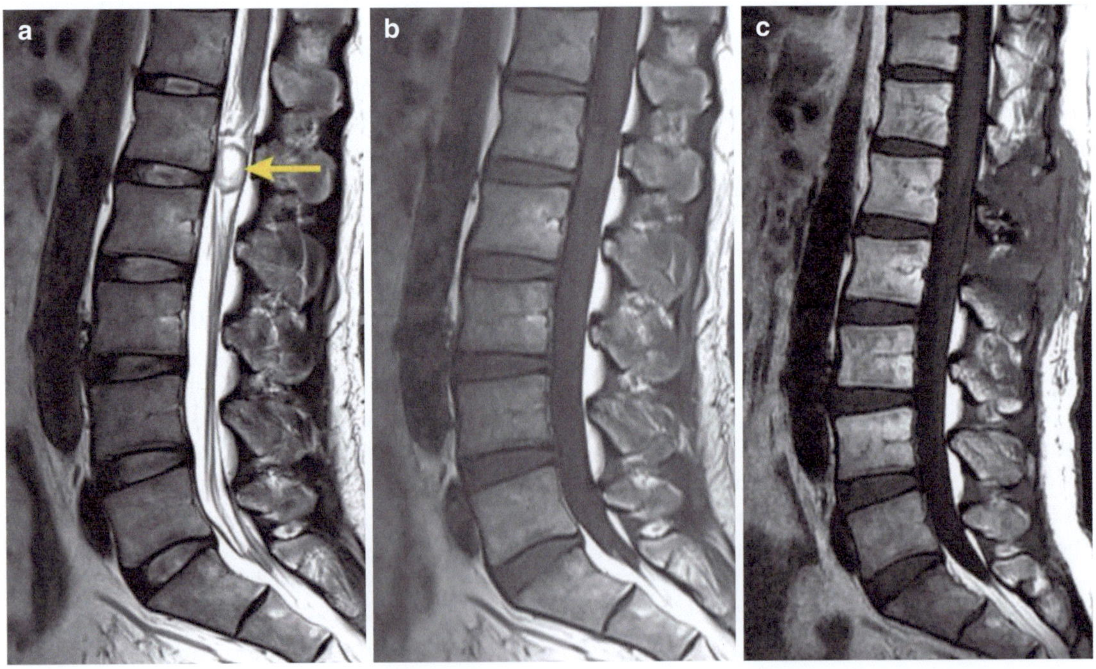

Fig. 10.12 Bone marrow depletion after radiation therapy. A 42-year-old male patient underwent surgery to remove an intradural carcinoid tumor (arrow, **a**, **b**: T2, T1-weighted images) and received a total of 50 gray of radiation therapy (T12-L3, **c**: T1-weighted image) 25 times. The thoracolumbar spine within the radiation exposure range is replaced by fat and shows high signal intensity on T1-weighted images

10.4.3 Multiple Myeloma

It is the most common primary malignant bone tumor in which plasma cells undergo monoclonal neoplastic proliferation in the marrow. It is characterized by bone destruction and the appearance of monoclonal immunoglobulin in serum and urine. It is common in the 60s, and it is very rare to occur in those under 40, <5%. The male to female ratio is about 2:1, and they complain of anemia, back pain, weakness, weight loss, and fever. About 5% of patients start with an isolated mass without invading the marrow, but most progress to plasma cell myeloma, multiple myeloma within 5 years. It is common in the vertebral body, ribs, skull, pelvic bones, and proximal limb bones [64].

Simple radiographic findings are characterized by extensive, well-defined punched out bone destruction lesions of relatively uniform size in the marrow cavity, which do not usually cause reactive bone sclerosis or periosteal reaction around the bone destruction. It destroys multiple vertebral bodies, causing compression fractures, but it is rare to invade the pedicle or posterior arch. Since multiple myeloma is a lesion of the marrow, it can occur anywhere in the skeletal system of the whole body, unlike metastatic bone tumors, it can also be found in the skeletal system of the knee joint or proximal knee joint, so it is necessary to examine the skeletal system of the whole body with X-ray pictures. The distal extremities of the primary bone should also be included in the examination. In about 15% of multiple myeloma cases, local bone destruction lesions are not present, and only severe osteopenia is observed, which may appear similar to severe osteoporosis, hyperparathyroidism, and metastatic bone destruction (Fig. 10.13).

In magnetic resonance imaging, multiple myeloma shows three types of invasive findings: focal, variegated, and diffuse (Fig. 10.14). Cases where the diffuse and focal types are mixed or appear normal are also observed [65, 66].

Among these, focal lesions are the most common and often appear as bone destruction in simple X-ray images. Against the background of normal bone marrow, they show low signal intensity in T1-weighted images, high signal intensity in T2-weighted images, and usually strong contrast enhancement. Diffuse homogeneous lesions account for about 25% of multiple myeloma cases, and the lesions are not well seen in simple X-ray images, and the prognosis is also poor. In more than 80% of patients with multiple myeloma, lytic bone lesions or osteopenia appear initially, so examining the skeletal system with simple imaging has been part of the staging of multiple myeloma for the past 20 years. However, to see lytic bone lesions in simple X-ray images, there must be a 30–50% decrease in bone, so it is not easy to detect lesions. The basic role of magnetic resonance imaging in patients with multiple myeloma is to evaluate patients with neurological symptoms. Immediate treatment is needed when there are local lesions in the spine and these lesions compress the spinal canal by spreading to the soft tissue. Also, if the focal lesions disappear or decrease in size or number in magnetic resonance imaging, or if there are no focal or diffuse lesions, it means there is a response to treatment. Also, if the signal intensity of the lesion decreases in T2-weighted images or the signal intensity of fat increases in T1-weighted images and there is no contrast enhancement or only peripheral contrast enhancement, it means there is a response to treatment. However, even if there is a response to treatment, the size of the lesion or the abnormal findings in the bone marrow may not change and remain, and abnormal findings may still be seen in cases where there are still active lesions or scars. Recently, it is expected that the response after treatment can be evaluated through the increase in apparent diffusion coefficients or changes in microcirculation using diffusion-weighted imaging or dynamic contrast-enhanced MRI [67, 68].

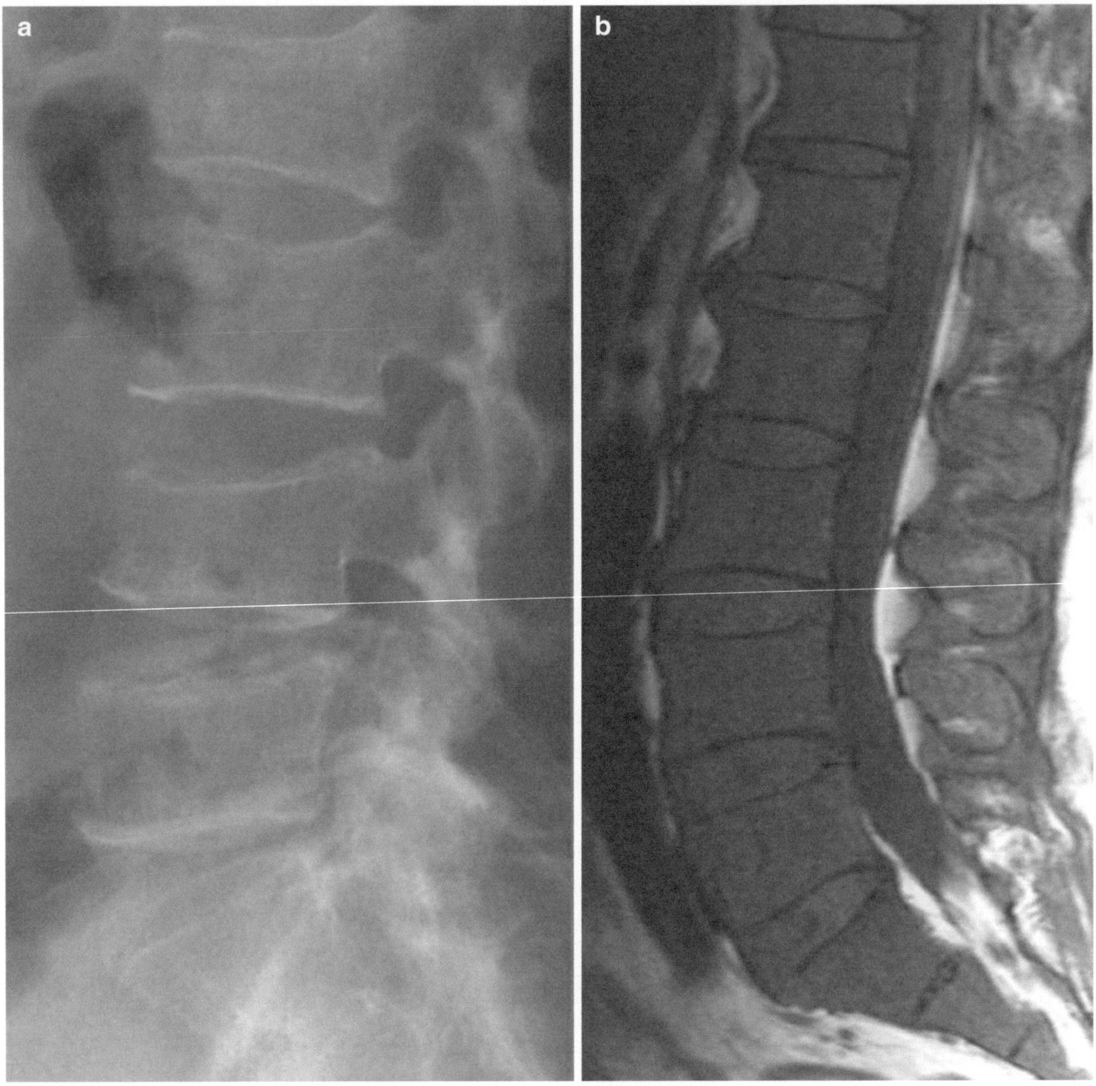

Fig. 10.13 Multiple myeloma with decreased bone density, not clearly destructive bone lesions. (**a**) A 41-year-old woman, on the lateral lumbar X-ray, shows a non-specific finding of overall decreased bone density compared to her age, which can be seen in the early stages of multiple myeloma. (**b**) On the lumbar T1-weighted image, not only the vertebral body but also the posterior part shows decreased bone marrow signal intensity compared to the adjacent disc, indicating diffuse bone marrow infiltration

18F-FDG-PET-CT is as effective as MRI in detecting multiple myeloma, and it is useful for detecting extraosseous masses. It has the advantage of being able to examine the whole body of the patient, making it useful for detecting multiple myeloma that has occurred outside the bone marrow and determining the stage. It is also more advantageous than whole-body MRI in evaluating the response after treatment. However, its high sensitivity can overestimate the stage or evaluate it as false positive [69, 70].

10.4.4 Leukemia

Leukemia is the most common malignant disease in children, characterized by acute and chronic tumors of myelogenous or lymphocytic white blood cells. Acute lymphocytic leukemia accounts for 75%, acute myelogenous leukemia for 15~20%, and chronic myelogenous leukemia for 5%. Symptoms include local or chronic bone pain, joint pain, joint effusion, fever, anemia, and recurring infections.

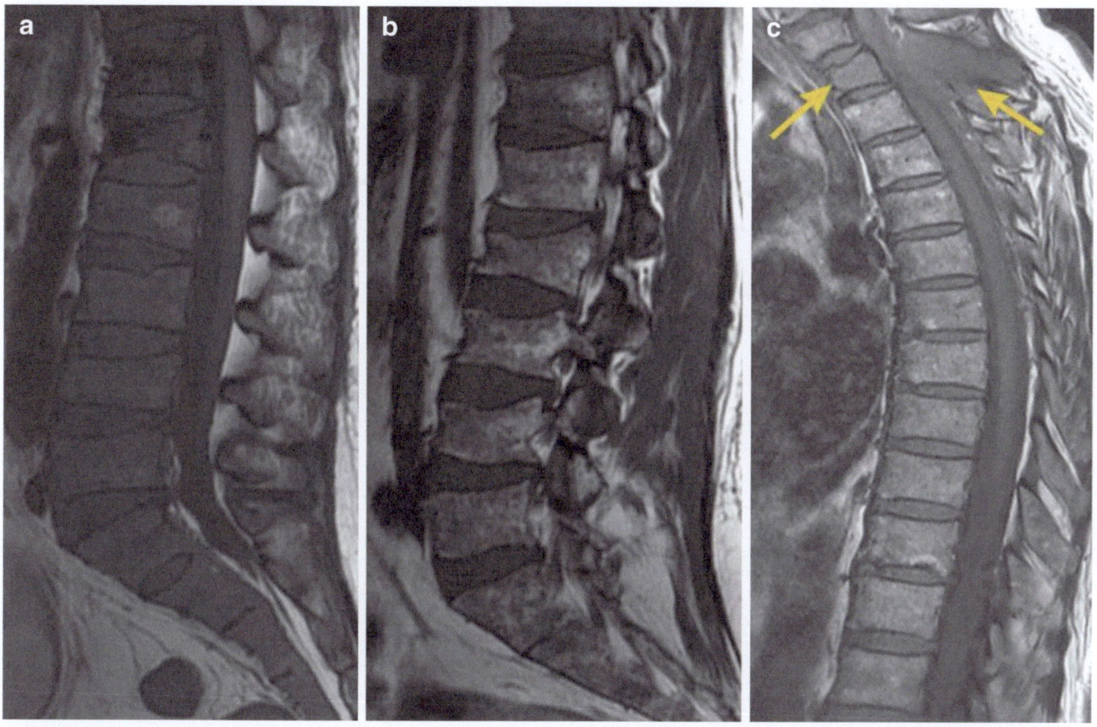

Fig. 10.14 Invasion patterns of multiple myeloma seen on MR T1-weighted images. The bone marrow signal intensity is uniformly decreased in the diffuse type (**a**), scattered small spots in the variegated type (**b**), and localized masses in the focal type (**c**, arrow)

Magnetic resonance imaging is very sensitive in depicting bone marrow lesions in leukemia patients. Although it usually invades the bone marrow chronically, it can also show various heterogeneous forms depending on cellularity (Fig. 10.15). Histological examination is essential for the diagnosis of leukemia or for its subclassification (Fig. 10.16). There have been studies on the role of bone marrow magnetic resonance imaging to alleviate the burden of having to perform bone marrow biopsy every time to evaluate the response to treatment. In cases where the treatment was responsive, the T1 relaxation time decreased and the fat ratio increased. However, there were also cases where there was no significant change in the T1 relaxation time of the bone marrow as the two processes of leukemia cell death and bone marrow regeneration occurred independently. It is expected that dynamic contrast-enhanced MR imaging or diffusion-weighted images, which utilize the fact that the speed or degree of contrast enhancement is affected by cellularity and vascular distribution, and the fact that lesions show high signal intensity and low apparent diffusion coefficient values, can provide information for evaluating the response after treatment [4, 52, 71, 72].

One of the side effects of leukemia, chloroma or granulocytic sarcoma, is a tumor composed of precursor cells of myelogenous white blood cells that has spread outside the bone marrow. It can invade any organ in the body, but it often occurs in the skin, bones, soft tissues of the head and neck, and lymph nodes, and when it spreads to the spinal canal, it compresses the spinal cord or nerves (Fig. 10.17). It is named for the blue color of the myeloperoxidase granules secreted by malignant myelogenous white blood cells [73, 74].

Like lymphoma, it can spread to soft tissues without clear bone destruction. On T1-weighted images, it shows low signal intensity similar to

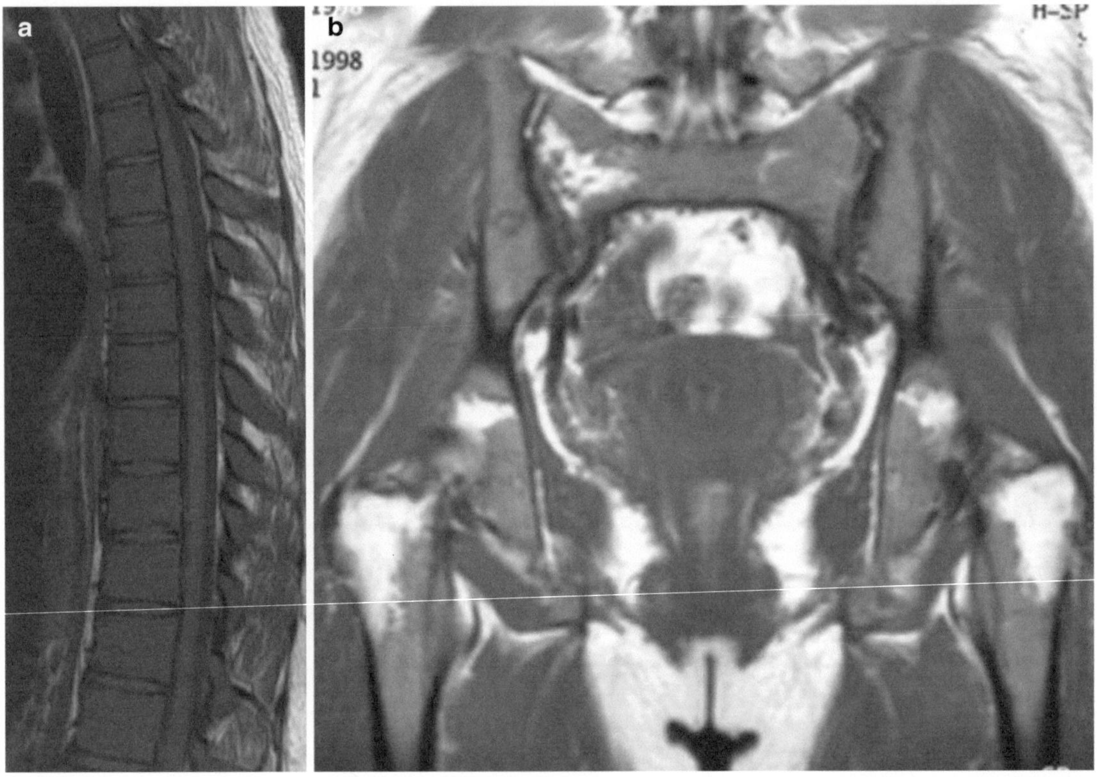

Fig. 10.15 MRI findings of acute myeloid leukemia. On T1-weighted images, the normal bone marrow signal intensity in adults is higher than that of the disc or muscle, but when immature white blood cells invade the bone marrow as in acute leukemia, the bone marrow signal intensity of the vertebral body (**a**) and pelvis (**b**) appears similar to or lower than the adjacent disc or muscle

muscle, moderate signal intensity on T2-weighted images, and homogeneous contrast enhancement, but in the case of large masses, necrosis may be accompanied in the center. There may also be a need to differentiate from complications such as osteomyelitis and hematoma, in which case chloroma can be differentiated by showing similar signal intensity to bone marrow on STIR images or contrast-enhanced images and having bone marrow invasion.

Differentiation from metastatic cancer, Langerhans cell histiocytosis, osteomyelitis, lymphoma, Ewing's sarcoma, etc. is necessary.

10.4.5 Lymphoma

Lymphoma is a condition where abnormal lymphocytes proliferate or deposit in lymphoid organs such as lymph nodes or spleen and can spread to the bones secondarily through the bloodstream or invade adjacent lymphomas that were in the lymph nodes or soft tissues often directly invade the bone, and it is not common for lymphomas to primarily occur in the bone. Hodgkin's lymphoma, non-Hodgkin's lymphoma, Burkitt's lymphoma, and mycosis fungoides are included in lymphomas, but they are generally classified as Hodgkin's lymphoma and non-Hodgkin's lymphoma. Non-Hodgkin's lymphoma is about three times more common than Hodgkin's lymphoma, but in the bone, non-Hodgkin's lymphoma accounts for the majority (94%). When a tumor is found in the bone and no lesions are found in the lymph nodes or internal organs within 6 months, it is diagnosed as primary bone lymphoma, which accounts for about 3–4% of primary malignant bone tumors.

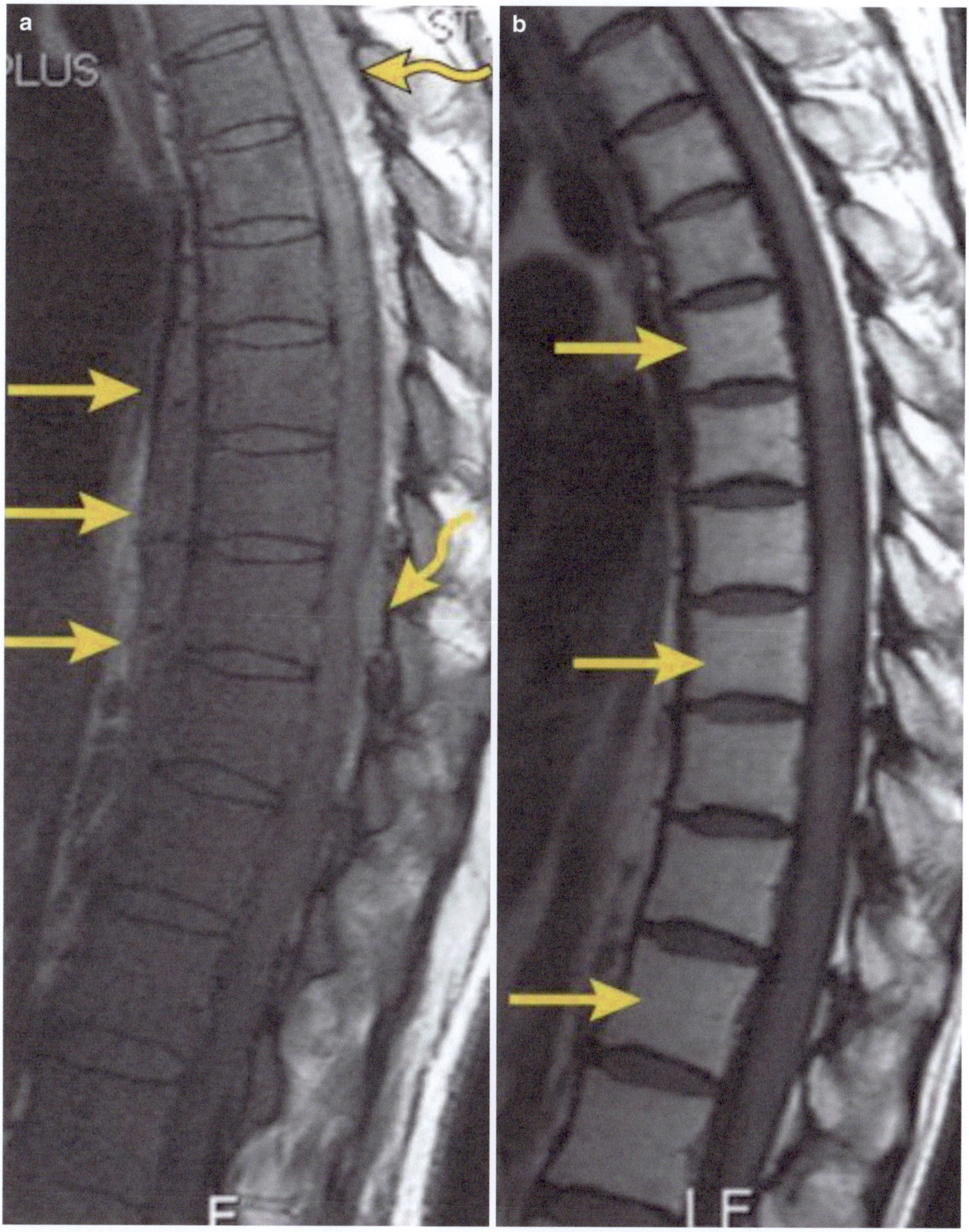

Fig. 10.16 Changes in MR signal intensity at the onset and after treatment of acute myeloid leukemia. (**a**) In the T1-enhanced image, the signal intensity of the thoracic vertebrae decreased to less than the adjacent disc, and there are tumors in the posterior epidural space (curved arrow) and the front of the vertebrae (arrow). (**b**) After chemotherapy and radiation therapy, the MR T1-enhanced image shows the disappearance of the anterior vertebrae and posterior epidural mass, and the conversion (arrow) to fatty bone marrow with a significant increase in the signal intensity of the bone marrow

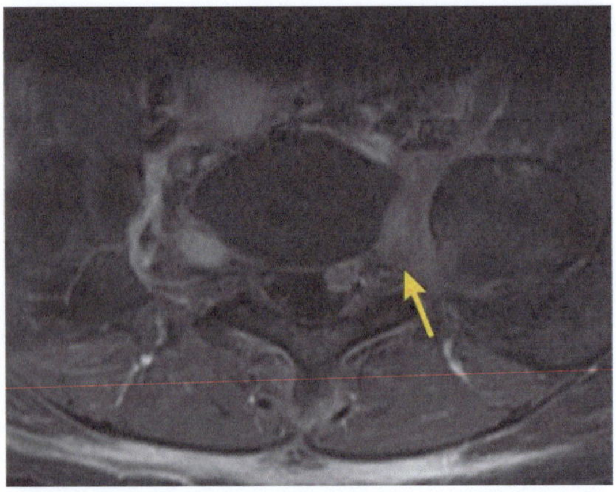

Fig. 10.17 Lumbar fat suppression contrast enhancement T1-enhanced image of chloroma. In patients with acute myeloid leukemia, the epidural mass is invading the L5-S1 nerve space (arrow)

The age distribution is 20–70 years old, with a peak incidence in the 50–60s, but it is also found in adolescents and young adults. The male to female ratio is about 1.8:1, and Hodgkin's lymphoma is more common in younger ages, 10–30 years old. There are usually no specific symptoms other than local pain, but sometimes it is discovered due to pathological fractures. It often invades the metaphysis and diaphysis of the long bones of the limbs such as the femur, tibia, humerus, pelvis, spine, skull, and scapula. In 10–40% of cases, multiple lesions are found in one bone or multiple bones at the same time. X-ray findings are characterized by moth-eaten or permeative bone destruction and a large soft tissue mass that is quite large compared to bone destruction. Sometimes, the tumor spreads to the soft tissue with almost no destruction of the cortical bone. Ivory bone appearance in the spine and flat bones is a finding that often appears in Hodgkin's lymphoma [75, 76]. Bone scans show moderate to strong uptake in most cases, and necrosis in the central area may also be seen. CT is useful for finding cortical bone destruction and periosteal reaction, but MRI is more sensitive for viewing the extent of the lesion and the accompanying soft tissue invasion. T1-weighted images (Fig. 10.18) show various findings of micronodular, punctate, or localized and usually show heterogeneous low signal intensity of bone marrow invasion, and T2-weighted images show heterogeneous various low, equal, and high signal intensities (Fig. 10.19) [77, 78]. The low signal intensity seen on T1- and T2-weighted images is thought to be due to fibrosis. After contrast administration, it usually shows heterogeneous strong enhancement. Especially, it shows a wrap-around appearance that creates a wide range of bone marrow invasion and adjacent soft tissue mass, even if the cortical bone destruction is not clear (Fig. 10.20). Soft tissue masses are found in about 75%, and they show a more homogeneous signal intensity than the lesions in the bone marrow, showing low signal intensity similar to adjacent muscles on T1-weighted images, high signal intensity on T2-weighted images, and micronodular enhancement. 18F-FDG-PET shows sensitive high FDG uptake in Hodgkin's lymphoma and high-grade non-Hodgkin's lymphoma [79]. In the case of small lymphocytic lymphoma or MALToma, FDG uptake is often low or not visible. Since the distribution pattern of lymphoma is heterogeneous, 18F-FDG-PET-CT, in addition to whole-body MRI, is useful in determining the staging with bone marrow biopsy and also in evaluating the response to treatment (Fig. 10.21).

Depending on the age of onset, it is necessary to differentiate from Ewing's sarcoma, osteomyelitis, metastatic neuroblastoma, Langerhans cell histiocytosis in children, osteosarcoma in adolescents, and metastatic cancer, fibrosarcoma, multiple myeloma, etc. in adults.

Primary Hodgkin's lymphoma in the bone is rare, accounting for about 6% of all lymphomas, but it invades the bone marrow in 5~32% of the disease progression and spreads hematogenously, resulting in poor prognosis. Bone marrow is invaded in 25~40% of Non-Hodgkin's lymphoma patients. Primary bone lymphoma corresponds to

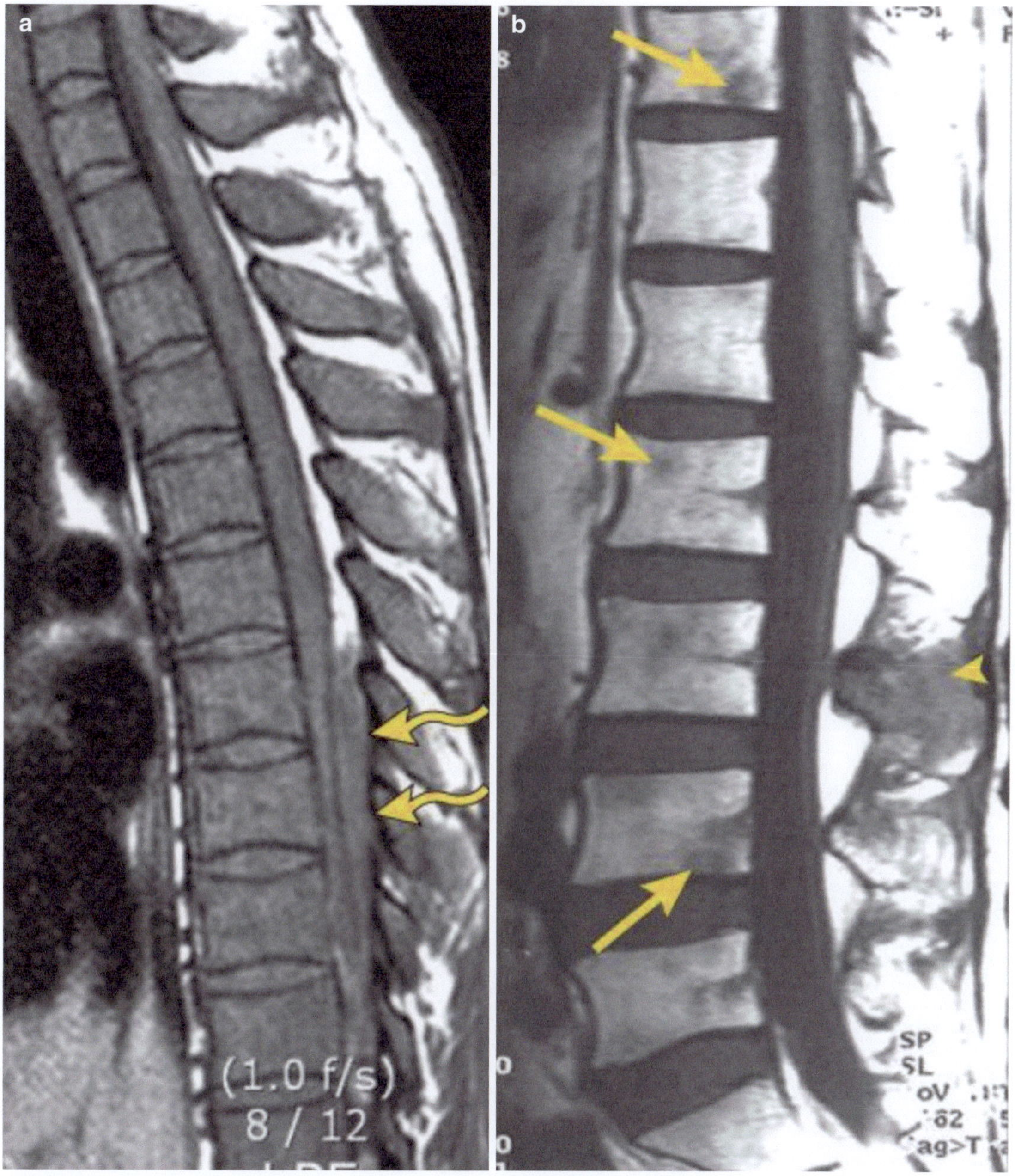

Fig. 10.18 MR T1 enhanced image of Non-Hodgkin's lymphoma. (**a**) Hypoplastic bone marrow invasion and posterior epidural mass (curved arrow) are visible. (**b**) There is localized bone destruction in the third lumbar spinous process (arrowhead) and a small tumor (arrow) with unclear boundaries in the vertebrae

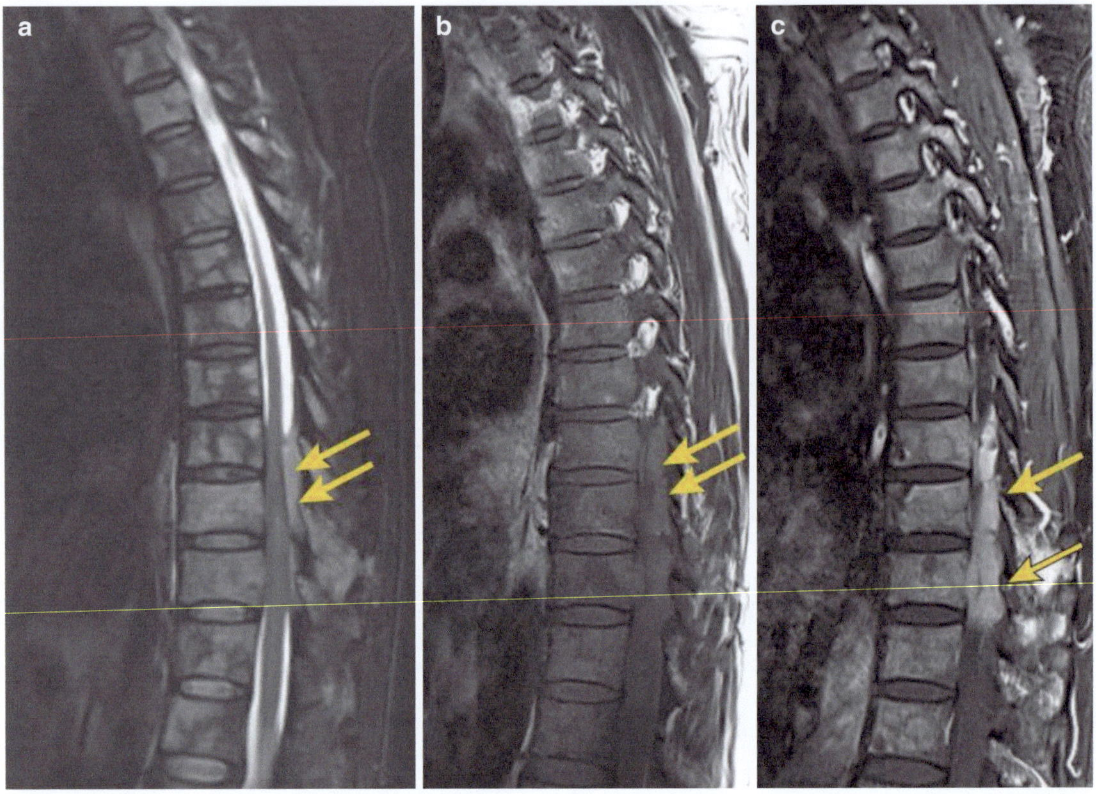

Fig. 10.19 A 56-year-old man, T cell lymphoma. (**a**) Fat saturation T2-enhanced image, (**b**) T1-enhanced image, (**c**) Fat saturation contrast enhancement T1-enhanced image shows a map-like heterogeneous bone marrow invasion. The spinal cord is compressed by the posterior epidural mass (arrow) located at T9~11

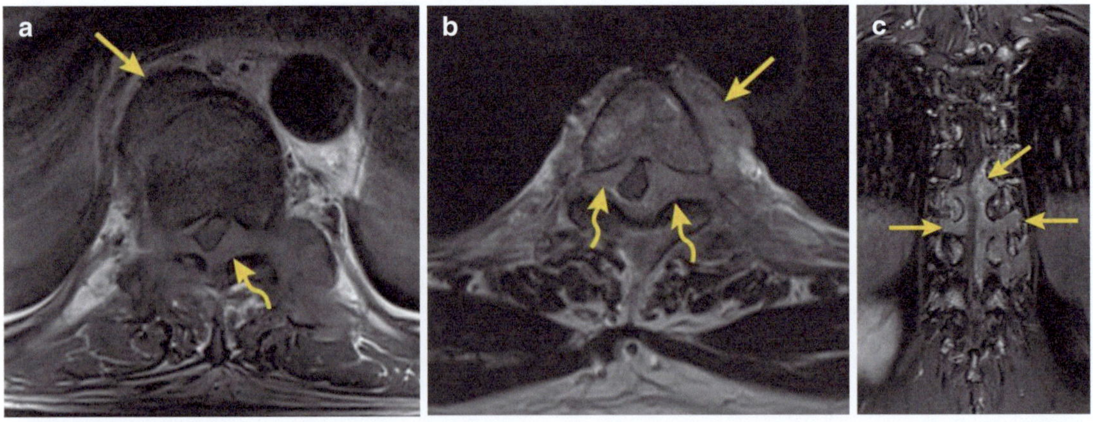

Fig. 10.20 MRI findings of lymphoma—wrap around. A large soft tissue tumor that seems to wrap around the bone while relatively preserving the cortical bone is seen around the vertebral body (arrow) and in the epidural space (curved arrow). This finding can also be seen in round cell tumors, such as Ewing's sarcoma or leukemia, in addition to lymphoma. [(**a**) T1-enhanced image, (**b**) T2-enhanced image, (**c**) Fat suppression contrast enhancement T1-enhanced image]

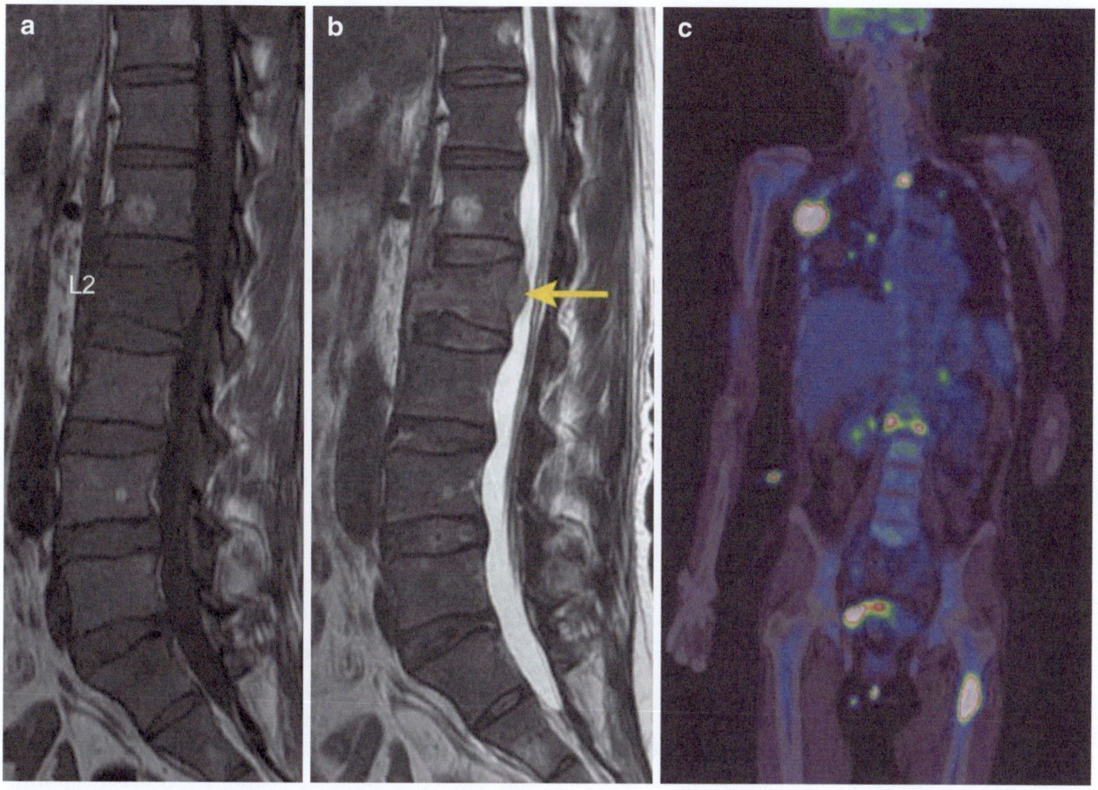

Fig. 10.21 The role of MRI and FDG-PET in staging lymphoma. In a 52-year-old female patient, hypoplastic bone marrow invasion, L2 compression fracture due to tumor, and anterior epidural mass (arrow) are seen in the T1-enhanced image (**a**) and T2-enhanced image (**b**). In FDG-PET (**c**), hypermetabolic foci are seen in the thoracic vertebrae, right third rib, and left femur in addition to L2

stage 1 in the Ann Arbor classification, but secondary bone invasion corresponds to stage 4, so it is very important to distinguish between primary and secondary lymphomas. The presence of bone marrow invasion is determined through a bone marrow biopsy, but since the bone marrow can be invaded unevenly, even if tissue is obtained from both iliac crests, lesions may not be found in about 20% of bone marrow biopsies. Therefore, bone marrow MR imaging is useful in evaluating the state of lymphoma bone marrow invasion and staging when performed in conjunction with tissue biopsy. If the treatment is responsive, the T1 relaxation time of the bone marrow is shortened, but if lymphoma invasion remains after treatment, fibrosis may occur in the bone marrow or in the case of reactive hypercellular marrow, the T1 relaxation time may be prolonged.

10.4.6 Myelofibrosis

Myelofibrosis refers to diseases that cause fibrosis in the bone marrow, where the fat cells and bone marrow cells of the bone marrow are replaced with reticulin and collagen, resulting in myeloid metaplasia in the spleen, liver, and lymph nodes.

Anemia and bleeding due to decreased platelets occur, the number of white blood cells is not constant, and erythroblasts or immature white blood cells may appear in the blood.

There are forms such as agnogenic myeloid metaplasia, where fibrosis occurs in the bone marrow as hepatosplenomegaly progresses without a preceding disease, and polycythemia vera or chronic granulocytic leukemia progresses to myelofibrosis. X-ray pictures show overall or localized osteosclerosis and cortical bone thinning. It shows bone hardening similar to that in metastatic prostate cancer, fluorosis, systemic mastocytosis, etc.

Characteristically, the signal intensity of the bone marrow is very low on T1- and T2-weighted images [80–82], and the signal intensity on STIR images varies depending on the degree of fibrosis rather than cellularity, and if fibrosis is not severe, the signal intensity increases (Fig. 10.22). If siderosis is deposited in the bone marrow due to transfusion, the signal intensity of the bone marrow can decrease on T1- and T2-weighted images. Extramedullary if hematopoiesis occurs, soft tissue masses form next to the liver and the vertebral body (Fig. 10.23). Extramedullary hematopoiesis often occurs at the seventh to twelfth thoracic levels and can be seen in congenital hemolytic anemia as well as in bone marrow fibrosis.

10.4.7 Bone Marrow Transplantation

Since the mid1950s, bone marrow transplantation has been performed as a curative treatment for various blood tumors, such as acute and chronic leukemia, lymphoma, multiple myeloma, aplastic anemia, and some solid cancers such as breast cancer, lung cancer, and testicular cancer.

The marrow to be transplanted is placed under various special stresses due to the pretreatment for transplantation and the transplantation itself. First, high-dose anticancer therapy and total body irradiation are performed as pretreatments to reduce the immune function of the recipient and to remove as many remaining cancer cells as possible and to prepare a space for the transplanted marrow to settle. Immediately after this, when the bone marrow cells are intravenously injected, the hematopoietic stem cells temporarily stay in the lungs or spleen and eventually find their place in the bone marrow cavity where engraftment occurs. About 3–4 weeks after transplantation, granulocytes appear in the peripheral blood. If high-dose chemotherapy or total body irradiation is performed as a pre-treatment for bone marrow transplantation, the signal intensity of the marrow decreases in MR T1-enhanced images due to increased water content caused by cell necrosis, edema, and bleeding in the bone marrow. In T2-enhanced images or STIR images, the signal intensity increases and T1 relaxation time also increases. Then, as the bone marrow edema disappears and the hematopoietic stem cells move into the bone marrow interstitium, cellularity increases. If engraftment is successful, the marrow appears as a low signal intensity in T1-enhanced images, and the signal intensity

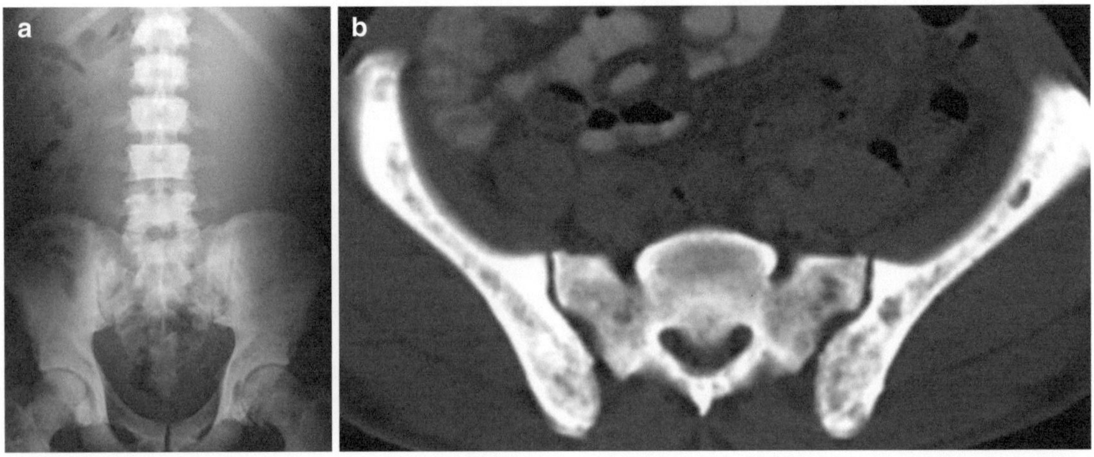

Fig. 10.22 Imaging findings of myelofibrosis. Increased bone density in the liver, lumbar spine, and pelvis is shown in the anterior abdominal X-ray (**a**) and pelvic CT (**b**). In the MR T1 (**c**), fat-saturated T2 (**d**) enhanced images, the signal intensity of the bone marrow is significantly reduced to a minimum

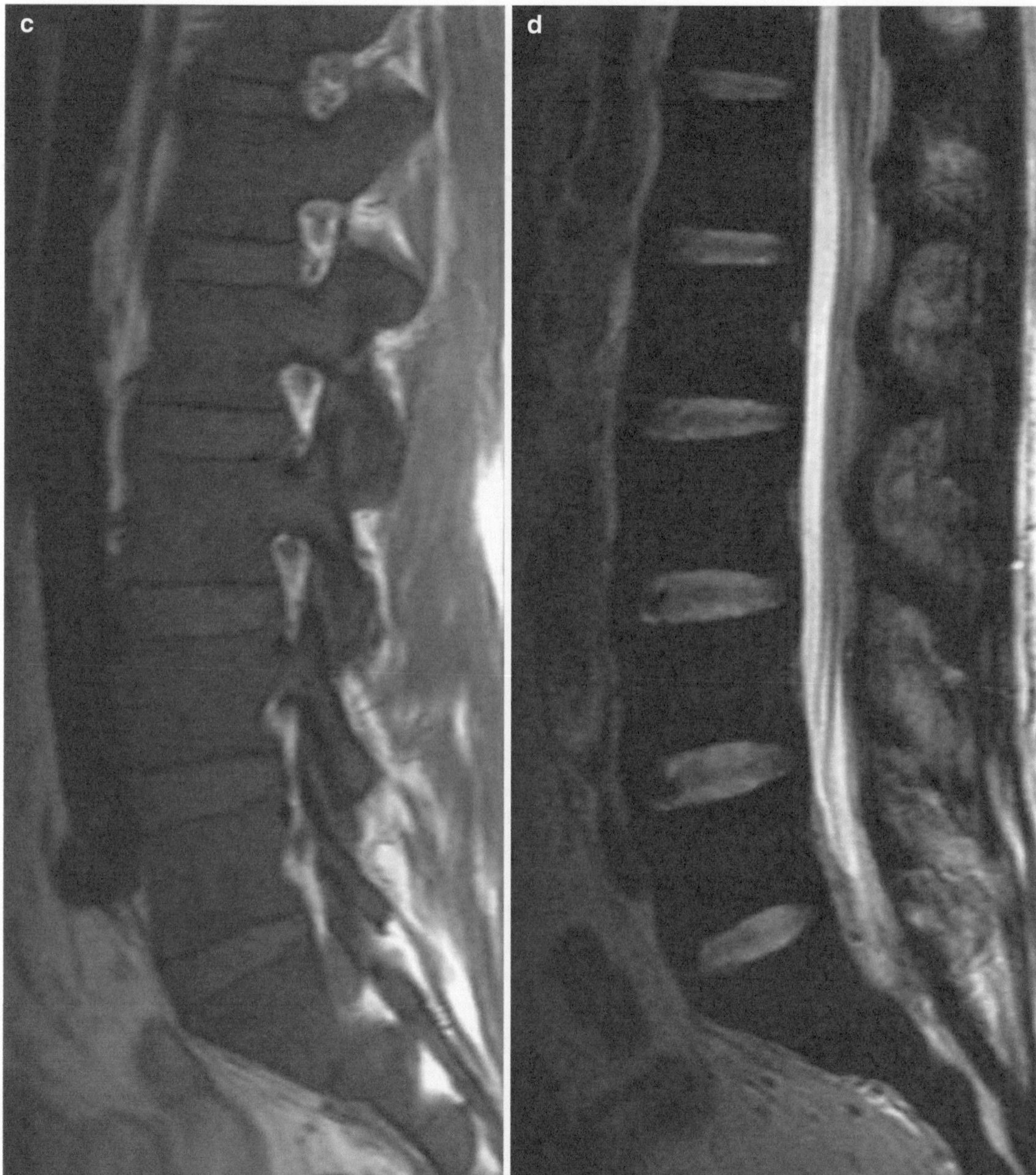

Fig. 10.22 (continued)

increases in water selective chemical shift images. On the other hand, if engraftment is delayed, fat cells remain undeposited and appear as a high signal intensity in T1-enhanced images and fat selective images.

After 6–8 weeks of transplantation, when the bone marrow is reorganized, partial fat deposition occurs in the bone marrow, and the signal intensity of the marrow appears heterogeneous due to the deposition of paramagnetic substances such as hemosiderin and fibrosis. It may be difficult to distinguish these low signal intensities seen in T1-enhanced images due to hematopoietic bone marrow from the recurrence of primary

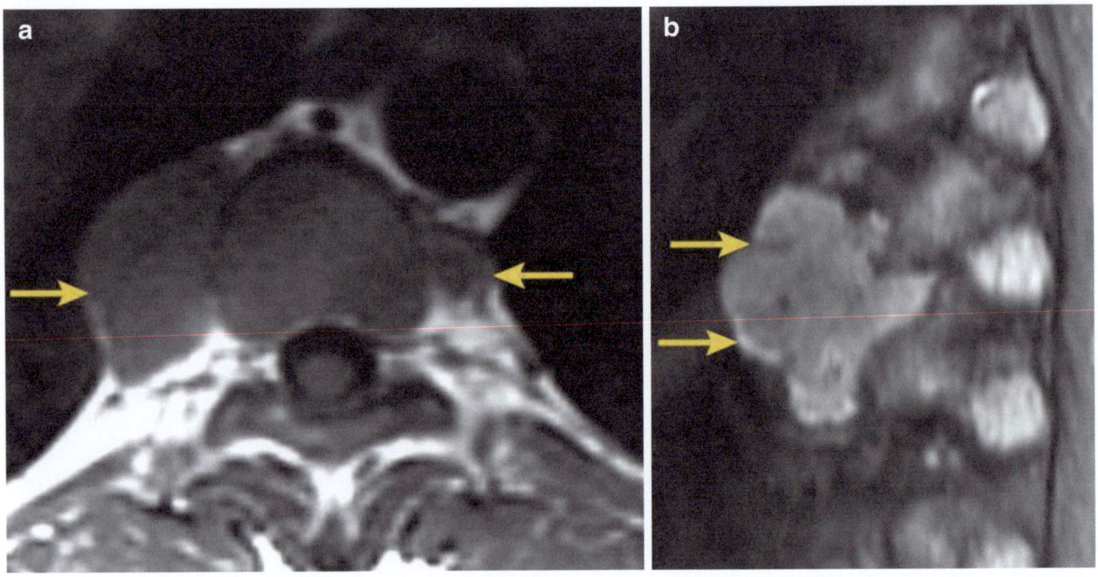

Fig. 10.23 Magnetic resonance imaging of extramedullary hematopoiesis. In the axial T1-enhanced image (**a**) and right parasagittal fat-suppressed T2-enhanced image (**b**), a soft tissue mass (arrow) is seen along the thoracic spine. The bone marrow has been fibrosed, and hematopoiesis has occurred in the liver, spleen, or next to the vertebral body

cancer, but it can be differentiated by the fact that the signal intensity does not increase much in STIR images. Also, because partial fat deposition occurs in the bone marrow, the signal intensity increases in T1-enhanced images compared to normal people, especially in the central part of the vertebral body, and T1 relaxation time decreases [83, 84]. Within 3 months after transplantation, the spinal marrow appears as a low signal intensity in the peripheral areas of the vertebral body, i.e., near the endplate, and as a high signal intensity in the central areas in T1-enhanced images. In STIR images, it shows a characteristic band-like signal intensity that reverses its signal intensity and gradually shows uniform signal intensity changes (Fig. 10.24).

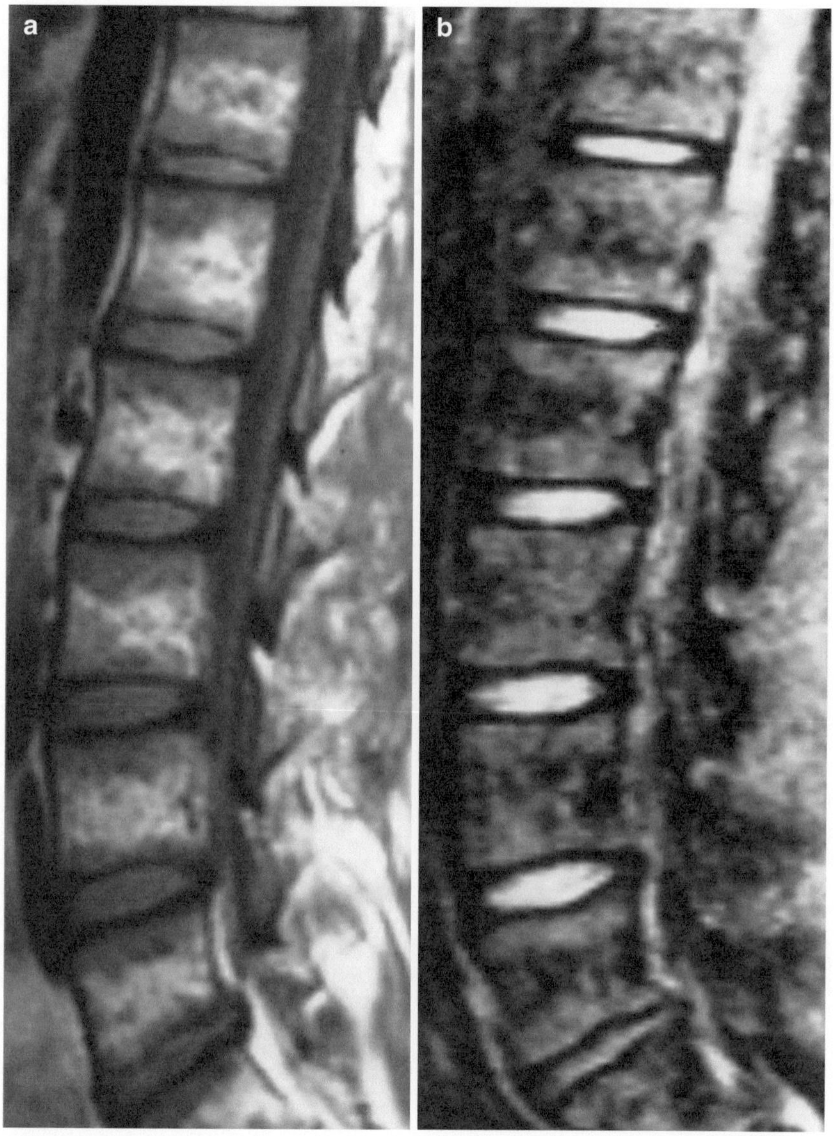

Fig. 10.24 Magnetic resonance imaging after bone marrow transplantation. After high-dose antihypertensive therapy or total body irradiation, hematopoietic stem cells are injected, and the hematopoietic cells are first attached near the endplate. In the T1-enhanced image (**a**), a horizontal band of low signal intensity is seen, and high signal intensity remains in the center for a long time, while in the STIR image (**b**), the signal intensity appears reversed

Bibliography

1. Tardivon AA, Vanel D, Munck JN, Boso J. Magnetic resonance imaging of bone marrow in lymphoma and leukemia. Leuk Lymphoma. 1997;25:55–68.
2. Vogler JB, Murphy WA. Bone marrow imaging. Radiology. 1988;168:679–93.
3. Steiner RM, Mitchell DG, Rao VM, Schweitzer. Magnetic resonance imaging of diffuse bone marrow disease. Radiol Clin North Am. 1993;31:383–409.
4. Olson DO, Shields AF, Scheurich CJ, Porter BA, Moss AA. Magnetic resonance imaging of the bone marrow in patients with leukemia, aplastic anemia and lymphoma. Investig Radiol. 1986;21:540–6.
5. McKinstry CS, Steiner RE, Young AT, Jones L, Swirsky D, Aber V. Bone marrow in leukemia and aplastic anemia: MRI imaging before, during, and after treatment. Radiology. 1987;162:701–7.
6. Hoane BR, Shields AF, Porter BA, Shulman HM. Detection of lymphomatous bone marrow involvement with magnetic resonance imaging. Blood. 1991;78:728–38.
7. Hartsock RJ, Smith EB, Petty CS. Normal variants with aging of the amounts of hematopoietic tissue in bone marrow from the outer iliac crest. Am J Clin Pathol. 1965;43:326–31.
8. Westerman MP. Bone marrow needle biopsy: an evaluation and critique. Semin Hematol. 1981;18:293–300.
9. Brookes M. Blood supply of long bones. Br Med J. 1963;2:1064–5.
10. Marenzana M, Timothy R. Arnett the key role of the blood supply to bone. Bone Research. 2013;1:203–15.
11. Brookes M, Harrison RG. The vascularization of the rabbit femur and tibio-fibula. J Anat. 1957;91:61–72.
12. Naveiras O, Nardi V, Wenzel PL, Hauschka PV, Fahey F, Daley GQ. Bone-marrow adipocytes as negative regulators of the haematopoietic microenvironment. Nature. 2009;460:259–63.
13. Zhou BO, Yu H, Yue R, et al. Bone marrow adipocytes promote the regeneration of stem cells and haematopoiesis by secreting SCF. Nat Cell Biol. 2017;19:891–903.
14. Moore SG, Dawson KL. Red and yellow marrow in the femur: age related changes in appearance at MR imaging. Radiology. 1990;175:219–23.
15. Ricci C, Cova M, Kang YS, et al. Normal age related patterns of cellular and fatty bone marrow distribution in the axial skeleton: MR imaging study. Radiology. 1990;177:83–8.
16. Vande Berg BC, Malghem J, Lecouvet FE, Maldague B. Normal bone marrow: dynamic aspects in magnetic resonance imaging. J Radiol. 2001;82:127–35.
17. Hajek PC, Baker LL, Goobar JE, et al. Focal fat deposition in axial bone marrow: MR characteristics. Radiology. 1987;162:245–9.
18. Małkiewicz A, Dziedzic M. Bone marrow reconversion – imaging of physiological changes in bone marrow. Pol J Radiol. 2012;77:45–50.
19. Tall MA, Thompson AK, Vertinsky T, Palka PS. MR imaging of the spinal bone marrow. Magn Reson Imaging Clin N Am. 2007;15:175–98.
20. Vande Berg BC, Malghem J, Lecouvet FE, Maldague B. Magnetic resonance imaging of the normal bone marrow. Skeletal Radiol. 1998;27:471–83.
21. Vande Berg BC, Lecouvet FE, Michaux L, Ferrant A, Maldague B, Malghem J. Magnetic resonance imaging of the bone marrow in hematological malignancies. Eur Radiol. 1998;8:1335–44.
22. Carroll KW, Feller JF, Tirman PF. Useful internal standards for distinguishing infiltrative marrow pathology from hematopoietic marrow at MRI. J Magn Reson Imaging. 1997;7:394–8.
23. Shah LM, Hanrahan CJ. MRI of spinal bone marrow: part I, techniques and normal age-related appearances. AJR Am J Roentgenol. 2011;197:1298–308.
24. Poulton TB, Murphy WD, Duerk JL, et al. Bone marrow reconversion in adults who are smokers: MR findings. AJR. 1993;161:1217–21.
25. Shellock FG, Morris E, Deutsch AL, Mink JH, Kerr R, Boden SD. Hematopoietic bone marrow hyperplasia: high prevalence on MR images of the knee in asymptomatic marathon runners. AJR. 1992;158:335–8.
26. Levine CD, Schweitzer ME, Ehrlich SM. Pelvic marrow in adults. Skeletal Radiol. 1994;23:343–7.
27. Ruzal-Shapiro C, Berdon WE, Cohen MD, Abramson SJ. MR imaging of diffuse bone marrow replacement in pediatric patients with cancer. Radiology. 1991;181:587–9.
28. Chan BY, Gill KG, Rebsamen SL, Nguyen JC. MR imaging of pediatric bone marrow. Radiographics. 2016;36:1911–30.
29. Cohen MD, Klatte EC, Baehner R, et al. Magnetic resonance imaging of bone marrow disease in children. Radiology. 1984;151(3):715–8.
30. Mirowitz SA, Apicella R, Reinus WR, Hammerman AM. MR imaging of bone marrow lesions: relative conspicuousness on T1-weighted, fat-suppressed T2-weighted and STIR images. AJR. 1994;162:215–21.
31. Guckel F, Brix G, Semmler W, et al. Systemic bone marrow disorders: characterization with proton chemical shift imaging. J Comput Assit Tomogr. 1990;14:954–9.
32. Rosen BR, Fleming DM, Kushner DC, et al. Hematologic bone marrow disorders: quantitative chemical shift MR imaging. Radiology. 1988;169:799–804.
33. Kellenberger CJ, Epelman M, Miller SF, Babyn PS. Fast STIR whole-body MR imaging in children. Radiographics. 2004;24:1317–30.
34. Disler DG, McCauley TR, Ratner LM, Kesack CD, Cooper JA. In phase and out-of-phase MR imaging of bone marrow: prediction of neoplasia based on the detection of coexistent fat and water. AJR. 1997;169:1439–47.
35. Erly WK, Oh ES, Outwater EK. The utility of in-phase/opposed phase imaging in differentiating malignancy

from acute benign compression fractures of the spine. AJNR Am J Neuroradiol. 2006;27:1183–8.
36. Ragab Y, Emad Y, Gheita T, et al. Differentiation of osteoporotic and neoplastic vertebral fractures by chemical shift {in-phase and out-of phase} MR imaging. Eur J Radiol. 2009;72:125–33.
37. Swartz PG, Roberts CC. Radiological reasoning: bone marrow changes on MRI. AJR. 2009;193(3 suppl):S1–S4; quiz, S5–S9.
38. Amano Y, Hayashi H, Kumazaki T. Gd-DTPA enhanced MRI of reactive hematopoietic regions in marrow. J Comput Assist Tomogr. 1994;18:214–7.
39. Saifuddin A, Bann K, Ridgway JP, Butt WP. Bone marrow blood supply in gadolinium-enhanced magnetic resonance imaging. Skeletal Radiol. 1994;23:455–7.
40. Baur A, Stäbler A, Bartl R, Lamerz R, Scheidler J, Reiser M. MRI gadolinium enhancement of bone marrow: age-related changes in normals and in diffuse neoplastic infiltration. Skeletal Radiol. 1997;26:414–8.
41. Weissleder R, Elizondo G, Wittenberg J, Rabito CA, Bengele HH, Josephson L. Ultrasmall superparamagnetic iron oxide: characterization of a new class of contrast agents for MR imaging. Radiology. 1990;175:489–93.
42. Seneterre E, Weissleder R, Jaramillo D, et al. Bone marrow: ultrasmall superparamagnetic ironoxide for MR imaging. Radiology. 1991;179:529–33.
43. Ahlawat S, Khandheria P, Subhawong TK, Fayad LM. Differentiation of benign and malignant skeletal lesions with quantitative diffusion weighted MRI at 3T. Eur J Radiol. 2015;84(6):1091–7.
44. Subhawong TK, Jacobs MA, Fayad LM. Diffusion-weighted MR imaging for characterizing musculoskeletal lesions. Radiographics. 2014;34(5):1163–77.
45. Herrmann J, Krstin N, Schoennagel BP, et al. Age-related distribution of vertebral bone-marrow diffusivity. Eur J Radiol. 2012;81(12):4046–9.
46. Chavhan GB, Alsabban Z, Babyn PS. Diffusion-weighted imaging in pediatric body MR imaging: principles, technique, and emerging applications. Radiographics. 2014;34(3):E73–88.
47. Atkin KL, Ditchfield MR. The role of whole-body MRI in pediatric oncology. J Pediatr Hematol Oncol. 2014;36(5):342–52.
48. Darge K, Jaramillo D, Siegel MJ. Whole-body MRI in children: current status and future applications. Eur J Radiol. 2008;68(2):289–98.
49. Schmidt GP, Reiser MF, Baur-Melnyk A. Whole-body imaging of the musculoskeletal system: the value of MR imaging. Skeletal Radiol. 2007;36:1109–19.
50. Padhani AR, Koh DM, Collins DJ. Whole-body diffusion-weighted MR imaging in cancer: current status and research directions. Radiology. 2011;261(3):700–18.
51. Kumar J, Seith A, Kumar A, et al. Whole-body MR imaging with the use of parallel imaging for detection of skeletal metastases in pediatric patients with small-cell neoplasms: comparison with skeletal scintigraphy and FDG PET/CT. Pediatr Radiol. 2008;38(9):953–62.
52. Kugel H, Jung C, Schulte O, Heindel W. Age- and sex-specific differences in the 1H-spectrum of vertebral bone marrow. J Magn Reson Imaging. 2001;13:263–8.
53. Rosen BR, Fileming DM, Kushner DG, et al. Hematologic bone marrow disorders: quantitative chemical shift MR imaging. Radiology. 1988;169:799.
54. Vande Berg BC, Michaux L, Scheiff JM, et al. Sequential quantitative MR analysis of bone marrow: differences during treatment of lymphoid versus myeloid leukemia. Radiology. 1996;201:519–23.
55. Vanel D, Dromain C, Tardivon A. MRI of bone marrow disorders. Eur Radiol. 2000;10:224–9.
56. Ishijima H, Ishizaka H, Horikoshi H, Sakurai M. Water fraction of lumbar vertebral bone marrow estimated from chemical shift misregistration on MR imaging: normal variations with age and sex. AJR. 1996;167:355–8.
57. Murphy DT, Moynagh MR, Eustace SJ, Kavanagh EC. Bone marrow. Magn Reson Imaging Clin N Am. 2010;18:727–35.
58. Griffith JF, Yeung DK, Antonio GE, et al. Vertebral marrow fat content and diffusion and perfusion indexes in women with varying bone density: MR evaluation. Radiology. 2006;241:831–8.
59. Kricun ME. Red-yellow marrow conversion: its effect on the location of some solitary bone lesions. Skeletal Radiol. 1985;14:10–9.
60. Fletcher BD, Wall JE, Hanna SL. Effect of hematopoietic growth factors on MR images of bone marrow in children undergoing chemotherapy. Radiology. 1993;189:745–51.
61. Poulton TB, Murphey WD, Duerk JL, Chapek CC, Feiglin DH. Bone marrow reconversion in adults who are smokers: MR imaging findings. AJR. 1993;161:1217–21.
62. Rao VM, Fishman M, Mitchell DG, et al. Painful sickle cell crisis: bone marrow pattern observed with MR imaging. Radiology. 1986;161:211–5.
63. Kaplan PA, Asleson RJ, Klassen LW, Duggan MJ. Bone marrow pattern in aplastic anemia: observations with 1.5 T MR imaging. Radiology. 1987;164:441–4.
64. Park JM, Lim GY, Kim EN, et al. Evaluation of severity in aplastic anemia by MR imaging. J Korean Radiol Soc. 1999;40:347–54.
65. Stevens SK, Morre SG, Kaplan ID. Early and late bone marrow changes after irradiation. AJR. 1990;154:745–50.
66. Winterbottom AP, Shaw AS. Imaging patients with myeloma. Clin Radiol. 2009;64:1–11.
67. Baur-Melnyk A, Buhmann S, Durr HR, Reiser M. Role of MRI for the diagnosis and prognosis of multiple myeloma. Eur J Radiol. 2005;55:56–63.
68. Moulopoulos LA, Dimopoulos MA, Alexanian R, Leeds NE, Libshits HI. Multiple myeloma:

MR patterns of response to treatment. Radiology. 1994;193:441–6.
69. Messiou C, Giles S, Collins DJ, et al. Assessing response of myeloma bone disease with diffusion-weighted MRI. Br J Radiol. 2012;85:e1198–203.
70. Dutoit JC, Vanderkerken MA, Verstraete KL. Value of whole body MRI and dynamic contrast enhanced MRI in the diagnosis, follow-up and evaluation of disease activity and extent in multiple myeloma. Eur J Radiol. 2013;82:1444–52.
71. Hanrahan CJ, Christensen CR, Crim JR. Current concepts in the evaluation of multiple myeloma with MR imaging and FDG PET/CT. Radiographics. 2010;30:127–42.
72. Lutje S, de Rooy JW, Croockewit S, Koedam E, Oyen WJ, Raymakers RA. Role of radiography, MRI and FDG-PET/CT in diagnosing, staging and therapeutical evaluation of patients with multiple myeloma. Ann Hematol. 2009;88:1161–8.
73. Shih TTF. Angiogenesis in hematological malignancy – evaluated by dynamic contrast-enhanced MRI. J Cancer Res Pract. 2016;3:97–103.
74. Cao W, Liang C, Chen Y, Wang C, Zhao C, Sun L. Role of diffusion-weighted imaging for detecting bone marrow infiltration in skull in children with acute lymphoblastic leukemia. Diagn Interv Radiol. 2016;22:580–6.
75. Neiman RS, Barcos M, Berad C, et al. Granulocytic sarcoma: a clinicopathologic study of 61 biopsied cases. Cancer. 1981;48:1426–37.
76. Seok JH, Park JM, Kim SK, Choi JE, Kim CC. Granulocytic sarcoma of the spine: MRI and clinical review. AJR Am J Roentgenol. 2010;194:485–9.
77. O'Neill J, Finlay K, Jurriaans E, Friedman L. Radiological manifestations of skeletal lymphoma. Curr Probl Diagn Radiol. 2009;38:228–36.
78. Ostrowski ML, Unni KK, Banks PM, et al. Malignant lymphoma of bone. Cancer. 1986;58:2646–4.
79. Mulligan ME, McRae GA, Murphey MD. Imaging features of primary lymphoma of bone. AJR Am J Roentgenol. 1999;173:1691–7.
80. Hermann G, Klein MJ, Abdelwahab IF, Kenan S. MRI appearance of primary non-Hodgkin's lymphoma of bone. Skeletal Radiol. 1997;26:629–32.
81. Wu LM, Chen FY, Jiang XX, Gu HY, Yin Y, Xu JR. 18F-FDG PET, combined FDG-PET/CT and MRI for evaluation of bone marrow infiltration in staging of lymphoma: a systematic review and meta-analysis. Eur J Radiol. 2012 Feb;81(2):303–11.
82. Charron D, Rober L, Couty MC, Binet J. Biochemical and histological analysis of bone marrow collagen in myelofibrosis. Br J Haematol. 1979;41:151–68.
83. Amano Y, Onda M, Amano M, Kumazaki T. Magnetic resonance imaging of myelofibrosis. STIR and gadolinium enhanced MR images. Clin Imaging. 1997;21:264–8.
84. Chun HJ, Park JM, Baek JH, et al. MR features of myelofibrosis: correlation with bone marrow biopsy findings. J Korean Radiol Soc. 1997;36:523–8.

Spinal and Spinal Cord Tumors 11

Eugene Lee

11.1 Diagnostic Methods for Spinal and Spinal Cord Tumors

11.1.1 Compartmental Approach to Tumors

The first step in the compartmental approach to spinal and spinal cord tumors is to determine whether the lesion is osseous (within the bone), extradural non-osseous (outside the dura), intradural extramedullary (within the dura, outside the spinal cord), or intramedullary (within the spinal cord) (Fig. 11.1). This approach is because the possible differential diagnosis and surgical approach for the tumor are influenced by the compartment location of the tumor. In most cases, it is not difficult to determine the compartment where these tumors are located on MRI, but in some cases, the boundaries are ambiguous, making diagnosis difficult. If the judgment of the compartment changes, the differential diagnosis itself changes. The following are radiological clues that can help localize the compartment in which the tumor is located for diagnosis.

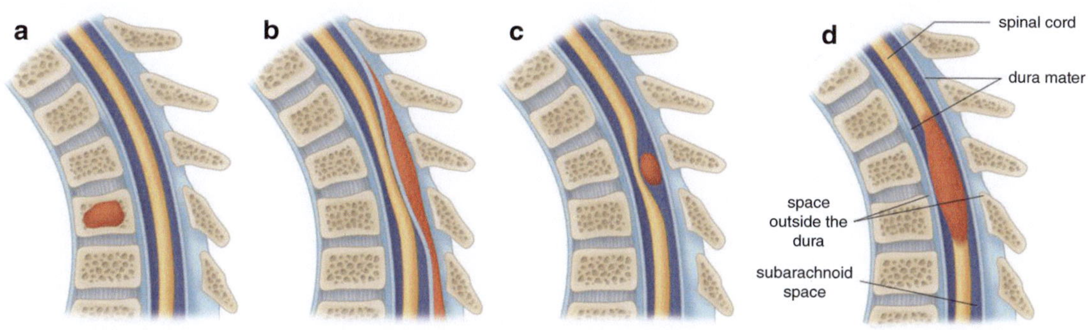

Fig. 11.1 Compartmental diagnostic approach to spinal tumors. Tumors occurring in the spine and spinal cord are divided into (**a**) osseous tumor, (**b**) extradural non-osseous tumor, (**c**) intradural extramedullary tumor, (**d**) intramedullary tumor according to their anatomical location, and such classification is most important in the differential diagnosis of the tumor

E. Lee (✉)
Department of Radiology, Seoul National University Bundang Hospital, Seongnam-si, Republic of Korea

© The Author(s), under exclusive license to Springer Nature Singapore Pte Ltd. 2025

H. S. Kang, J. W. Lee (eds.), *Spinal Imaging*, https://doi.org/10.1007/978-981-95-1386-4_11

11.1.2 Extradural vs. Intradural Tumor

The main findings suggesting a spinal extradural non-osseous tumor are external compression of the dural sac and tumor extension through the neural foramen. However, in severe cases of such tumor compression, it can be difficult to distinguish on MRI whether these findings are due to severe compression by an extradural tumor or compression by an intradural tumor. In such cases, the clue to distinguish between the two lies in the shape of the subarachnoid space at the edge of the tumor. If compression occurs due to an extradural tumor, the subarachnoid space between the dura and the spinal cord is lost at the edge of the tumor due to compression, whereas in the case of an intradural tumor, the dura is pushed out by the internal tumor, compressing the spinal cord and widening the subarachnoid space at the edge of the tumor (Fig. 11.2). However, if the size of the intradural extramedullary tumor is large and the spinal cord compression is very severe and the cerebrospinal fluid (CSF) is hardly visible, such differentiation can be difficult, and this also applies to the differentiation from the intramedullary tumor below (Fig. 11.3).

11.1.3 Intradural Extramedullary vs. Intramedullary Tumor

An important clue in distinguishing between intradural extramedullary tumors and intramedullary tumors is the outer contour of the spinal cord at the tumor boundary. In the case of an intradural extramedullary tumor, the outer contour of the spinal cord at the point of contact with the tumor is compressed by the tumor and sinks in, thereby widening the subarachnoid space. On the other hand, in the case of an intramedullary tumor, the outer contour of the spinal cord protrudes convexly due to the internal tumor, thereby narrowing the subarachnoid space. Sometimes, intramedullary tumors that grow protruding outward can have a similar shape to intradural extramedullary tumors, making diagnosis difficult, especially when they occur in the lower thoracic

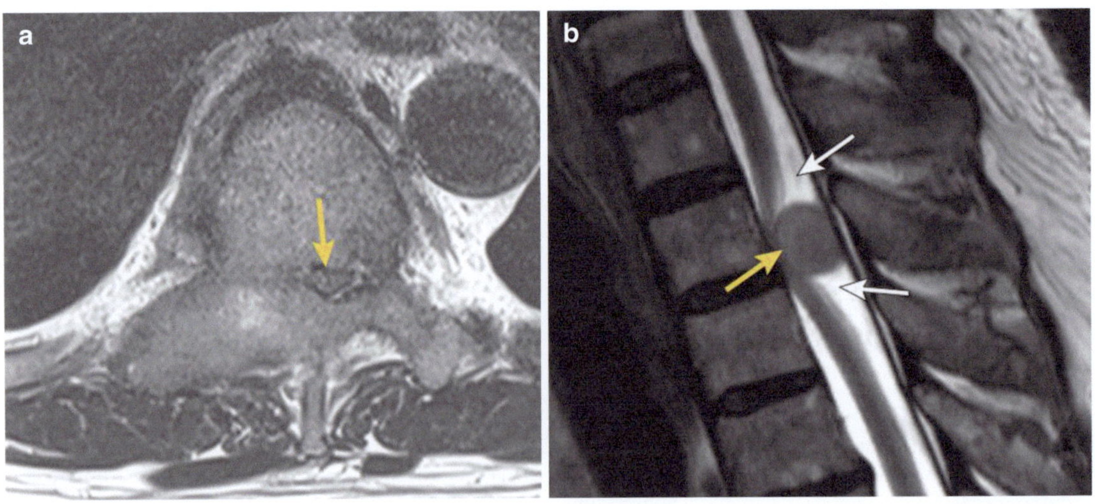

Fig. 11.2 Comparison of extradural tumor and intradural tumor. (**a**) Example of metastasis that occurred in a 59-year-old male patient. The metastatic tumor that invaded the spine is expanding into the epidural space, causing severe spinal cord compression in the extradural space (arrow). Due to this compression, CSF is not visible in the subarachnoid space. (**b**) Example of a meningioma that occurred in a 69-year-old male patient (yellow arrow). The tumor is located in the intradural extramedullary space and is compressing the spinal cord at the T2 location, displacing it forward. In the case of an intradural extramedullary tumor, the subarachnoid space can be seen expanding at the edge of the tumor (white arrow)

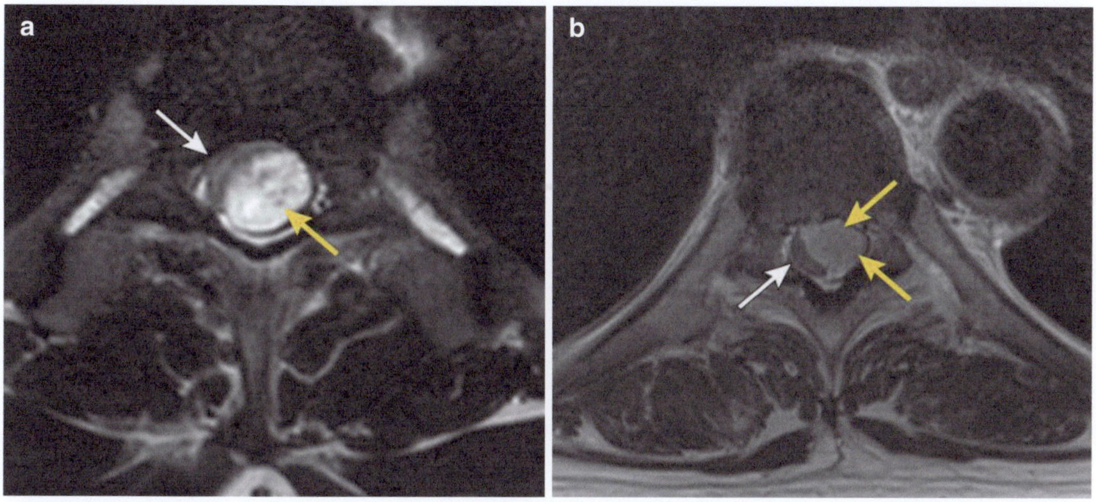

Fig. 11.3 Spinal cord compression and loss of CSF space due to intradural extramedullary tumor. (**a**) Example of a schwannoma (yellow arrow) that occurred at the T2/3 location in a 39-year-old male patient. (**b**) Example of a meningioma (yellow arrow) that occurred at the T9 location in a 66-year-old female patient. Both cases show severe spinal cord compression (white arrow) and loss of CSF space. In case (**a**), the T2 signal intensity of the spinal cord is increased, indicating the occurrence of compressive myelopathy

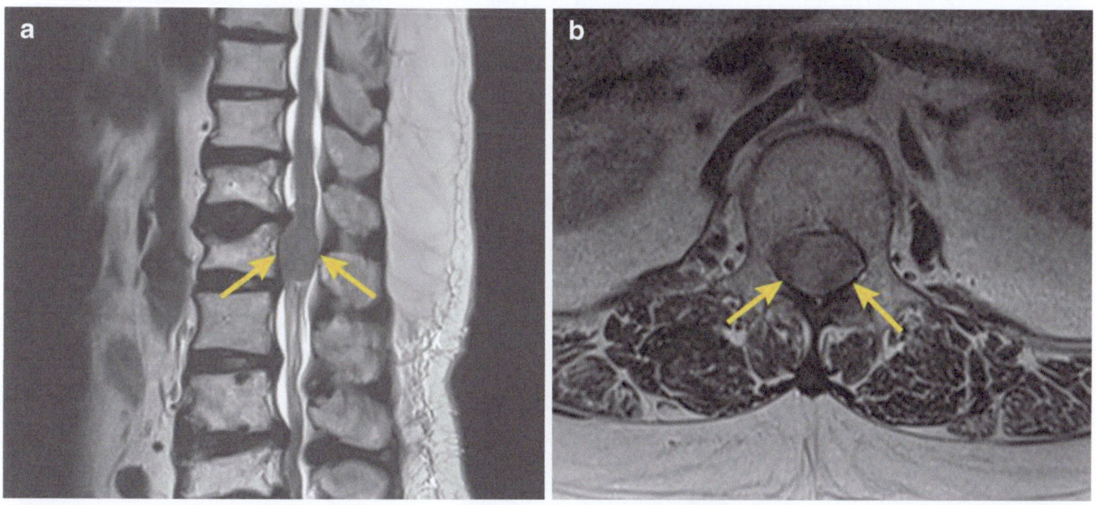

Fig. 11.4 There is a tumor protruding into the intradural space at the conus medullaris. In the MR T2-weighted sagittal (**a**) and axial (**b**) images, the lesion has unclear boundaries with the spinal cord, making it difficult to distinguish between an intradural extramedullary tumor and an intramedullary tumor. The patient is a 72-year-old woman who was confirmed to have an intradural extramedullary meningioma after surgery

spine and conus medullaris (Fig. 11.4). In such cases, MR axial images should be carefully examined. If the image can show that part of the intramedullary tumor is continuous with the spinal cord, it can be concluded that the tumor originates from the spinal cord, but it is often difficult.

11.1.4 Pathological Approach

For an accurate diagnosis of spinal and spinal cord tumors, it is necessary to understand pathologically how the components of the tumor appear in the image, which is also an essential element for a reasonable differential diagnosis.

Through a pathological approach, the differential diagnosis can be reduced and a more likely diagnosis can be made with a compartmental diagnosis.

11.1.4.1 Fatty Component

First, if the fatty component inside the tumor is clear in the image, the types of differential diagnoses can be limited. The fat component shows high signal intensity in both MR T1 enhanced images and T2 enhanced images, and low signal intensity in fat-suppressed MR techniques. The most common tumor containing a fat component is a hemangioma, and if there is a tumor containing a fatty component within the vertebral body, it is the most likely diagnosis (Fig. 11.5). On the other hand, what should be noted is that unlike osseous hemangiomas, most hemangiomas occurring in the epidural space do not show the signal intensity of fat. If a tumor containing fat is seen in the epidural space, the most likely diagnosis is angiolipoma. On the other hand, the most common tumor containing fat that occurs in the paravertebral muscle is lipoma or liposarcoma.

11.1.4.2 Red Marrow Component

Local or widespread red marrow hyperplasia can appear similar to the imaging findings of bone metastasis. Red marrow hyperplasia appears as intermediate signal intensity on MR T1 enhanced images, and mild enhancement appears in this area. The MR T1 signal intensity of this red marrow is similar to or slightly brighter than the signal intensity of the disc, which is a differential point from other malignant tumor diseases (Fig. 11.6). A similar signal intensity can be seen in multiple myeloma, but in the case of multiple myeloma, it often shows much stronger enhancement and the MR T1 signal intensity is often lower.

11.1.4.3 Vascular Component

The vascular component inside the tumor shows strong enhancement as seen in the venous structure in MRI. In most cases, this vascular component shows high signal intensity on MR T2 enhanced images, but it can show low signal intensity in areas where there is bleeding inside the tumor. Common vascular tumors originating

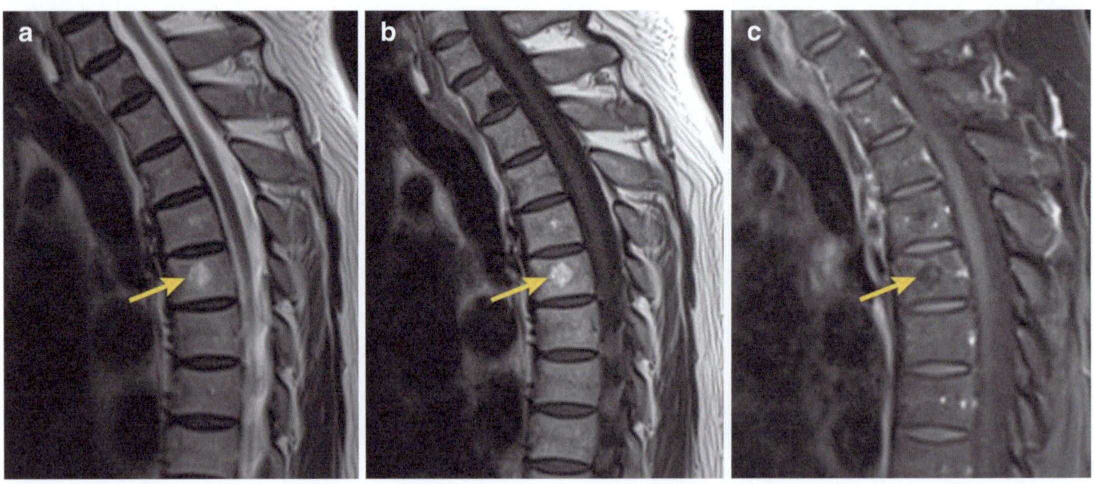

Fig. 11.5 Example of a hemangioma that occurred in the T5 vertebral body of a 78-year-old male patient. There is a tumor showing high signal intensity in both MR T2-weighted images (**a**) and T1-weighted images (**b**), suggesting an internal fatty component. In the fat-suppressed T1 contrast-enhanced image (**c**), the lesion appears as a low signal intensity compared to the surrounding bone marrow due to the suppression of the fat component inside, and there are also parts that are partially enhanced. This is a typical finding of a hemangioma

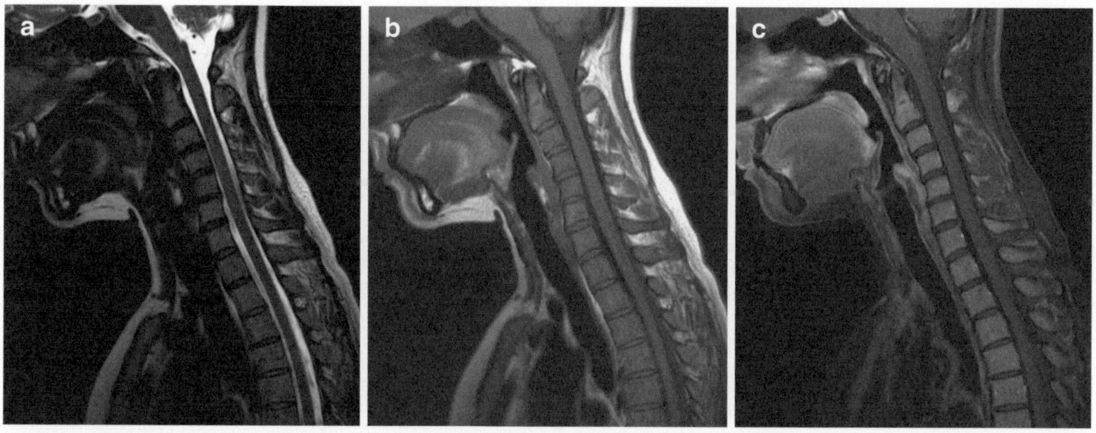

Fig. 11.6 Example of diffuse red marrow hyperplasia seen in a 39-year-old female patient. In the MR T2-weighted image (**a**), no distinct abnormal findings can be found in the bone marrow, but in the T1-weighted image (**b**), the signal intensity of the bone marrow is generally decreased and shows a similar degree to the disc. In the fat-suppressed contrast-enhanced T1-weighted image (**c**), this bone marrow shows mild enhancement, which is consistent with red marrow

from bony vertebrae include hemangioma, telangiectatic osteosarcoma, and aneurysmal bone cyst. The most common vascular tumors occurring in the epidural space are hemangioma and angiolipoma. On the other hand, the most common vascular tumor occurring in the intradural extramedullary space is paraganglioma, and the most common tumor occurring in the intramedullary is hemangioblastoma.

11.1.4.4 High Cellularity

If the tumor has high cellularity, it shows intermediate signal intensity on MR T2 enhanced images and is enhanced, and it can be seen that the T2 signal intensity is somewhat lower compared to tumors with low cellularity (Fig. 11.7). These findings are often observed in lymphoma and meningioma and are also observed in metastatic tumors or sarcomas with high cellularity.

11.1.4.5 Hemorrhagic Component

The hemorrhagic component inside the tumor can show various MR signal intensities depending on the stage of the hemorrhage, chronic repetitive hemorrhage in the tumor. It appears as an accumulation of internal or surrounding hemosiderin, which is seen as a dark signal intensity on MR T1- and T2-weighted images (Fig. 11.8). This signal intensity is further emphasized on gradient echo images due to the susceptibility blooming artifact.

11.1.4.6 Calcification/Ossification

Calcification/ossification within the tumor is better seen on CT than on MR images, appearing as high attenuation on CT. In most cases, calcification is represented as low signal intensity on MR T1- and T2-weighted images, but can also appear in various signal intensities. If ossification occurs and normal bone marrow is formed inside, it appears as high signal intensity due to the fatty bone marrow component. Tumor calcification can be seen in chondrosarcoma or meningioma (Fig. 11.9), and ossification can be seen in osteoid osteoma/osteoblastoma or osteosarcoma (Fig. 11.10).

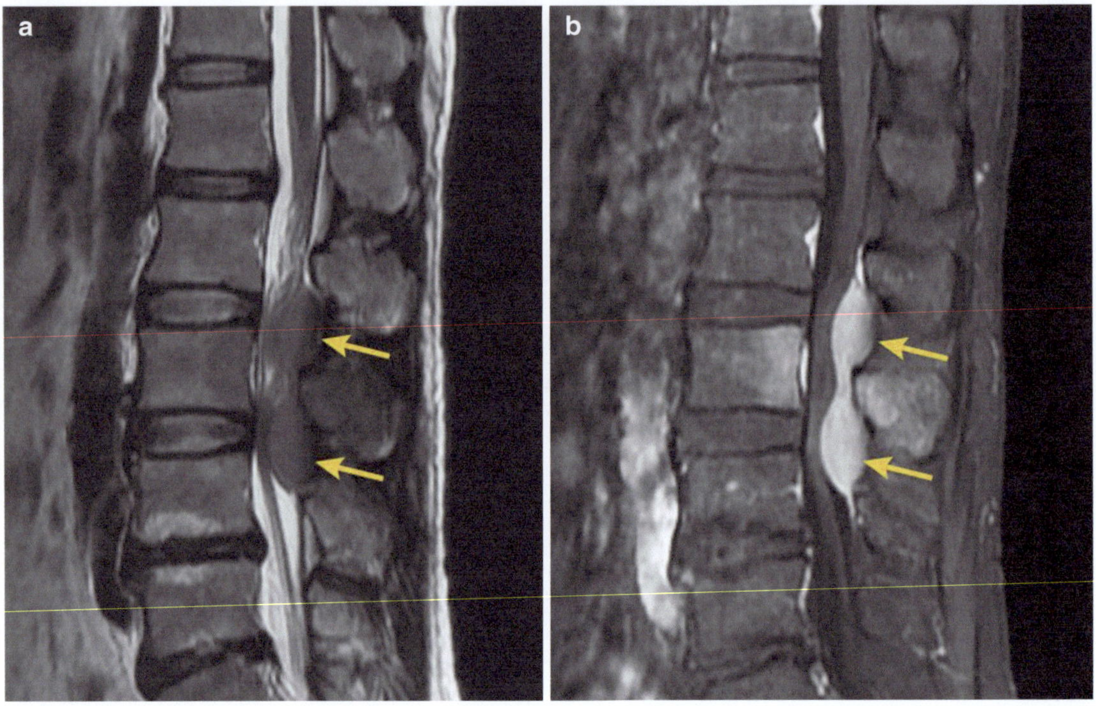

Fig. 11.7 In a patient with B-lymphoblastic lymphoma, a tumor is seen mainly in the epidural space of L2-3-4 on MR T2 enhanced images (**a**), and the low T2 signal intensity suggests high cellularity (arrow). This high cellularity portion shows good enhancement when contrast-enhanced (**b**) (arrow)

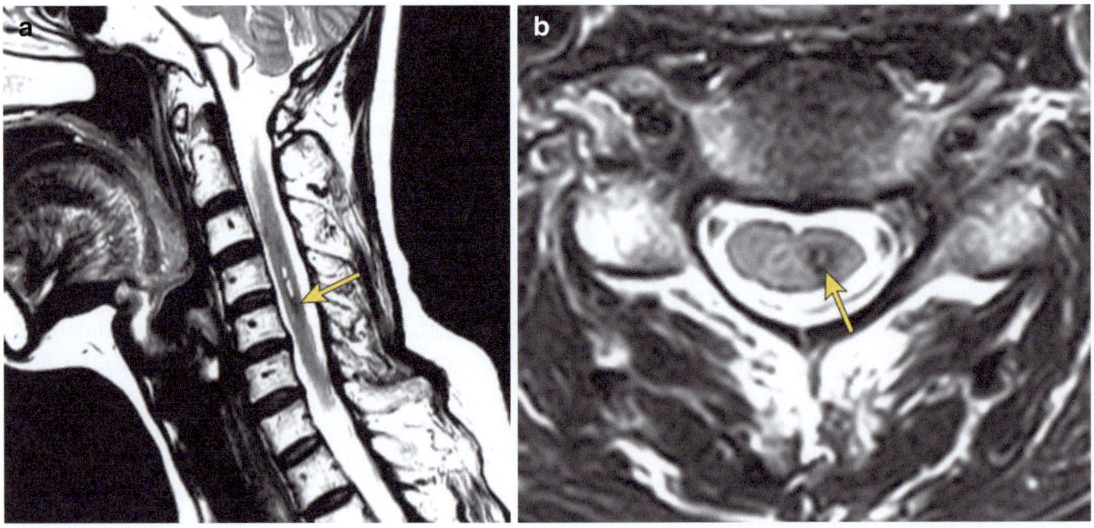

Fig. 11.8 Example of an intramedullary cavernous hemangioma that occurred in a 55-year-old female patient. Hemosiderin deposition showing a dark signal is seen in the area marked with an arrow in both T2-weighted sagittal (**a**) and axial (**b**) images, which is a characteristic of the tumor. The findings suggest a long-standing internal repetitive hemorrhage

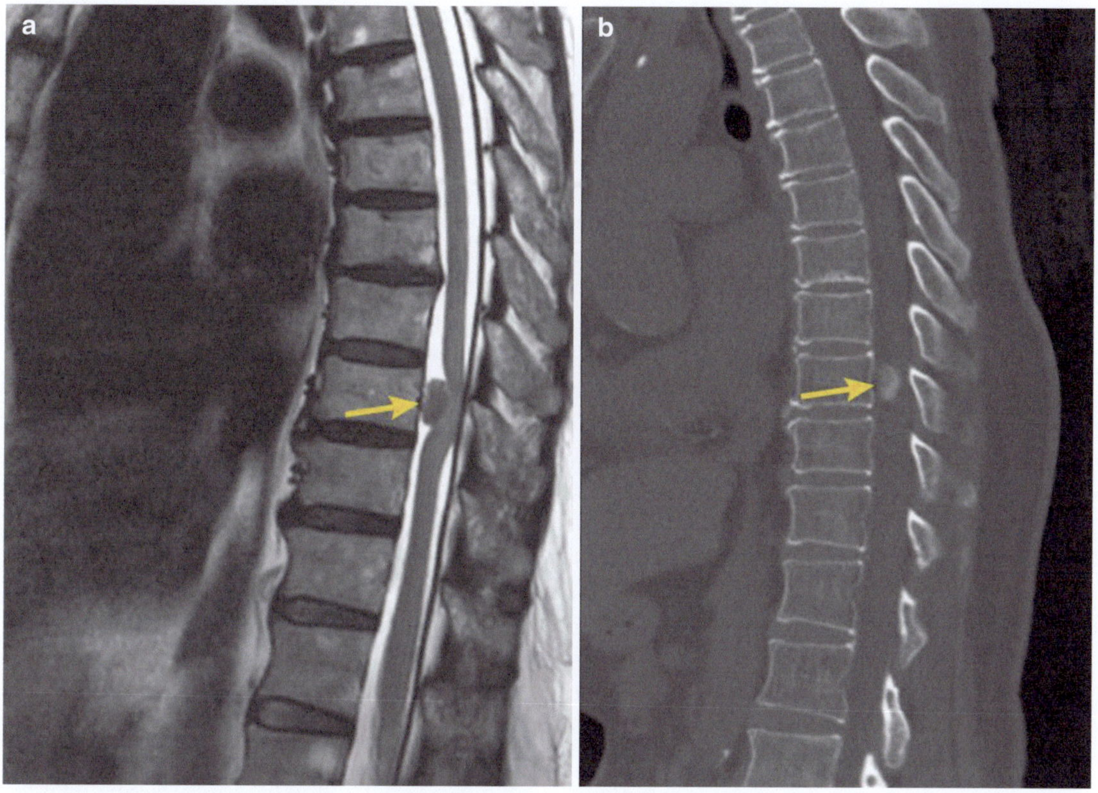

Fig. 11.9 An example of calcified meningioma that occurred at the T9 level in a 72-year-old female patient. There is a tumor showing somewhat low signal intensity on MR T2-weighted images (**a**) in the anterior intradural extramedullary space at the T9 level, and it is severely compressing the spinal cord. On the preoperative CT scan (**b**), the tumor shows high attenuation of calcification

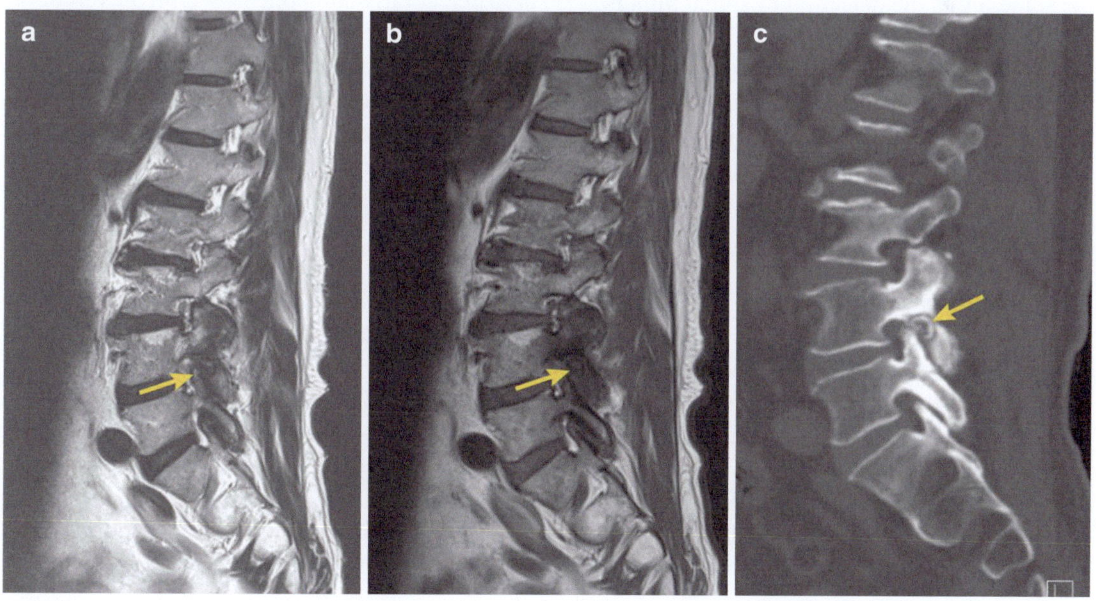

Fig. 11.10 An example of osteoid osteoma that occurred in a 66-year-old male patient who visited with low back pain as the main complaint. A lesion thought to be a nidus showing about 1.2 cm of ossification (yellow arrows) in the left inferior articular process of the L4 vertebrae is observed (**a**, **b**), and it is more clearly observed on CT (**c**)

11.2 Osseous Tumor

Most osseous tumors occurring in the spine are metastases or hematologic malignancies, and it is not difficult to diagnose if the patient has been previously diagnosed with cancer or has multiple lesions. However, if there is no history of cancer diagnosis or only one lesion, although rare, primary osseous tumor must be considered.

11.2.1 Imaging Diagnosis Method

The imaging diagnosis of spinal tumors, like osseous tumors in the limbs, should take into account age, location, lesion boundaries, presence or absence of calcification, bone expansion, soft tissue mass formation, and signal intensity on MRI. Especially, the clinical findings, history, and whether the lesion is single or multiple are very important because metastasis or hematologic malignancy is common. However, this chapter does not cover bone marrow lesions.

11.2.1.1 Plain Radiography

Plain radiography can only diagnose when there is 50~70% of bone destruction, so its sensitivity is low [1]. The complex anatomical structure of the spine limits the detection of spinal tumors.

11.2.1.2 Computed Tomography (CT)

CT is useful for observing calcification and destruction of the bony cortex, but it has lower sensitivity than MRI for observing lesions in the bone marrow, epidural space, and paravertebral space, and nerve compression [2].

11.2.1.3 Bone Scintigraphy

Technetium-99m methylene diphosphonate (Tc-MDP) scintigraphy can detect bony abnormalities throughout the body in a single test, so it is commonly used to test for metastasis, but its specificity is low. It is effective in detecting lesions that have invaded the bony cortex, but it cannot see invasion of the spinal canal and formation of soft tissue mass [2].

11.2.1.4 Magnetic Resonance Imaging (MRI)

MRI is more sensitive than bone scan in detecting primary bone tumors and metastases occurring in the spine. It is also the best imaging diagnostic method that shows the relationship with bone marrow and surrounding soft tissues, and nerves, and it is also easy for initial diagnosis and follow-up after treatment. However, it is less effective in observing calcification and destruction of the bony cortex. Its sensitivity is lower than that of CT. The sequences commonly used in MRI are T1-weighted images, fast spin echo T2-weighted images, fat-suppressed T2-weighted images or STIR images, and contrast-enhanced fat-suppressed T1-weighted images. Tumors mainly show moderate or low signal intensity that contrasts well with the high signal intensity of the surrounding fatty bone marrow in T1-weighted images. On the other hand, in T2-weighted images, both the fatty bone marrow and the tumor often appear as high signal intensity, which is used more for detecting spinal nerve compression, neuropathy, intradural lesions, etc. than for finding lesions. Fat-suppressed T2-weighted images or STIR images can suppress the signal intensity of the surrounding fatty bone marrow of the lesion, increase the contrast of the lesion, and help detect fatty components within the tumor. In contrast-enhanced fat-suppressed T1-weighted images, contrast enhancement is often well done compared to the surrounding fatty bone marrow with suppressed signal intensity, and it is also useful for observing the spread to surrounding soft tissues or extradural space [2].

11.2.2 The Most Common Spinal Osseous Tumor

11.2.2.1 Hemangioma

Hemangioma is the most common benign tumor of the spine, and according to autopsy studies, it was found in about 11% of all cases [3]. Histologically, it consists of vessels covered with endothelium along with non-vascular tissues (fat, muscle, fibrous tissue, bone). It is divided into various forms (capillary, cavernous, arteriovenous, venous), among which the capillary type is the most common. About 25% to 30% are multiple and most commonly occur in the thoracic spine, but can occur anywhere. The incidence increases with age and is most common between the ages of 30 and 50. On plain radiographs, the vertical trabeculae are thickened, which is called a "corduroy appearance." If you look at these thickened vertical trabeculae on the CT axial section, they appear as multiple osteosclerotic spots, which are called "polka dot signs" (Fig. 11.11). The low attenuation part that forms the background of such polka dot signs can be fatty stroma or vascular tissue. In MRI, it is observed as high signal intensity in T1- and T2-weighted images due to the fatty component. Polka dot signs or corduroy appearance can be observed as low signal intensity on axial or sagittal, coronal MRI (Fig. 11.11). The vascular part of the tumor is observed as high signal intensity in T2-weighted images, reflecting slow blood flow and can also appear in a twisted shape. Most are often found incidentally without symptoms, and rarely can cause neurological symptoms or radiating pain by aggressively spreading to the posterior element or surrounding spinal soft tissues (Fig. 11.12) [4]. Large hemangiomas can weaken the vertebral body and cause pathologic fractures (Fig. 11.12) [5]. If there are no symptoms, treatment is not necessary, and if there are symptoms, endovascular embolization, vertebrectomy, sclerotherapy, and vertebroplasty can be performed [5].

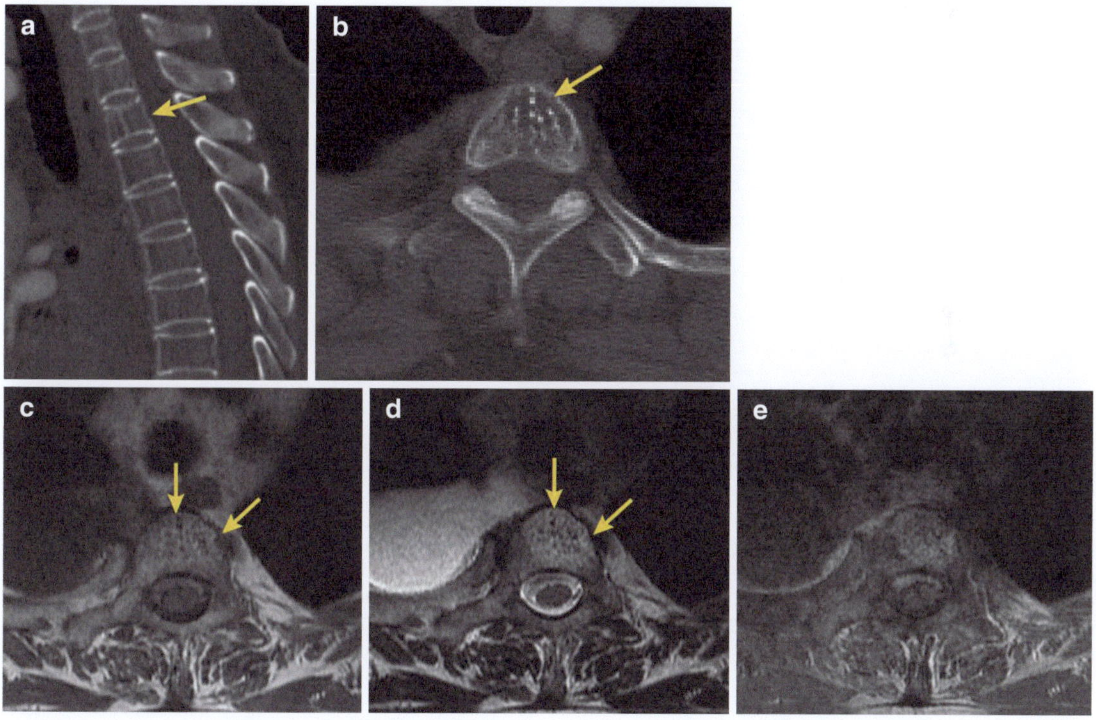

Fig. 11.11 CT and MRI findings of hemangioma. On the CT sagittal image (**a**), the vertical trabeculae are thickened, showing a "corduroy appearance." The thickened vertical trabeculae appear as multiple osteosclerotic spots on the CT axial image (**b**), which is called the "polka dot sign." Multiple osteosclerotic spots of low signal intensity are also observed on MR T1 (**c**) and T2 (**d**) enhanced images. The low attenuation part forming the background of these on CT shows high signal intensity on MR T1 and T2 enhanced images and shows weak enhancement on fat-suppressed contrast-enhanced T1 enhanced images (**e**), indicating fat tissue and slow-flow vascular tissue components

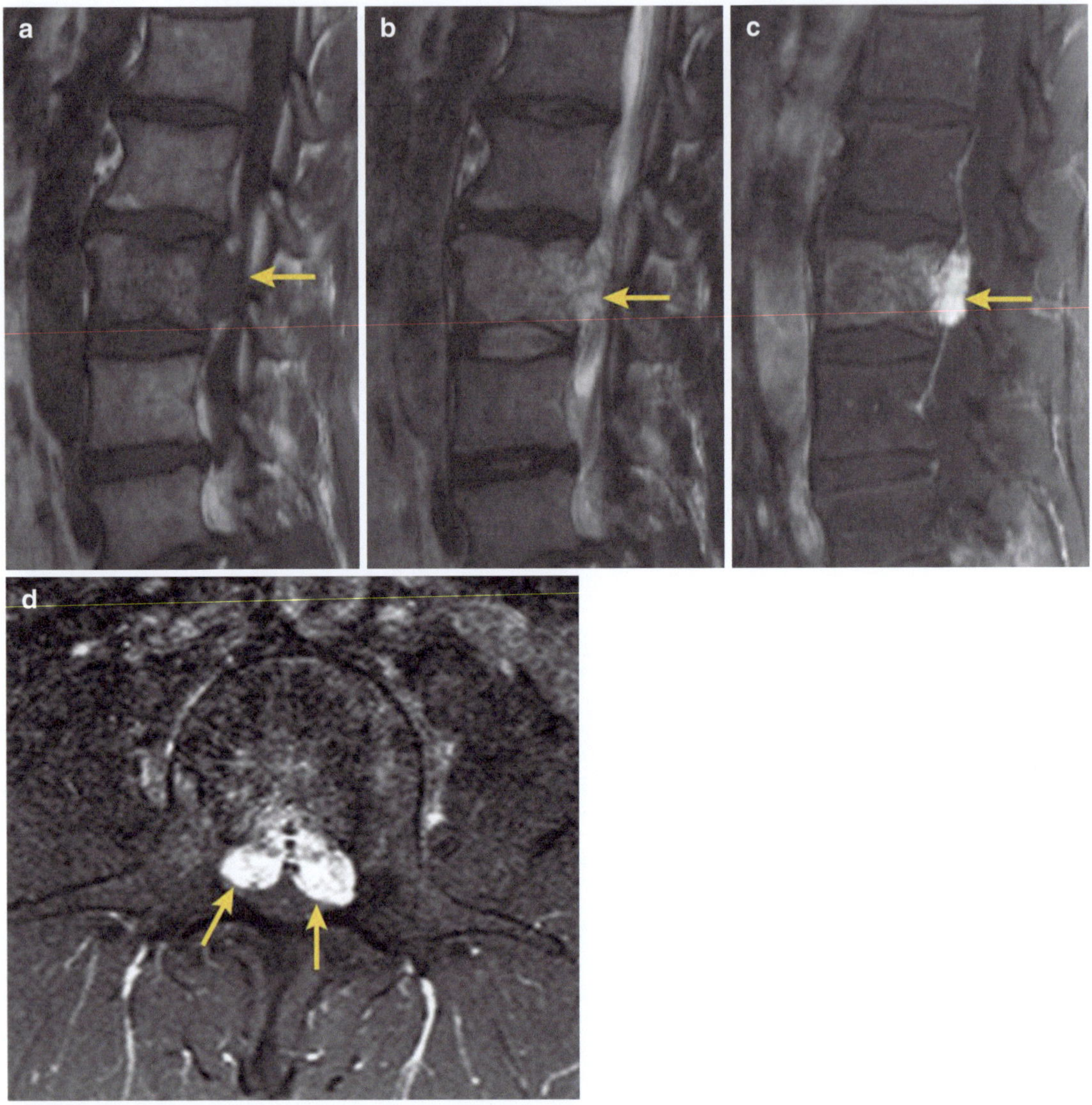

Fig. 11.12 MRI findings of aggressive hemangioma. There is a hemangioma that shows high signal intensity overall on MR T1 enhanced images (**a**) and T2 enhanced images (**b**) in the L3 vertebral body and shows weak enhancement on contrast-enhanced fat-suppressed T1 enhanced images (**c**, **d**). There is a lesion (arrow) that shows low signal intensity on T1 enhanced images and high signal intensity on T2 enhanced images in the adjacent epidural space, and shows very good enhancement, suggesting that the hemangioma has invaded. A pathologic compression fracture is also present

11.2.2.2 Metastasis

Metastasis is the most common malignant tumor occurring in the spine. Most malignant tumors originating from other parts can metastasize to the spine, but in women, breast cancer and lung cancer, and in men, prostate cancer and lung cancer are particularly prone to metastasize to the spine [6]. The most common sites are the thoracic spine (about 70%), lumbar spine (20%), and cervical spine (10%) in that order [6]. Any part of the spine can be metastasized, but it is most common in the vertebral body, and in 30% of cases, it metastasizes in multiple places [7]. Clinically, it is accompanied by severe pain, and if it compresses the spinal cord, there can be loss of visceral organ function or decreased motor/sensory function [7]. It mainly occurs in the medullary bone and appears as osteolytic (70%), osteoblastic (9%), and a mixed form of the two lesions (21%). In the case of osteolytic metastasis, it can be diagnosed on plain radiography only when there is 50~70% of bone destruction, so the sensitivity is low [1]. On CT, it appears as multiple osteolytic lesions of various sizes, and the boundaries may be clear or unclear, and unlike benign lesions that grow slowly, the sclerotic rim of the lesion is not visible (Figs. 11.13) [7]. Sometimes it destroys the cortical bone and invades the surrounding soft tissues or epidural space of the spine [7]. On MRI, it mainly appears as moderate or low signal on T1-weighted images, and low or high signal intensity on T2-weighted images, and most of them are well enhanced [7]. Osteoblastic metastasis is common especially in breast cancer and prostate cancer, and it often appears as a reactive increase in bone formation activity rather than the tumor cells themselves [7]. On magnetic resonance imaging, it shows low signal on both T1- and T2-weighted images, and enhancement is heterogeneous or only on the periphery, and it varies depending on the degree of sclerosis of the lesion (Fig. 11.14).

11.2.2.3 Multiple Myeloma

Multiple myeloma is the second most common hematologic malignancy after non-Hodgkin's lymphoma, characterized by the proliferation of monoclonal plasma cells in the bone marrow. It is most commonly found in the vertebral body and is often referred to as the most common primary malignant tumor occurring in the spine. The most common age of onset is between 50 and 60. Clinical symptoms include weight loss, fatigue, bone pain, and recurrent infections. About 70% can have spinal compression fractures, which can be malignant compression fractures caused by multiple myeloma invading the bone marrow, but about 33~67% show the same imaging findings as benign compression fractures, either due to secondary osteoporosis caused by increased bone resorption or due to therapeutic drugs such as steroid therapy [2, 8, 9]. Fractures occur in 87% between T6 and L4, which is the same distribution as fractures due to osteoporosis [2]. Plain radiographs and CT show punched-out osteolytic lesions, overall osteopenia, fractures, and rarely osteoblastic lesions [4]. About 20% are normal on plain films [7]. On MRI, it varies depending on the stage and degree of bone marrow involvement, and as the stage is higher and bone marrow involvement progresses, abnormal signal intensity is shown and enhancement also increases [10]. There are five major patterns observed, the first of which is seen as the signal intensity of normal fatty marrow. It is observed in about 28% and is the early stage of myeloma. The bone marrow involvement suggests <20% [11, 12]. It is mainly seen in low-stage multiple myeloma, but can also be seen in stage III multiple myeloma [11]. Second, it is localized and observed in about 30%, showing low signal intensity on T1-weighted images, high signal intensity on fat-suppressed T2-weighted or STIR images, and high signal intensity on contrast-enhanced fat-suppressed T1-weighted images (Fig. 11.15a) [11]. Third, it appears as a diffuse pattern on T1-weighted images, showing homogeneous signal intensity compared to the intervertebral disc and is enhanced (Fig. 11.15b, c) [11]. It is often seen in high-stage cases. Fourth, the bone marrow appears as a heterogeneous, mottled or "salt and pepper pattern," showing multiple small low signal intensities on T1-weighted images (Fig. 11.15d) [11]. The reason for the mottled appearance is due to the mixture of multiple small fatty marrow and infiltrating malignant plasma cells, as the malignant plasma cell suppresses hematopoiesis. It is observed in about 3% and is often seen in low-stage cases. Fifth, bone marrow involvement and local lesions are observed together in about 11% of cases [13].

A detailed overview of multiple myeloma is covered in the bone marrow disease chapter. Also, refer to the bone marrow disease chapter for plasmacytoma, the initial stage of multiple myeloma.

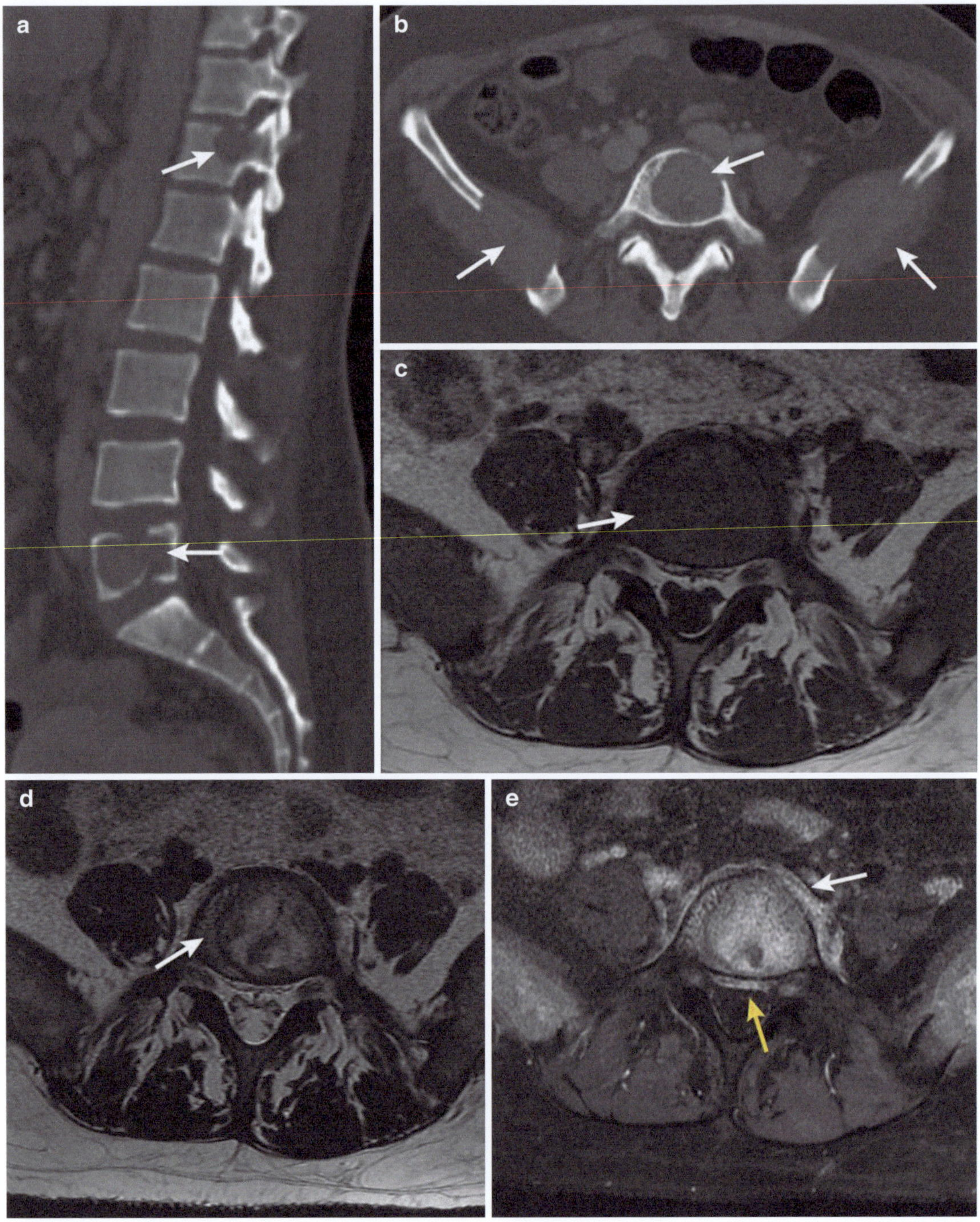

Fig. 11.13 Osteolytic metastasis of breast cancer. On CT images, there are osteolytic metastases (**a**, arrow) in the T12 and L5 vertebral bodies, and there is a malignant compression fracture in L5. The sclerotic rim of the lesion is not visible. There are also osteolytic metastases in both iliac bones. (**b**, arrow) is present, destroying the cortex and forming a soft tissue mass. The lesion shows low signal intensity on MR T1 enhanced image (**c**), high signal intensity on T2 enhanced image (**d**), and strong enhancement on fat-suppressed contrast-enhanced T1 enhanced image (**e**). Such lesions are extending into the paravertebral space (white arrow) and epidural space (yellow arrow)

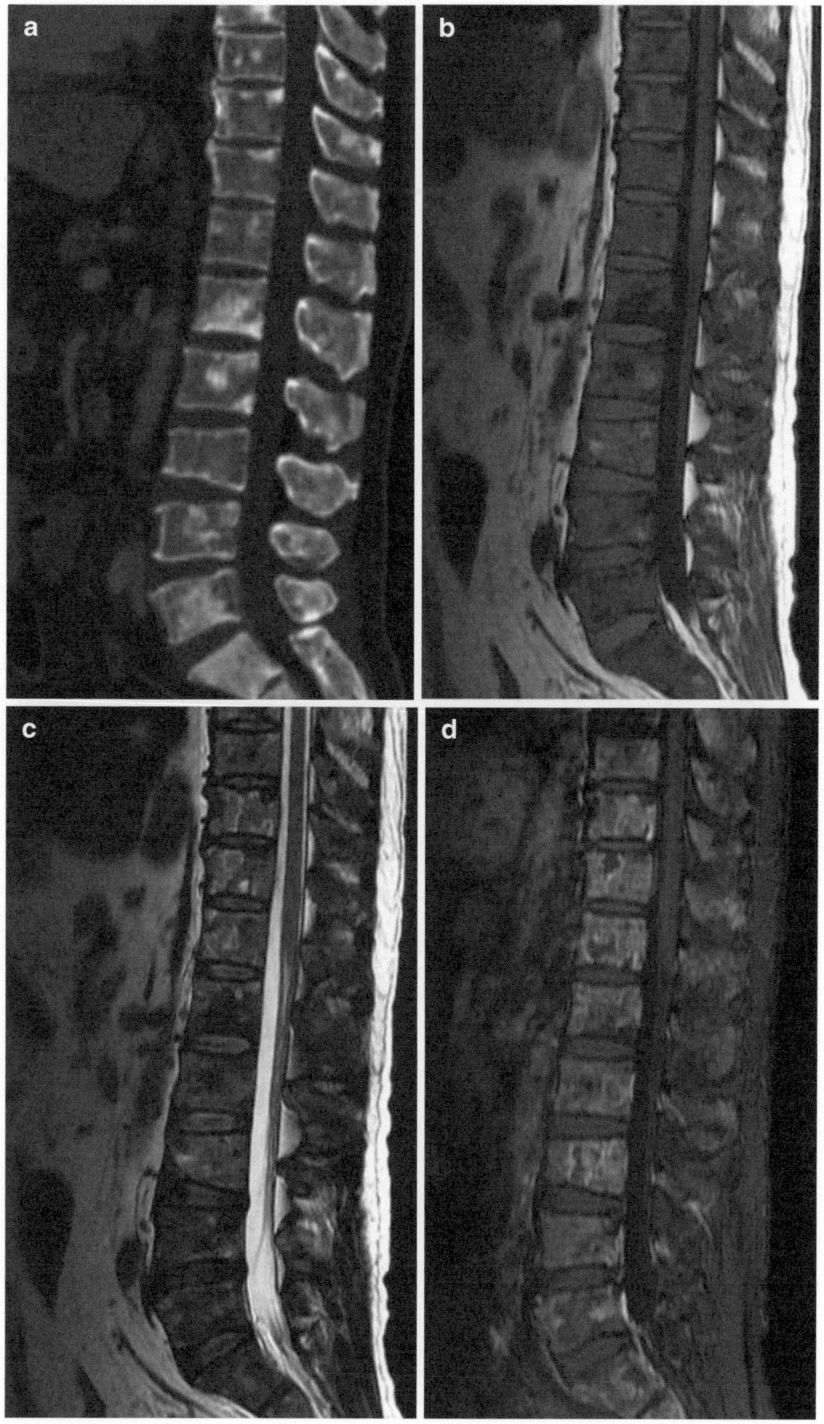

Fig. 11.14 Osteoblastic metastasis of prostate cancer. Multiple poorly defined osteoblastic metastases are present on CT image (**a**). Osteoblastic metastases show low signal intensity on both MR T1 (**b**) and T2 (**c**) enhanced images, and enhancement on fat-suppressed contrast-enhanced T1 enhanced image (**d**) is heterogeneous or peripheral enhancement is observed

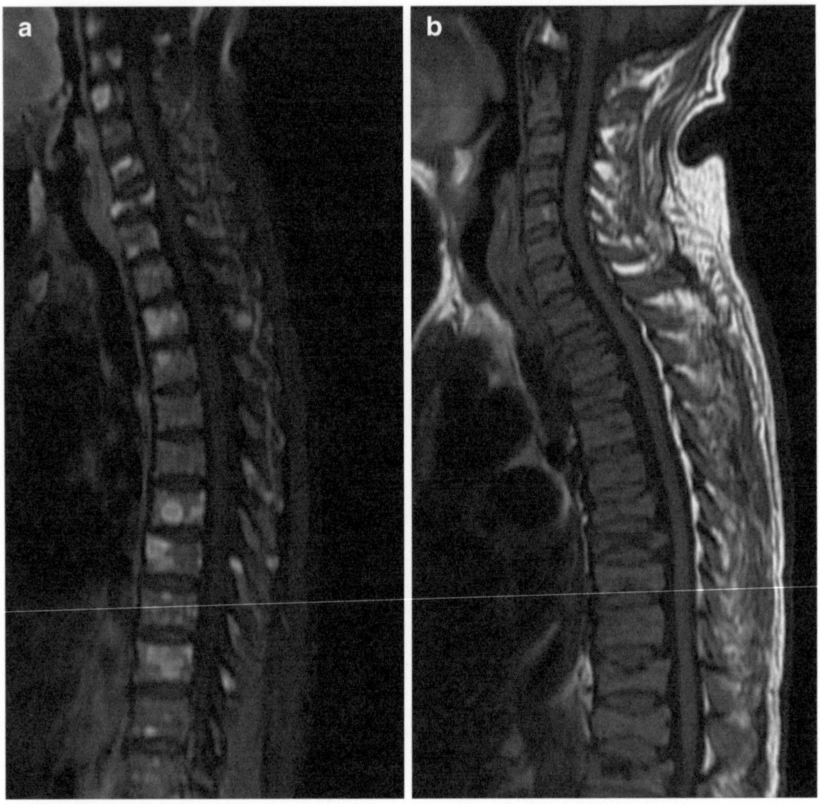

Fig. 11.15 Various patterns of multiple myeloma. (**a**) As an example of localized type, multiple well-defined enhancing lesions are observed on fat-suppressed contrast-enhanced T1 enhanced sagittal image. (**b**, **c**) As an example of diffuse type, bone marrow appears as diffuse type with the same signal intensity as the disc on T1 enhanced image (**b**) and shows homogeneous enhancement on contrast-enhanced fat-suppressed T1 enhanced image (**c**). Multiple pathologic compression fractures are observed in the thoracic spine. (**d**) Example of "salt and pepper pattern." On T1 enhanced image, multiple small fatty marrow and malignant plasma cell infiltrations are mixed like sprinkling salt and pepper. Pathologic compression fractures are observed at T10 and L3

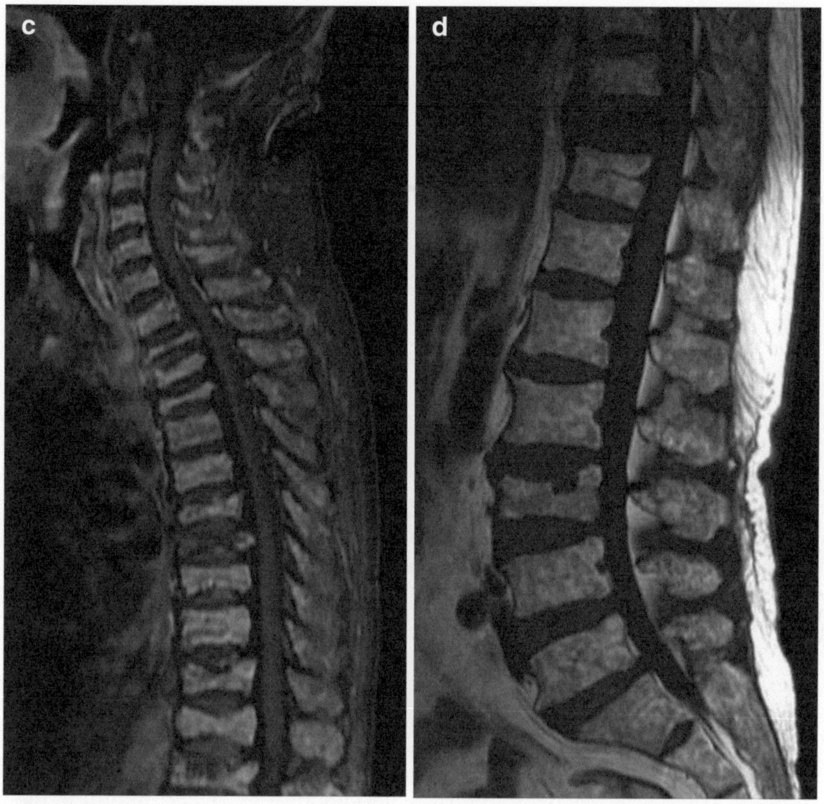

Fig. 11.15 (continued)

11.2.3 Spinal Primary Benign Osseous Tumor

11.2.3.1 Bone Island (Enostosis)

Bone Island, or enostosis, is a common benign tumor of the spine. Histologically, it is dense cortical bone within the medullary bone. It is often discovered incidentally as it is mostly asymptomatic. The common sites are between T1 and T7, and L2 and L3. It is observed as radiodense on both plain radiographs and CT. It is usually round or oval in shape and ranges in size from 2 mm to 2 cm. It shows irregular and sharp boundaries along the surrounding normal trabeculae. It is usually located like an island within the medullary bone, but sometimes it is located on the inner surface of the cortical bone. It usually shows similar radionuclide uptake to the surrounding bone on bone scan, but in large cases, uptake may slightly increase. On MRI, it appears as low signal intensity on both T1-weighted and T2-weighted images and does not enhance (Fig. 11.16) [3]. Diagnosis is not difficult as it usually shows typical imaging findings, but diseases to be differentiated include other tumors that can show osteosclerosis, namely osteoblastic metastases, osteoid osteoma, low-grade osteosarcoma, etc. Especially, differentiation from osteoblastic metastasis is important. Basically, Bone Island does not enhance, but in the case of osteoblastic metastasis, enhancement is often seen in the peripheral portion of the lesion, which is an important differential point. Also, in large cases, it may be difficult to differentiate from osteoblastic

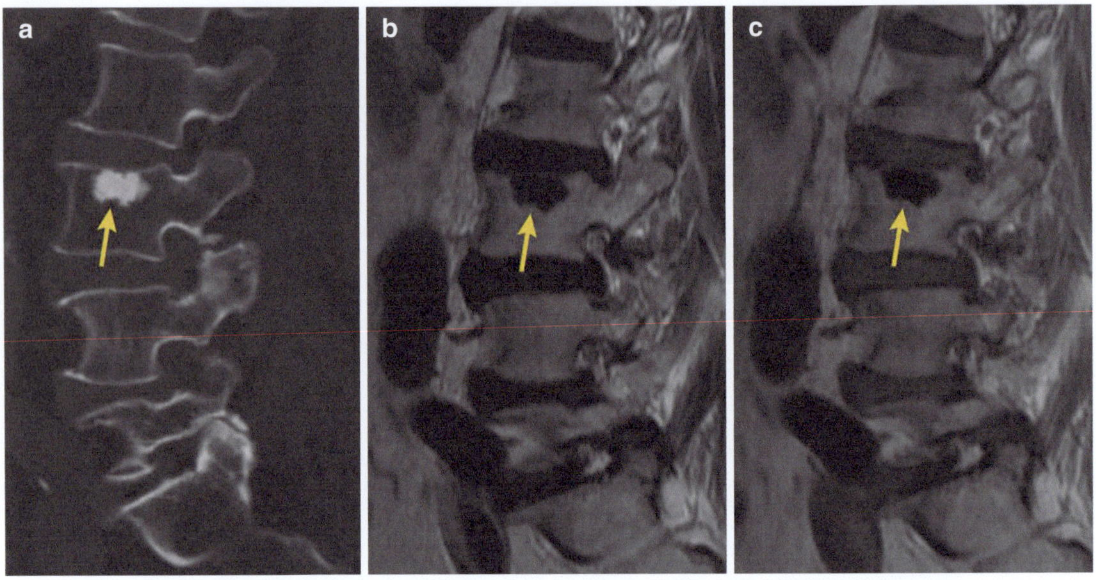

Fig. 11.16 Findings of bone island on CT and MR. On CT, a radiodense lesion with irregular and sharp boundaries following the surrounding normal trabeculae is observed below the endplate (**a**). It shows very low signal intensity on both MR T1 enhanced image (**b**) and T2 enhanced image (**c**)

metastasis, but Bone Island shows almost normal or slightly increased uptake on bone scan, which is a differential point. If the size has increased by 25–50% within 6 months to 1 year, the possibility of malignancy cannot be ruled out, so bone A biopsy should be considered [3]. Other diseases related to Bone Island include osteopoikilosis, osteopathia striata, and melorheostosis.

11.2.3.2 Osteoid Osteoma

Osteoid osteoma accounts for about 11% of all confirmed primary osseous tumors of the spine. Histologically, there is a nidus composed of small vascular tissue and osteoid matrix within the fibrous tissue, with a diameter of about 1.5~2 cm or less, and it shows various degrees of osteosclerosis and sclerosis of the cortical bone around it. About 10% of all osteoid osteomas occur in the spine. It can be suspected when there is scoliosis accompanied by severe pain, and it can also show local pain, radiating pain, and gait disturbance. The pain characteristically worsens at night and is alleviated by nonsteroidal anti-inflammatory drugs (NSAIDs). The most common age of onset is young adults in their teens to 20s, and it is more common in men (2:1~3:1) [14]. The most common sites are the lumbar (59%), cervical (27%), thoracic (12%), and sacral (2%) in order, and about 93% occur mainly in the posterior element (pedicles, superior and inferior articular processes, lamina, transverse, and spinous processes), and rarely occur in the vertebral body [14, 15]. Because it is small in size, the nidus is radiolucent and occurs in the posterior element, it is often not well seen in simple radiographs. On CT, the nidus is well seen and sometimes accompanied by calcification/ossification in the center (Fig. 11.10). This central calcification/ossification needs to be differentiated from the sequestrum caused by dead bone tissue caused by multiple myeloma, osteoblastic metastasis, lymphoma, Langerhans cell histiocytosis (LCH), etc. It also accompanies various degrees of sclerosis of the surrounding bone, especially when sclerosis is caused in the pedicle, it needs to be differentiated from osteoblastic metastasis, bone island, chronic inflammation/infection, lymphoma, and reactive sclerosis due to instability of the spine. On bone scan, the nidus shows very strong radionuclide uptake and the surrounding tissue shows a "double uptake scintigraphic pattern" with less strong but still

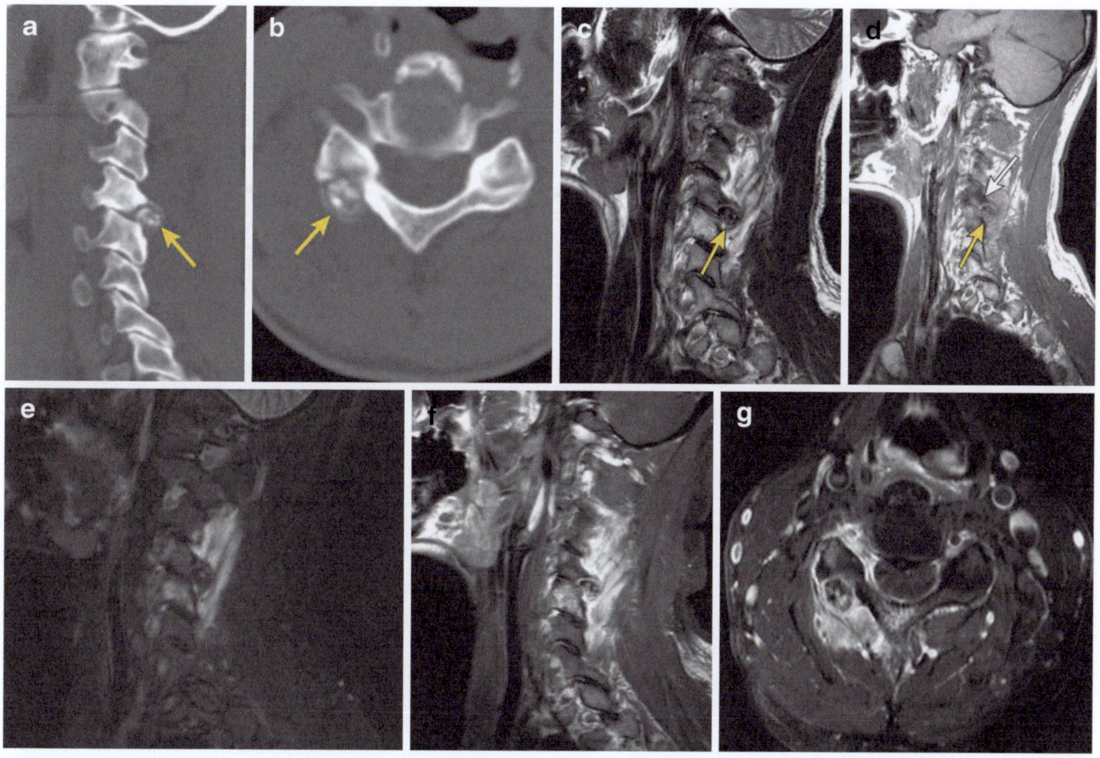

Fig. 11.17 Example of osteoid osteoma originating from the neck of a 51-year-old male patient. On CT sagittal and axial images (**a**, **b**), there is an exophytic bony lesion from the right inferior articular process of C4, and a lesion thought to be a nidus showing internal calcification/ossification. Such nidus shows heterogeneous low signal intensity on MR T2 (**c**) and T1 (**d**) enhanced images, causing sclerosis in the surrounding bony structure (**d**, white arrow). Severe bone and soft tissue swelling around such lesions is observed on fat-suppressed T2 enhanced image (**e**) and fat-suppressed contrast-enhanced T1 enhanced image (**f**, **g**)

increased radionuclide uptake. On MRI, the nidus appears variably depending on the degree of calcification/ossification, showing low or moderate signal intensity on T1-weighted images and moderate or increased signal intensity on T2-weighted images. If the edema of the surrounding bone marrow or soft tissue is very severe, the nidus may not be well seen and may be mistaken for other aggressive osseous tumors or infectious spondylitis (Fig. 11.17). If there is chronic edema in the surrounding soft tissue, muscle atrophy and fatty degeneration increase. Treatment varies, but although it responds to NSAIDs, complete removal is necessary for complete cure. Radiofrequency ablation is commonly used in the upper extremities, but surgical removal is preferred in the spine due to the risk of nerve damage from heat conduction [3, 14, 15].

11.2.3.3 Osteoblastoma

Osteoblastoma is a rare tumor, also known as a giant osteoid osteoma. It accounts for 1% of surgically confirmed primary osseous tumors. Histologically, it is similar to osteoid osteoma, but the difference is that it is larger than 1.5 cm. The trabeculae and fibrovascular tissue are intertwined. The most common site of occurrence is the posterior element of the spine (85%), and it often invades the vertebral body (42%). However, it is rare for it to occur primarily in the vertebral body. It can occur at any age, but it is common in young adults between their teens and 20s, and slightly more common in men (2:1). There may be dull pain and, although rare, neurological symptoms such as sensory abnormalities or paralysis. In imaging, it can appear in three patterns: first, like an osteoid osteoma, there is a

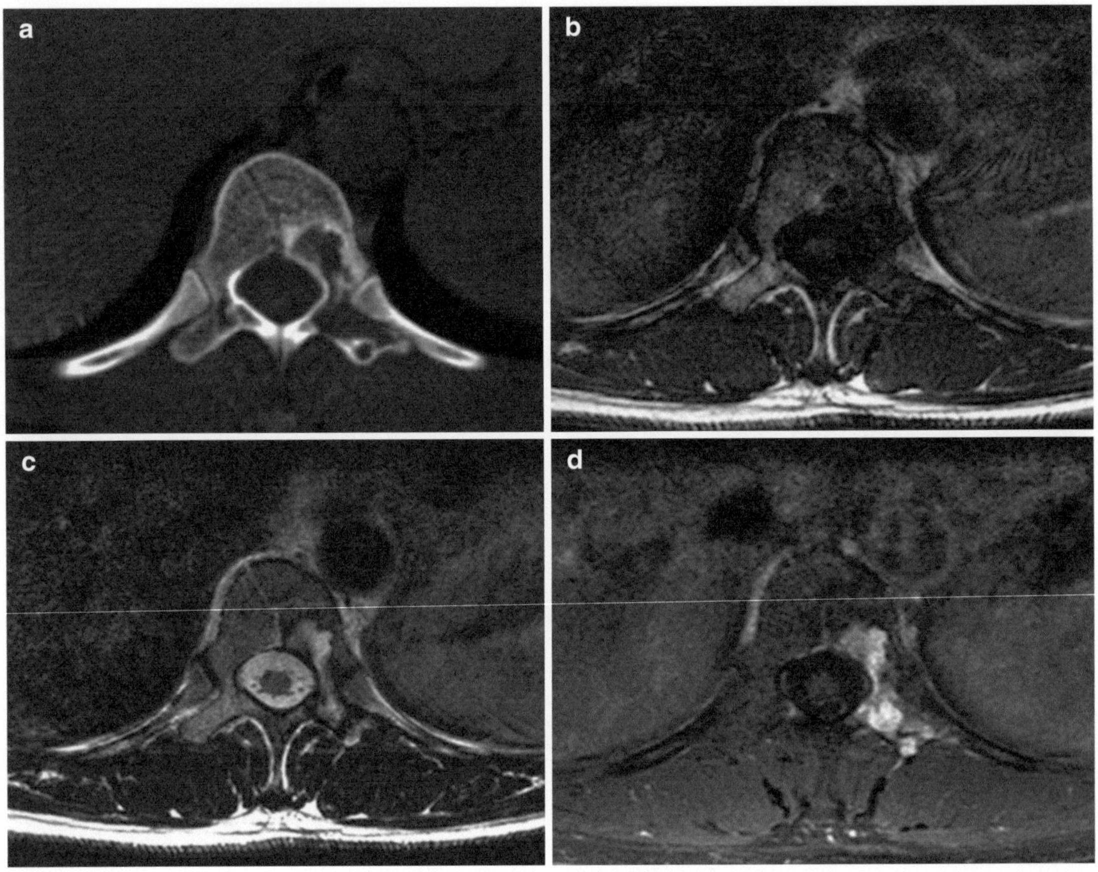

Fig. 11.18 CT and MRI findings of osteoblastoma. In the CT image (**a**), there is an osteolytic lesion that expands the bone and has small calcifications inside. The perimeter of the osteolytic lesion shows sclerotic changes. In the MR T1-weighted image (**b**), it shows low and moderate signal intensity, and in the T2-weighted image (**c**), it shows high signal intensity along with low signal intensity at the calcification site. In the fat-suppressed contrast-enhanced T1-weighted image (**d**), it shows heterogeneous enhancement, and there is almost no edema in the surrounding soft tissue or bone marrow

radiolucent nidus in the center and it is accompanied by osteosclerosis. However, the nidus is larger than the nidus of osteoid osteoma (1.5~2 cm). Second, it expands the bone and shows many small calcifications and a peripheral sclerotic rim within the lesion. In the spine, this second pattern is the most common (Fig. 11.18). The third pattern is when the tumor expands and destroys the bone, invades the surrounding soft tissue, and is accompanied by calcification. This appears very aggressive, and the calcification can look like chondroid calcification [16, 17]. On a bone scan, it shows strong uptake like osteoid osteoma. On CT, calcification, bone expansion, and remodeling can be observed, and a sclerotic rim can be seen around the lesion (Fig. 11.18). On MRI, it appears in various ways and there are no characteristic findings. On T1-weighted images, it shows low or moderate signal intensity, and on T2-weighted images, it shows various signal intensities (Fig. 11.18). There is expansive remodeling of the bone and soft tissue, and the edema of the surrounding bone marrow and soft tissue is less than that of osteoid osteoma. Aneurysmal bone cyst (ABC) changes can be accompanied in about 10~15% of cases, and in these cases, T1-weighted images show low signal intensity, T2-weighted images show very high signal intensity, and there are many fluid-fluid levels. Surgical resection is the treatment method and about 10~15% of cases recur. If it appears aggressive on imaging, it is often histologically aggressive as well, and in these cases, it can recur up to 50%, can invade important surrounding organs, and although rare, malignant transformation or metastasis is possible [3, 16].

11.2.3.4 Aneurysmal Bone Cyst

A primary aneurysmal bone cyst is histologically a multilocular space filled with blood, separated by thin septa, and unlike vascular channels, it lacks an endothelium [3]. The internal septum is composed of giant cells, fibrous tissue, and reactive bone. It occurs in the spine in 12~30% of all cases, with the thoracic spine being the most common, and the lumbar and cervical spine being rare. It is rare in the sacrum, but if it occurs in the first and second sacrum, it is difficult to distinguish from a giant cell tumor. It typically occurs in young patients under 20 and is slightly more common in women [18]. It mainly occurs in the posterior element and often spreads to the vertebral body (75~90%). Back pain is a common clinical symptom, and it can also cause neurological symptoms by pressing on the spinal nerves or nerve roots. On plain radiographs, it appears as an osteolytic lesion that expands and remodels the bone [18]. On a bone scan, it is like a giant. The cell tumor also shows increased isotope intake in the transformation part, like the donut sign. In MRI or CT, it is characteristic that the fluid-fluid level due to internal bleeding and precipitation is observed in the entire tumor as a single or multiple. In MR T1 and T2 enhanced images, an increased signal intensity due to methemoglobin is seen in the fluid, and there is a characteristic peripheral rim that appears as a low signal intensity in all signal intensities, suggesting an intact or thickened periosteal membrane [19]. During contrast enhancement, mainly the lesion's periphery and internal septum are enhanced (Fig. 11.19). If there is a solid component that is enhanced in addition to the fluid-fluid level inside the tumor, it is likely to be a secondary aneurysmal bone cyst that originated from other tumors such as giant cell tumor or osteoblastoma. The treatment of aneurysmal bone cysts that occur in the spine is often difficult because they are often adjacent to the surrounding spinal nerves and nerve roots. The recurrence rate is about 20~30% and the recurrence rate is high if the resection is incomplete [18, 20]. Surgical treatment is curettage and bone grafting [21]. Other attempts include endovascular embolization, sclerotherapy, and percutaneous placement of polymethylmethacrylate [18–20, 22].

11.2.3.5 Benign Notochordal Cell Tumor (BNCT)

The benign notochordal cell tumor is a new term recently proposed, referring to benign notochordal tissue creating a tumorous lesion in the spine. It is understood as a spectrum of tumorous lesions originating from notochordal cells, with benign lesions being benign notochordal cell tumors, malignant lesions being chordomas, and the distinction between the two is mostly based on radiological findings. Notochordal cells can exist in the nucleus pulposus until the second decade. These notochordal cells can move to the vertebral body through tiny cracks in the vertebral body endplate and can proliferate in the bone marrow [23]. Clinically, many cases are asymptomatic and are often found incidentally during other tests. On CT, sclerosis may or may not be seen in the lesion, and although it is mostly located within the vertebral body, some cases have been reported where it extends to the cortex or involves the entire vertebral body, appearing as ivory vertebrae. Trabecular or cortical destruction is not seen. On MR T1 enhanced images, it appears as a well-defined tumor showing low signal intensity, located mainly in the midline of the vertebral body, and it is characteristic that it does not enhance on contrast-enhanced T1 enhanced images (Fig. 11.20) [24]. It also does not show diffusion restriction on diffusion-enhanced images. There is no bony destruction or extension

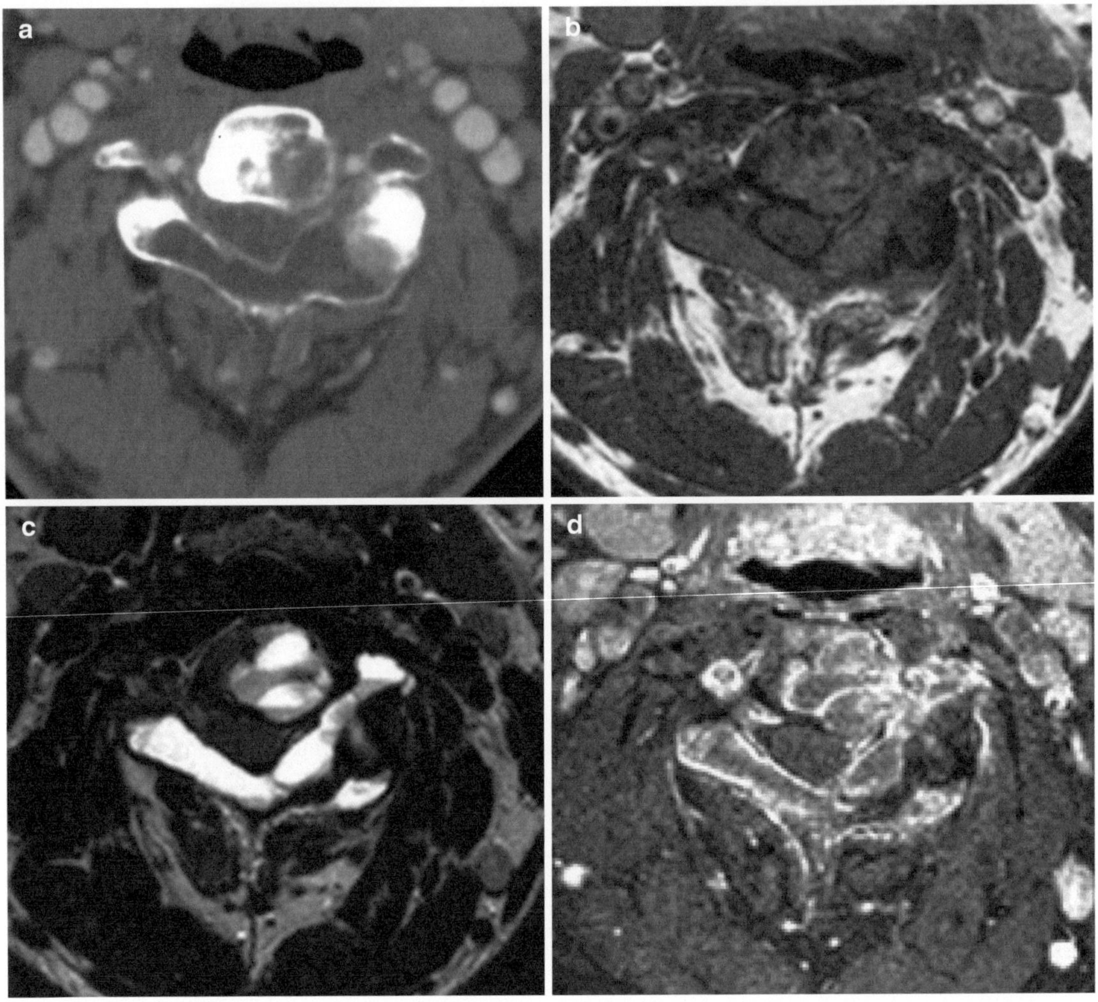

Fig. 11.19 CT and MRI findings of aneurysmal bone cyst. In the CT image (**a**), there is an osteolytic lesion that expands and reshapes the bone in the posterior element of the vertebra, and the vertebral body is also partially invaded. In the MR T1-weighted image (**b**) and T2-weighted image (**c**), a fluid-fluid level due to internal bleeding and deposition is observed in all directions throughout the entire tumor. The outer boundary of the lesion appears as low signal intensity in all signal intensities, suggesting an intact or thickened periosteal membrane. In the contrast-enhanced fat-suppressed T1-weighted image (**d**), the surrounding tissue and internal septum are enhanced

into soft tissue, and the lack of change in long-term follow-up examinations is important in the diagnosis of benign notochordal cell tumors. Some believe that long-term follow-up examinations are necessary as it is known that malignant transformation into chordoma is possible in some cases.

11.2.3.6 Giant Cell Tumor (GCT)

Giant cell tumor is a common benign osseous tumor in the upper limb bones, and about 7~15% of the total occur in the spine [3]. Histologically, it is typical to see a lot of osteoclast giant cells mixed in the mononuclear spindle cell stroma, but there can also be hemosiderin due to previous

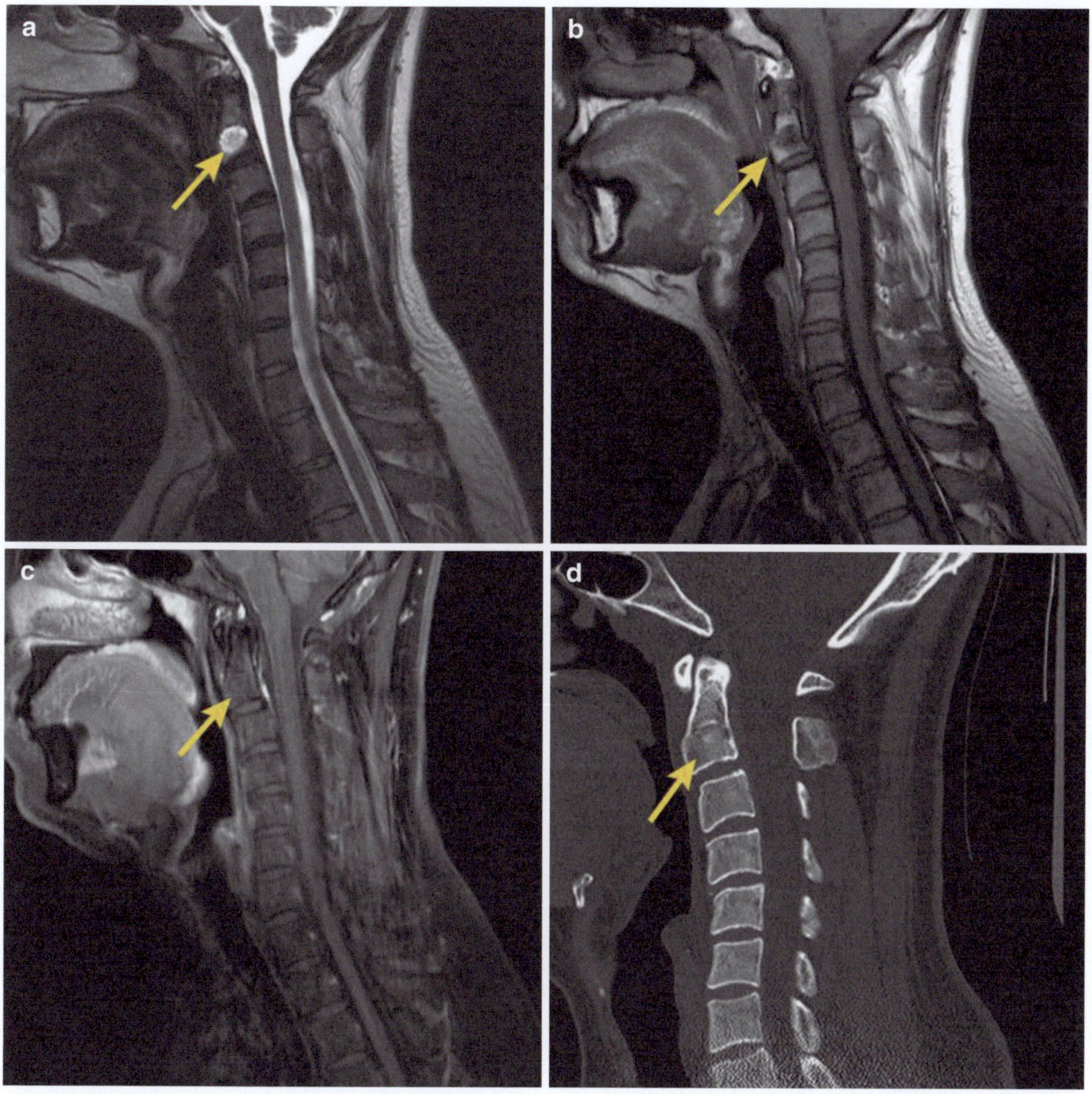

Fig. 11.20 Example of a benign notochordal cell tumor (BNCT) in a 30-year-old male patient. There is a well-defined tumor in the C2 vertebral body, located in the midline. It shows high signal intensity in the T2-weighted image (**a**), low signal intensity in the T1-weighted image (**b**), and no enhancement in the fat-suppressed contrast-enhanced T1-weighted image (**c**), which is consistent with BNCT. This lesion shows subtle sclerosis in the CT image (**d**)

bleeding, and there may be few giant cells. Fibrous tissues with collagen components may be present in larger amounts in certain areas [3]. It commonly accompanies secondary aneurysmal bone cystic (ABC) changes. The most common site is the sacrum, followed by the thoracic spine, cervical spine, and lumbar spine [25, 26]. It is most common between the ages of 10 and 30, and slightly more common in men than women (3:2). It can be accompanied by symptoms such as radiating pain, muscle weakness, and sensory abnormalities. It can also grow very quickly during pregnancy due to hormonal stimulation. It primarily shows osteolysis and bulging (enlarge-

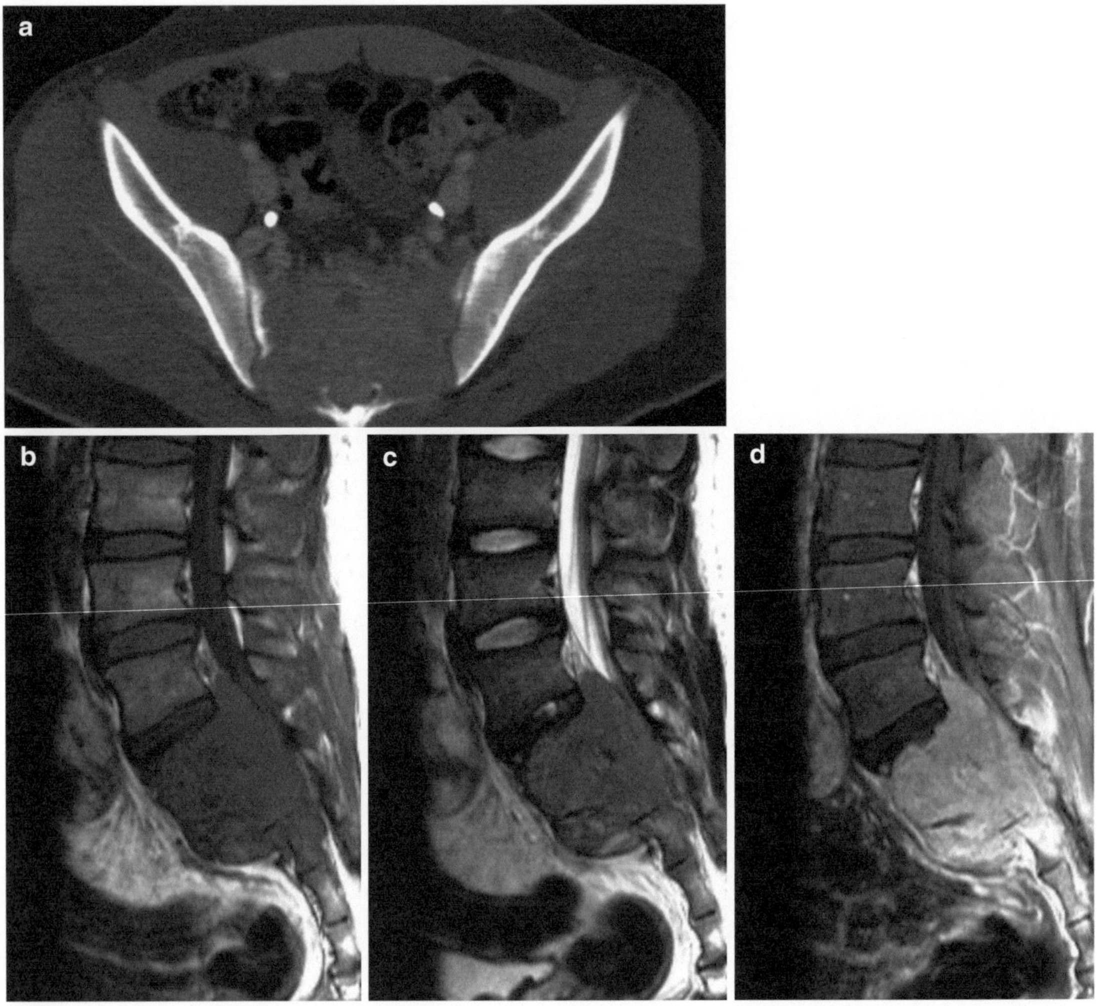

Fig. 11.21 CT and MRI findings of giant cell tumor. In the CT image (**a**), an osteolytic soft tissue mass is observed in the neural foramen, sacral body, and sacral ala of the first and second vertebrae. Both MR T1-weighted image (**b**) and T2-weighted image (**c**) show low or moderate signal intensity, and strong enhancement is seen after contrast injection (**d**). Invasion into part of the adjacent disc and central canal is also observed

ment), and does not usually accompany calcification inside (Fig. 11.21). When it occurs in the sacrum, it is most common in the first and second sacral vertebrae, and often invades the sacral neural foramen, sacral body and ala, and sacroiliac joint [27]. In the rest of the spine, it often occurs in the vertebral body, causing pathologic compression fractures or spreading to the posterior element or surrounding soft tissues. Although rare, it can also invade the disc or adjacent spine. On a bone scan, it shows a peripheral increased uptake called a donut sign, or a generally increased uptake. On MRI, most cases show low or moderate signal intensity on both T1- and T2-weighted images (90~95% of lesions), which is very rare in other bone tumors (Fig. 11.21). Enhancement is heterogeneous, and there may be areas that do not enhance due to internal necrosis. If ABC change is accompanied, it shows a fluid-fluid level on CT or MRI. This area lacks diagnostic tissue and should be avoided during biopsy. Treatment is primarily curettage or cryosurgery, or bloc resection and bone graft. Partial resection may be performed due to peripheral neurological

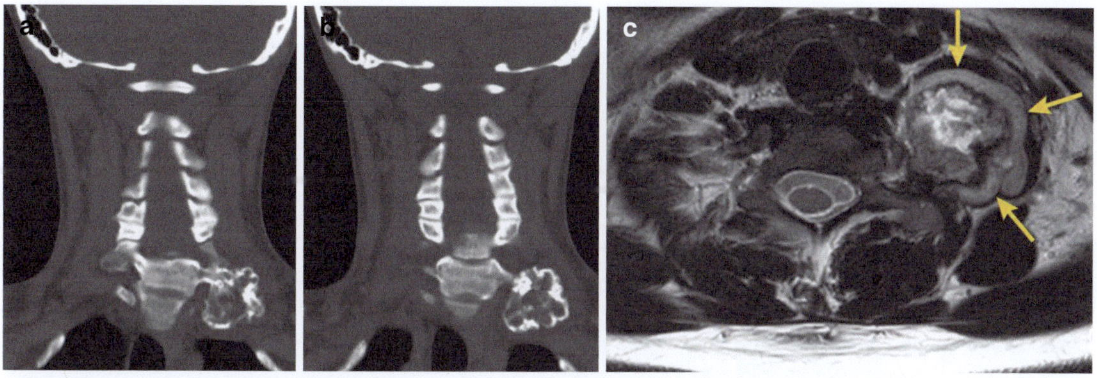

Fig. 11.22 Example of osteochondroma occurring in a 24-year-old female patient. (**a**, **b**) There is an exophytic mass connected to the spine on the Lt. side of C7, which is consistent with osteochondroma. (**c**) In the MR T2-weighted image, the cartilage cap (arrow) surrounding the tumor is observed as high signal intensity

relationships, and radiation therapy may be performed, but there is a disadvantage that secondary sarcoma can occur due to radiation. About 2~25% may recur locally, and this is not related to imaging findings or histological findings [28]. Signs suggesting recurrence are new bone destruction or newly formed soft tissue tumors, and in rare cases of recurrence in soft tissues, peripheral calcification/ossification may be accompanied. Two to five percent may metastasize to the lungs, and more than half of these have benign histological findings. Malignant giant cell tumors account for about 5~7% of giant cell tumors [25, 26, 28–31].

11.2.3.7 Osteochondroma (Exostosis)

Osteochondroma is a rare benign tumor in the spine, with a frequency of about 1% when occurring singly in the spine and accounting for 4% of all spinal tumors [3]. It can occur singly (solitary exostosis) or in multiple forms due to heredity (hereditary multiple exostoses), but even in these cases, only 7~9% occur in the spine. Histologically, it is a protruding bone that is connected to both the medullary bone and the cortical bone, and the cartilage covers the end of the protruding bone. Osteochondroma can occur anywhere in the spine, but it is most common in the cervical spine (especially C2). In the case of solitary, it is usually found between the ages of 20 and 30, and in the case of hereditary multiple exostoses, it is found at a younger age. Osteochondromas that point towards the back are more common than those that point towards the spinal canal or neural foramen. Osteochondromas are often detected early because they press on nerves or the spinal cord, causing neurological symptoms to appear quickly (Fig. 11.22) [32–34]. Unlike osteochondromas that occur in the upper body, it is often difficult to see in simple imaging due to the complex anatomical structure of the spine. In MRI, characteristic connected medullary bone, cortical bone, and bone protrusions showing the same signal intensity are visible. In T1 enhanced images, a medium or low signal intensity cartilage cap is seen covering the protruding end of the bone like a hat. In T2 enhanced images, a high signal intensity cartilage cap is seen. If this cartilage cap is thicker than 1.5 cm, malignant transformation to chondrosarcoma should be suspected [3]. Most can be cured by surgical resection, and symptoms improve in about 89% of patients. Although rare, recurrence can occur if the resection is incomplete [21, 32–34].

11.2.4 Spinal Primary Malignant Osseous Tumor

11.2.4.1 Chordoma

Chordoma is the most common primary malignant osseous tumor in the spine of adults, excluding hematologic malignancy. It is known to

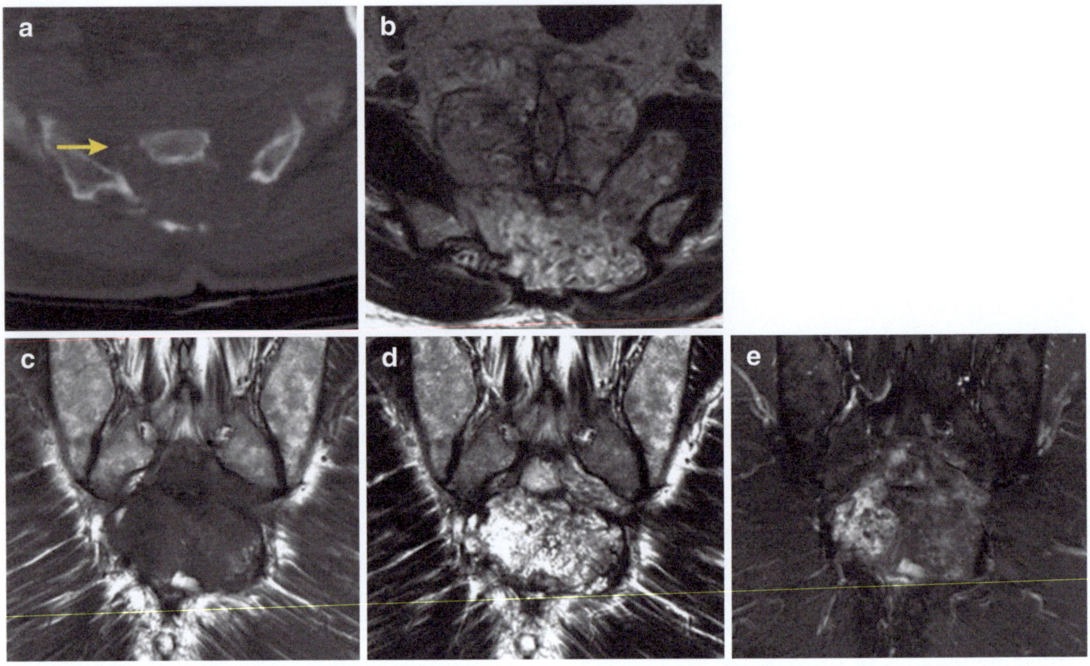

Fig. 11.23 CT and MRI findings of chordoma. In the CT image (**a**), an osteolytic lesion is destroying and expanding the sacrum's central canal and neural foramen, and calcification within the lesion is observed. In the MR T2 enhanced axial image (**b**), similar to CT, it is forming a soft tissue mass in the presacral area while expanding the central canal and neural foramen. In the oblique coronal image taken parallel to the axis of the sacrum, the lesion shows low signal intensity in the T1 enhanced image (**c**), high signal intensity in the T2 enhanced image (**d**), and heterogeneous enhancement in the periphery in the contrast-enhanced fat-suppressed T1 enhanced image (**e**). There is a high signal intensity area in the T1 enhanced image (**c**) that is thought to be a hemorrhage

originate from notochordal remnants extended from Rathke's pouch of the coccyx. About 50% occur in the sacrum, 35% in the clivus, and 15% in the rest of the movable spine (especially the cervical spine). Unlike giant cell tumors, when it occurs in the sacrum, it originates from the lower part (S3, S4) [35–39]. It usually occurs in the center of the vertebral body and rarely in a paracentral location slightly away from the center, following the spine from the surrounding tissues of the spine, which is called "parachordoma" [3]. It is most common in the 40s and occurs most frequently between the ages of 30 and 60. The most common imaging finding is bone destruction, and bony sclerosis is seen in about 15% of cases originating from the movable spine segment. Tumor calcification is observed in about 64% of simple imaging and CT [40]. Invasion into the surrounding soft tissues is common and can also spread to the sacroiliac joint (SI joint) [41]. On T1-weighted MRI, it shows low or medium signal intensity and very high signal intensity on T2-weighted images, which is due to its high water content, similar to the nucleus pulposus of the disc (Fig. 11.23) [41]. When it occurs in the spheno-occipital region or within the skull, it may show increased signal intensity on T1-weighted images due to its high protein content, which is rare in the spine [39, 40, 42]. Lobular margins and areas with hemorrhage are also occasionally observed (Fig. 11.23). During contrast enhancement, enhancement is mainly observed in the thick periphery and septum. These findings are similar to chondrosarcoma, but they appear more prominently. The location of the tumor determines whether complete resection is possible, which is related to the patient's prognosis. In cases that occur in the sacrococcygeal region, the survival rate is higher than in other locations because complete resection is often possible [3].

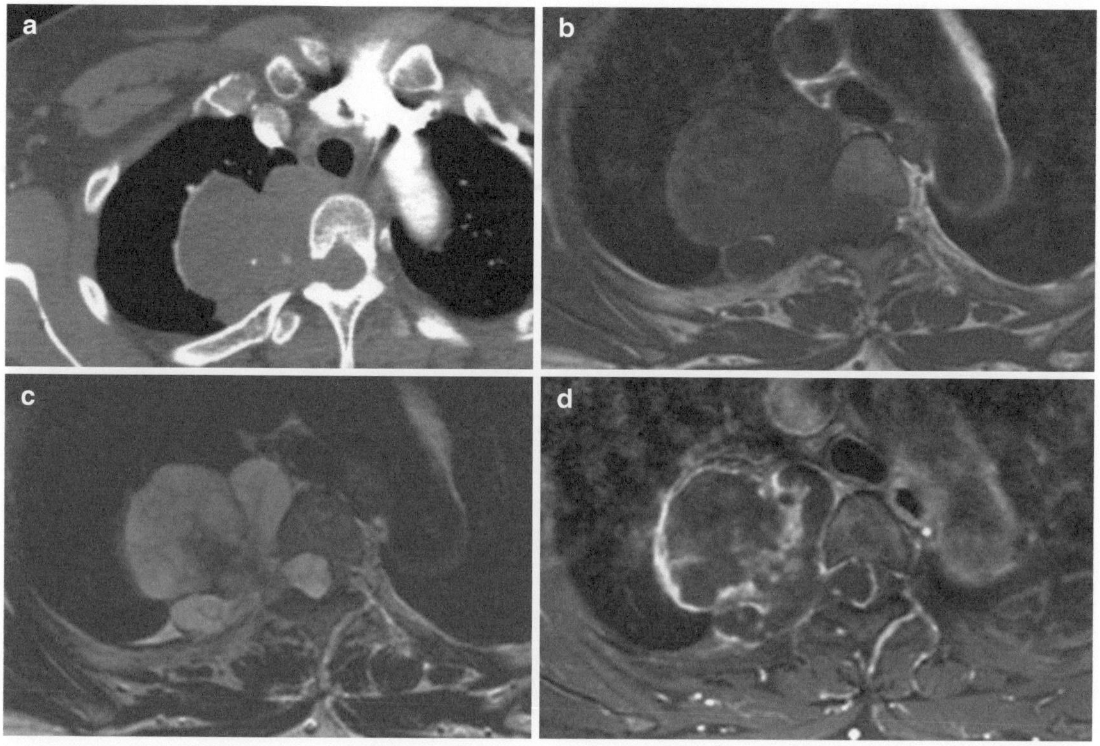

Fig. 11.24 CT and MRI findings of chondrosarcoma. In the CT image (**a**), there is a low attenuation mass that destroys the right pedicle of the thoracic vertebra and invades the central canal and right thoracic cavity through the neural foramen, and there is calcification inside. The mass appears as low signal intensity in the MR T1 enhanced image (**b**), high signal intensity in the T2 enhanced image (**c**), and shows enhancement in the periphery and septum in the fat-suppressed contrast-enhanced T1 enhanced image (**d**)

11.2.4.2 Chondrosarcoma

Chondrosarcoma accounts for 7–12% of all primary malignant tumors that occur in the spine of adults, and the frequency of occurrence in the spine among all chondrosarcomas is about 3–12% [43]. Histologically, lobular articular cartilage is it is divided by a fibrovascular septum and may contain mucous tissue. Most chondrosarcomas are low grade. They can occur anywhere, but are most common in the thoracic spine and can also occur in the vertebral body, but are more common in the posterior element (40%). The average age is 45 and it is two to four times more common in men than women. Symptoms include pain, palpable mass, and neurological symptoms. On plain radiography and CT, "ring and arc calcification" like cartilaginous calcification is observed along with bone destruction findings [43, 44]. On MR T1-weighted images, it appears as low signal intensity, and on T2-weighted images, it appears as high signal intensity. The boundary of the articular cartilage is best seen on T2-weighted images (Fig. 11.24). On contrast enhancement, both CT and MRI show enhancement in the periphery and septum. The part showing calcification of the stroma appears as low signal intensity in all pulse sequences, but is better seen on CT than MRI. Treatment is recommended for surgical resection if possible, and if complete resection is impossible due to the location or size of the lesion, about 74% may die due to recurrence. Chemotherapy or radiation therapy does not have a good prognosis in chondrosarcoma [3].

11.2.4.3 Osteosarcoma

Osteosarcoma occurring in the spine is relatively rare, accounting for 0.6–4% of all osteosarcomas and about 5% of all primary malignant tumors occurring in the spine [45]. It occurs at a slightly older age (30s) than those occurring in the limbs and is more common in men [45]. Symptoms include pain and palpable mass, and about 70–80% have neurological symptoms [45]. Tumor-induced bone turn-over increases, raising the level of serum alkaline phosphatase. It can occur anywhere, but is most common in the thoracolumbar segments. When it occurs in the spine, it is pathologically mostly high grade, and the osteoblastic type is the most common, but there can also be chondroblastic type and fibroblastic type. If osseous calcification is severe, the vertebral body may appear white. Bone scan shows very increased uptake. MRI is very useful for determining the extent of the lesion, soft tissue invasion, mass formation, and the relationship with the spinal cord and nerve root (Fig. 11.25). Areas with a lot of bone formation

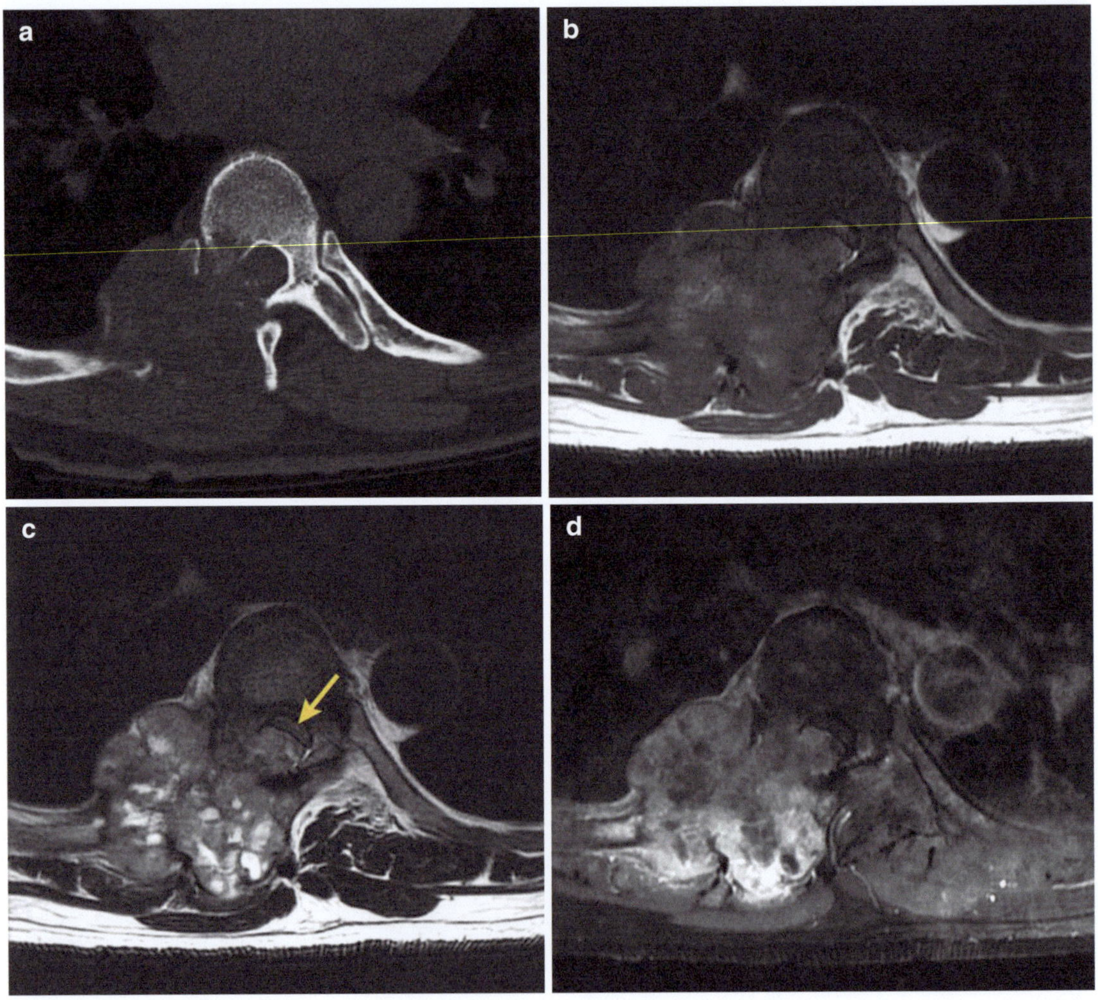

Fig. 11.25 CT and MRI findings of osteosarcoma. In the CT image (**a**), an ill-defined osteolytic mass that invades the right vertebral body's posterior element and rib, forms a soft tissue mass, and calcification is observed. It appears as heterogeneous signal intensity in the MR T1 enhanced image (**b**) and heterogeneous signal intensity in the T2 enhanced image (**c**). Inside, there is a high signal intensity in the T1 enhanced image and a secondary ABC change with a multilocular septum in the T2 enhanced image. It invades the surrounding soft tissue as in CT and extends to the central canal, compressing the spinal cord (**c**, arrow). In the fat-suppressed contrast-enhanced T1 enhanced image (**d**), the internal solid portion is strongly enhanced, and the part with secondary ABC change is not enhanced

show low signal intensity in all sequences. Complete resection is often impossible due to the location of the lesion and soft tissue mass, and the prognosis is poor despite chemotherapy and radiation therapy, usually dying within 1 year of diagnosis [3, 45].

11.2.4.4 Ewing Sarcoma and Primitive Neuroectodermal Tumor (PNET)

Ewing sarcoma and primitive neuroectodermal tumor (PNET) are often classified together because they are histologically, radiologically, and clinically very similar. These types of tumors are the most common primary malignant tumors occurring in the spine in children and adolescents, excluding hematologic malignancies. They are slightly more common in males [46–49]. About 3–10% of all Ewing sarcoma and PNET primary origins occur in the spine, and it is more common for them to metastasize to the spine from elsewhere. The common sites of occurrence are the sacrum and coccyx, and it can also occur in the lumbar, thoracic, and very rarely, cervical spine [46–49]. Necrosis within the tumor is common, and it can appear in various shapes on plain radiography and CT, most often as very aggressive osteolytic lesions, causing malignant compression fractures or appearing as flat vertebrae (vertebra plana). It is characteristic that it can involve multiple compartments like hematologic malignancies, and accordingly, it can invade the vertebral body, spinal canal, and soft tissues well, forming a large soft tissue mass around the spine (Fig. 11.26) [46–49]. At this time, the formation of a soft tissue mass may have little to no destruction of the cortical bone, which is also a finding observed in other small round cell tumors such as leukemia, multiple myeloma, and lymphoma. Bone scans typically show increased uptake. On MRI, it appears non-specifically, with equal signal intensity on T1-weighted images and equal/high signal intensity on T2-weighted images (Fig. 11.26) [46–49]. Due to the location of the tumor and the formation of a large soft tissue mass, surgical removal is often impossible, and chemotherapy and radiation therapy are the main treatments [46–49]. The most influential factor in prognosis is the location of the tumor.

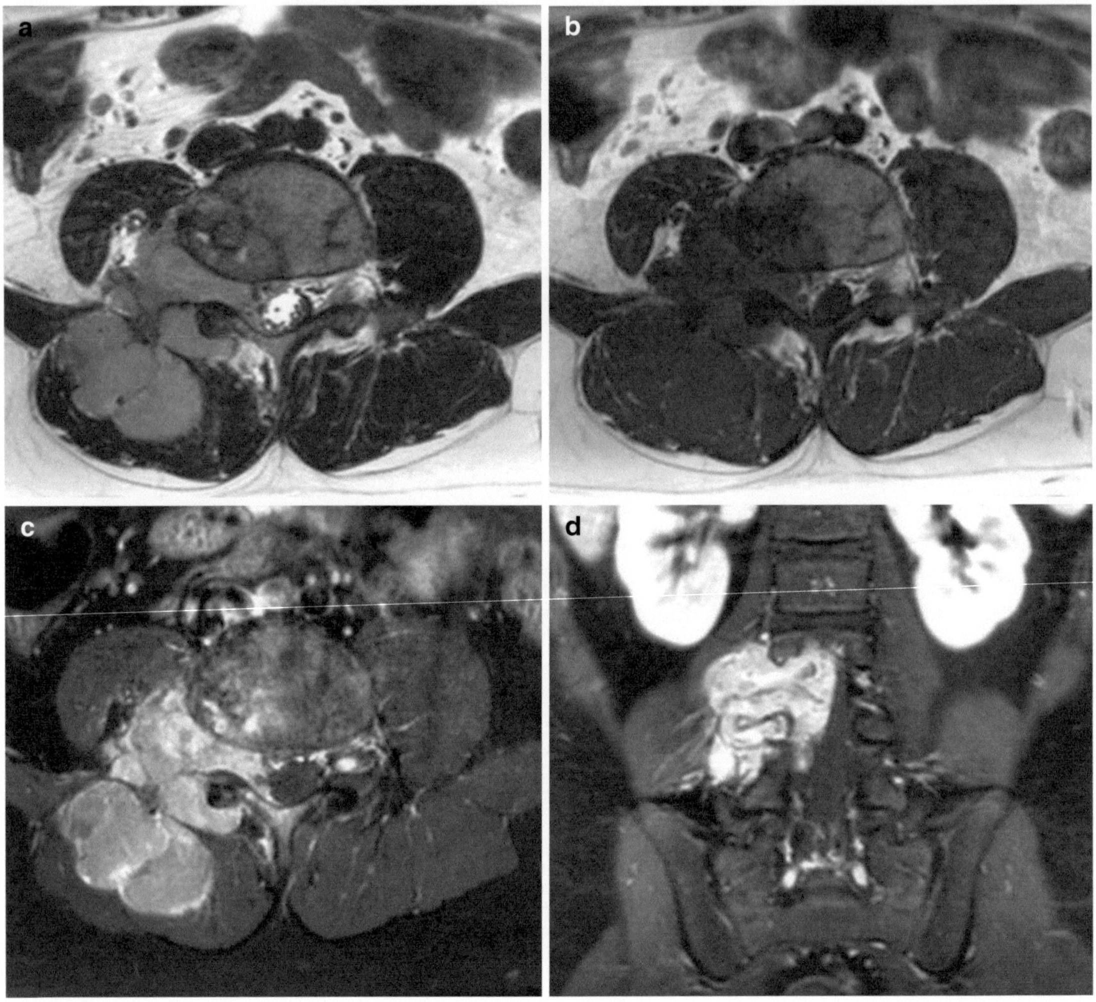

Fig. 11.26 An example of Ewing sarcoma in an 8-year-old male pediatric patient. In the MR T2-weighted image (**a**, **b**), a tumor showing high signal intensity and low signal intensity in the T2-weighted image is showing multi-compartment involvement through the vertebral body, epidural space, and paravertebral space. Such a mass is very well enhanced in the fat-suppressed contrast-enhanced T1-weighted image (**c**, **d**). The boundary of the tumor that compromises the central canal and extends to the neural foramen and paravertebral space is well seen in the contrast-enhanced T1-weighted coronal image (**d**)

11.3 Extradural Non-osseous Tumor

11.3.1 Common Extradural Non-osseous Tumor

11.3.1.1 Peripheral Nerve Sheath Tumor (Schwannoma, Neurofibroma)

Peripheral nerve sheath tumors (schwannoma, neurofibroma) that occur in this area are the most common tumors not only in this area but also in the intradural extramedullary (IDEM) space. They can originate only in the extradural space, extend from the intradural space to the extradural space, or be located only in the intradural space. These two tumors will be described together in the next chapter (intradural extramedullary tumor), and in this chapter, we intend to show extradural schwannoma (Fig. 11.27) and neurofibroma (Fig. 11.28).

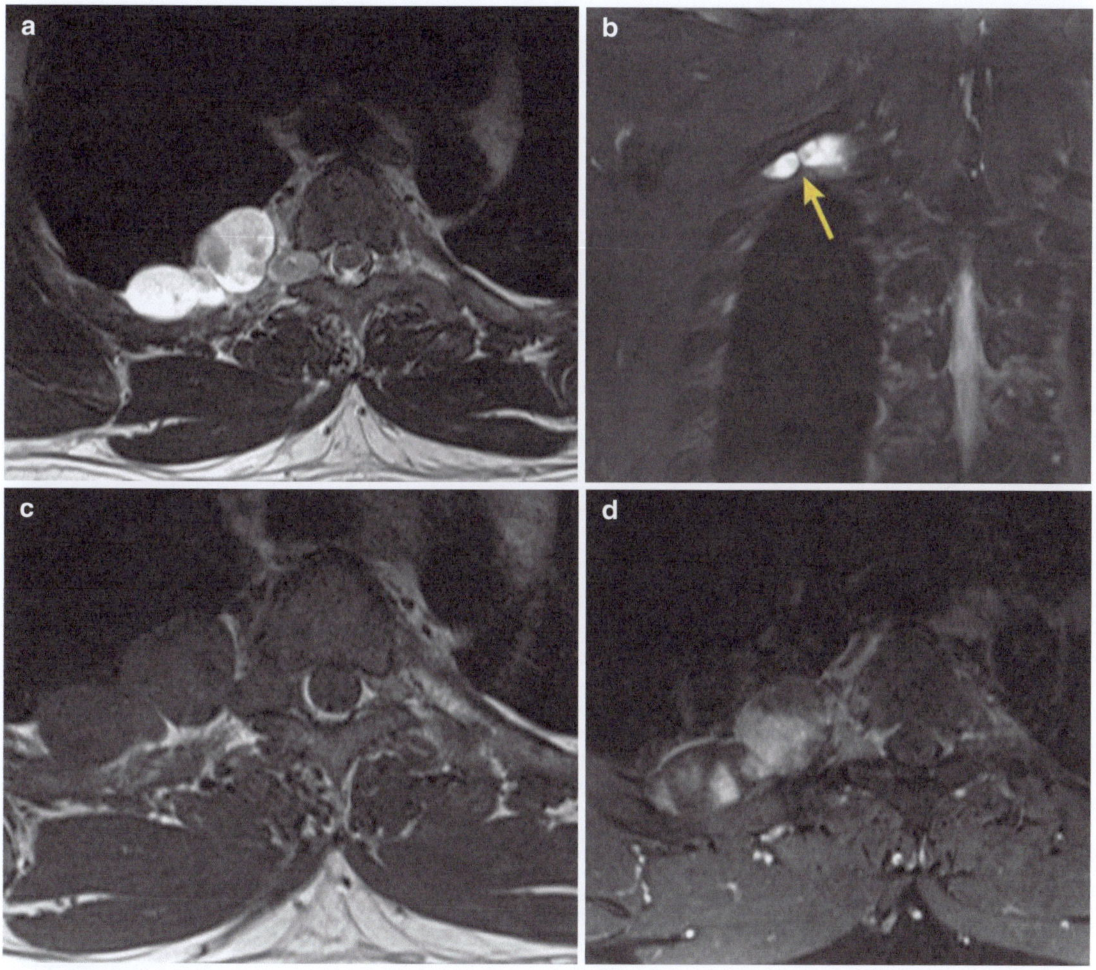

Fig. 11.27 An example of extradural schwannoma originating from the thoracic vertebra. In the MR T2-weighted image (**a**), a lobular contour mass showing high signal intensity is seen. It is extending from the right neural foramen to the intercostal space (**b**). T1-weighted image (**c**) shows a low signal intensity and fat-suppressed contrast enhancement. T1-weighted image (d) shows contrast enhancement in the periphery and the solid portion inside the tumor

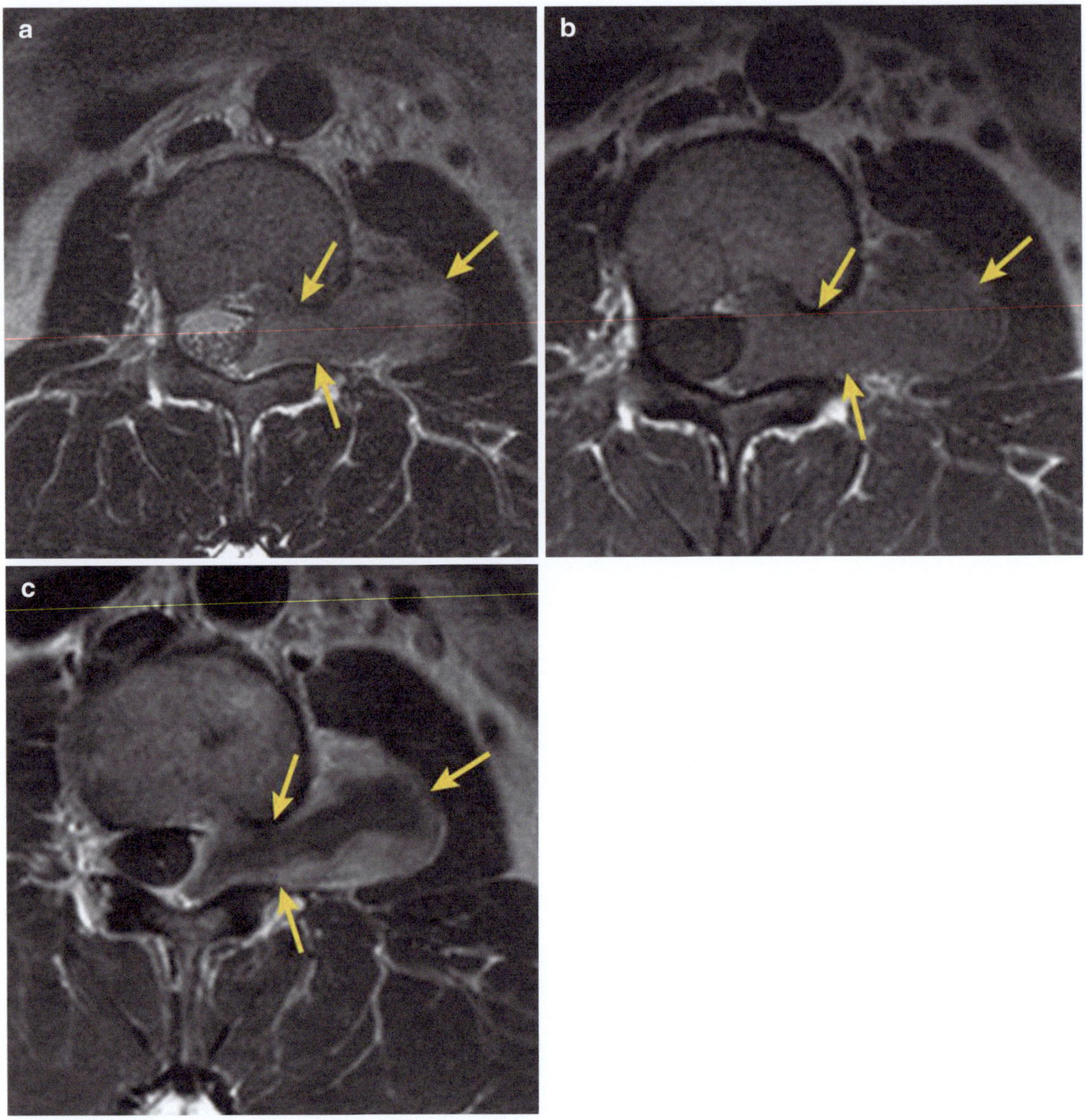

Fig. 11.28 An example of extradural neurofibroma. In the MR T2 enhanced image, a dumbbell-shaped mass with mixed low and high signal intensity is seen along the left neural foramen (**a**, arrow). This appears as a low signal intensity lesion in the T1 enhanced image and is accompanied by erosion at the back of the vertebral body (**b**). The tumor shows contrast enhancement along its outer edge in the contrast-enhanced T1 enhanced image (**c**). The dural sac is pushed aside, but no tumor extension into the intradural space is seen

11.3.2 Other Extradural Non-osseous Tumor

11.3.2.1 Angiolipoma

This is a rare tumor that occurs in the epidural space, but its image finding is characteristic. It mainly occurs in people in their 40s and 50s and is more common in women than in men. It usually occurs in the dorsal (posterior) epidural space of the thoracic spine. As can be seen from the name of the tumor, it contains both fatty and vascular components, and these two findings appear on CT and MRI. The fatty component shows low attenuation on CT, and on MRI, it shows high signal intensity on both T1- and T2-weighted images and fat suppression on fat

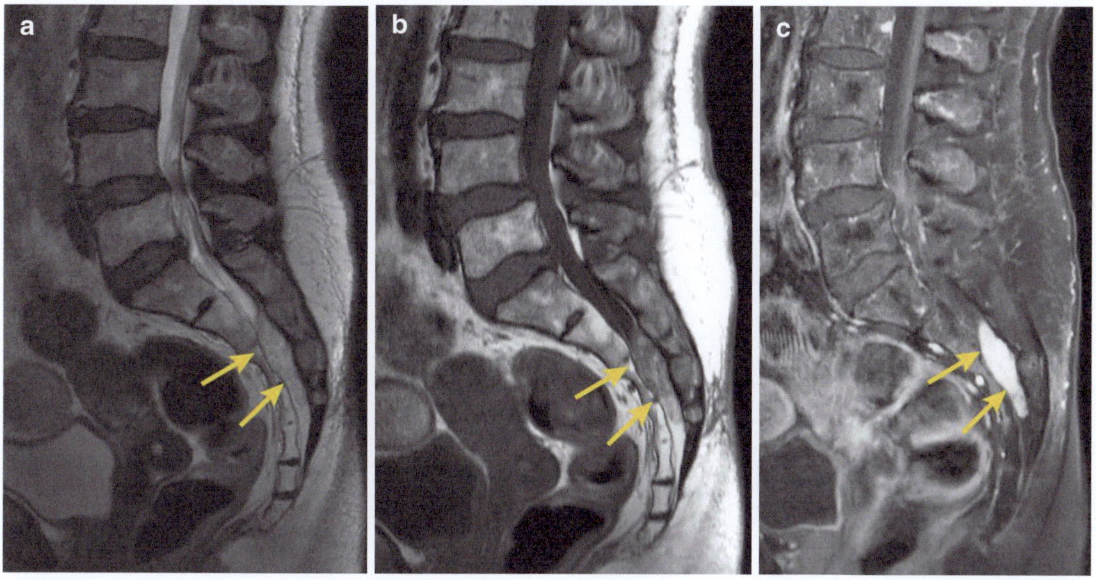

Fig. 11.29 Angiolioma originating from the sacral epidural space. There is a well-defined tumor with a lobular contour in the epidural space at the S2-3-4 level. In the MR T2 (**a**) and T1 (**b**) enhanced images, it shows high signal intensity due to the fatty component, and a somewhat lower signal intensity mixed in due to the vascular component inside. The tumor shows very strong contrast enhancement in the fat-suppressed contrast-enhanced T1 enhanced image (**c**)

suppression sequences. Due to the vascular component, it shows very strong enhancement on fat-suppressed contrast-enhanced T1-weighted images (Fig. 11.29). Most of them have good boundaries and appear as a lobular contour. Some infiltration angiolipomas have been reported, and in these cases, infiltration findings into surrounding structures can be seen.

11.4 Intradural Extramedullary Tumor

11.4.1 Common Intradural Extramedullary Tumor

11.4.1.1 Peripheral Nerve Sheath Tumor (Schwannoma, Neurofibroma)

This is the most common primary tumor occurring in the spine and at the same time, it is the most common tumor in the intradural extramedullary space, accounting for about 70~75%. It mainly includes schwannoma and neurofibroma. Schwannoma is composed of nerve sheaths. Originating from Schwann cells, neurofibromas are tumors composed of peripheral nerves, Schwann cells, and fibroblasts. They are common in people aged 30–60, with no gender difference. Most appear as single lesions, but peripheral nerve sheath tumors that occur multifocally at a younger age may be a sign of neurofibromatosis type 1 or 2 [50]. They are often accompanied by symptoms such as pain or radiating pain in the lower extremities, and they usually grow very slowly. Typical schwannomas do not recur, but those associated with neurofibromatosis or melanotic schwannoma may. If the size increases rapidly or the pain suddenly worsens, the possibility of malignant transformation should be considered, especially in patients with neurofibromatosis, as the likelihood of malignant transformation is high. Contrast-enhanced MRI is most useful for diagnosis. As a well-defined solid tumor, it most commonly occurs in the thoracic region. On MR T1-weighted images, it shows a signal intensity similar to the adjacent spinal cord, slightly higher signal intensity on T2-weighted images,

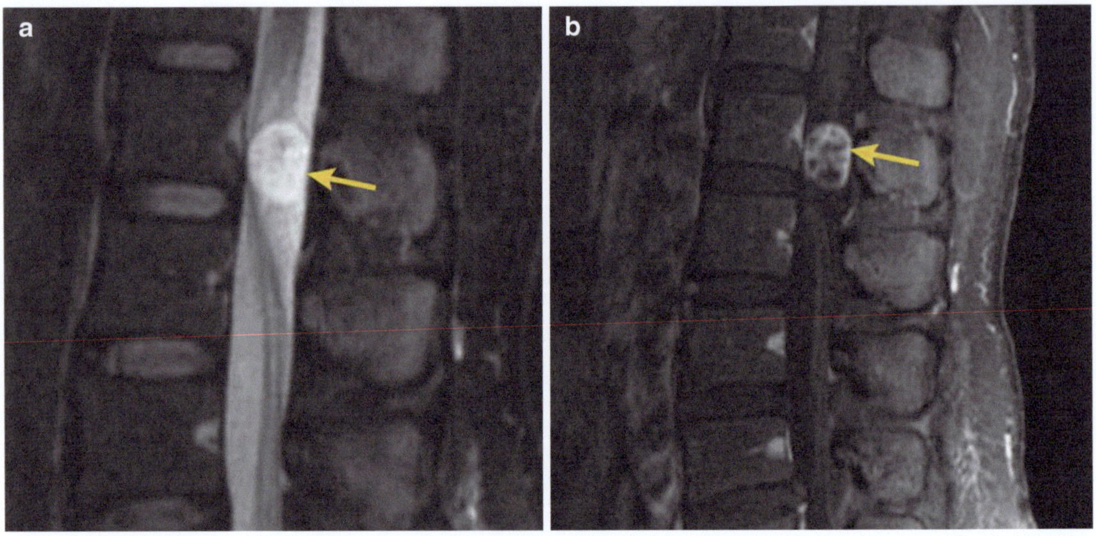

Fig. 11.30 An example of a peripheral nerve sheath tumor (schwannoma). In the T2 enhanced image, there is a relatively homogeneous high signal intensity intradural extramedullary tumor with good boundaries, which is pushing the adjacent spinal cord forward and the surrounding CSF space appears widened above and below (**a**, arrow). In the fat-suppressed contrast-enhanced T1 enhanced image, it shows heterogeneous contrast enhancement and clear boundaries (**b**)

and various patterns of contrast enhancement. As a well-defined solid tumor, schwannomas often show a mixture of Antoni A, which has a dense cellular composition, and Antoni B, which has a loose cellular composition, usually showing a mixed signal intensity on T2-weighted images. They often show cystic changes internally, but hemorrhage or calcification is rare (Figs. 11.30 and 11.31). The degree of contrast enhancement varies, and if there are many internal cystic changes, it tends to enhance towards the periphery. About 15% of schwannomas grow into the adjacent neural foramen, showing the so-called dumbbell shape appearance, and due to their slow growth, they can cause bone remodeling in the adjacent vertebrae, thinning the adjacent pedicle or widening the neural foramen, and causing scalloping of the vertebral body (Fig. 11.32). They often appear as multiple nodules hanging on the cauda equina [51]. Tumors distributed along multiple nerve roots on both sides across multiple segments are relatively common plexiform neurofibromas in neurofibromatosis type 1. The outer part composed of myxoid material shows high signal intensity on T2-weighted images, and the central part due to the included nerve tissue shows low signal intensity, which is a relatively characteristic appearance of neurofibroma, the "target sign," but it is difficult to distinguish small single lesion neurofibromas from schwannomas. Treatment is surgical resection, and radiosurgery is performed if there is concern about functional damage due to nerve damage.

11.4.1.2 Meningioma

Meningioma is the second most common tumor in the intradural extramedullary space after peripheral nerve sheath tumor, commonly occurring in middle-aged women over 40. It can present symptoms such as radiating pain in the lower extremities and sensory abnormalities. Meningiomas originate from meningothelial cells (arachnoid cap cells), fibroblasts, or trabecular cells that make up the arachnoid membrane, and they grow very slowly. Most are single lesions, but multiple meningiomas can occur in patients with neurofibromatosis type 2, and other tumors such as schwannomas and ependymomas are also common. They usually cause sensory or motor dysfunction, and gait. It is discovered

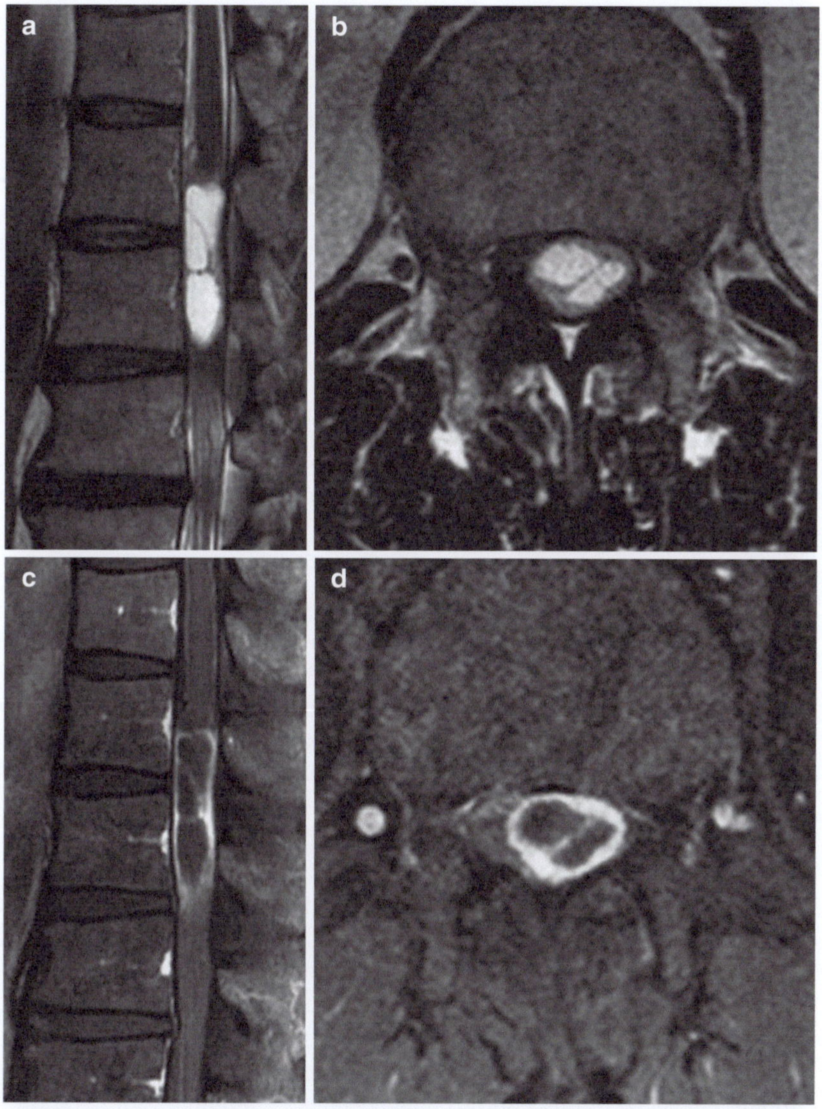

Fig. 11.31 An example of schwannoma with cystic degeneration. In the MR T2 enhanced sagittal image, a long lesion of high signal intensity composed of multiple cysts is located in the intradural space (**a**), and in the T2 enhanced axial image, there is a slightly lower signal intensity outer wall on the outside of the lesion (**b**) and the spinal cord is pushed to the right. In the fat-suppressed contrast-enhanced T1 enhanced sagittal image (**c**) and axial image (**d**), a band of contrast enhancement can be seen along the peripheral margin of the tumor and the septum inside, and most of the mass shows a cystic change that does not enhance

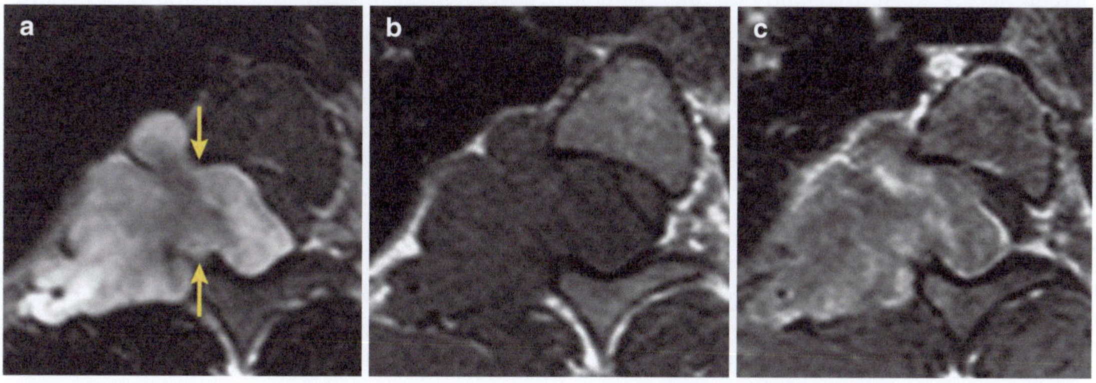

Fig. 11.32 An example of a peripheral nerve sheath tumor (neurofibroma). In the MR T2 enhanced image, a mass mainly showing high signal intensity is spread from the central canal to the peripheral tissues, causing the adjacent neural foramen to widen (**a**, arrow). In the T1 enhanced image, it appears as a low signal intensity lesion (**b**). The mass inside the tumor is unevenly enhanced in the contrast-enhanced T1 image (**c**)

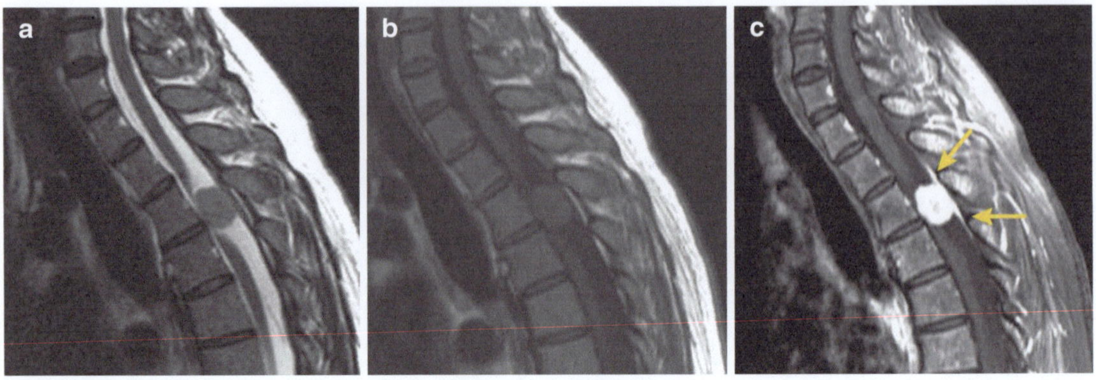

Fig. 11.33 MRI findings of Meningioma. In the MR T2 enhanced image, there is a mass with a slightly higher signal intensity than the adjacent spinal cord (**a**), the CSF space is expanded above and below the mass, and the spinal cord is pushed forward, which is consistent with the findings of an intradural extramedullary tumor. In the T1 enhanced image, it shows a similar signal intensity to the adjacent spinal cord (**b**). In the fat-suppressed contrast-enhanced T1 image, it shows strong enhancement, and the "dural tail sign" is well seen, which shows a long band-like enhancement along the adjacent dura (**c**, arrow)

through symptoms such as disability and pain and occurs in middle-aged women in their 40s and 50s. In contrast-enhanced MRI, it is observed as a mass with good boundaries and a lobulated appearance. It shows a slightly higher signal intensity compared to the adjacent spinal cord in T1 and T2 enhanced images, and it generally shows a relatively uniform signal intensity. Characteristically, it is usually firmly attached to the dura on the ventral side, often showing a dural tail sign ("dural tail sign") along this connection (Fig. 11.33). In about 1~5% of cases, calcification inside or on the surface of the tumor is also accompanied in CT scans (Fig. 11.34). It is very strongly enhanced during contrast enhancement, and it occurs most frequently in the thoracic spine. Most have good boundaries and are round or ovoid in shape, and often show a plaque shape (en plaque). It can cause bone hyperostosis (hyperostosis) in adjacent bones, but unlike peripheral nerve sheath tumors, it does not accompany bone remodeling. Compared to Schwannoma, it is characterized by a slightly lower, uniform signal intensity in T2 enhanced images, and only 2~4% show cystic degeneration, and the dural tail sign and calcification findings help in differentiation. Meningiomas have very rich blood vessels inside and can also show flow-void findings inside. Therefore, angiography and embolization are performed before surgery to reduce the risk of bleeding during surgery [52, 53]. The treatment is to remove it surgically, and radiosurgery is performed if there is concern about functional damage due to nerve damage.

11.4.2 Other Intradural Extramedullary Tumors

11.4.2.1 Intradural Lipoma

Intradural lipoma is a kind of hamartomatous lesion that occurs when mesenchymal cells differentiate into adipose tissue during the normal development process of the neural tube closing. Intradural lipomas can be divided into those that occur in the cervical-thoracic or lumbosacral regions and those that occur in the filum terminale. Most lipomas occur along the filum terminale, which can be associated with spinal dysraphism, leading to the so-called tethered cord syndrome and associated characteristic cutaneous stigma. In 84% of intradural lipomas, they appear in forms associated with lipomyelomeningocele or myelomeningocele. Intradural lipomas that do not accompany spinal dysraphism are usually found in their 10s and 20s due

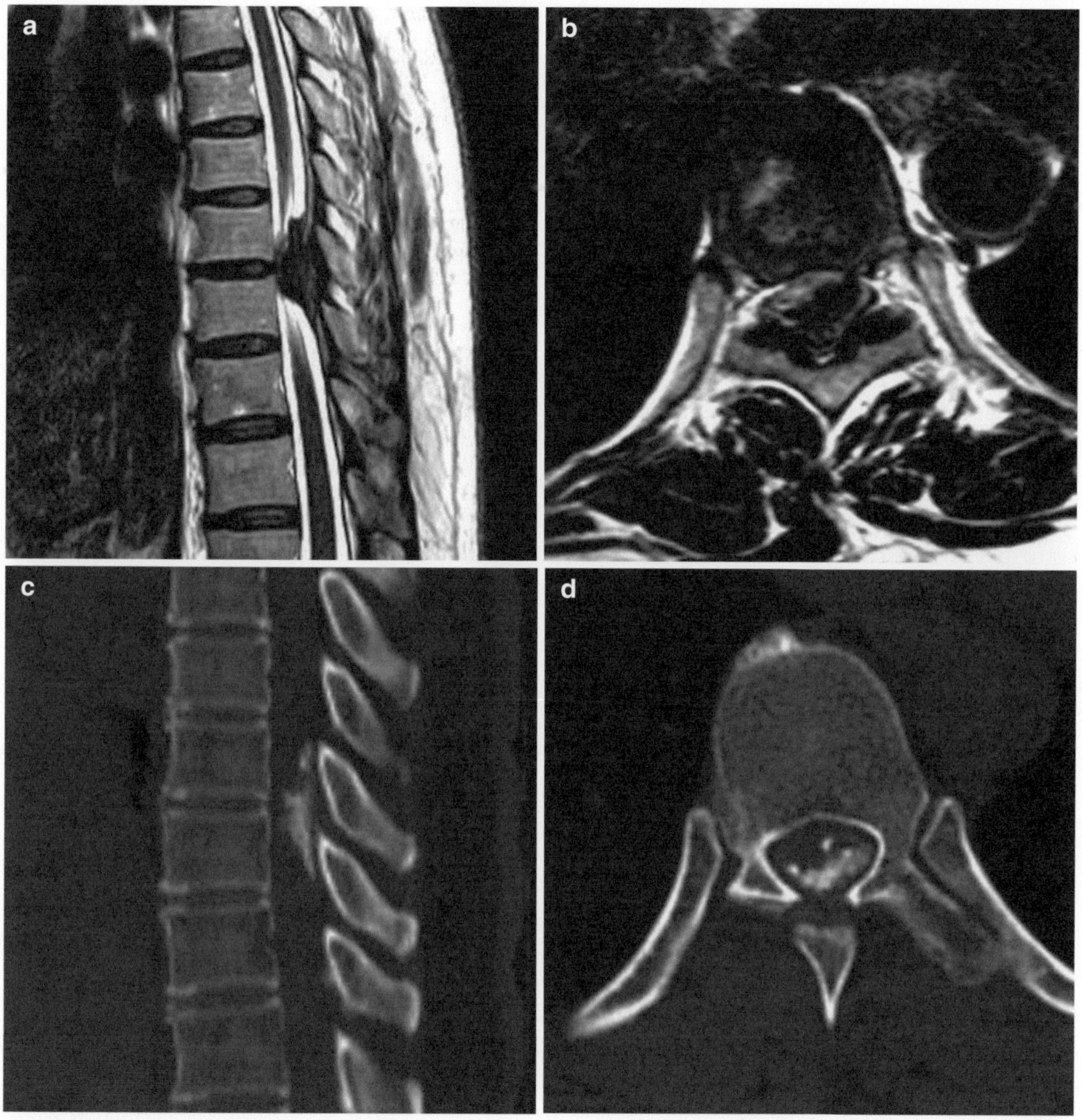

Fig. 11.34 Example of calcified meningioma. In the MR T2 enhanced sagittal image, a triangular mass with a very low signal intensity is attached to the posterior dura (**a**), causing the spinal cord to be pushed forward and severely compressed. In the T2 enhanced axial image, a lesion with a very low signal intensity is located at the back of the spinal cord (**b**). In CT, it can be confirmed that there is a lot of calcification in most of the lesions (**c**, **d**)

to pain, sensory disorders, and neurological symptoms. Intradural lipomas are common in women, whether or not they are associated with spinal dysraphism, and symptoms can worsen during pregnancy. They are most common in the thoracic spine (30%) and are also common in the cervical spine. They usually appear on the dorsal side of the spinal cord (73%), and are rare on the ventral side of the spinal cord. On MRI, it appears as a mass composed of homogeneous high signal intensity fat in T1 enhanced images and does not enhance. Various degrees of spinal dysraphism findings and expansion of the central canal or neural foramen may also be seen. In the fat-suppressed MRI sequence, the internal fat signal disappears, showing a dark signal intensity

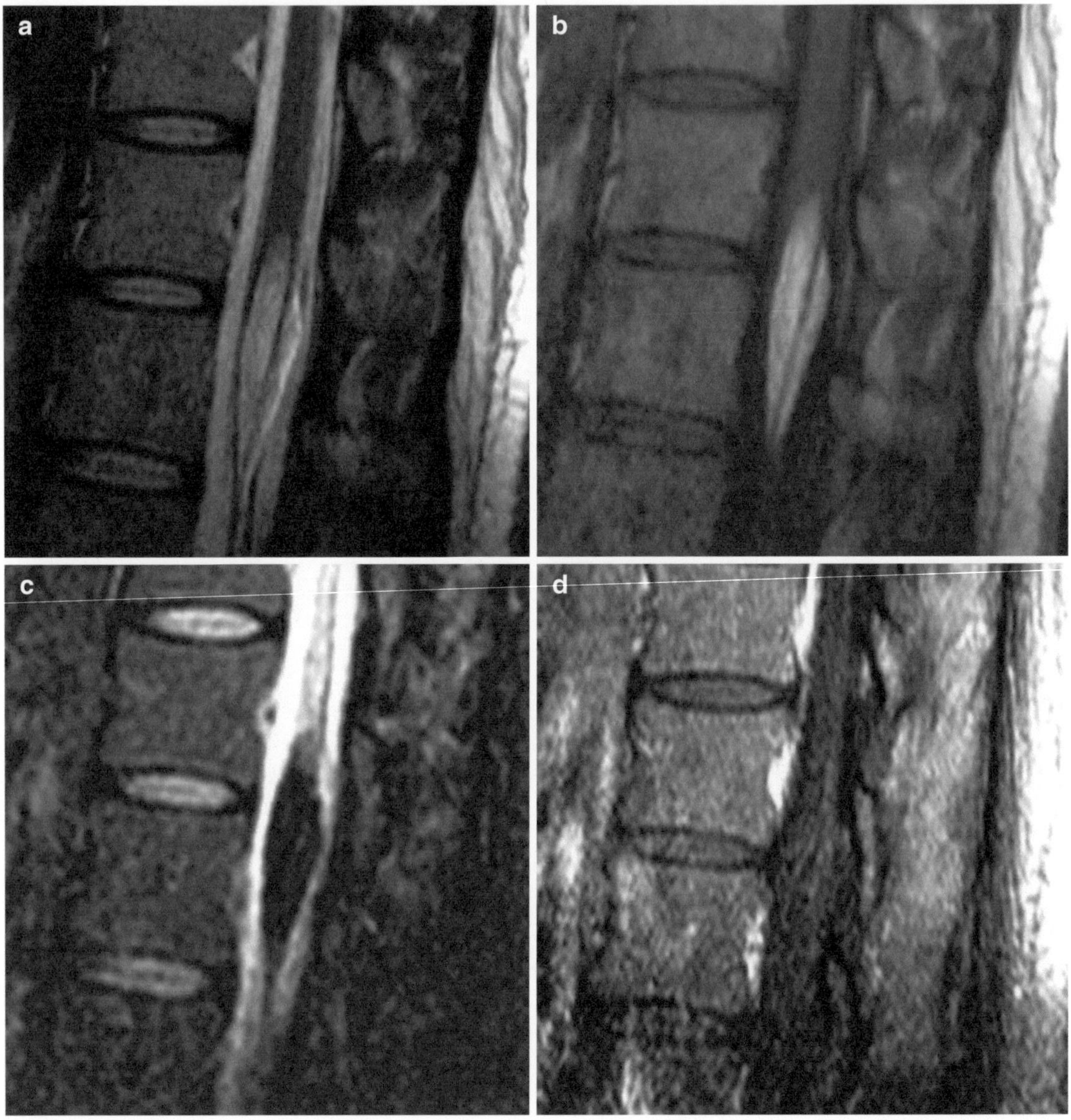

Fig. 11.35 MRI findings of intradural lipoma. In the MRI of a 26-year-old female patient who visited the hospital with back pain, there is a long lesion containing a fatty component that shows high signal intensity in both MR T2 enhanced (**a**) and T1 enhanced (**b**) images, and it includes a long band shape inside, which is thought to be a nerve stem included in the lesion. In addition, a chemical shift artifact occurring between fat and CSF behind the lesion is seen (**a**). In the fat-suppressed T2 enhanced image, the fat inside is completely suppressed and appears as a dark lesion (**c**), and it does not enhance (**d**)

like CSF (Fig. 11.35). There is no enhancement at all [54]. It is treated with surgery, but it is difficult to completely remove it because it usually contains nerves inside. In the case of intradural lipoma that causes symptoms, it is difficult for the symptoms to disappear naturally, so resection is necessary.

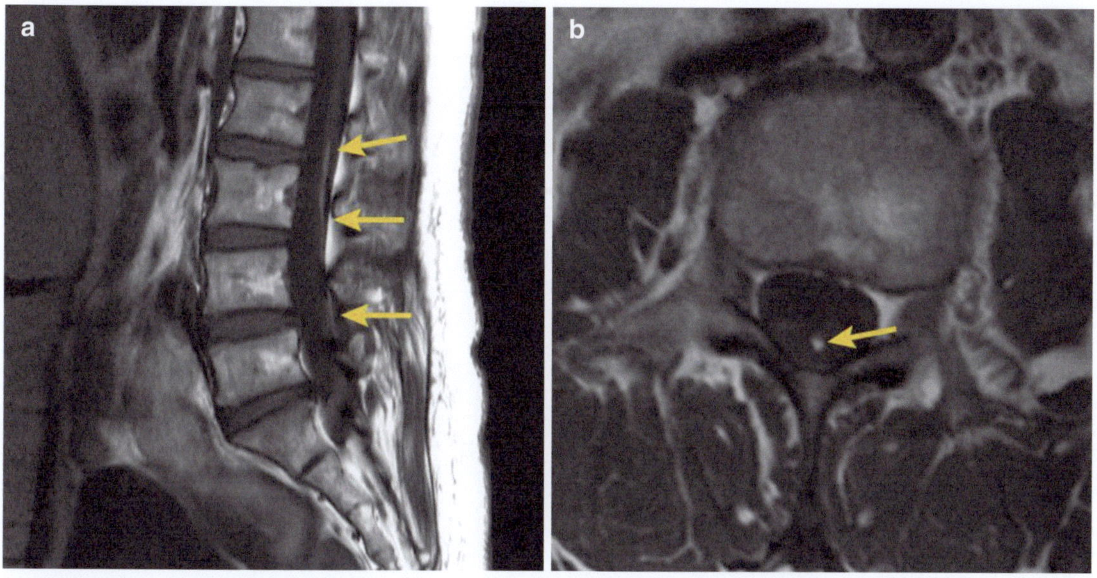

Fig. 11.36 Example of Filum terminale lipoma. In the MR T1 enhanced sagittal (**a**) and axial (**b**) images, due to the fat the lesion appears as a high signal intensity within the central canal and is extending downwards following the course of the filum terminale (arrow)

11.4.2.2 Myxopapillary Ependymoma

Unlike typical intramedullary ependymoma, myxopapillary ependymoma falls into the category of intradural extramedullary tumors and occurs around the conus of the lumbar spine, filum terminale, and cauda equina (Fig. 11.36). It can occur at all ages and tends to occur in slightly younger ages (30s to 40s) compared to ependymoma, and it is more common in men than women. It usually spans the length of 2–4 vertebral body segments and can fill the intradural space of the lumbar spine. It often grows slowly and often accompanies bone remodeling of adjacent bones. On MRI, a well-defined, large lobular mass grows in the craniocaudal direction and is located in the middle of the central canal. Most show a lot of cystic changes and various degrees of enhancement, and strong enhancement is common in most cases (Fig. 11.37) [55]. It often shows high signal intensity on T1 enhanced images due to the high mucin content inside, and hemosiderin deposition due to hemorrhage is also common. Before hemorrhage, it shows high signal intensity on T2 enhanced images. Due to the abundant blood vessels, flow-voids can be seen, and superficial siderosis showing dark signals on the surface of the spinal cord or cerebellum due to repeated hemorrhages can also appear. Especially in children, the presence of leptomeningeal seeding should be carefully examined. Some also accompany calcification.

11.4.2.3 Paraganglioma

Paraganglioma is a tumor that originates from chromaffin cells that make up the autonomic nervous system. It is a type of extra-adrenal pheochromocytoma, but it usually does not secrete catecholamines, and only about 1–3% are known to secrete norepinephrine, epinephrine, etc. It is also called a glomus tumor, extra-adrenal pheochromocytoma, or chemodectoma. It mainly occurs in middle-aged adults between the ages of 40 and 50 and often occurs in the conus medullaris or filum terminale of the lumbar spine. It grows very slowly and the prognosis varies depending on the location of the tumor. Symptoms can include back or leg pain, sensory or motor abnormalities, and urinary or bowel disorders. In terms of imag-

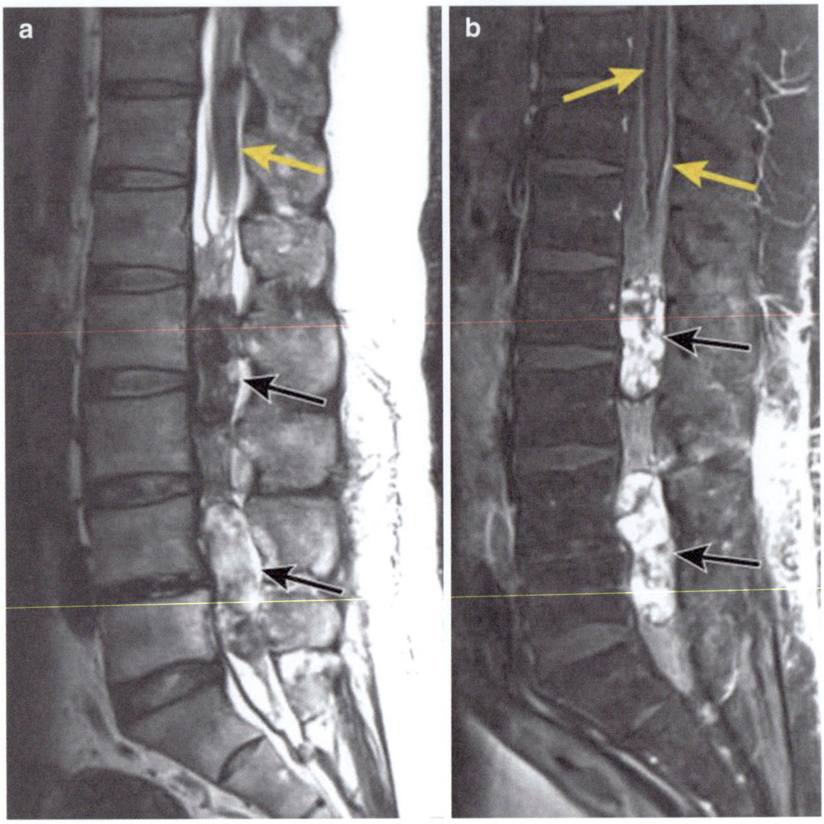

Fig. 11.37 Example of myxopapillary ependymoma. In the MR T2-weighted image, there are two large heterogeneous high signal-low signal intensity bulky masses that occupy almost the entire central canal in the lumbar spine (black arrow), and superficial siderosis of low signal intensity along the conus medullaris is accompanied (yellow arrow) (**a**). The mass (black arrow) shows uneven and strong enhancement in the fat-suppressed contrast-enhanced T1-weighted sagittal image (**b**), and the findings of superficial siderosis along the conus medullaris are well seen as in the T2-weighted image (yellow arrow)

ing findings, it is almost identical to a single myxopapillary ependymoma. On MRI, it is a well-defined mass located in the cauda equina, showing low signal intensity on T1 enhanced images and high signal intensity on T2 enhanced images, and is characterized by strong enhancement. There are many vessels showing multiple flow-void signs inside and around the mass, giving a "salt and pepper" appearance (Fig. 11.38). The size of the mass varies up to over 5 cm, but it is usually large and often accompanies bone remodeling of adjacent bones. Many cases accompany cystic changes showing very high signal intensity on T2 enhanced images, and due to frequent hemorrhages, many cases accompany hemosiderin deposition inside and around the mass. It is removed by surgery. Angiography and embolization are sometimes performed first to reduce bleeding during surgery [56]. If completely resected, the recurrence rate is known to be <5%.

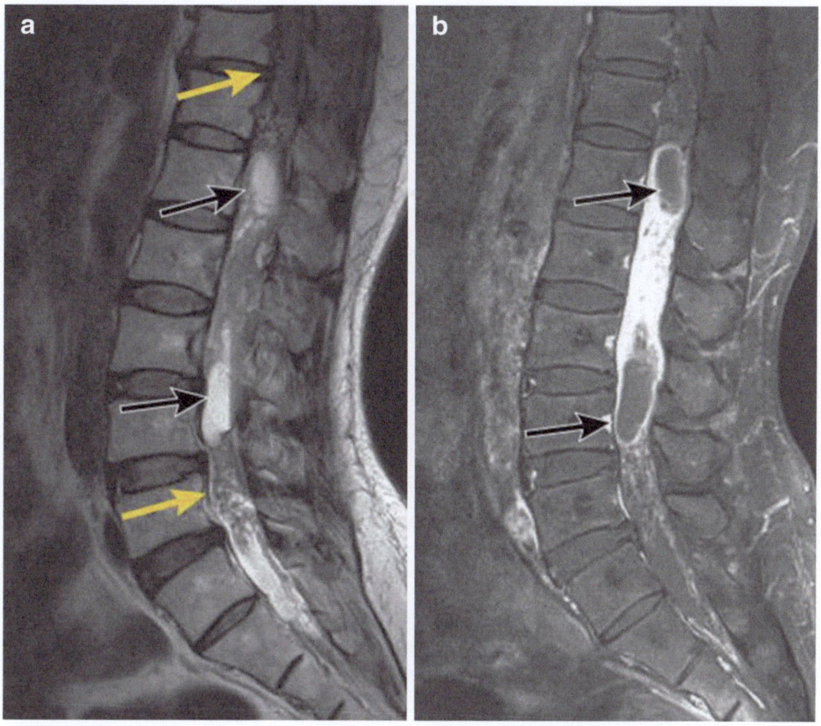

Fig. 11.38 Paraganglioma. On the lumbar T2 enhanced image, a wide-ranging lesion of high and low signal intensity fills the entire central canal, accompanied by cystic changes inside (**a**, black arrow). There are low signal intensity flow-voids above and below the lesion, indicating the presence of abundant vessels around the mass (yellow arrow). On the fat-suppressed contrast-enhanced T1 enhanced image, the mass appears as a long lesion with mostly very strong enhancement, accompanied by non-enhancing cystic changes inside (**b**)

11.5 Intramedullary Tumor

11.5.1 Common Intramedullary Tumor

11.5.1.1 Ependymoma

Ependymoma is a tumor originating from the ependymal cells of the central canal, and it is the most common intramedullary tumor in adults, accounting for about 60%. It is most common in middle-aged men and histologically includes myxopapillary ependymoma, subependymoma, and anaplastic ependymoma. It usually appears as a single mass, but in patients with neurofibromatosis type 2, it can show multiple masses or be accompanied by schwannoma or meningioma. Although it is a malignant tumor, it grows very slowly, so neurological symptoms often appear late, taking an average of 2.5 years to manifest. Characteristically, it can cause superficial siderosis by repeatedly causing microhemorrhages on the surface, which can lead to cranial nerve disorders. Most are well-defined, hemorrhagic, and strongly enhancing masses located in the middle of the spinal cord, and the corresponding part of the spinal cord shows relatively symmetrical hypertrophy. It is most common in the cervical area and can also occur in the thoracic area and, rarely, in the conus medullaris. Most invade a long area spanning 3–4 vertebral body segments, and in about 20%, the central canal is enlarged. Slow-growing tumors can also be accompanied by bone remodeling of adjacent bones. Due to its characteristic of frequent hemorrhage, about 20–64% show a "hemosiderin cap sign" with low signal intensity hemosiderin deposition above and below the lesion (Fig. 11.39). Cystic changes are common, and about 50–90% show cystic changes located inside the mass or at both ends, or an enlarged central canal. In addition, there is widespread spinal cord edema above and below the lesion. Calcification within the lesion is rare [57]. The enhancement pattern is very diverse, and most show strong enhancement, while cases with minimal or no enhancement are rare. If resected surgically, complete resection is possible in about 85% of cases, but if complete resection is difficult or recurrence occurs, radiation

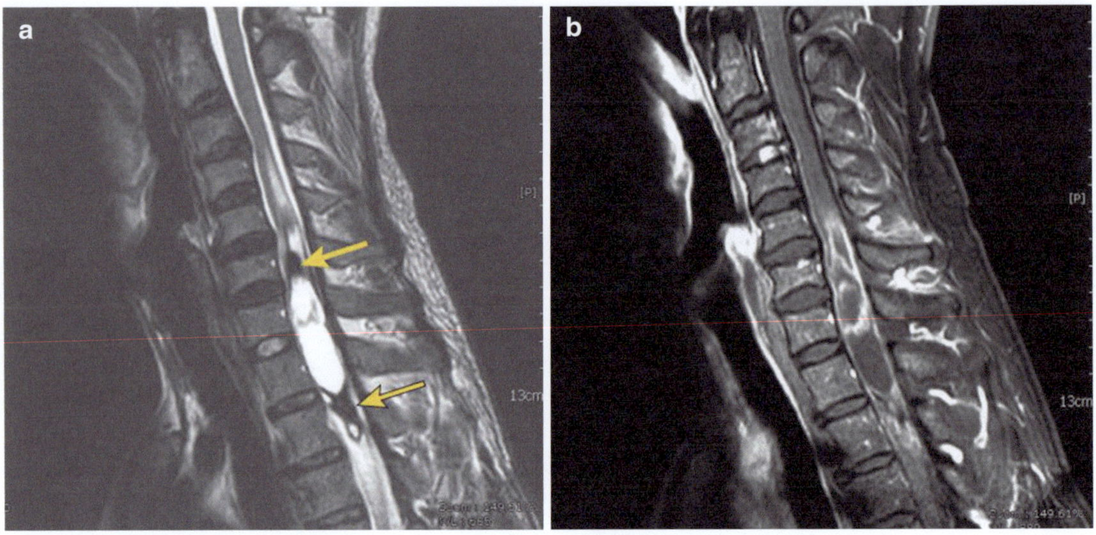

Fig. 11.39 MRI findings of ependymoma. On the MR T2 enhanced image, there is a mass including a wide-ranging high signal intensity intratumoral cyst, showing a "hemosiderin cap sign"'of low signal intensity along the top and bottom of the lesion (**a**, arrow). There is extensive high signal intensity spinal cord edema (cord edema) along the spinal cord above and below the lesion. On the fat-suppressed contrast-enhanced T1 enhanced image, it enhances unevenly along the inside and outside of the mass (**b**)

therapy or chemotherapy is performed. Metastasis is rare and the 5-year survival rate is about 85%.

11.5.1.2 Astrocytoma

Astrocytoma is a tumor originating from astrocytes and histologically includes pilocytic astrocytoma (WHO grade I), diffuse astrocytoma (WHO grade II), anaplastic astrocytoma (WHO grade III), and glioblastoma multiforme (WHO grade IV). It is the second most common intramedullary tumor in adults after ependymoma, and in children, it is the most common intramedullary tumor, especially pilocytic astrocytoma. It progresses slowly, showing symptoms such as pain, sensory and motor disorders, and bowel and bladder disorders. It usually appears in children or young adults, especially accounting for 60% of intramedullary tumors occurring in children. In MRI examinations, it usually shows low signal intensity in T1 enhanced images and high signal intensity in T2 enhanced images. The degree of contrast enhancement varies, and in some cases, there is almost no contrast enhancement (20~30%), but usually, the corresponding spinal cord is bulging as an infiltrative tumor that is slightly enhanced in part (Figs. 11.40, 11.41, and 11.42). It mainly occurs in the cervical area and also in the thoracic area. It usually shows a long shape over 3~4 segments of the vertebral body, and although it is less frequent than ependymoma, it often shows cystic changes inside the tumor. It is also a slowly growing tumor that often involves bone remodeling of the surrounding bone tissue. Unlike ependymoma, it tends to show an eccentric location in the spinal cord, and hemorrhage is rare. Also, unlike ependymoma, it grows by infiltrating the surrounding spinal cord tissue, so most of the time, a biopsy is performed by surgery, but complete resection is often difficult due to nerve tissue damage [58]. Rarely, it may show findings mixed with high signal intensity in T1 enhanced images due to methemoglobin deposition accompanied by hemorrhage. Since it is usually a low-grade tumor histologically, the 5-year survival rate is about 80%, so the prognosis is generally good. However, the prognosis worsens as the WHO grade histologically increases.

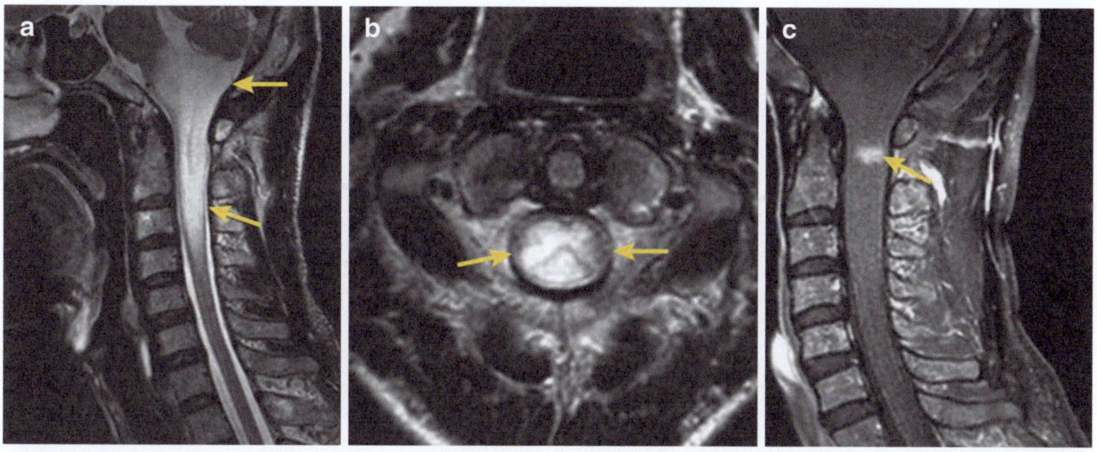

Fig. 11.40 Pilocytic astrocytoma. On the MR T2 enhanced sagittal image, a high signal intensity lesion is seen occupying a wide range from the medulla oblongata to the cervical spinal cord area (**a**, arrow), accompanied by extensive edema of the spinal cord. On the T2 enhanced axial image, this lesion occupies the entire length of the spinal cord (**b**, arrow), and on the fat-suppressed contrast-enhanced T1 enhanced sagittal image, only part of the entire lesion shows enhancement (**c**, arrow)

11.5.1.3 Hemangioblastoma

The cellular origin of hemangioblastoma is unclear, but it is the third most common intramedullary tumor. It is also called capillary hemangioma. It usually occurs in young adults and tends to occur mainly in the dorsal column of the spinal cord, often showing sensory abnormalities, especially loss of proprioception. It is a highly vascular tumor that often accompanies acute subarachnoid hemorrhage, chronic microhemorrhage, etc. It is usually a single lesion (68%), but if it is multiple, there is a possibility of von Hippel-Lindau syndrome. It shows sensory abnormalities, motor function abnormalities, pain, etc. and 95% of symptomatic cases are accompanied by syrinx. In the case of von Hippel-Lindau syndrome, there is often one main lesion that causes symptoms. It is prevalent in the 30s, and in the case of von Hippel-Lindau syndrome, it appears at a younger age. In contrast-enhanced MRI, it appears as a mass showing strong contrast enhancement, and several feeding arteries with serpentine flow-void can be seen inside and around the lesion. It is located subpially and often accompanied by syrinx around it in T1 and T2 enhanced images (40~55%). It is common in the thoracic spine and is also found in the cervical spine. Due to venous congestion and edema, the spinal cord area where the mass is located usually appears enlarged. Because there is a high possibility of bleeding during resection, it is common to treat the feeding artery with embolization through angiography before surgery (Fig. 11.43) [59]. Most of them undergo embolization before surgery and treat symptoms. The tumor mass is surgically removed, and procedures such as gamma knife are performed when there are too many lesions, as in von Hippel-Lindau syndrome (Fig. 11.44). Malignant transformation does not occur.

11.5.2 Other Intramedullary Tumor

11.5.2.1 Cavernous Hemangioma

Also known as cavernous malformation, cavernous angioma, and cryptic vascular malformation, it is a lesion composed of elongated capillaries and sinusoidal vessels. There is no normal spinal cord nerve tissue inside, and there are no feeding arteries or draining veins. It is known to occur due to excessive secretion of various substances

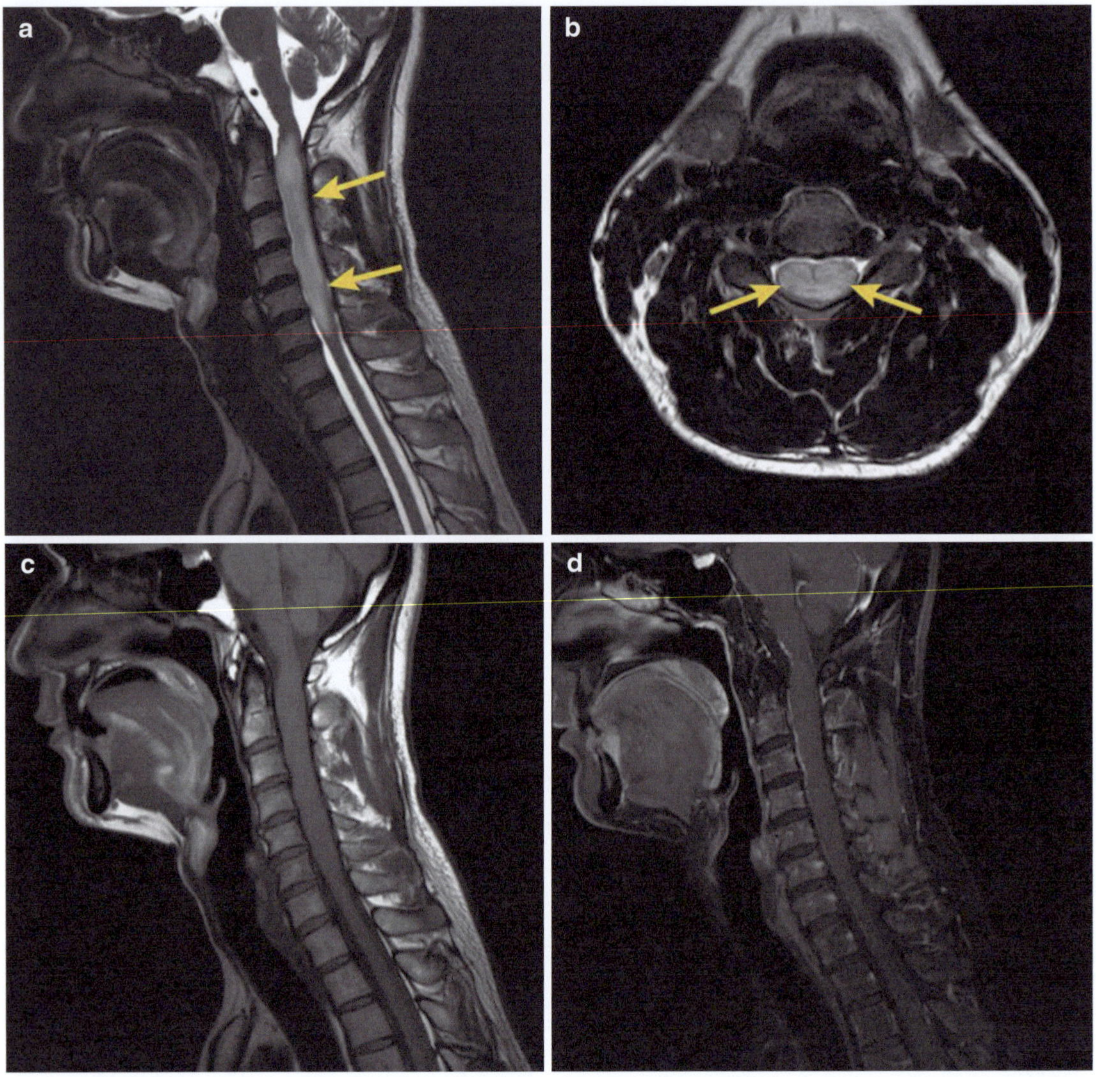

Fig. 11.41 Anaplastic astrocytoma. On the MR T2-weighted image, a high signal intensity bulky mass is invading the spinal cord from C1/2 to C6 (**a**, **b**). The mass appears as isointense on the T1 -weighted image (**c**), and although it is a WHO grade 3 anaplastic astrocytoma, enhancement is not clearly visible (**d**)

(VEGF, BFGF, TGFα, etc.) that induce immature vascular endothelial hyperplasia and vascular proliferation. It is most common in the thoracic region of middle-aged people and also occurs well in the cervical region. It is also called a cross-sectional vascular malformation (cavernous malformation). Cavernous hemangioma is rare in the spine, and only about 3~5% are found in the spine. The size is a few millimeters, but often lesions larger than 1 cm are found. Usually, acute spinal cord hemorrhage occurs repeatedly, causing acute neurological deficits. It usually shows sensory and motor ataxia, progressive paralysis symptoms, and may have recurring neurological loss symptoms that improve and worsen, or neurological symptoms may gradually progress, or neurological symptoms may suddenly worsen within a few hours or days. It is common in women in their 20s to 50s, and 10~30% have multiple lesions or a family history. On MR T2 enhanced images, it appears as a well-defined lesion, with a low signal intensity band on the out-

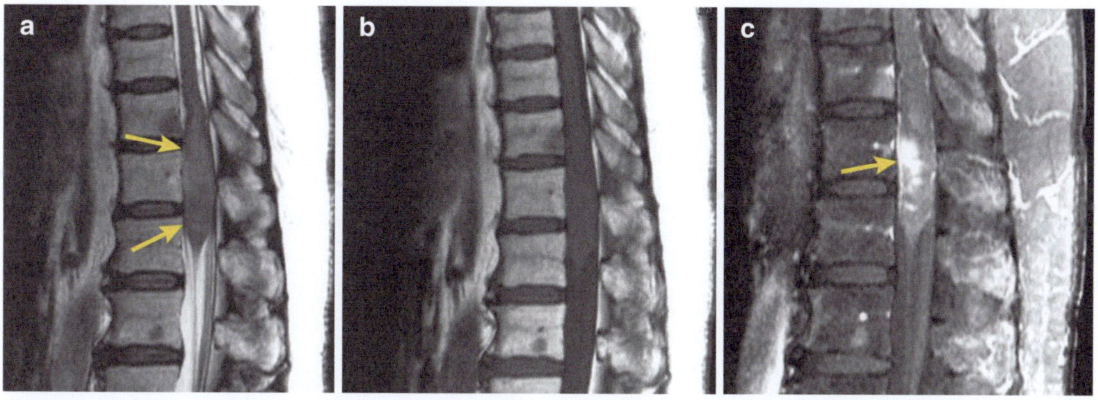

Fig. 11.42 Glioblastoma multiforme. In the MR T2 enhanced image, there is a lesion with heterogeneous signal intensity in the conus medullaris, showing slightly higher signal intensity than the adjacent normal spinal cord, and the corresponding conus medullaris is expanded (**a**, arrow). This lesion shows similar signal intensity to the spinal cord in the T1 enhanced image (**b**), and in the fat-suppressed contrast-enhanced T1 enhanced image, it shows heterogeneous enhancement and is not well distinguished from the normal spinal cord above (**c**, arrow)

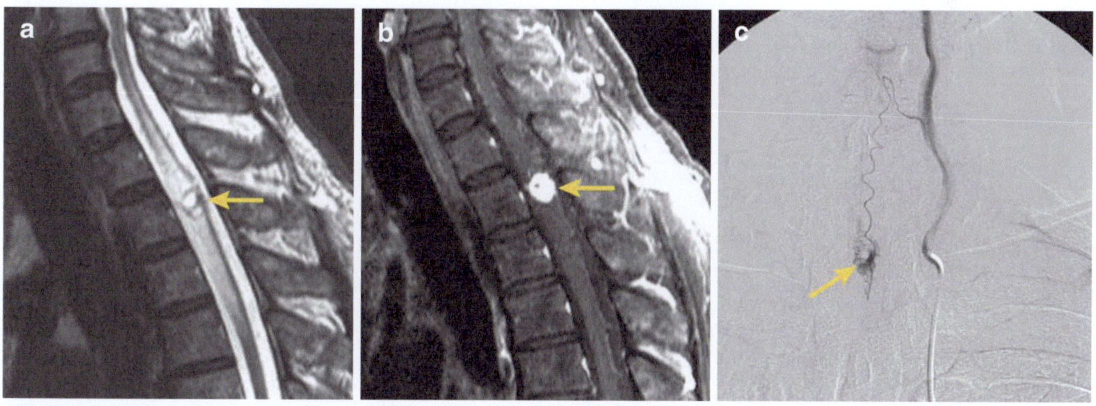

Fig. 11.43 MRI and angiography of hemangioblastoma. On the MR T2 enhanced image, there is an intramedullary tumor showing almost the same high signal intensity as water (**a**, arrow), accompanied by extensive high signal intensity spinal cord edema along the adjacent spinal cord. On the contrast-enhanced T1 enhanced image, it appears as a well-defined mass showing very strong enhancement (**b**, arrow). In angiography, a tumor receiving blood supply from the posterior spinal artery originating from the left vertebral artery is observed (**c**, arrow)

side and heterogeneous high signal intensity locules with a fluid-fluid level inside, showing a popcorn appearance (Fig. 11.45). The outer low signal intensity band is known to be half, and the inside is due to the deposition of by-products from repeated hemorrhages at different times, showing heterogeneous signal intensity on T1 and T2 enhanced images. If the size is very small, it is not easy to find on T1 and T2 enhanced images, and it can be found only as a small low signal intensity lesion on T2 enhanced images without surrounding spinal cord edema. On T2* gradient echo images, the susceptibility artifact due to the by-products of repeated hemorrhages is strongly visible ("blooming effect"), making it easier to find small lesions. Contrast enhancement is often minimal or absent. Also, in angiography, it is easy to show false negative findings because cavernous hemangioma is a lesion with very slow blood flow and does not accompany abnormal arteries or veins [60]. Symptomatic cavernous hemangioma is treated as a principle, and surgical removal is

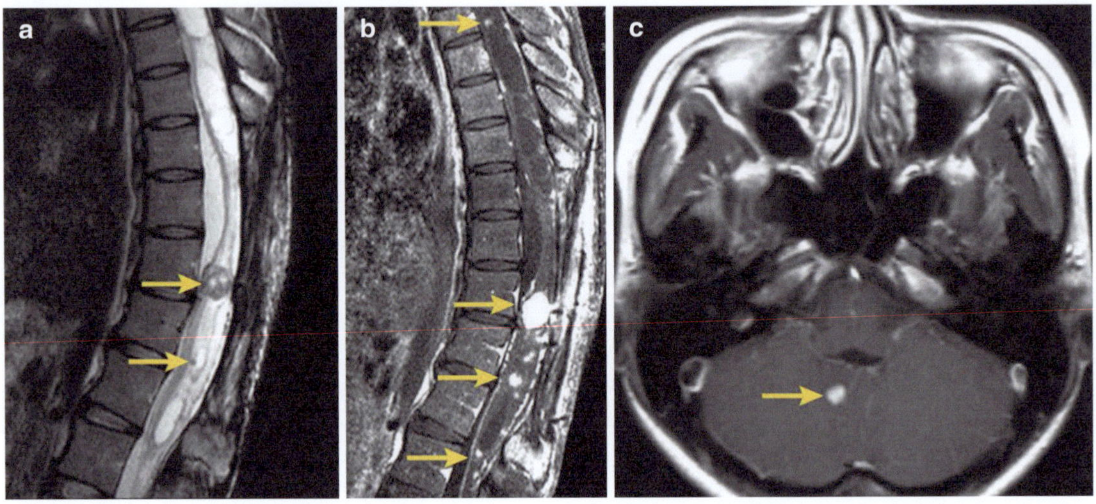

Fig. 11.44 Multiple hemangioblastomas in a patient with von Hippel-Lindau syndrome. In the MR T2 enhanced image, multiple tumors are located in the intramedullary space, and extensive cystic change is accompanied in the adjacent spinal cord (**a**, arrow). In the contrast-enhanced T1 enhanced image, these tumors show very strong enhancement, and the extensive cystic change in the spinal cord is not enhanced (**b**). In the brain MR contrast-enhanced T1 enhanced image, there is a small tumor in the cerebellum that is enhanced (**c**, arrow), and it was diagnosed as von Hippel-Lindau syndrome

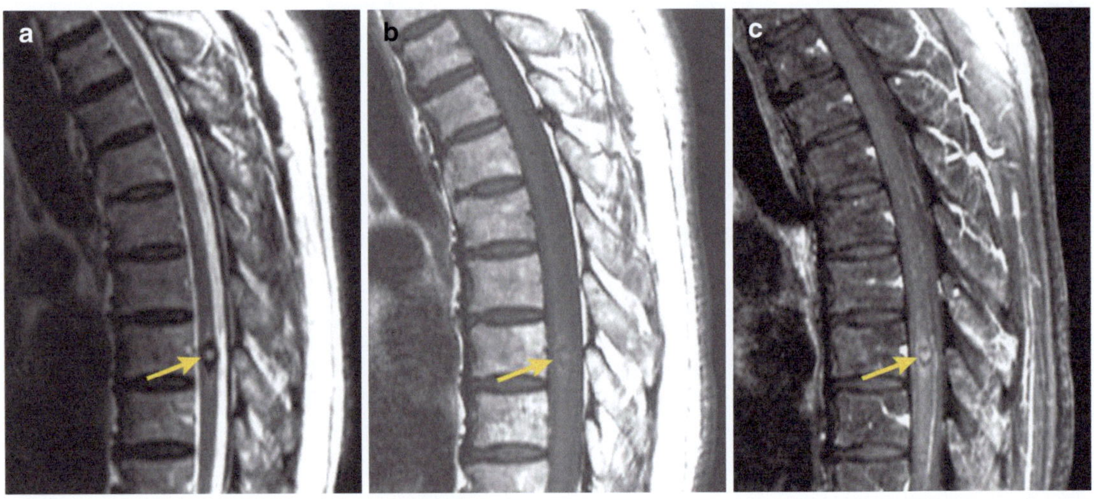

Fig. 11.45 MRI findings of cavernous hemangioma. In the MR T2 enhanced image, a small intramedullary mass is seen at the T9 position, surrounded by a low signal intensity band on the outside and showing high signal intensity inside (**a**, arrow). This lesion also shows a low signal intensity band on the outside and high signal intensity inside in the T1 enhanced image, and it is considered to be a lesion surrounded by hemosiderin deposition, with the inside accompanied by subacute stage hemorrhage (**b**, arrow), and at the time of enhancement, it shows moderate pial enhancement on the outside of the lesion and spinal cord (**c**)

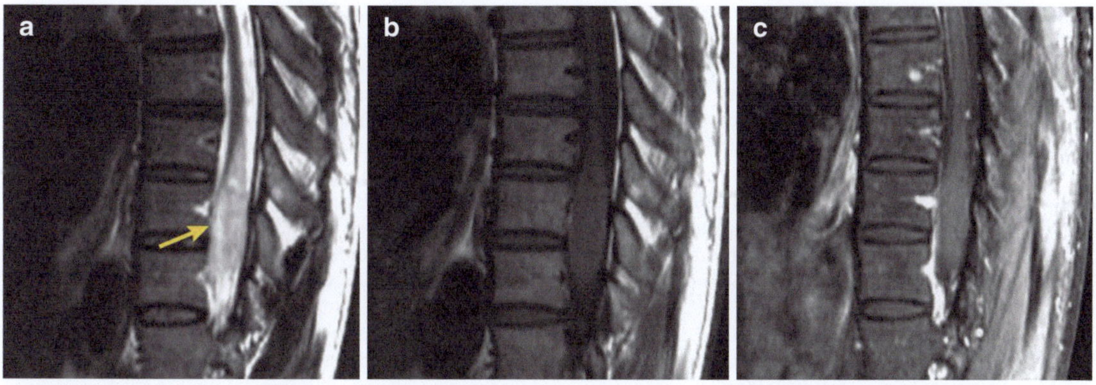

Fig. 11.46 MRI findings of ganglioglioma. In the MR T2 enhanced image, there is a mass showing relatively homogeneous high signal intensity at the conus medullaris, and the corresponding spinal cord is enlarged (**a**, arrow). In the T1 enhanced image, it shows similar signal intensity to the adjacent normal spinal cord (**b**) and shows mild homogeneous enhancement (**c**)

the standard treatment. The lesion itself can show various aspects such as growing or shrinking on its own, and 1~5% of the lesions cause symptoms through hemorrhage annually.

11.5.2.2 Ganglioglioma

Ganglioglioma is a combination of neuromal elements and glial cells. It is a very rare tumor with mixed features. It is also called Gangliocytoma, Ganglioneuroma, and Neuroastrocytoma. It is a well-defined, slowly growing tumor with symptoms that progress gradually over several years. It is a benign tumor mixed with neuronal and glial components, and most are classified as WHO grade 1. It may be accompanied by cystic changes and calcification, but internal hemorrhage or necrosis is rare. It is usually found in young patients in their 20s, with 80% being under 30. It often occurs in the cervical spine (67%) and then frequently in the thoracic spine. It presents with symptoms such as lower back pain, lower limb muscle weakness, paralysis, bowel and bladder disorders, and gait disorders, and it takes an average of 7–8 years for symptoms to appear because it is a very slowly growing tumor. It is often a long lesion that invades more than eight vertebral body segments, and there are often lesions throughout the cross-section of the spinal cord. It is often located eccentrically on the cross-section. On MRI, it is common to have accompanying cystic changes or syrinx. The degree of contrast enhancement varies and may not be enhanced at all (Fig. 11.46) [61]. It may show heterogeneous low signal intensity on T1-weighted images and usually shows high signal intensity on T2-weighted images (60%). It shows heterogeneous contrast enhancement and does not enhance in about 15%. Compared to Ependymoma or Astrocytoma, intratumoral cystic changes are more common, and contrast enhancement can be seen inside the cystic change. There is almost no spinal cord swelling around the tumor. The principle is to remove it surgically, and the prognosis varies depending on the extent of resection. Compared to those that occur in the brain, spinal gangliogliomas have a higher recurrence rate, and radiation therapy is sometimes performed in cases of recurrence or histologically malignant cases.

Bibliography

1. Donthineni R. Diagnosis and staging of spine tumors. Orthop Clin North Am. 2009;40(1):1–7.
2. Wald JT. Imaging of spine neoplasm. Radiol Clin North Am. 2012;50(4):749–76.

3. Vidal JA, Murphey MD. Primary tumors of the osseous spine. Magn Reson Imaging Clin N Am. 2007;15(2):239–55. vii
4. Laredo JD, Assouline E, Gelbert F, Wybier M, Merland JJ, Tubiana JM. Vertebral hemangiomas: fat content as a sign of aggressiveness. Radiology. 1990;177(2):467–72.
5. Acosta FL Jr, Dowd CF, Chin C, Tihan T, Ames CP, Weinstein PR. Current treatment strategies and outcomes in the management of symptomatic vertebral hemangiomas. Neurosurgery. 2006;58(2):287–95; discussion-295.
6. Gasbarrini A, Cappuccio M, Mirabile L, et al. Spinal metastases: treatment evaluation algorithm. Eur Rev Med Pharmacol Sci. 2004;8(6):265–74.
7. Van Goethem JW, van den Hauwe L, Ozsarlak O, DeSchepper AM, Parizel PM. Spinal tumors. Eur J Radiol. 2004;50(2):159–76.
8. Lecouvet FE, Vande Berg BC, Maldague BE, et al. Vertebral compression fractures in multiple myeloma. Part I. Distribution and appearance at MR imaging. Radiology. 1997;204(1):195–9.
9. Winterbottom AP, Shaw AS. Imaging patients with myeloma. Clin Radiol. 2009;64(1):1–11.
10. Libshitz HI, Malthouse SR, Cunningham D, MacVicar AD, Husband JE. Multiple myeloma: appearance at MR imaging. Radiology. 1992;182(3):833–7.
11. Baur-Melnyk A, Buhmann S, Durr HR, Reiser M. Role of MRI for the diagnosis and prognosis of multiple myeloma. Eur J Radiol. 2005;55(1):56–63.
12. Moulopoulos LA, Dimopoulos MA, Smith TL, et al. Prognostic significance of magnetic resonance imaging in patients with asymptomatic multiple myeloma. J Clin Oncol. 1995;13(1):251–6.
13. Alyas F, Saifuddin A, Connell D. MR imaging evaluation of the bone marrow and marrow infiltrative disorders of the lumbar spine. Magn Reson Imaging Clin N Am. 2007;15(2):199–219.
14. Greenspan A. Benign bone-forming lesions: osteoma, osteoid osteoma, and osteoblastoma. Clinical, imaging, pathologic, and differential considerations. Skeletal Radiol. 1993;22(7):485–500.
15. Azouz EM, Kozlowski K, Marton D, Sprague P, Zerhouni A, Asselah F. Osteoid osteoma and osteoblastoma of the spine in children. Report of 22 cases with brief literature review. Pediatr Radiol. 1986;16(1):25–31.
16. Kroon HM, Schurmans J. Osteoblastoma: clinical and radiologic findings in 98 new cases. Radiology. 1990;175(3):783–90.
17. Lucas DR, Unni KK, McLeod RA, O'Connor MI, Sim FH. Osteoblastoma: clinicopathologic study of 306 cases. Hum Pathol. 1994;25(2):117–34.
18. Kransdorf MJ, Sweet DE. Aneurysmal bone cyst: concept, controversy, clinical presentation, and imaging. AJR Am J Roentgenol. 1995;164(3):573–80.
19. Beltran J, Simon DC, Levy M, Herman L, Weis L, Mueller CF. Aneurysmal bone cysts: MR imaging at 1.5 T. Radiology. 1986;158(3):689–90.
20. Mankin HJ, Hornicek FJ, Ortiz-Cruz E, Villafuerte J, Gebhardt MC. Aneurysmal bone cyst: a review of 150 patients. J Clin Oncol. 2005;23(27):6756–62.
21. Roblot P, Alcalay M, Cazenave-Roblot F, Levy P, Bontoux D. Osteochondroma of the thoracic spine. Report of a case and review of the literature. Spine (Phila Pa 1976). 1990;15(3):240–3.
22. Mohit AA, Eskridge J, Ellenbogen R, Shaffrey CI. Aneurysmal bone cyst of the atlas: successful treatment through selective arterial embolization: case report. Neurosurgery. 2004;55(4):982.
23. Yamaguchi T, Suzuki S, Ishiiwa H, Shimizu K, Ueda Y. Benign notochordal cell tumors: a comparative histological study of benign notochordal cell tumors, classic chordomas, and notochordal vestiges of fetal intervertebral discs. Am J Surg Pathol. 2004;28(6):756–61.
24. Nishiguchi T, Mochizuki K, Ohsawa M, et al. Differentiating benign notochordal cell tumors from chordomas: radiographic features on MRI, CT, and tomography. AJR Am J Roentgenol. 2011;196(3):644–50.
25. Turcotte RE, Biagini R, Sim FH, Unni KK. Giant cell tumor of the spine and sacrum. Chir Organi Mov. 1990;75(1 Suppl):104–7.
26. Bidwell JK, Young JW, Khalluff E. Giant cell tumor of the spine: computed tomography appearance and review of the literature. J Comput Tomogr. 1987;11(3):307–11.
27. Chhaya S, White LM, Kandel R, Wunder JS, Ferguson P, Agur A. Transarticular invasion of bone tumours across the sacroiliac joint. Skeletal Radiol. 2005;34(12):771–7.
28. Seider MJ, Rich TA, Ayala AG, Murray JA. Giant cell tumors of bone: treatment with radiation therapy. Radiology. 1986;161(2):537–40.
29. Schwimer SR, Bassett LW, Mancuso AA, Mirra JM, Dawson EG. Giant cell tumor of the cervicothoracic spine. AJR Am J Roentgenol. 1981;136(1):63–7.
30. Smith J, Wixon D, Watson RC. Giant-cell tumor of the sacrum. Clinical and radiologic features in 13 patients. J Can Assoc Radiol. 1979;30(1):34–9.
31. Mirra JM, Rand F, Rand R, Calcaterra T, Dawson E. Giant-cell tumor of the second cervical vertebra treated by cryosurgery and irradiation. Clin Orthop Relat Res. 1981;(154):228–33.
32. Palmer FJ, Blum PW. Osteochondroma with spinal cord compression: report of three cases. J Neurosurg. 1980;52(6):842–5.
33. Govender S, Parbhoo AH. Osteochondroma with compression of the spinal cord. A report of two cases. J Bone Joint Surg Br. 1999;81(4):667–9.
34. Ratliff J, Voorhies R. Osteochondroma of the C5 lamina with cord compression: case report and review of the literature. Spine (Phila Pa 1976). 2000;25(10):1293–5.
35. Bianchi PM, Marsella P, Masi R, et al. Cervical chordoma in childhood: clinical statistical contribution. Int J Pediatr Otorhinolaryngol. 1989;18(1):39–45.

36. Eriksson B, Gunterberg B, Kindblom LG. Chordoma. A clinicopathologic and prognostic study of a Swedish national series. Acta Orthop Scand. 1981;52(1):49–58.
37. Healey JH, Lane JM. Chordoma: a critical review of diagnosis and treatment. Orthop Clin North Am. 1989;20(3):417–26.
38. Wippold FJ 2nd, Koeller KK, Smirniotopoulos JG. Clinical and imaging features of cervical chordoma. AJR Am J Roentgenol. 1999;172(5):1423–6.
39. Firooznia H, Golimbu C, Rafii M, Reede DL, Kricheff II, Bjorkengren A. Computed tomography of spinal chordomas. J Comput Tomogr. 1986;10(1):45–50.
40. de Bruine FT, Kroon HM. Spinal chordoma: radiologic features in 14 cases. AJR Am J Roentgenol. 1988;150(4):861–3.
41. Sung MS, Lee GK, Kang HS, et al. Sacrococcygeal chordoma: MR imaging in 30 patients. Skeletal Radiol. 2005;34(2):87–94.
42. Rosenthal DI, Scott JA, Mankin HJ, Wismer GL, Brady TJ. Sacrococcygeal chordoma: magnetic resonance imaging and computed tomography. AJR Am J Roentgenol. 1985;145(1):143–7.
43. Shives TC, McLeod RA, Unni KK, Schray MF. Chondrosarcoma of the spine. J Bone Joint Surg Am. 1989;71(8):1158–65.
44. Hirsh LF, Thanki A, Spector HB. Primary spinal chondrosarcoma with eighteen-year follow-up: case report and literature review. Neurosurgery. 1984;14(6):747–9.
45. Barwick KW, Huvos AG, Smith J. Primary osteogenic sarcoma of the vertebral column: a clinicopathologic correlation of ten patients. Cancer. 1980;46(3):595–604.
46. Grubb MR, Currier BL, Pritchard DJ, Ebersold MJ. Primary Ewing's sarcoma of the spine. Spine (Phila Pa 1976). 1994;19(3):309–13.
47. Kornberg M. Primary Ewing's sarcoma of the spine. A review and case report. Spine (Phila Pa 1976). 1986;11(1):54–7.
48. Ilaslan H, Sundaram M, Unni KK, Dekutoski MB. Primary Ewing's sarcoma of the vertebral column. Skeletal Radiol. 2004;33(9):506–13.
49. Subbarao K, Jacobson HG. Primary malignant neoplasms. Semin Roentgenol. 1979;14(1):44–57.
50. Egelhoff JC, Bates DJ, Ross JS, Rothner AD, Cohen BH. Spinal MR findings in neurofibromatosis types 1 and 2. AJNR Am J Neuroradiol. 1992;13(4):1071–7.
51. Friedman DP, Tartaglino LM, Flanders AE. Intradural schwannomas of the spine: MR findings with emphasis on contrast-enhancement characteristics. AJR Am J Roentgenol. 1992;158(6):1347–50.
52. Liu WC, Choi G, Lee SH, et al. Radiological findings of spinal schwannomas and meningiomas: focus on discrimination of two disease entities. Eur Radiol. 2009;19(11):2707–15.
53. Lee JW, Lee IS, Choi KU, et al. CT and MRI findings of calcified spinal meningiomas: correlation with pathological findings. Skeletal Radiol. 2010;39(4):345–52.
54. Kabir SM, Thompson D, Rezajooi K, Casey AT. Nondysraphic intradural spinal cord lipoma: case series, literature review and guidelines for management. Acta Neurochir. 2010;152(7):1139–44.
55. Wippold FJ 2nd, Smirniotopoulos JG, Moran CJ, Suojanen JN, Vollmer DG. MR imaging of myxopapillary ependymoma: findings and value to determine extent of tumor and its relation to intraspinal structures. AJR Am J Roentgenol. 1995;165(5):1263–7.
56. Sousa J, O'Brien D, Crooks D. Paraganglioma of the filum terminale. J Clin Neurosci. 2005;12(5):584–5.
57. Sun B, Wang C, Wang J, Liu A. MRI features of intramedullary spinal cord ependymomas. J Neuroimaging. 2003;13(4):346–51.
58. Abel TJ, Chowdhary A, Thapa M, et al. Spinal cord pilocytic astrocytoma with leptomeningeal dissemination to the brain. Case report and review of the literature. J Neurosurg. 2006;105(6 Suppl):508–14.
59. Imagama S, Ito Z, Wakao N, et al. Differentiation of localization of spinal hemangioblastomas based on imaging and pathological findings. Eur Spine J. 2011;20(8):1377–84.
60. Hegde A, Mohan S, Tan KK, Lim CC. Spinal cavernous malformations: magnetic resonance imaging and associated findings. Singapore Med J. 2012;53(9):582–6.
61. Lotfinia I, Vahedi P. Intramedullary cervical spinal cord ganglioglioma, review of the literature and therapeutic controversies. Spinal Cord. 2009;47(1):87–90.

Non-neoplastic Spinal Cord Diseases

12

Guen Young Lee

Most non-neoplastic spinal cord diseases are often compressive spinal cord diseases due to trauma or degenerative changes. However, when various neurological diseases with spinal cord dysfunction are shown without such preseading causes and radiological abnormalities are shown, neoplastic or non-neoplastic spinal cord diseases are considered. Neoplastic spinal cord diseases are covered in Chap. 11, and here we will describe non-neoplastic spinal cord diseases.

12.1 Differential Diagnosis of Non-neoplastic Spinal Cord Diseases

To diagnose non-neoplastic spinal cord diseases, the following four things should be considered. The first is the speed of symptom onset, and depending on whether the symptoms occur in one of the four patterns of hyperacute, acute, subacute, and chronic, the differential diseases can vary greatly. For example, if the patient's symptoms occur and progress rapidly in 1–2 h, spinal cord ischemia/infarct should be considered first. On the other hand, if symptoms appear and worsen over 2–3 days, possibilities such as multiple sclerosis and optic-spinal myelitis should be considered, and if symptoms appear and worsen slowly over several months or years, vascular spinal cord lesions, neoplastic diseases of the spinal cord, metabolic diseases, etc. can be considered (Fig. 12.1). The second consideration is how the disease appears over time (disease course), whether it is monophasic, whether it repeats improvement and worsening over time (relapsing or progressive), how much recovery is there with treatment (complete, partial, or no recovery), or whether there is no change from the initial state or continuous change (stable or fluctuating). In the case of multiple sclerosis, many patients often show a pattern of alternating improvement and deterioration, generally worsening over time, and this clinical pattern can aid in diagnosis. Thirdly, there are findings from magnetic resonance imaging. The size of the lesion, especially the length of the lesion in the sagittal image, the anatomical location where the lesion is mainly invaded in the axial image, the asymmetry or eccentricity, the degree of contrast enhancement, etc. can help in differential diagnosis. For example, neuromyelitis optica typically presents as a long lesion of three or more spinal segments with strong contrast enhancement (Fig. 12.2). Fourthly, other tests and clinical findings should also be considered in addition to radiological examinations. If a vascular spinal disease like a dural arteriovenous fistula is suspected, it can be confirmed through angiography, and if neuromyelitis optica is suspected, it can be confirmed through an aquaporin-4 antibody test [1, 2].

G. Y. Lee (✉)
Department of Radiology, Chung-Ang University College of Medicine, Seoul, Republic of Korea

© The Author(s), under exclusive license to Springer Nature Singapore Pte Ltd. 2025
H. S. Kang, J. W. Lee (eds.), *Spinal Imaging*, https://doi.org/10.1007/978-981-95-1386-4_12

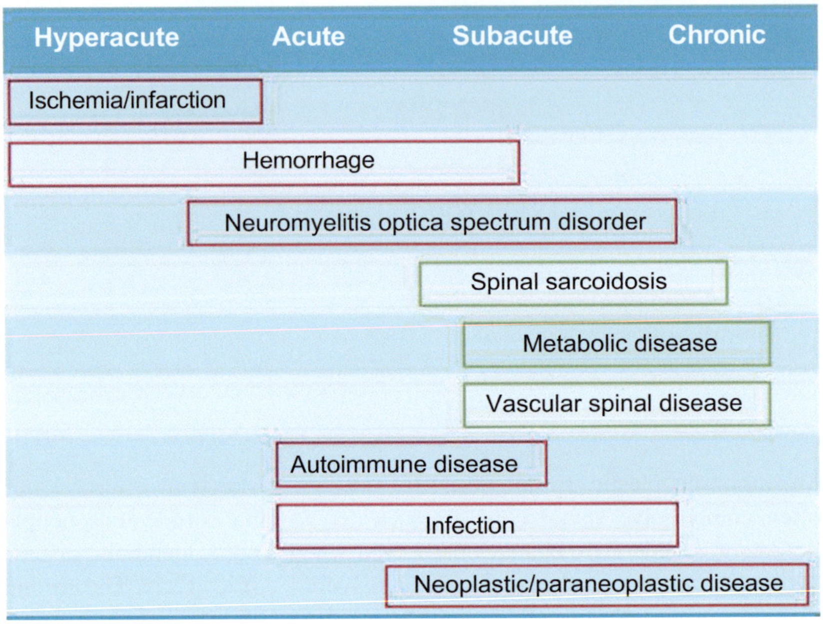

Fig. 12.1 Differentiation of non-tumorous spinal disease according to the speed of symptom onset. Excluding compressive myelopathy, the most common cause of spinal lesions due to degenerative changes or trauma, non-tumorous spinal diseases can be differentiated as follows when the speed of symptom onset is divided into four categories—hyperacute, acute, subacute, chronic

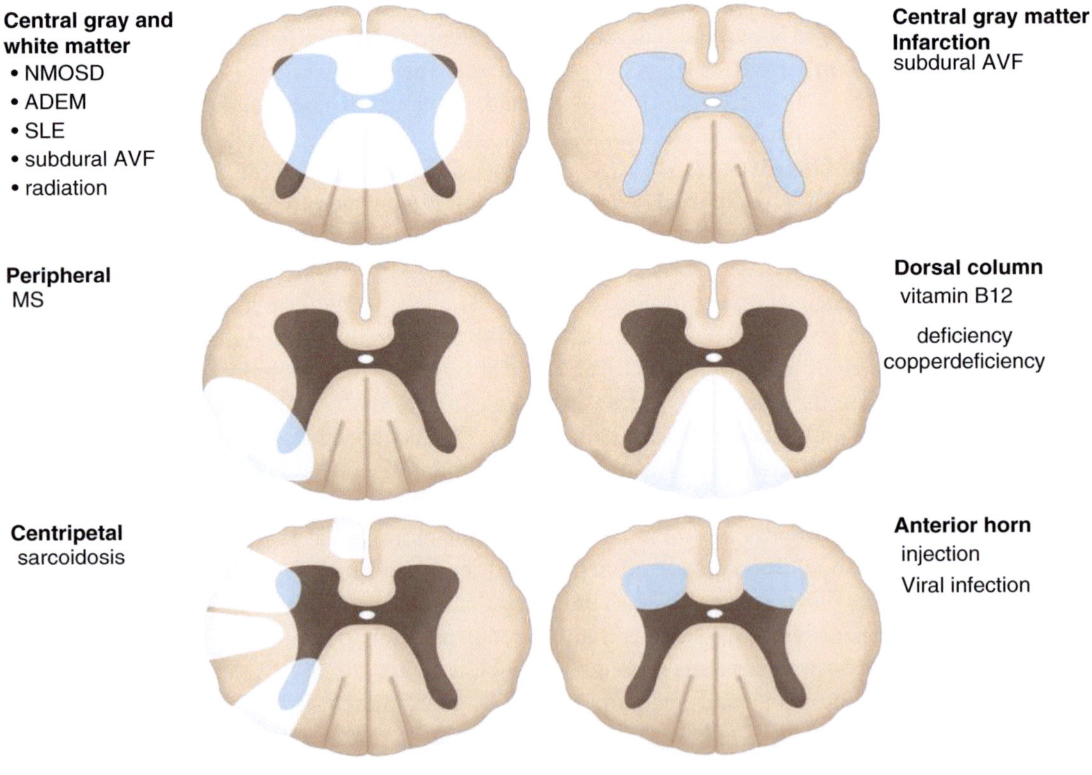

Fig. 12.2 Differentiation of non-tumorous spinal disease according to the location and shape of the lesion in the axial image of magnetic resonance imaging. *NMOSD* neuromyelitis optica spectrum disorder, *ADEM* acute demyelinating encephalomyelitis, *SLE* systemic lupus erythematosus, *AVF* arteriovenous fistula, *MS* multiple sclerosis

12.2 Inflammatory Diseases (Inflammation of the Spinal Cord)

Noninfectious inflammatory diseases of the spinal cord are broadly divided into autoimmune, immune-mediated, and paraneoplastic myelopathy. Generally, inflammatory spinal diseases present as acute sensory or motor dysfunction over a period of days or weeks, often accompanied by autonomic dysfunction of the bladder or bowel. These diseases are often difficult to diagnose based solely on imaging findings and often require consideration of the clinical course, test findings, and brain MRI examinations [3].

12.2.1 Acute Transverse Myelitis

Acute transverse myelitis is a clinical term for an acute inflammatory disease that invades the spinal cord. In the past, it referred only to the idiopathic form, but it is also used to refer to inflammatory diseases that invade both sides of the spinal cord, causing motor, sensory, and autonomic abnormalities on both sides, even if the cause is known [4]. It usually presents with bilateral sensory abnormalities, resulting in pain, loss of temperature sensation, symptoms of paralysis (paraplegia, quadriplegia), back or leg pain, urinary dysfunction, bowel dysfunction, and stiffness. Symptoms usually worsen rapidly within a few days of onset. It is most common in adolescents or young adults, especially between the ages of 10–19 and 30–39. Acute transverse myelitis needs to be differentiated from other diseases with similar symptoms, especially spinal compression due to degenerative changes, and other cases that can cause similar spinal lesions—previous radiation exposure, spinal ischemia or infarction, spinal vascular malformations, sarcoidosis, Sjogren's disease, systemic lupus erythematosus and other connective tissue diseases, multiple sclerosis, and central nervous system infections—should be ruled out. The mechanism of onset is not yet established, but it is thought to be due to immune response disorders.

In magnetic resonance imaging, abnormal findings may not be found for several hours or days after the onset of symptoms, but usually appear as high signal intensity lesions on T2-weighted images, located in the central cord of the spinal cord in cross-sectional images, occupying most of the cross-section of more than two-thirds of the spinal cord, and often appearing as long lesions that invade more than twice the height of the vertebral body in sagittal images, usually spanning 3–4 vertebrae. The spinal cord area where the lesion is located generally shows edema and is often accompanied by various degrees of contrast enhancement, often skewed to one side, often requiring differentiation from tumors. Contrast enhancement is very diverse, with no contrast enhancement seen in 40–50%, and contrast enhancement is more common in the subacute phase than in the initial phase. It most commonly occurs in the thoracic spinal cord and occurs in the cervical area in about 10% (Figs. 12.3 and 12.4). Unlike multiple sclerosis, it usually does not recur [5].

Treatment is with high-dose intravenous steroid pulse therapy, and the course varies, with about 30% of patients left with permanent disabilities.

Differential diagnoses include multiple sclerosis, neuromyelitis optica, intramedullary tumors, spinal cord ischemia/infarction, and spinal dural fistula.

12.2.2 Multiple Sclerosis

Multiple sclerosis is the most common chronic demyelinating inflammatory disease that affects the central nervous system—brain and spinal cord—and its clinical course is very diverse, but it tends to recur. It is thought to be caused by damage to the brain's myelin due to a cellular immune autoimmune response.

It is more common in women than in men (2:1) and usually occurs in the 20s to 40s. Smoking, vitamin D status, Epstein-Barr virus, etc. are known risk factors and show various prevalence rates by country. Most patients (90%) have brain lesions, and cases where only the spi-

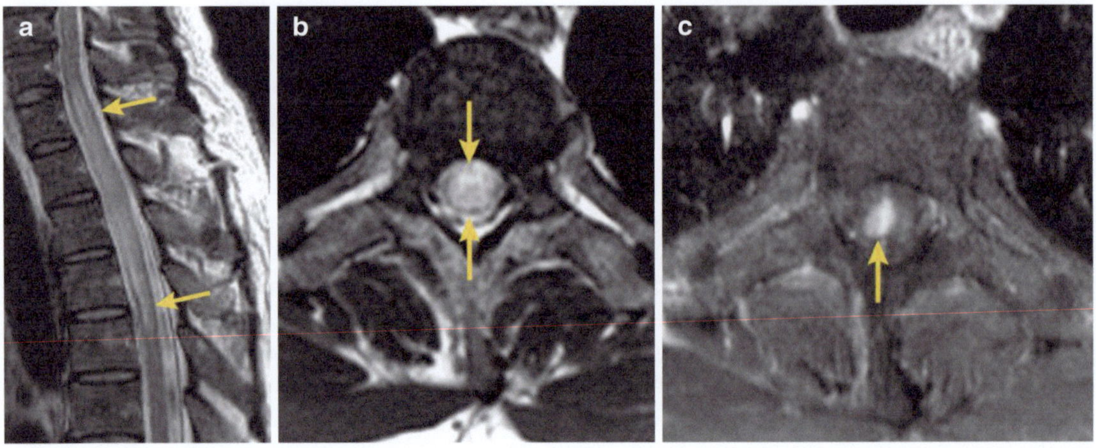

Fig. 12.3 Acute transverse myelitis. In the T2-weighted sagittal image, a long high signal intensity lesion is located within the spinal cord across 4–5 spinal segments, accompanied by spinal cord edema (**a**, arrow). In the T2-weighted axial image, this lesion invades the entire cross-section of the spinal cord (**b**, arrow), and some parts show moderate enhancement (**c**, arrow)

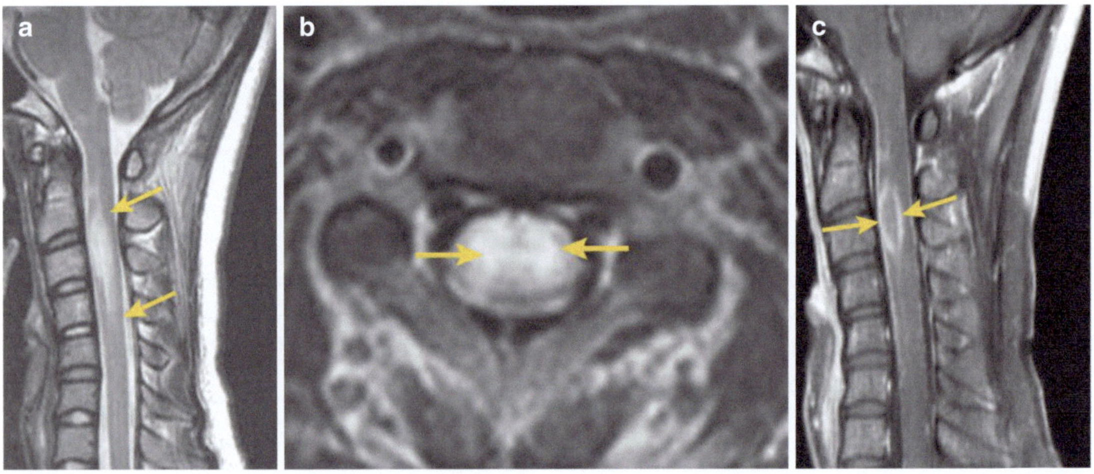

Fig. 12.4 Acute transverse myelitis. In the T2-weighted sagittal image, a long high-signal-intensity lesion is present from the second to the fourth cervical vertebrae, accompanied by corresponding spinal cord edema (**a**, arrow). In the T2-weighted axial image, the lesion invades almost the entire cross-section of the spinal cord, and there are high signal intensity lesions in both the white matter and gray matter (**b**, arrow). During enhancement, a band-like enhancement is accompanied in front and behind the lesion (**c**, arrow)

nal cord is affected alone are about 10–20%. Spinal cord lesions are seen in 80–90% of patients and are most common in the cervical area. Over a period of several days to weeks, various symptoms such as sensory abnormalities, muscle weakness, bowel and bladder disorders, and gait disorders are seen, and usually unilateral spinal cord lesions are seen, resulting in sensory and motor abnormalities in one arm and leg. Spinal cord lesions may not cause symptoms. Clinical findings are very diverse, and although they may occur as a single episode and then improve, they can also show a fulminant pattern that worsens very quickly.

Magnetic resonance imaging is the most important radiological diagnostic method, and spinal cord and brain magnetic resonance imaging are performed together. At the time of diagnosis, brain lesions are mostly found, usually around the ventricles (periventricular, subcallosal), brainstem, and cerebellum. It is common in the cerebellar white matter. Two-thirds of spinal cord lesions occur in the cervical region, showing high signal intensity on T2-weighted images and various degrees of enhancement. Most lesions are small, half or less of the total spinal cord area on axial images, and are wedge-shaped, pointing towards the central canal. This is mainly located on the outside of the spinal cord, especially on the dorsolateral side, invading the dorsal column or lateral column white matter. On sagittal images, the size usually does not exceed the height of two vertebral bodies, and various degrees of peripheral spinal cord tissue edema may be accompanied (Fig. 12.5) [6]. The size usually increases around 4 weeks and then decreases over 6–8 weeks as the surrounding edema improves. Various forms of enhancement can be seen, and enhancement is usually good in the acute-subacute phase, clear for 1–2 months, and almost no enhancement after 3 months. In the chronic phase, there is no enhancement and spinal cord atrophy is accompanied.

Cerebrospinal fluid examination can show mild inflammatory findings (0–50 cells, mild elevation in protein), an increase in oligoclonal band and IgG, but about 15% show normal findings.

Treatment includes oral or intravenous steroids, plasmapheresis, and administration of interferon β. The clinical course is very diverse, often recurring with improvement and deterioration (relapsing remitting or secondary progressive), worsening from the beginning (primary progressive), or continuing to worsen while recurring (progressive relapsing).

Differential diagnosis includes intramedullary tumors, acute transverse myelitis, and neuromyelitis optica.

12.2.3 Neuromyelitis Optica (NMO)

Neuromyelitis optica is a demyelinating disease that accompanies optic neuritis and acute transverse myelitis, also known as Devic's syndrome,

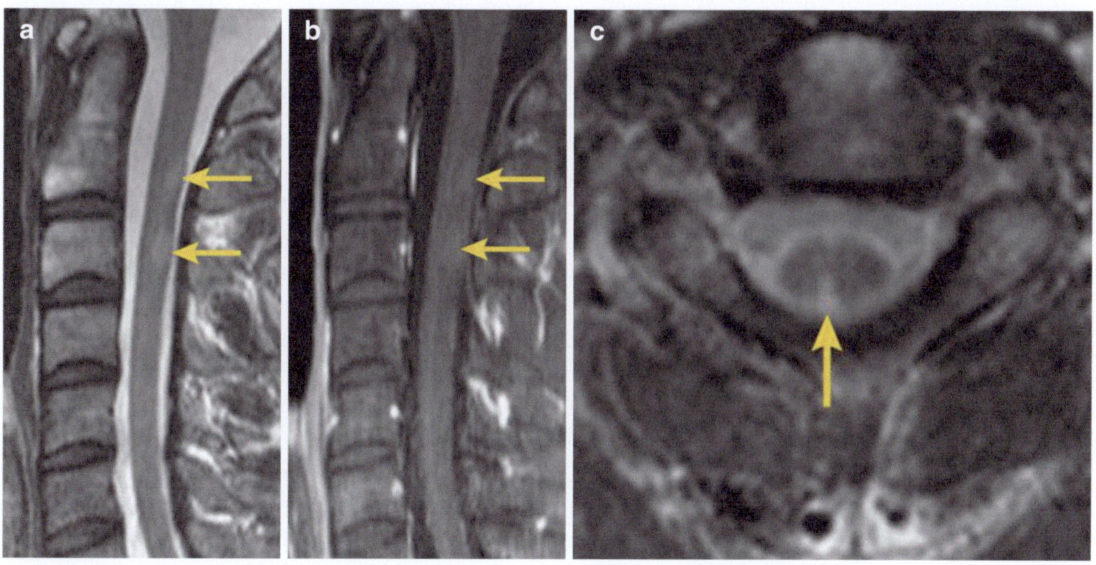

Fig. 12.5 Multiple sclerosis. A 25-year-old male patient who had been showing repeated sensory abnormalities and muscle weakness for several years, with alternating improvements and deteriorations in symptoms. In the T2-weighted sagittal image, there is a high signal intensity lesion at the back of the spinal cord at the second/third cervical vertebrae (**a**, arrow), showing slight enhancement (**b**, arrow). These lesions are slightly shifted to the right at the back of the spinal cord in the T2-weighted axial image (**c**, arrow)

Devic's disease, Devic neuromyelitis optica, and optic-spinal multiple sclerosis. It is an inflammatory disease caused by autoimmunity that invades the nerve myelin of the optic nerve and spinal cord, and brain parenchymal lesions are limited. Neurological damage is greater than in patients with multiple sclerosis. Recurrence is common. It is more common in adult women in their 30s and 40s (8–9:1) and more common in Africans. It can show visual impairment due to optic neuritis and muscle weakness, bowel and bladder disorders due to myelitis. Bilateral optic neuritis can occur with myelitis or sequentially. About one third of patients may have respiratory failure due to extensive cervical myelitis. Compared to multiple sclerosis, the age of onset is higher, it is more common in women, the clinical course is worse, and painful paroxysmal tonic spasm is more common.

The mechanism of neuromyelitis optica is autoimmunity against the aquaporin-4 protein. Explained as a response, proteins of the aquaporin family are substances that constitute water channels located in the cell membrane, participating in water movement through the cell membrane. Among them, aquaporin-4 protein is particularly distributed in the cell membrane water channels located in the brain and is mainly located in the foot process of astrocytes surrounding the cerebral capillary endothelium. Recently, an antibody against aquaporin-4 (AQP4-IgG) has been discovered and is being used as a useful serum test for diagnosing optic neuritis, with a sensitivity of 76% and a specificity of 94%. Autoimmune diseases such as autoimmune thyroiditis, myasthenia gravis, and Sjogren syndrome can be accompanied in patients with optic neuritis, and there may also be a history of previous viral infection. Recently, it is collectively referred to as "NMO-spectrum disorders NMOSDs," including patients who are AQP4-IgG negative and clinically show symptoms of optic neuritis, and some of them show positive antibodies against myelin oligodendrocyte glycoprotein (MOG) [7, 8].

85% of patients show long spinal lesions and abnormal contrast enhancement lesions of the optic nerve. On magnetic resonance imaging, it appears as a very long expansile pattern of spinal lesions showing high signal intensity on T2-weighted images, more than 3–4 vertebrae high, in the form of longitudinally extensive transverse myelitis (LETM), and in cross-sectional images, it invades most of the spinal cross-section, usually invading both gray and white matter in the center of the spinal cross-section. Often accompanied by edema and unclear boundaries, ring-shaped contrast enhancement (Fig. 12.6). In the chronic phase, spinal atrophy is accompanied by a nonspecific hyperintense spot remaining on T2-weighted images. Optic nerve lesions can be seen on one or both sides and may be accompanied by contrast enhancement. Initially, it was thought that brain lesions were rare in patients with optic neuritis, but brain lesions similar to multiple sclerosis can be accompanied in 10–30% of patients with optic neuritis, and are common in areas near the thalamus, hypothalamus, or brainstem, third ventricle or fourth ventricle where there are many aquaporin proteins. These brain nerve lesions usually do not accompany symptoms, and especially in children, there are many cases accompanied by such asymptomatic brain lesions [9]. According to the guidelines announced in 2015, the diagnosis of NMOSDs in adults is possible through (1) at least one or more core clinical findings, (2) positive AQP4-IgG serum test, (3) exclusion of other diseases, and the core clinical findings refer to one of the following six: (1) optic neuritis, (2) acute myelopathy, (3) area postrema syndrome (unexplained hiccups or nausea, vomiting symptoms), (4) acute brainstem syndrome, (5) symptomatic narcolepsy or acute diencephalic clinical syndrome showing NMOSD-typical diencephalic MRI lesions, and (6) symptomatic cerebral syndrome showing NMOSD-typical brain lesion [8].

Treatment involves intravascular steroid injections or immunosuppressant administration, and optic neuritis and myelitis often recur, similar to multiple sclerosis, with a variety of clinical courses. The prognosis is worse than multiple sclerosis and often recurs during pregnancy. It is known that the prognosis is not good if there are

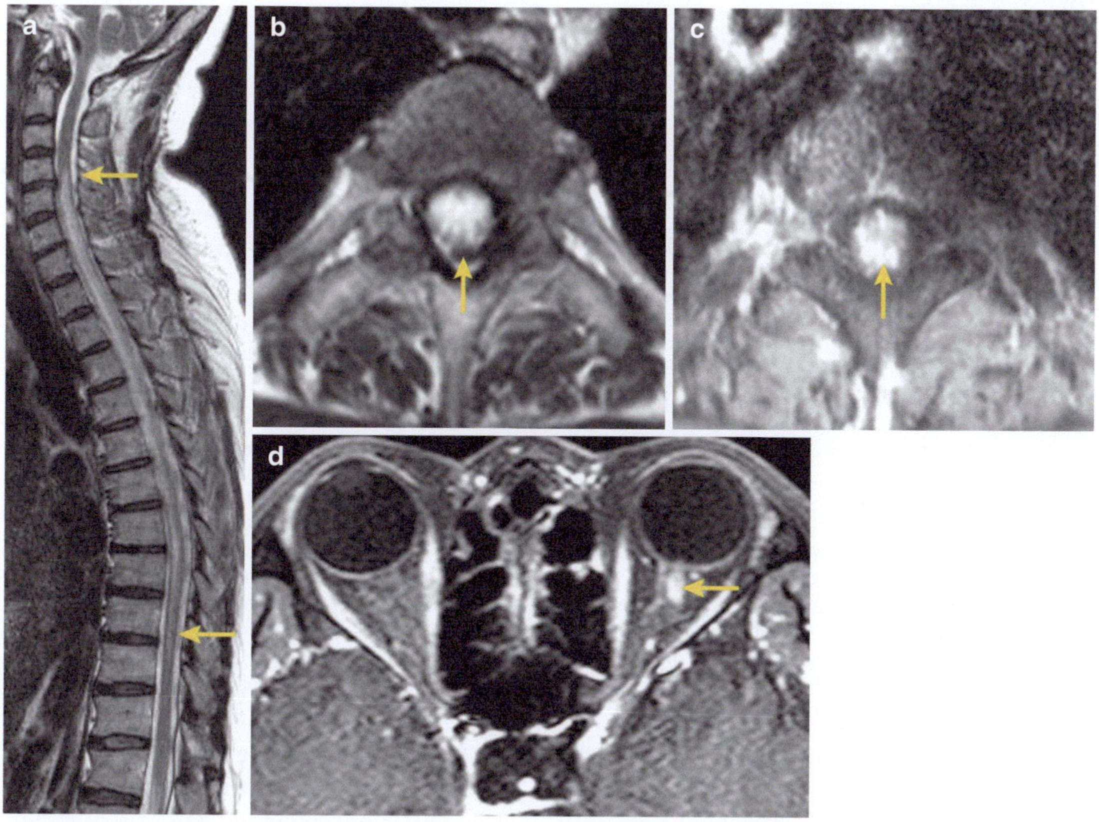

Fig. 12.6 Neuromyelitis optica. In the T2-weighted sagittal image, there is a very long high signal intensity lesion in the spinal cord from the fourth cervical vertebra to the tenth thoracic vertebra (**a**, arrow). In the T2-weighted axial image, it invades the entire cross-section of the spinal cord (**b**, arrow), showing relatively strong enhancement (**c**, arrow). In the brain contrast-enhanced MRI performed due to abnormal vision in the left eye, there was strong enhancement along the left optic nerve (**d**, arrow), and the patient was diagnosed with neuromyelitis optica due to positive findings for the antibody against aquaporin-4 (NMO-IgG)

many brain lesions at the time of diagnosis. Differential diagnoses include multiple sclerosis, idiopathic acute transverse myelitis, viral myelitis, spinal cord dural fistula, spinal cord-intramedullary tumors, etc.

12.2.4 Spinal Sarcoidosis

Sarcoidosis is an idiopathic inflammatory granulomatous disorder that affects multiple organs. Neurological involvement is reported in about 5~10% of patients, and in half of these cases, the first symptoms are neurological. It is common in middle-aged adults, similar to optic neuritis and myelitis, but shows a much longer subacute symptom onset of about a month. The symptom onset period and the degree of neurological damage vary greatly, and sensory abnormalities are common as it mainly invades the dorsal subpial area of the spinal cord [10]. On MRI, similar to optic neuritis and myelitis, it appears as a long high signal intensity lesion in more than three segments of the vertebral body on sagittal T2-weighted images, a finding of longitudinally extensive transverse myelitis (LETM). During contrast enhancement, it shows sheet-like or plaque-like enhancement along the surface of the spinal cord, and when it spreads centripetally into the spinal cord, it shows a wedge-like pattern of enhancement (Fig. 12.7). On the sagittal plane, linear dorsal subpial

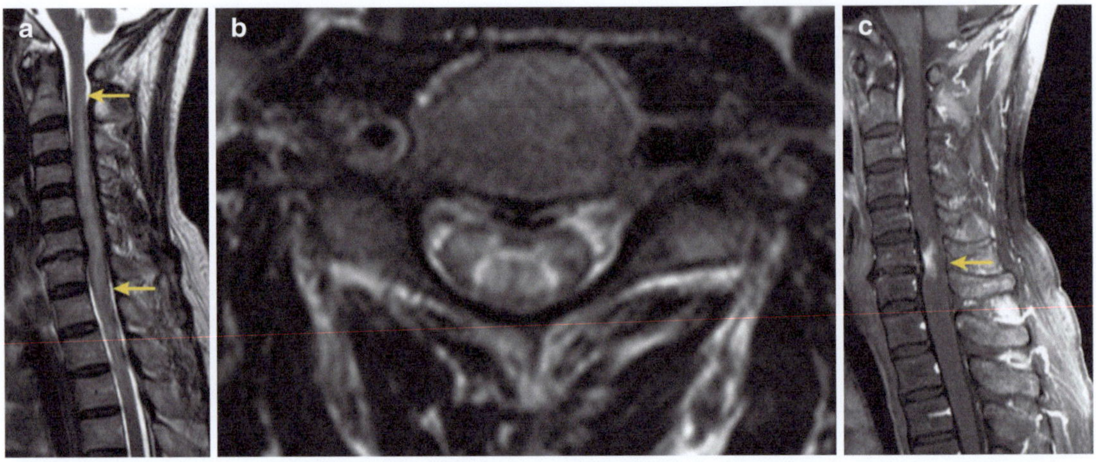

Fig. 12.7 Spinal sarcoidosis. A 62-year-old female patient who showed gradually worsening upper limb muscle weakness and sensory abnormalities for 2 weeks. In the T2-weighted sagittal image, there is a long high signal intensity spinal cord lesion (**a**, arrow), which mainly invaded the central part of the spinal cord's white matter on the T2 enhanced axial image (**b**). On the contrast-enhanced T1 enhanced sagittal image, enhancement is seen in the central part of the spinal cord at the sixth cervical vertebra (**c**, arrow). The angiotensin-converting enzyme (ACE) level was significantly increased to 113 U/L in the blood test, and bilateral jugular lymph node enlargement was accompanied. Through lymph node biopsy, it was pathologically confirmed as sarcoidosis. (Courtesy of Pf. Min A Yoon, Department of Radiology, Asan Medical Center, Seoul, Korea)

enhancement is seen, and when accompanied by central canal enhancement, it shows a characteristic "trident sign." This characteristic enhancement pattern is thought to occur as granulomatous inflammation first occurs in the leptomeninges and gradually progresses inward along the perivascular space to the parenchyma [11]. The angiotensin-converting enzyme (ACE) level is also tested in serum and cerebrospinal fluid, which can help in differential diagnosis with higher specificity than sensitivity. For diagnosis, it is important to look for signs of sarcoidosis in other organs, check for abnormalities in the skin, lymph nodes, and lungs, and often accompany thoracic lymph node enlargement at the time of diagnosis. PET/CT or chest CT scans are performed for this purpose, and diagnosis is possible by confirming noncaseating granuloma in pathological tissue after biopsy. Treatment involves intravascular steroid injections or immunosuppressant administration, and clinical and radiological follow-up examinations are recommended every 3 months for follow-up.

12.2.5 Myelin Oligodendrocyte Glycoprotein Antibody (MOG-IgG) Associated CNS Demyelinating Disease

Initially, the antibody against myelin oligodendrocyte glycoprotein (MOG-IgG) was noted as a serum biomarker related to recurrence in patients with multiple sclerosis, but now it is associated with acute disseminated encephalomyelitis (ADEM), single/recurrent optic neuritis, single/recurrent myelitis, AQP4-IgG seronegative NMOSD, and other atypical CNS demyelinating diseases are known to be related. In pediatric patients, there is known relapsing ADEM associated with MOG-IgG, and in cases of AQP4-IgG seronegative NMOSD, early relapses often appear in the form of optic neuritis, myelitis, and brainstem encephalitis, which are related to the distribution of MOG. It is also known that such inflammatory processes can be initiated by infections or vaccinations.

MOG-IgG associated CNS demyelinating disease shows similar imaging findings to AQP4-

IgG seropositive NMOSD, which can be accompanied by a similar discontinuous second lesion while showing longitudinally extensive transverse myelitis (LETM) findings. It often involves the conus, and enhancement is minimal or not well done like ADEM. A positive MOG-IgG test is a distinguishing point from AQP4-IgG seropositive NMOSD and other diseases [12].

12.2.6 Acute Disseminated Encephalomyelitis (ADEM)

ADEM is a rare disease that mainly occurs in children but can also appear in adults. It is an idiopathic CNS demyelinating disease that clinically and pathologically has similarities to some cases of multiple sclerosis. Pathologically, perivenous sleeves of demyelination are characteristic, and diffuse cortical microglial activation is also characteristic. Common predisposing factors include respiratory or gastrointestinal infections, and a history of vaccination. Compared to multiple sclerosis, it often presents as encephalopathy with decreased consciousness, headache, and nystagmus. Serum MOG-IgG is found in about 50% of patients and if it continues to be high, it can be a sign of recurrence. It is typically monophasic and responds well to steroid treatment. If it recurs, the possibility of recurrent ADEM, MOG-IgG associated CNS demyelinating disease, AQP4-IgG seropositive NMOSD, etc. should be considered.

On MRI, it is characteristic to show lesions with high signal intensity on T2-weighted images in deep gray matter such as the basal ganglia, thalamus, or white matter, and enhancement may or may not be well done. About one third of patients have spinal cord lesions, which appear as long high signal intensity lesions as seen in MOG-IgG associated CNS demyelinating disease (Fig. 12.8).

Treatment usually involves high-dose steroid treatment, and immunosuppressive treatment is not done when a monophasic course is observed [13].

12.2.7 Guillain-Barre Syndrome

This is a disease that mainly occurs in children, adolescents, or young adults, also known as acute inflammatory demyelinating polyradiculoneuropathy (AIDP). It is a phenomenon where acute inflammatory demyelination occurs in the peripheral nerve, nerve root, cranial nerve, etc. due to an autoimmune reaction caused by an infectious disease or vaccination. The characteristic symptom is sudden bilateral symmetrical flaccid paralysis, which shows a gradually ascending pattern ("ascending paralysis"), usually peaking about 4 weeks after symptom onset. It is rare, but it can also be accompanied by sensory impairment, abnormal sensation, tingling sense, etc. It is thought to be a demyelination disease caused by autoimmune or viral mechanisms, and about 70% of patients have factors that can trigger such immune responses, usually viral infectious diseases (*Campylobacter jejuni* infection) just before symptom onset. Other factors include influenza vaccination, recent surgical history, etc. The autoimmune response caused by this is considered the main mechanism of occurrence, and it can often go up to the brainstem and invade, causing respiratory paralysis that may require a ventilator in severe cases, and cranial nerves can also be invaded, causing facial nerve paralysis or ophthalmoparesis. In magnetic resonance imaging contrast enhancement, it is characteristic to show smooth leptomeningeal enhancement along the cauda equina and conus medullaris, especially along the ventral nerve stem (Fig. 12.9). This finding should be differentiated from leptomeningeal seeding seen in cancer patients, which usually shows leptomeningeal enhancement with significant nodularity [14]. The conus medullaris usually shows normal findings, and the nerve root may appear slightly swollen. Initially, intravenous immunoglobulin treatment or plasma exchange treatment is performed. Most patients gradually improve within 2–3 months, but about half have symptoms for up to a year, and 5–10% have permanent disabilities. There are rare cases of recurrence, and about 8% die from respiratory

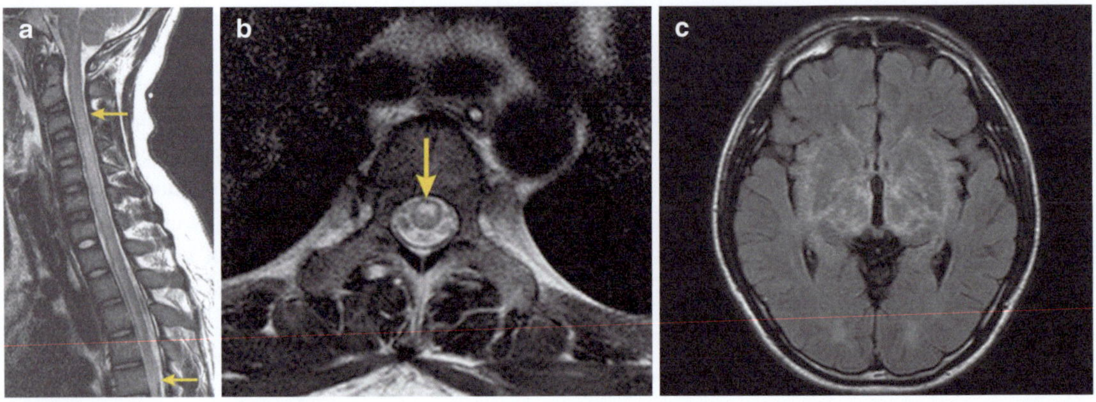

Fig. 12.8 Acute disseminated encephalomyelitis (ADEM). A 16-year-old male patient with fever, chills, headache, and sore throat has a very long high signal intensity lesion in the spinal cord from the third cervical vertebra to the fifth thoracic vertebra on the T2 enhanced sagittal image (**a**, arrow), which invaded the front part of the spinal cord on the T2 enhanced axial image (**b**, arrow). There are extensive high signal intensity lesions in the basal ganglia and thalamus on the brain MRI FLAIR image (**c**)

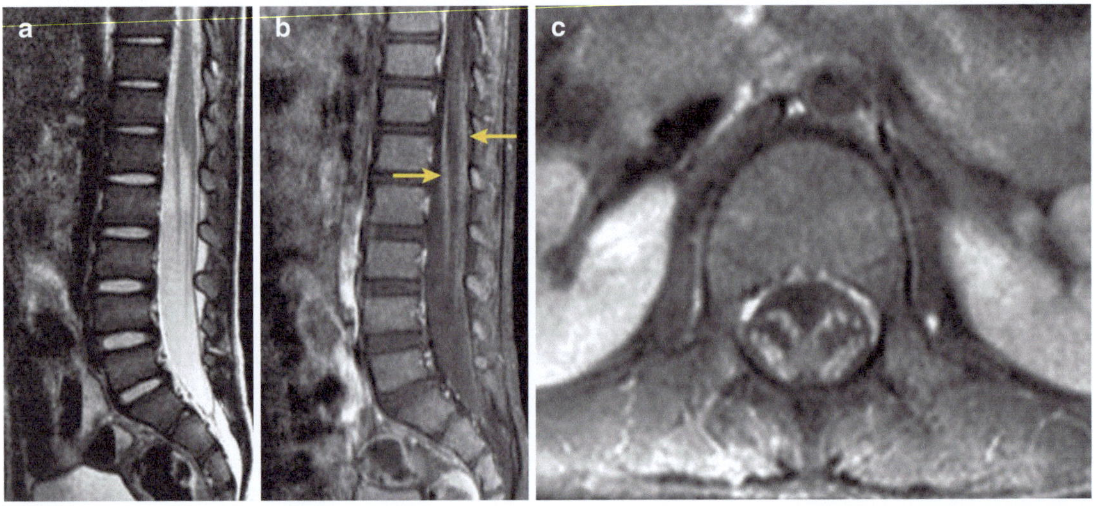

Fig. 12.9 Guillain-Barre syndrome. In a 5-year-old male patient with lower limb weakness and sensory abnormalities, the spinal cord cone (conus medullaris) appears slightly thicker on the lumbar spine MRI T2 enhanced image (**a**) and shows thick enhancement along the cauda equina and conus medullaris on the contrast-enhanced T1 enhanced sagittal image (**b**, arrow). This enhancement finding is clear on the T1 enhanced axial image from both the ventral and dorsal sides (**c**)

failure. Differential diagnosis includes Miller-Fisher syndrome, a variant of Guillain-Barre syndrome, vasculitis-related neuritis such as polyarteritis nodosa or Churg-Strauss syndrome, acute transverse myelitis, bacterial or granulomatous meningitis, carcinomatous or lymphomatous meningitis, vincristine-related chemical arachnoiditis, anterior lumbar radiculopathy caused by intrathecal chemotherapy, post-radiation radiculopathy, etc.

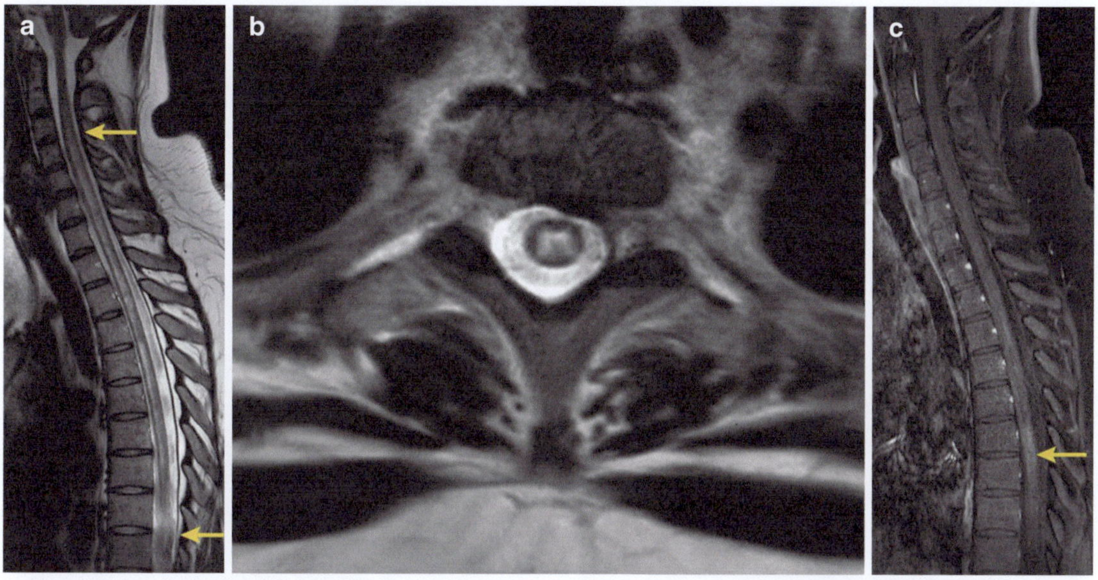

Fig. 12.10 Systemic lupus erythematosus (SLE). A 24-year-old female patient diagnosed with systemic lupus erythematosus (SLE) 3 years ago, has a very long high signal intensity lesion in the spinal cord from the third cervical vertebra to the ninth thoracic vertebra on the MRI T2 enhanced image due to the symptom of losing strength in both legs since the day before (**a**, arrow). It mainly invaded the white matter of the spinal cord on the T2 enhanced axial image (**b**). On the contrast-enhanced T1 enhanced axial image, only the spinal cord lesion at the sixth to seventh thoracic vertebrae shows slight enhancement (**c**, arrow)

12.2.8 Spinal Cord Disease Related to Systemic Inflammatory Disease

Acute spinal lesions can occur in systemic lupus erythematosus (SLE), Sjogren's syndrome, mixed connective tissue disorder, Behcet disease, sarcoidosis, etc. These lesions all appear as expansile LETM forms with various contrast enhancements on MRI (Fig. 12.10). However, each has a different mechanism of occurrence. SLE myelitis is known to cause spinal lesions due to thrombotic events caused by antiphospholipid antibodies rather than inflammatory reactions, while Behcet disease can cause spinal lesions due to systemic vasculitis. In the case of sarcoidosis, as mentioned earlier, spinal lesions occur due to granulomatous reactions [15, 16].

12.3 Infectious Spinal Diseases (Infectious Disease of Spinal Cord)

Infections of the spinal cord and spinal nerves can be caused by various factors such as viruses, bacteria, parasites, and fungi, which are different from postinfectious myelopathy that occurs due to the autoimmune mechanism after infection. In developed countries, such direct infection-induced spinal diseases are rare, but they can cause various motor disorders and sensory damage by causing inflammation not only in the spinal cord but also in the spinal nerves.

Bacterial infections of the spinal cord usually occur due to the spread of bacterial meningitis or infections of adjacent vertebrae or discs. Rarely, an intramedullary abscess can also occur. Nonspecific bacteria such as Aspergillus,

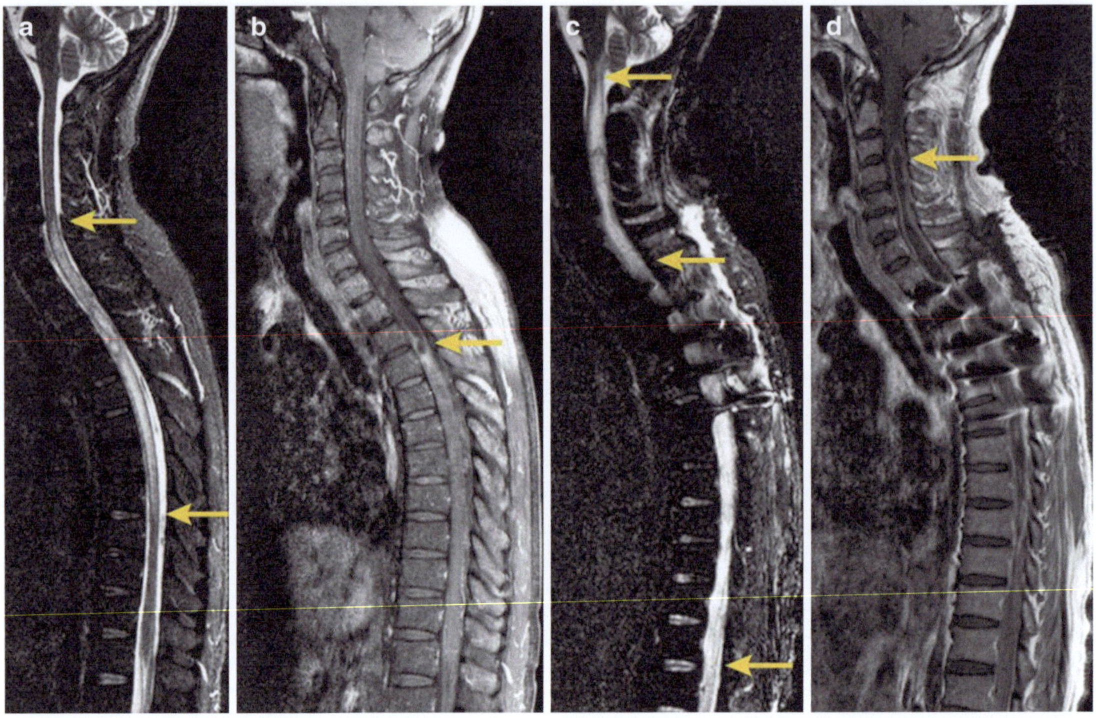

Fig. 12.11 Bacterial infection of spinal cord-intramedullary cord abscess. A 57-year-old male patient who visited the hospital with gradually progressing weakness and sensory loss in both legs from 3 to 4 months ago, on the T2 enhanced sagittal image at the time of admission, from the fifth cervical vertebra to the ninth thoracic vertebra. A long high signal intensity spinal lesion is seen extending to (**a**, arrow), and a cystic portion showing peripheral enhancement along the lesion at the thoracic 2–4 site is seen in the contrast-enhanced T1-weighted sagittal image (**b**, arrow). A week later, a follow-up examination after surgery shows a high signal intensity lesion spreading upwards to the medulla oblongata in the T2-weighted sagittal image (**c**, arrow) and an enlarged intramedullary abscess extending upwards to the cervical 3 in the contrast-enhanced T1-weighted sagittal image (**d**, arrow). Pus was confirmed in the spinal cord during the second surgery. (Courtesy of Pf. So Young Park, Department of Radiology, Kyung Hee University Hospital at Gangdong, Seoul, Korea)

Candida, Norcardia, Actinomyces can cause acute necrotizing myelitis (Fig. 12.11).

Common causative viruses include enterovirus (EV-D68, EV-71, poliovirus), herpesvirus (varicella-zoster virus, cytomegalovirus, herpes simplex), arbovirus (arthropod-borne virus, including West Nile virus). Poliovirus invades the lower motor neuron, causing acute flaccid paralysis, which has decreased significantly as vaccines have become widespread. On MRI, it is characterized by high signal intensity lesions along the anterior horn cell in T2-weighted images [17]. Varicella-zoster virus, the causative virus of chickenpox in pediatric patients, can lie dormant in nerve cells for decades, reactivate to cause herpes zoster, or spread along the nerve root to cause radiomyelitis. On MRI, lesions can be confirmed in the dorsolateral spinal cord and adjacent nerve root entry part [18].

Parasitic infections such as cysticercosis, schistosomiasis, and echinococcus are very rare outside of endemic areas, and these parasitic infections can appear as acute or chronic spinal lesions (Fig. 12.12) [19].

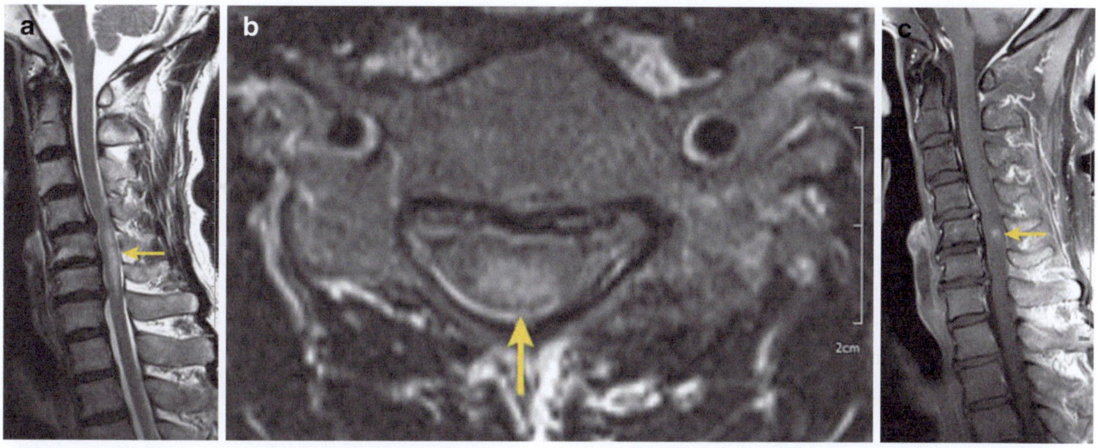

Fig. 12.12 Parasite infection of spinal cord-Toxocara canis myelitis. A 65-year-old male patient who visited the hospital with symptoms of pain and weakness in both upper limbs that started a month ago, shows a high signal intensity spinal lesion at the cervical 5–6 site in the cervical T2-weighted sagittal image (**a**, arrow), which is widely invading the gray and white matter in the T2-weighted axial image (**b**, arrow). After contrast enhancement, it is slightly enhanced only at the cervical 5 site in the T1-weighted sagittal image (**c**, arrow)

12.4 Metabolic Diseases (Metabolic Disease of Spinal Cord)

The representative metabolic diseases that occur in the spinal cord are caused by vitamin B12 deficiency and copper deficiency.

12.4.1 Subacute Combined Degeneration

This is a common spinal lesion in vitamin B12 deficiency, most commonly caused by pernicious anemia. It usually occurs in middle-aged people in their 60s. The main cause is the destruction of the parietal cells of the gastric mucosa due to an abnormal immune system, which leads to achlorhydria, atrophic gastritis, and a decrease in the action of the intrinsic factor, resulting in vitamin B12 absorption disorder in the gastrointestinal tract. Vitamin B12 absorption disorders can also occur due to previous gastric or small intestine resection surgery, fish tapeworm (*Diphyllobothrium latum*) infection, Crohn's disease, celiac disease, bacterial overgrowth in blind loops after previous intestinal operation, etc. After anesthesia or inhalation of nitrous oxide (N_2O, laughing gas), when the action of vitamin B12 is inhibited and methylmalonic acid is deposited, myelin toxicity occurs, or in cases of transcobalamin II deficiency, the same imaging findings as subacute combined degeneration are shown. Vitamin B12 (cobalamin) is mainly absorbed through meat consumption, so it can also be deficient in strict vegetarians.

It usually appears in middle-aged people in their 40s to 70s and is more common in men. Most of them complain of gradually progressing upper limb sensory abnormalities, tingling sense, sensory ataxia, position and vibration sensory disorders, stiffness, etc. and usually worsen bilaterally, symmetrically, and from the periphery to the center over weeks or months. Rarely, motor disorders and urinary disorders are accompanied. In the blood test findings, it is accompanied by macrocytic anemia and the level of vitamin B12 in the serum is reduced.

It mainly causes degeneration by selectively invading the dorsal column of the cervical-thoracic region, and the lateral column also shows degeneration. On T2-weighted images, it is typical to see a very long high signal intensity along the back of the spinal cord, and the lesion seen along the dorsal column in the cross-sectional image is characterized by an inverted V shape ("inverted V") or inverted rabbit ear shape ("inverted rabbit ears"). The spinal cord in the area generally appears slightly swollen. Mild enhancement may appear along the dorsal column (Fig. 12.13) [20].

If left untreated, it is difficult to improve on its own, and it improves with the administration of vitamin B12, but the course varies, and the already destroyed nerve tissue is difficult to recover.

Differential diagnoses include HIV vacuolar myelopathy, infectious myelitis caused by Varicella-Zoster or Herpes, and inflammatory myelitis such as multiple sclerosis, acute disseminated encephalomyelitis, and acute transverse myelitis.

12.4.2 Copper Deficiency Spinal Disease (Copper Deficiency)

Copper is a cofactor that acts on important electron transfers in essential enzyme reactions in bone marrow and nervous system functions. In 2001, Schleper and Stuerenburg first reported spinal disease due to copper deficiency after gastrointestinal resection [21]. Copper deficiency can cause megaloblastic anemia and pancytopenia similar to patients with pernicious anemia, and neurologically, it can show symptoms similar to subacute combined degeneration seen in vitamin B12 deficiency. Sensory ataxia and spasticity due to disorders of the posterior column and lateral column can cause walking disorders.

The cause of copper deficiency is usually digestive and absorption disorders, and copper is mainly absorbed in the duodenum and stomach, so gastrointestinal resection is a common cause. In addition, celiac disease and inflammatory bowel disease also cause absorption disorders. Often, excessive intake of zinc increases the expression of the chelator metallothionein in intestinal enterocytes, which is more than zinc. The absorption of copper is prevented due to its stronger adsorption with zinc, causing it to be excreted in the feces [22].

In magnetic resonance imaging findings, it appears very similar to subacute combined degeneration as a high signal intensity lesion invading the dorsal column of the cervical spinal cord in T2-weighted images, and the lateral column can also be invaded. Enhancement is usually not observed [23].

The diagnosis is made by confirming a decrease in serum copper and ceruloplasmin levels, and an increase in zinc levels can be helpful

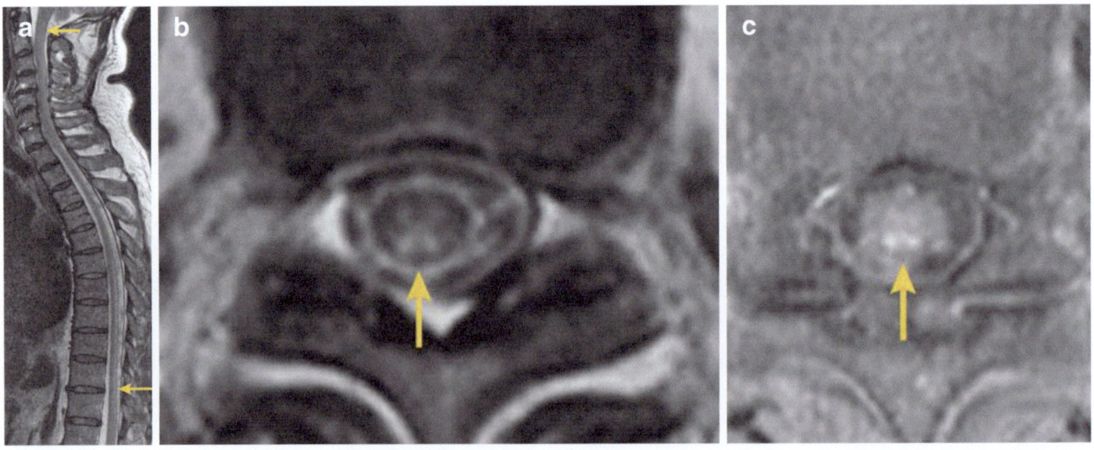

Fig. 12.13 Subacute combined degeneration. A long high signal intensity spinal lesion is seen from the cervical 2 to the thoracic 11 in the T2-weighted sagittal image, especially prominent at the back of the thoracic site (**a**, arrow). Because it selectively invades the dorsal, lateral column of the spinal cord, it shows an "inverted V sign" at the back of the spinal cord in the T2-weighted axial image (**b**, arrow) and often enhances (**c**, arrow). It was diagnosed as subacute combined degeneration due to the finding of low vitamin B12 levels in the blood test

in diagnosis. Treatment is oral intake of copper, and it may be necessary to limit zinc intake.

12.5 Vascular Diseases (Vascular Disease of the Spinal Cord)

Vascular-related diseases occurring in the spinal cord can be broadly divided into ischemia or infarction and vascular malformation, and here we will mention based on representative magnetic resonance imaging findings.

12.5.1 Spinal Cord Ischemia, Infarction

Ischemia or infarction occurring in the spinal cord often occurs in the thoracolumbar or conus medullaris, and the exact incidence is not known. Atherosclerosis of the spinal artery is rare, and due to multiple anastomoses, spinal cord ischemia and infarction are very rare compared to the cerebrum. The spinal cord is basically supplied from various levels of segmental arteries, such as the vertebral artery, ascending cervical artery, deep cervical artery, intercostal artery, lumbar artery, and sacral artery, and receives nutritional supply from one anterior spinal artery and two posterior spinal arteries that come out from the radicular arteries branched from them. The anterior spinal artery supplies the central gray matter and adjacent part of the white matter while stretching up and down in the middle of the front of the spinal cord, and the two posterior spinal arteries mainly receive supply from the vertebral artery or posterior inferior cerebellar artery and run up and down in pairs on the back of the spinal cord, mainly supplying the outer and back one third of the spinal cord. The two posterior spinal arteries have many anastomoses with each other (Fig. 12.14). The thoracolumbar spinal cord is supplied from the great radicular artery or the artery of Adamkiewcz, which is a major radiculomedullary artery, which usually originates from the segmental artery between the ninth and twelfth thoracic vertebrae on the left side (75%) and shows a characteristic hairpin-shaped bend on angiography.

Spinal cord ischemia and infarction occur without knowing the exact cause in more than 50% of cases, and known causes include dissection or embolism due to atherosclerosis of the aorta, aortic aneurysm, septicemia, arterial dissection or direct injury due to trauma, vasculitis, and injury due to epidural steroid injection. Spinal cord ischemia/infarction often occurs in the upper thoracic region, which is considered the boundary area of adjacent arterial blood, and was previously often referred to as watershed

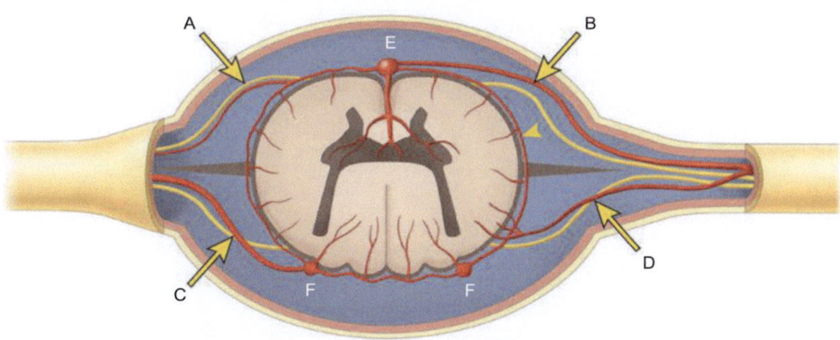

Fig. 12.14 Arterial supply of spinal cord. The spinal artery branches into anterior and posterior branches within the neural foramina, which then become (1) radicular artery (**a**) distributing to the nerve root and dura, (2) anterior radiculomedullary artery (**b**) distributing to the anterior cord parenchyma with the anterior spinal artery (ASA)(E), (3) posterior radiculomedullary artery (**c**) distributing to the posterior cord parenchyma with the posterior spinal arteries (PSAs)(F), (4) radiculopial artery (**d**) distributing to the cord's pial surface, (5) ASA distributing to two-thirds of the anterior spinal cord, (6) two PSAs distributing to one third of the posterior spinal cord. Also, the vasa corona (white arrowheads) forms a rich anastomotic network along the surface of the spinal cord. However, there are no vessels within the deep spinal cord parenchyma connecting the ASA and the two PSAs

infarction. The mechanisms of spinal cord ischemia or infarction have been explained, but it is now also explained as the intervertebral disc cartilage being rapidly forced into the spinal blood vessels due to spinal trauma, obstructing the blood flow.

Neurological damage varies depending on the location of the spinal cord ischemia or infarction. If the front part of the spinal cord is mainly damaged (anterior spinal syndrome), paralysis, loss of pain and temperature sensation, and bowel and bladder disorders are shown. If the back of the spinal cord is damaged (posterior spinal syndrome), symptoms such as loss of vibration sensation and loss of position sense are shown. The characteristic clinical features of spinal cord ischemia and infarction are that symptoms occur very rapidly and progress quickly, showing significant neurological loss within a few hours. It usually occurs in middle-aged people over 50, and there is no difference between men and women.

On T2-weighted magnetic resonance imaging, it usually appears as a high signal intensity lesion that invades the front two-thirds of the spinal cord, and high signal intensity lesions can be seen across the entire cross-section of the spinal cord. About 50% may not show clear magnetic resonance imaging findings within 24 h of symptom onset. Characteristically, on T2-weighted images, it shows a high signal intensity lesion in the shape of an "owl's eye" along the gray matter of the spinal cord ("owl eye appearance"). It rarely invades the posterior one third of the spinal cord or the entire cross-section of the spinal cord. It usually occurs longitudinally over one or more segments of the vertebral body. In rare cases of accompanying hemorrhage (hemorrhagic conversion), it is accompanied by high signal intensity on T1-weighted images. In the acute phase, it does not enhance, but subacute spinal infarction around 1~3 weeks can show various enhancements. In cases where a specific segmental artery is invaded, it may also be accompanied by infarction of the adjacent vertebral bone. Recently, it has been reported that performing diffusion-weighted imaging together is useful for diagnosis, but susceptibility artifacts often occur, which can easily degrade the quality of the image (Figs. 12.15 and 12.16). Magnetic resonance angiography (MR angiography) is also performed, but it is not necessarily possible to diagnose spinal cord ischemia and infarction because the anterior spinal artery is not well

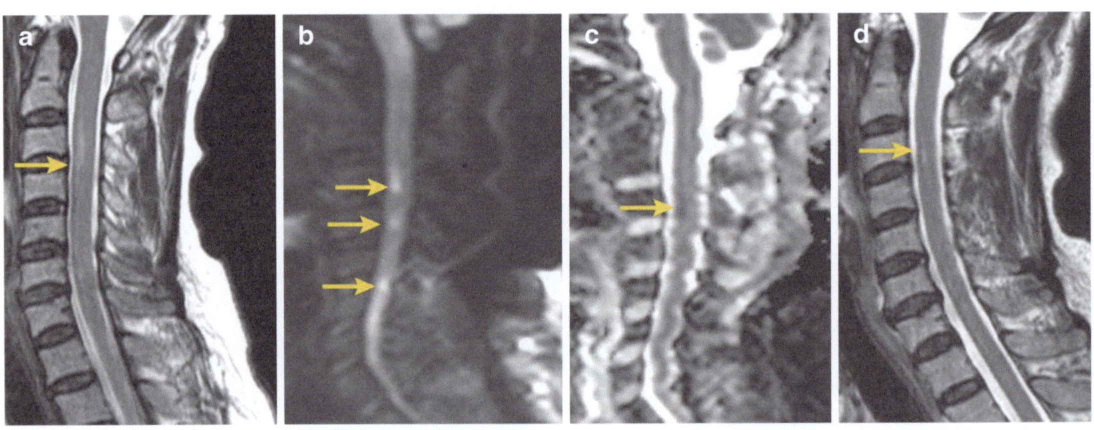

Fig. 12.15 Spinal cord ischemia, infarction. A 48-year-old male patient who visited the hospital with sudden sensory abnormalities and muscle weakness showed a long, indistinctly bordered high signal intensity lesion along the front of the cervical spinal cord in the T2 enhanced sagittal image (**a**, arrow). These lesions appear as high signal intensity in the diffusion-weighted image (**b**, arrow), with a decreased apparent diffusion coefficient (ADC), resulting in a low signal intensity (**c**, arrow). These findings are consistent with acute spinal cord ischemia and infarction, and most of the high signal intensity lesions disappeared in the T2 enhanced sagittal image taken 2 months after treatment, but a slight lesion remained at the cervical 3 site (**d**)

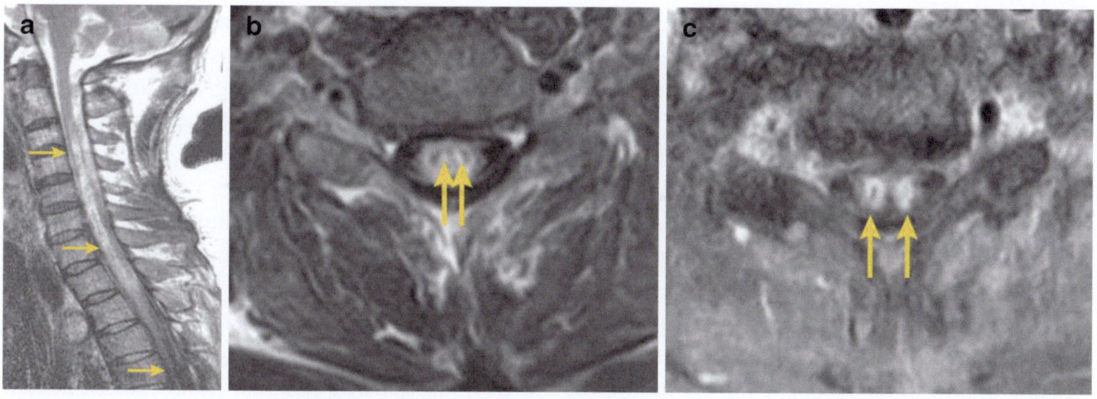

Fig. 12.16 Subacute spinal cord ischemia, infarction. A patient admitted with Type A aortic dissection complained of muscle weakness and sensory disorders. Approximately 20 days after admission, a long high signal intensity lesion was found along the entire length of the cervical-thoracic spinal cord in the T2 enhanced sagittal image of the MRI examination (**a**, arrow). In the T2 enhanced axial image, it appears as a "owl eye appearance" gray matter lesion (**b**, arrow). After contrast enhancement, it shows enhancement outside the "owl eye appearance" gray matter lesion in the fat-suppressed T1 enhanced axial image (**c**, arrow). Thus, subacute spinal infarction can show significant contrast enhancement

seen, and it is often useful for differential diagnosis of other conditions such as dural arteriovenous fistula [24, 25].

Treatment includes administration of anticoagulants such as heparin and aspirin, administration of steroids, etc., but the prognosis is not good as neurological damage remains depending on the intensity of neurological symptoms at the time of initial discovery and the part of the spinal cord involved.

Differential diagnoses include multiple sclerosis, acute transverse myelitis, neuromyelitis optica, viral myelitis, dural fistula, spinal tumors, etc.

12.5.2 Spinal Vascular Lesions

Vascular-related diseases of the spinal cord include arteriovenous malformation, cavernous hemangioma, and arteriovenous fistula are among the many classifications of vascular malformations that occur in the spine [26]. Generally, they are divided into four types: Type 1 is dural arteriovenous fistula, Type 2 is spinal cord arteriovenous malformation (glomus type), Type 3 is juvenile-type arteriovenous malformation (intramedullary or extramedullary) that occurs in children, and Type 4 is intradural perimedullary arteriovenous fistula. Here, we will describe them as dural arteriovenous fistulas that occur in the dura mater and spinal cord arteriovenous malformations that occur inside or around the spinal cord (spinal cord arteriovenous glomus malformation, perimedullary arteriovenous fistula).

12.5.2.1 Dural Arteriovenous Fistula

An abnormal connection between the radiculomeningeal artery and radicular vein leads to venous congestion in the spinal cord due to retrograde flow into the perimedullary vessel, causing neurological deficits due to congestive myelopathy. It is the most common vascular malformation in the spinal cord and is usually common in middle-aged men. The radiculomeningeal artery, which supplies the nerve root and meninges, is located around the nerve root with the radicular vein. It is commonly found in the thoracolumbar region (T5–L3) and often invades the adjacent nerve foramen or dural root sleeve. Arterial blood is supplied from the dural branch of the adjacent radicular artery, and the expanded intradural vein directly flows into the spinal cord pia mater vein.

The cause is not exactly known, but it is believed to occur when abnormally increased venous pressure due to a thrombus originating from the extradural vein is transmitted to the pia mater vein. This pressure eventually transfers to the spinal cord, causing spinal cord ischemia due to increased venous pressure.

Most show a progression of loss of motor ability in the lower or upper limbs, accompanied by symptoms such as back pain and bowel and bladder disorders. It is common for the level of arteriovenous shunt and clinically visible neurological deficits not to match. It is common in middle-aged men and accounts for the majority (80%) of vascular malformations occurring in the spinal cord.

It is common in the spinal cord area from the thoracic vertebrae to the conus. The characteristic finding is a pia mater vein that is abnormally expanded and covered with a spinal cord that shows high signal intensity on T2-weighted images and is abnormally elongated. On T2-weighted axial MRI, a wide central high signal intensity due to spinal cord edema over several segments can be seen, surrounded by a low signal intensity band due to deoxygenated blood-filled capillaries, accompanied by various contrast enhancements (Figs. 12.17 and 12.18). Venous hypertensive myelopathy caused by local blood pressure increase due to venous congestion can be seen extending outward from the spinal cord on T2-weighted images. It also shows a low signal strength. The elongated draining vein across multiple segments appears as a structure showing flow-void, especially well seen near the conus. During contrast enhancement, the elongated veins show strong contrast enhancement on the surface of the spinal cord, and the inside of the spinal cord also accompanies patchy slight contrast enhancement. Magnetic resonance angiography or selective angiography using contrast enhancement is also used for diagnosis. Catheter angiography is the most important test for diagnosis, and it can identify the exact location of the arteriovenous shunt and the location and origin of the anterior spinal artery, and through this, embolization can be performed [27, 28].

Treatment includes surgical treatment and embolization through angiography, but the success rate varies from 25% to 75%, and the clinical prognosis is not good. If left untreated, symptoms progress, leading to poor prognosis such as causing limb paralysis, and often leave serious neurological damage as they slowly progress over several years.

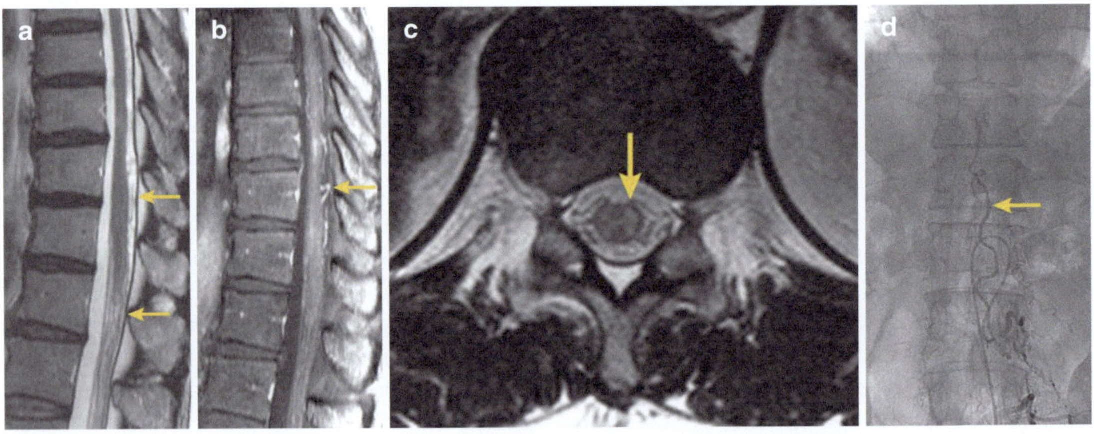

Fig. 12.17 Dural arteriovenous fistula. In the T2 enhanced sagittal image, a tortuous lesion is seen along the back of the conus medullaris (**a**, arrow), and in the contrast-enhanced T1 enhanced image, it is observed as enhanced dilated vessels (**b**, arrow). In the T2 enhanced axial image, a high signal intensity lesion is accompanied inside the skewed conus medullaris to the left, suggesting a concomitant ischemic lesion of the spinal cord (**c**, arrow). In the angiography, an abnormal vessel supplied through the left segmental artery initiated at the lumbar 1 position is seen (**d**, arrow). A diagnosis of dural arteriovenous fistula was made

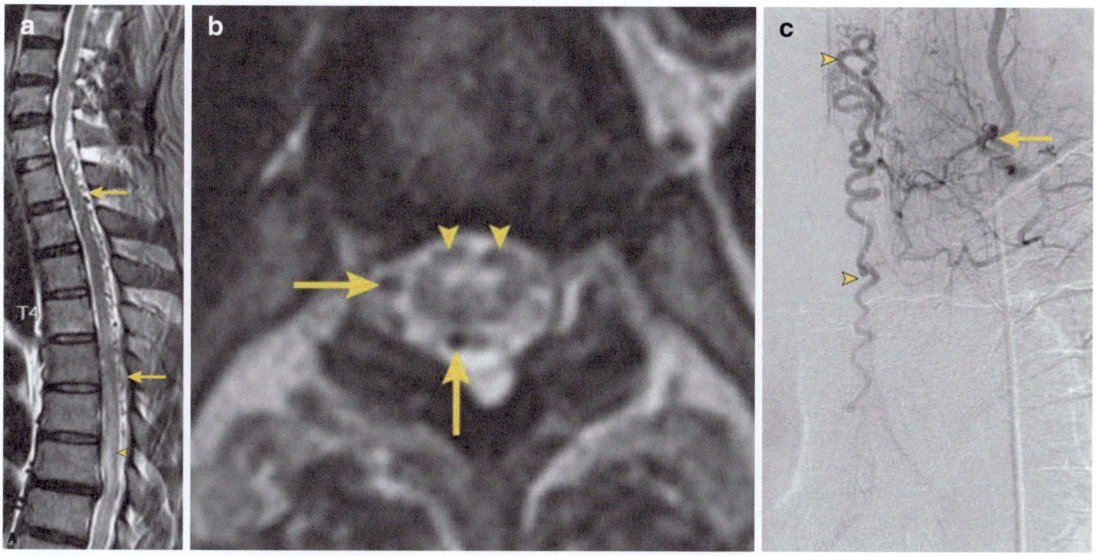

Fig. 12.18 Dural arteriovenous fistula. In the T2 enhanced sagittal image, a lesion resembling a tangled thread, showing flow-void along the back of the cervical and thoracic spinal cord, is visible (**a**, arrow). Below the sixth thoracic vertebra, there is a distinct spinal lesion of high signal intensity, thought to be due to ischemic changes in the spinal cord (arrowhead). In the T2 enhanced axial image, the ischemic lesion of the spinal cord appears in an "owl eye appearance" (arrowhead), surrounded by tortuous vessels showing flow-void (**b**, arrow). In angiography, this abnormal vascular lesion is supplied through an abnormal vessel supplied by the left segmental artery originating at the first thoracic vertebra (**c**, arrow). It was diagnosed as a dural arteriovenous fistula

Differential diagnoses include cerebrospinal fluid flow artifact (CSF flow artifact), intramedullary cord tumor, spinal cord arteriovenous malformation, etc.

12.5.2.2 Spinal Cord Arteriovenous Malformation

Also known as Glomus type or plexiform arteriovenous malformation, it accounts for 15–20% of all spinal cord arteriovenous malformations. An abnormal direct connection occurs between the anterior spinal artery or posterior spinal artery, which are the direct nutrient arteries of the spinal cord, and the intrinsic vein plexus on the surface of the spinal cord, and it has a nidus in the spinal cord. Due to such a direct arteriovenous shunt, the inside and surroundings of the lesion show a very fast blood flow speed, and it is common to accompany aneurysms (20–44%). Eventually, venous pressure rises, and various pathological symptoms occur due to ischemia caused by arterial blood supply disorders by nutrient arteries, spinal cord compression by enlarged blood vessels, and subarachnoid hemorrhage caused by ruptured aneurysms. It is common in patients in their 10s and 20s and often causes acute intramedullary or subarachnoid hemorrhage, causing sudden neurological deficits. Symptoms may worsen during pregnancy.

It commonly occurs in the cervical or thoracic spinal cord. It occurs alone, but it also occurs in relation to Klippel-Trenaunay-Weber syndrome and Rendu-Osler-Weber syndrome.

On magnetic resonance imaging, abnormal elongated blood vessels are observed as multiple flow voids in T2-weighted images, which appear as various signal intensities in T1-weighted images depending on the speed and direction of blood flow (Fig. 12.19). The corresponding spinal cord area appears swollen, and if spinal cord edema, ischemia, gliosis, etc. are mixed or residues from bleeding accumulate, various high signal intensities are seen in T2-weighted images. It appears. In T2* gradient echo images, the susceptibility artifacts caused by the by-products of hemorrhage are strongly visible, making it easier to know whether there is bleeding. During contrast enhancement, the internal nidus, spinal cord,

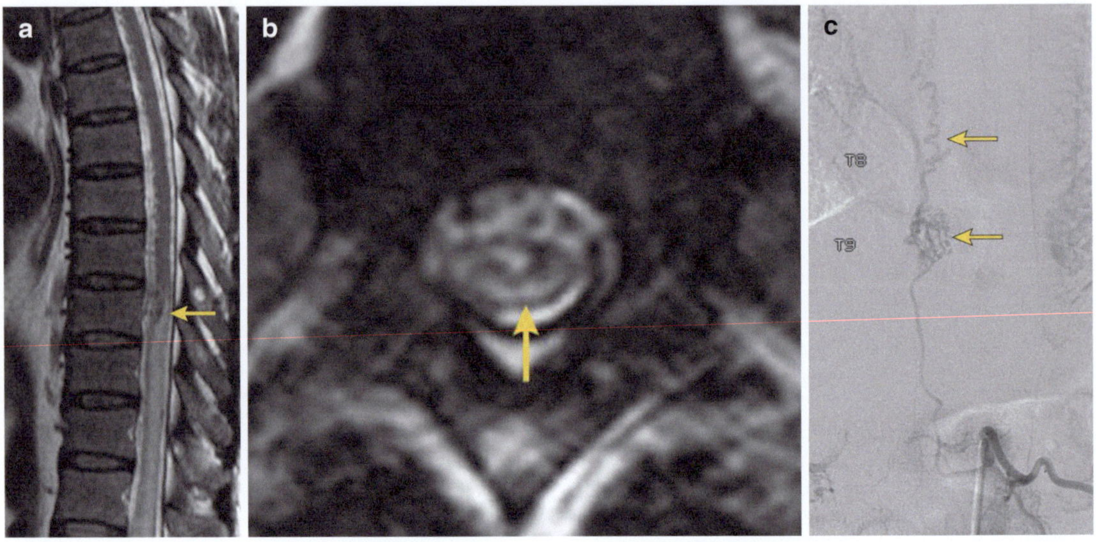

Fig. 12.19 Spinal cord arteriovenous malformation. In the T2 enhanced sagittal image, a low signal intensity lesion showing flow-void, shaped like a band or string of beads, is attached directly in front of the spinal cord, and below this, it forms a mass at the ninth thoracic vertebra (**a**, arrow). Further down, there is extensive high signal intensity spinal cord edema. In the T2 enhanced axial image performed at the ninth thoracic vertebra, the flow-void concentrated in front of the spinal cord and the high signal intensity edema of the spinal cord are more distinct (**b**, arrow). In angiography, the mass seen at the ninth thoracic vertebra is being nourished like a thread through a branch of the left eleventh intercostal artery, and an extended draining vein is seen upwards (**c**, arrow). It was diagnosed as a glomus type arteriovenous malformation of the spinal cord

and adjacent enlarged vessels are variously and strongly enhanced. It is difficult to accurately distinguish the detailed types of spinal cord arteriovenous malformations with magnetic resonance imaging, but it is possible to evaluate the relationship with accompanying spinal cord edema, hemorrhage, and adjacent meninges. The degree of contrast enhancement varies, and in the case of slow-flow arteriovenous malformations, diagnosis can be aided by performing contrast-enhanced magnetic resonance imaging together. Recently, magnetic resonance angiography has been helpful in diagnosing the feeding arteries of arteriovenous malformations, but so far, selective angiography is considered an important procedure that enables accurate diagnosis of detailed types and embolization of the corresponding feeding arteries [29, 30].

The prognosis is generally better than other arteriovenous malformations, and it is a principle to immediately treat spinal arteriovenous malformations with symptoms. It is common to perform surgical resection after endovascular embolization.

Differential diseases include ependymoma, astrocytoma, hemangioblastoma, paraganglioma, cavernous hemangioma, and type 3 or 4 arteriovenous fistula/malformation.

12.5.2.3 Cavernous Hemangioma

Also known as cavernous malformation, cavernous angioma, cryptic vascular malformation, it is a lesion composed of enlarged capillaries and sinusoidal vessels, with no normal spinal cord nerve tissue inside, and unlike arteriovenous malformations, there are no feeding arteries or draining veins. It is known to occur due to excessive secretion of various substances (VEGF, BFGF, TGFα, etc.) that induce immature endothelial cell proliferation and angiogenesis, and it is most common in the thoracic region and also occurs well in the cervical region. It is also called cavernous malformation. It is common in middle-aged adults and is often found in the thoracic region. Usually, acute intraspinal hemorrhage occurs repeatedly, causing acute repetitive neurological deficits. It is rare for cavernous hemangiomas to occur in the spinal cord, and only about

3~5% are found in the spinal cord. The size is often several millimeters, and lesions over 1 cm are also found.

Usually, sensory and motor ataxia, progressive paralysis symptoms are shown, neurological loss symptoms that repeat improvement and deterioration may occur, neurological symptoms may gradually progress, and neurological symptoms may suddenly worsen within a few hours or days. It is common in women in their 20s to 50s, and 10~30% have multiple lesions. It is visible or there is a family history.

On the T2-weighted magnetic resonance image, it appears as a well-defined lesion, with a low signal intensity band on the outside and heterogeneous high signal intensity locules inside, which show a popcorn appearance, characterized by fluid-fluid levels (Fig. 12.20). The outer low signal intensity band is known to be caused by the magnetic artifact of hemosiderin deposited due to repeated hemorrhage, and the inside is deposited with waste products caused by repeated hemorrhage at different times, showing heterogeneous signal intensity in T1- and T2-weighted images. In very small cases, it is not easy to find in T1- and T2-weighted images, and it can be found only as a small low signal intensity lesion in T2-weighted images without surrounding spinal cord edema. In T2* gradient echo images, the magnetic artifacts caused by waste products from repeated hemorrhages are strongly visible, making it easier to find small lesions due to the so-called blooming effect. Contrast enhancement is often minimal or absent. Also, in angiography, it is easy to show negative findings because cavernous hemangiomas are lesions with very slow blood flow and do not accompany abnormal arteries or veins unlike arteriovenous malformations [31].

The principle is to treat symptomatic cavernous hemangiomas, and surgical removal is the

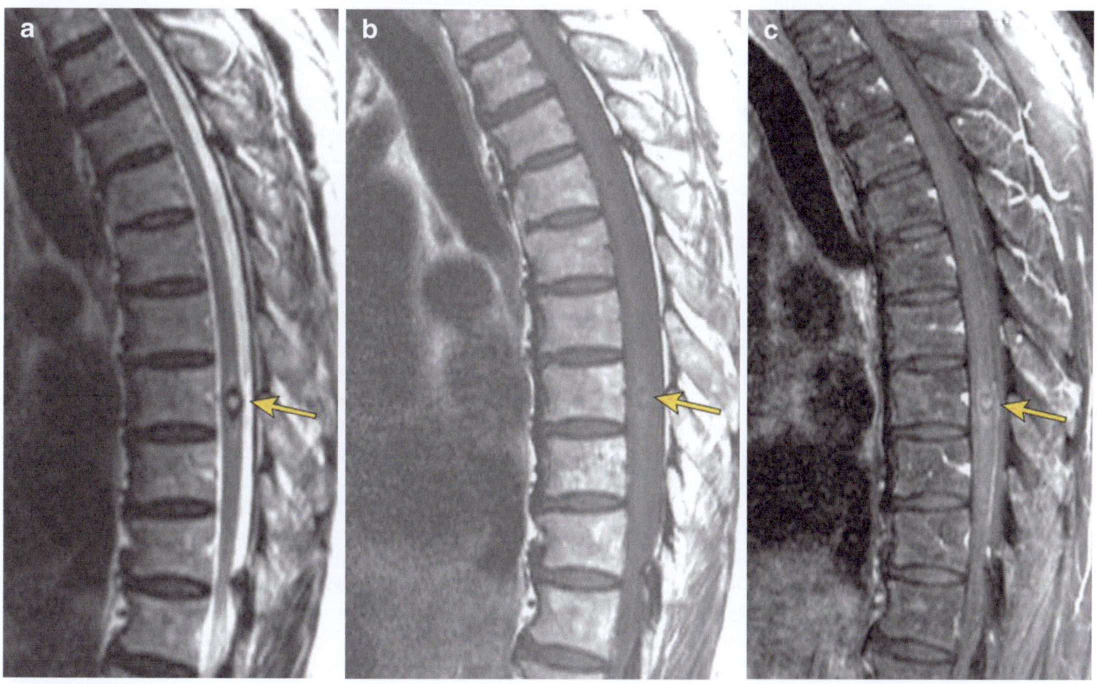

Fig. 12.20 Cavernous hemangioma. In the T2 enhanced sagittal image, a small mass is seen at the ninth thoracic vertebra within the spinal cord, surrounded by a low signal intensity band on the outside and showing high signal intensity inside (**a**, arrow). This lesion also shows a low signal intensity band on the outside and high signal intensity inside in the T1 enhanced sagittal image, suggesting a lesion surrounded by hemosiderin deposition, with the inside accompanying subacute stage hemorrhage (**b**, arrow), and moderate pial enhancement is seen on the outside of the lesion and spinal cord during contrast enhancement (**c**, arrow). It was diagnosed as a cavernous hemangioma with mixed findings of hemosiderin deposition due to repeated hemorrhage and hemorrhage at various stages

standard treatment. The lesion itself can grow, shrink spontaneously, and show various aspects, and 1~5% of the lesions cause symptoms through hemorrhage annually.

Differential diagnoses include ependymoma, astrocytoma, hemangioblastoma, intramedullary metastasis, spinal arteriovenous malformation, multiple sclerosis, etc.

Bibliography

1. Mariano R, Flanagan EP, Weinshenker BG, Palace J. A practical approach to the diagnosis of spinal cord lesions. Pract Neurol. 2018;18(3):187–200.
2. Kranz PG, Amrhein TJ. Imaging approach to myelopathy: acute, subacute, and chronic. Radiol Clin North Am. 2019;57(2):257–79.
3. DeSanto J, Ross JS. Spine infection/inflammation. Radiol Clin North Am. 2011;49(1):105–27.
4. Transverse Myelitis Consortium Working Group. Proposed diagnostic criteria and nosology of acute transverse myelitis. Neurology. 2002;59(4):499–505.
5. Merine D, Wang H, Kumar AJ, Zinreich SJ, Rosenbaum AE. CT myelography and MR imaging of acute transverse myelitis. J Comput Assist Tomogr. 1987;11(4):606–8.
6. Hickman SJ, Miller DH. Imaging of the spine in multiple sclerosis. Neuroimaging Clin N Am. 2000;10(4):689–704, viii.
7. Sato DK, Callegaro D, Lana-Peixoto MA, et al. Distinction between MOG antibody-positive and AQP4 antibody-positive NMO spectrum disorders. Neurology. 2014;82(6):474–81.
8. Wingerchuk DM, Banwell B, Bennett JL, et al. International consensus diagnostic criteria for neuromyelitis optica spectrum disorders. Neurology. 2015;85(2):177–89.
9. Pessôa FM, Lopes FC, Costa JV, Leon SV, Domingues RC, Gasparetto EL. The cervical spinal cord in neuromyelitis optica patients: a comparative study with multiple sclerosis using diffusion tensor imaging. Eur J Radiol. 2012;81(10):2697–701.
10. Flanagan EP, Kaufmann TJ, Krecke KN, et al. Discriminating long myelitis of neuromyelitis optica from sarcoidosis. Ann Neurol. 2016;79(3):437–47.
11. Zalewski NL, Krecke KN, Weinshenker BG, et al. Central canal enhancement and the trident sign in spinal cord sarcoidosis. Neurology. 2016;87(7):743–4.
12. Hyun J-W, Woodhall MR, Kim S-H, et al. Longitudinal analysis of myelin oligodendrocyte glycoprotein antibodies in CNS inflammatory diseases. J Neurol Neurosurg Psychiatry. 2017;88(10):811–7.
13. Pohl D, Alper G, Van Haren K, et al. Acute disseminated encephalomyelitis: updates on an inflammatory CNS syndrome. Neurology. 2016;87(9 Suppl 2):S38–45.
14. Byun WM, Park WK, Park BH, Ahn SH, Hwang MS, Chang JC. Guillain-Barré syndrome: MR imaging findings of the spine in eight patients. Radiology. 1998;208(1):137–41.
15. Téllez-Zenteno JF, Remes-Troche JM, Negrete-Pulido RO, Dávila-Maldonado L. Longitudinal myelitis associated with systemic lupus erythematosus: clinical features and magnetic resonance imaging of six cases. Lupus. 2001;10(12):851–6.
16. West TW, Hess C, Cree BA. Acute transverse myelitis: demyelinating, inflammatory, and infectious myelopathies. Semin Neurol. 2012;32(2):97–113.
17. Malzberg MS, Rogg JM, Tate CA, Zayas V, Easton JD. Poliomyelitis: hyperintensity of the anterior horn cells on MR images of the spinal cord. AJR Am J Roentgenol. 1993;161(4):863–5.
18. Yokota H, Yamada K. Viral infection of the spinal cord and roots. Neuroimaging Clin N Am. 2015;25(2):247–58.
19. Thurnher MM, Olatunji RB. Infections of the spine and spinal cord. Handb Clin Neurol. 2016;136:717–31.
20. Ravina B, Loevner LA, Bank W. MR findings in subacute combined degeneration of the spinal cord: a case of reversible cervical myelopathy. AJR Am J Roentgenol. 2000;174(3):863–5.
21. Schleper B, Stuerenburg HJ. Copper deficiency-associated myelopathy in a 46-year-old woman. J Neurol. 2001;248(8):705–6.
22. Schwendimann RN. Metabolic, nutritional, and toxic myelopathies. Neurol Clin. 2013;31(1):207–18.
23. Ramalho J, Nunes RH, da Rocha AJ, Castillo M. Toxic and metabolic myelopathies. Semin Ultrasound CT MR. 2016;37(5):448–65.
24. Thurnher MM, Bammer R. Diffusion-weighted MR imaging (DWI) in spinal cord ischemia. Neuroradiology. 2006;48(11):795–801.
25. Alblas CL, Bouvy WH, Lycklama À Nijeholt GJ, Boiten J. Acute spinal-cord ischemia: evolution of MRI findings. J Clin Neurol. 2012;8(3):218–23.
26. Spetzler RF, Detwiler PW, Riina HA, Porter RW. Modified classification of spinal cord vascular lesions. J Neurosurg. 2002;96(2 Suppl):145–56.
27. Krings T, Lasjaunias PL, Hans FJ, et al. Imaging in spinal vascular disease. Neuroimaging Clin N Am. 2007;17(1):57–72.
28. Pattany PM, Saraf-Lavi E, Bowen BC. MR angiography of the spine and spinal cord. Top Magn Reson Imaging. 2003;14(6):444–60.
29. Eddleman CS, Jeong H, Cashen TA, et al. Advanced noninvasive imaging of spinal vascular malformations. Neurosurg Focus. 2009;26(1):E9.
30. Turowski B, Za nella FE. Interventional neuroradiology of the head and neck. Neuroimaging Clin N Am. 2003;13(3):619–45.
31. Hegde A, Mohan S, Tan KK, Lim CC. Spinal cavernous malformations: magnetic resonance imaging and associated findings. Singapore Med J. 2012;53(9):582–6.

Spinal Alignment Disorders 13

Ho-Joong Kim

13.1 General Concept

Changes in spine alignment begin with degenerative changes. Therefore, changes in spine alignment that do not cause symptoms can be seen as a normal aging phenomenon. However, alignment disorders that exceed the physiological range require a lot of energy in daily life movements, so the ideal alignment of the spine is an essential element in minimizing muscle energy consumption. In the sagittal plane, the curvatures of the spine (lordosis of the cervical region, kyphosis of the thoracic region, lordosis of the lumbar region), straight alignment in the coronal plane, balanced tension of the ligamentous tissue, and activation of the muscles around the spine are factors that enable an erect position without pain [1]. According to the "Cone of Economy" proposed by Jean Dubousset, if the center of the body is located at the center of the cone, an ergonomically ideal erect posture can be maintained, but as it deviates from the center of the Cone, more energy is needed to maintain an erect posture (Fig. 13.1). As a result, when the center of the body moves outside the cone, it is difficult to maintain posture, so external support such as a cane is needed [2].

Interest in alignment disorders of the spine, a degenerative disease of the spine, has not been long. Radiological analysis and concepts of adult spinal deformities began to emerge in the 2000s, and as the average age is gradually increasing and the number of elderly patients with spinal diseases is increasing, interest in this is gradually increasing.

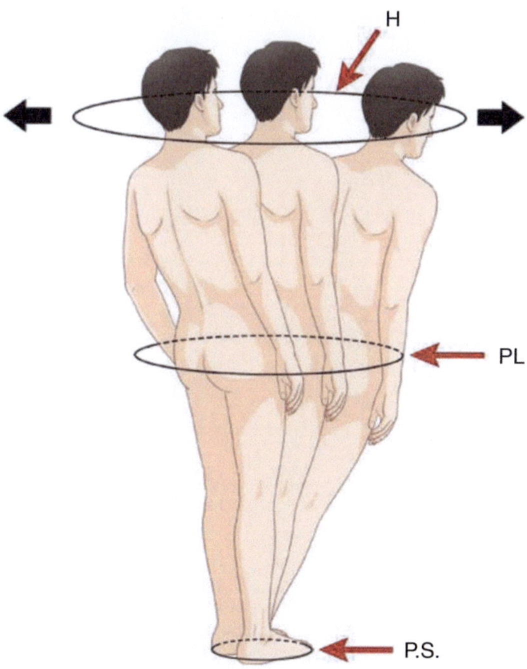

Fig. 13.1 Cone of economy. When the center of the body is located within the cone, it can maintain a stable and painless standing posture. *H* head, *P-L* pelvic level, *P-S* polygon of sustentation

H.-J. Kim (✉)
Department of Orthopedic Surgery, Seoul National University College of Medicine, Seoul, Republic of Korea

© The Author(s), under exclusive license to Springer Nature Singapore Pte Ltd. 2025

H. S. Kang, J. W. Lee (eds.), *Spinal Imaging*, https://doi.org/10.1007/978-981-95-1386-4_13

13.2 Sagittal Imbalance: Kyphosis

The most representative sagittal imbalance is the posterior deformation of the spine. There are three main causes of posterior deformation of the spine. The first is due to degenerative changes in the spine and weakening of the muscles around the spine, and Takemitsu and others named this disease lumbar degenerative kyphosis (Fig. 13.2). The second cause is due to spinal fractures. When osteoporotic spinal compression fractures associated with old age occur multiple times, even if the fractures are fused, they remain as posterior deformities, and these posterior deformities become risk factors for other vertebral fractures (Fig. 13.3). The third is due to surgery. In the 1970s and 1980s, when there was a lack of awareness of sagittal balance, there were many cases of flat back deformity after spinal fusion surgery (Fig. 13.4).

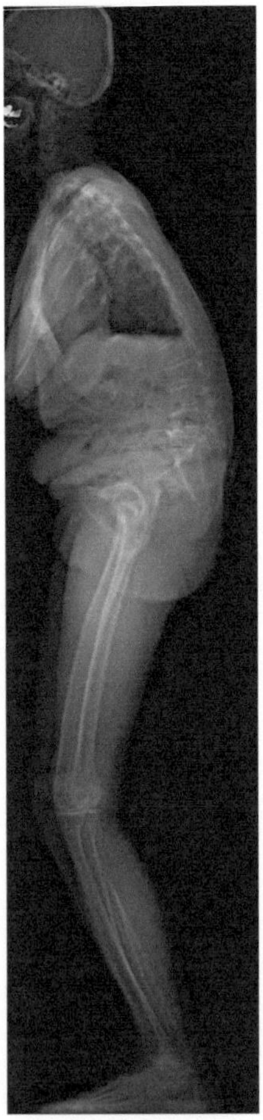

Fig. 13.2 Full-body standing lateral EOS image of a patient with lumbar degenerative kyphosis

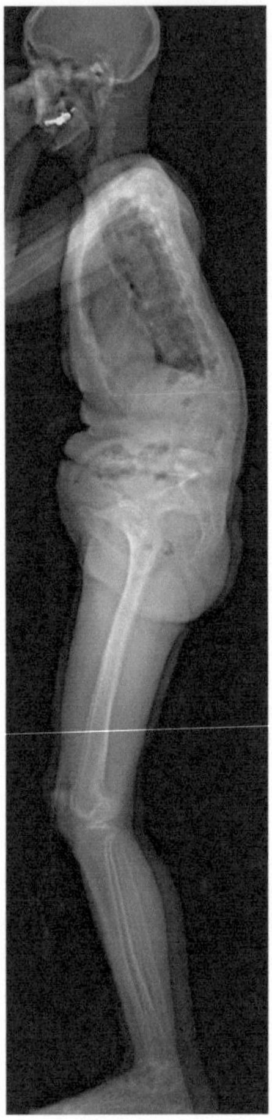

Fig. 13.3 Full-body standing lateral EOS image of a patient with sagittal imbalance associated with lumbar fracture

13.2.1 Spinopelvic Parameter

The reason why the spinopelvic parameter is important in sagittal balance is According to the spinal-pelvic index, each individual's sagittal balance is determined. Important spinal-pelvic indices include lumbar lordosis, pelvic incidence, pelvic tilt, sacral slope, and sagittal vertical axis (Fig. 13.5) [3, 4].

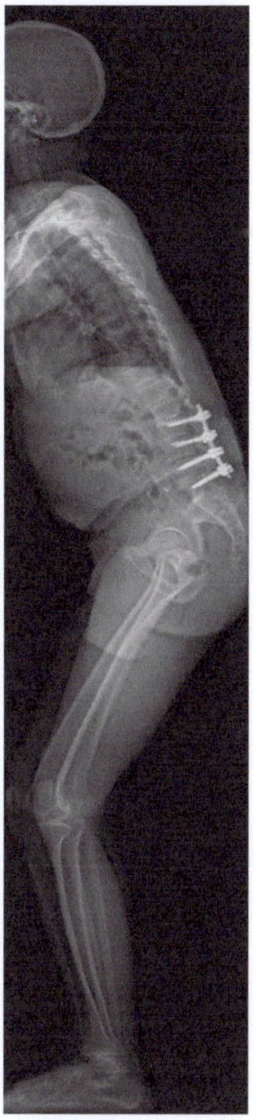

Fig. 13.4 Full-body standing lateral EOS image of a patient with sagittal imbalance after lumbar fusion surgery

13.2.1.1 Pelvic Tilt

The pelvic tilt is the angle formed by a line connecting the center of the femoral head and the center of the upper sacral endplate with the vertical line (Fig. 13.5). Unlike pelvic incidence, pelvic tilt and sacral slope change depending on the position and posture of the spine and pelvis. A high pelvic tilt means that the pelvis is more retroverted, and a low pelvic tilt means that the pelvis is anteverted. Importantly, such an anteverted pelvis brings the axis of the body weight (the endplate of the spine) closer to the axis of the lower body weight (the hip joint) in the pelvis, reducing the torque of the bilateral vectors that must be neutralized by muscle contraction, making muscle energy use more efficient.

13.2.1.2 Sacral Slope

The sacral slope is the angle formed by a line connecting the upper sacral endplates and the horizontal line (Fig. 13.5). If the value is low, it is called a vertical sacrum, and if the value is high, it is called a horizontal sacrum. The sacral slope is closely related to the lumbar lordosis, and if the sacral slope increases, the lumbar lordosis also increases.

13.2.1.3 Pelvic Incidence

Pelvic incidence is defined as the angle formed by a line connecting the axis of the hip joint and the center of the first sacral promontory and a line perpendicular to the first sacral promontory, which is a morphological variable that shows a

Fig. 13.5 Spinal pelvic parameters. *PI* pelvic incidence, *LL* lumbar lordosis, *SS* sacral slope, *SVA* sagittal vertical axis, *PT* pelvic tilt

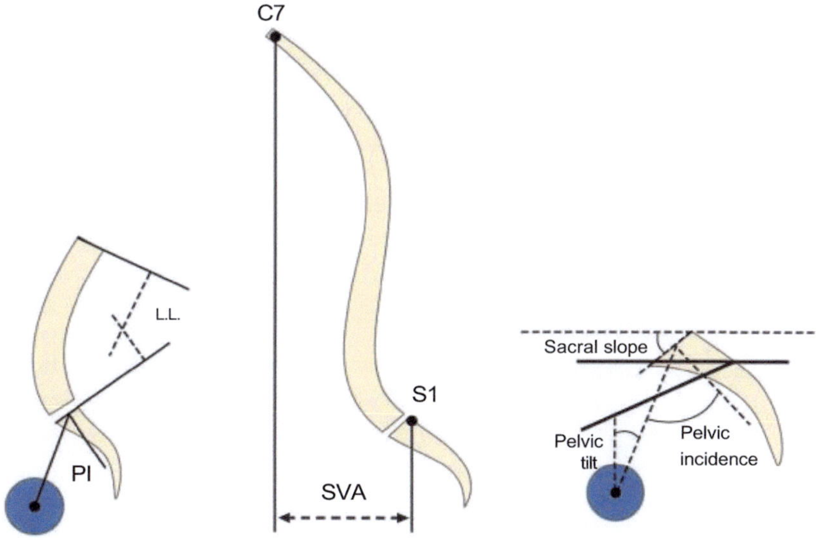

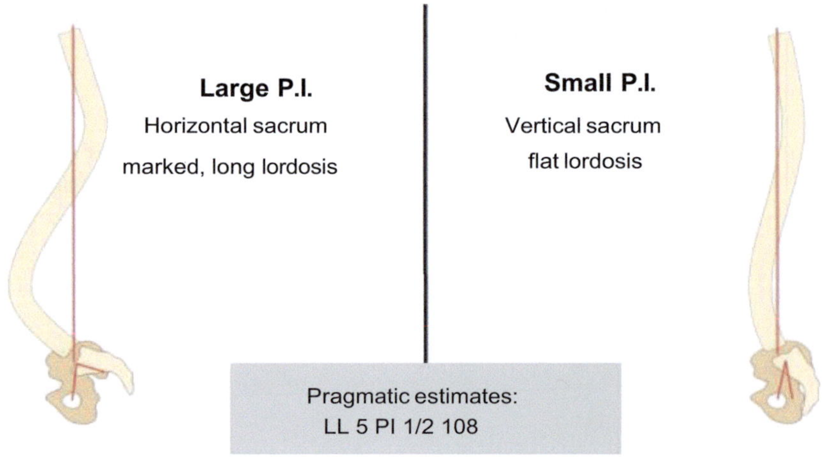

Fig. 13.6 Large PI and long lordosis vs. small PI and flat lordosis. *PI* pelvic incidence, *LL* lumbar lordosis

unique shape for each individual (Fig. 13.5). Mathematically, it is the sum of the pelvic tilt and sacral slope (PI = PT + SS). Pelvic incidence is not an intuitively understandable measure, but it signifies the clinical anterior–posterior size of the pelvis, which is an important factor determining the lumbar lordosis [5, 6]. Pelvic incidence tends to increase from age 4 to 18, which is due to the increase in pelvic tilt and lumbar lordosis to maintain appropriate sagittal curvature with growth. Generally, the pelvic index stabilizes after adulthood and is known not to change depending on the position of the pelvis. Unlike other spinal-pelvic indices, pelvic incidence does not change depending on the posture of the body and is known to have a unique value for each individual after adulthood, but recent studies suggest that it increases somewhat with age [7]. In other words, a high pelvic incidence means a large anterior–posterior size of the pelvis, and physiologically, the lumbar lordosis forms a much larger curvature than when the pelvic incidence is small (Fig. 13.6). For example, there is a racial difference in pelvic incidence, with Hispanics having a larger pelvic incidence than Asians, which is linked to differences in lumbar lordosis [8].

13.2.2 Body Compensation

Whenever the body's sagittal plane tilts forward (kyphosis) for any reason, the body's compensation mechanism (body compensation) is activated. The first compensatory action that occurs is the retroversion of the pelvis (Fig. 13.7). As the pelvis rotates backwards around the femoral head, the body's center of gravity moves back to the center (Fig. 13.7). Therefore, if there is an imbalance in the sagittal plane, the pelvic tilt value will increase, and the sacral slope will decrease accordingly. As previously mentioned, the pelvic incidence is the sum of the pelvic tilt and sacral slope, so the pelvic incidence does not change. However, in such compensatory actions, the pelvic incidence has a very important meaning. According to Roussouly and others, people with a large pelvic incidence have a greater ability to compensate because they can retrovert the pelvis to a greater extent in response to posterior deformities of the spine. On the other hand, those

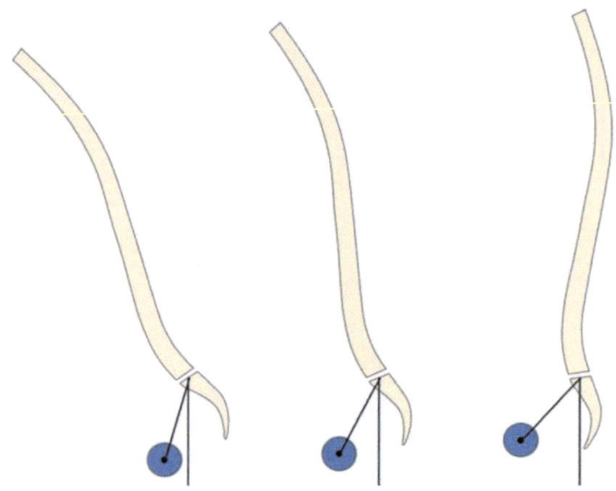

Fig. 13.7 Body compensation by retroversion of pelvis

Fig. 13.8 Schematic comparison of the difference in the ability to compensate for sagittal imbalance depending on the size of the PI

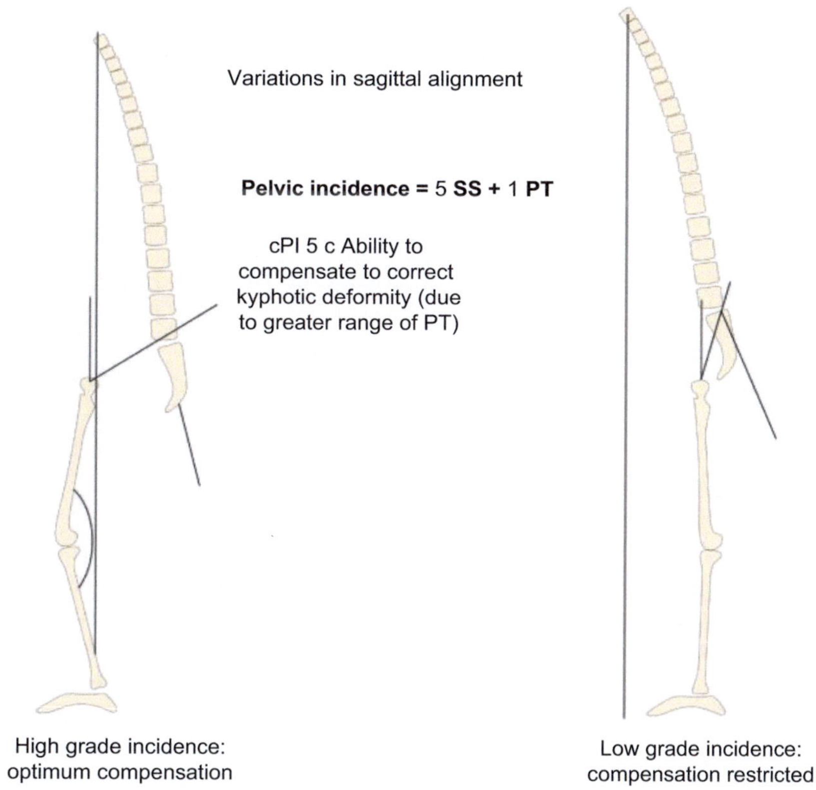

with a small pelvic incidence have a reduced ability to compensate due to the opposite mechanism (Fig. 13.8) [5].

If the balance in the sagittal plane is not achieved even with such pelvic compensation, the compensatory action of the lower limbs is activated [5]. By extending the hip joint and flexing the knee joint during walking, the body's balance is limited from shifting forward, and forward vision is possible (Fig. 13.9). However, this series of processes increases the energy consumption of the muscles, leading to inefficient walking, and as a result, most patients with sagittal imbalance experience walking disorders.

Then, the question of "how can clinically significant sagittal imbalance be defined?" has been a controversial issue in the past. According to

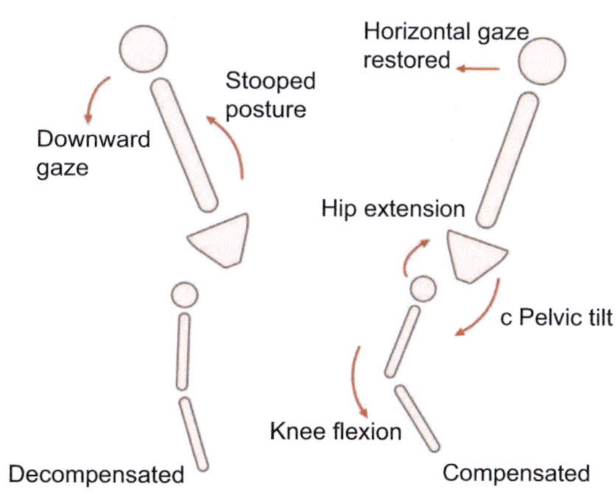

Fig. 13.9 In the case of a small PI (right picture), the pelvis can be maximally Even with retroversion, it cannot fully compensate for sagittal imbalance. *PI* pelvic incidence, *PT* pelvic tilt, *SS* sacral slope

recent studies [1, 6, 9–11], it can be considered clinically significant sagittal imbalance if radiologically the following conditions are met.

Sagittal vertical axis: 5 cm
Pelvic tilt: 20°
Pelvic incidence 2 lumbar lordosis: 10°

These definitions are important criteria in deciding when to perform surgical treatment and how much correction to make in surgical treatment.

13.2.3 Natural Course and Choice of Treatment

Adult spinal deformity, especially sagittal imbalance, includes a very heterogeneous group of diseases, making it difficult to know the exact natural course. Even if they show similar radiological findings, patients' subjective symptoms and quality of life can vary greatly. Also, surgical treatment for such diseases is among the largest spine surgeries, and the fact that it mainly targets elderly patients also makes it difficult to decide on a treatment method. There may be disagreements among spine specialists who specialize in surgical or non-surgical treatment, but based on several recent research results, it can be summarized as follows [12].

The complication rate of treatment for adult spinal deformity with sagittal imbalance is reported to be about 30% for surgical treatment and 10% for non-surgical treatment.

The occurrence of such complications significantly affects the outcome of treatment, and especially in the case of surgical treatment, the frequency of complications is higher, so if complications occur, it has a more negative impact on the outcome.

However, on the other hand, such ventral imbalance makes it difficult to achieve the effect of treatment by conservative treatment, and surgical treatment can solve various disabilities and pain caused by the disease.

Comparing surgical treatment and non-surgical treatment, the group that underwent surgical treatment showed improvement in high-level symptoms, and even if complications occurred after surgical treatment, patients who received surgical treatment overall were able to achieve better results than the group that received non-surgical treatment.

13.2.4 Lumbar Degenerative Kyphosis

Takemitsu and others named it lumbar degenerative kyphosis for kyphosis caused by degenerative changes in the lumbar spine and divided it into four types (Fig. 13.10) [13].

- Type 1: degenerative flat back, which shows little lumbar lordosis and marked loss of thoracic kyphosis
- Type 2: slight lumbar kyphosis with slight lordosis in thoracic spine
- Type 3: increased lumbar kyphosis with varying degree of thoracic lordosis
- Type 4: enlarged thoracic kyphosis which extends downward through lower lumbar region

Types 1 and 2 maintain an upright position at the beginning of walking, but as walking continues, the body gradually bends forward, and Types 3 and 4 lean forward from the beginning of walking.

13.2.4.1 Pathophysiology

The weakening of the lumbar extensor muscles is thought to be the main cause. Especially, it is thought that the disease occurs when the lumbar extensor muscles weaken and the instability of the lumbar spine increases due to degenerative changes, as it mainly occurs in people who live a lot of crouching life in Asian countries such as Korea and Japan. However, it is often found that it occurs even when the lumbar extensor muscles weaken regardless of actual instability.

13.2.4.2 Clinical Symptoms

The most prominent clinical symptom is first, the stooping of the trunk. Especially after starting to

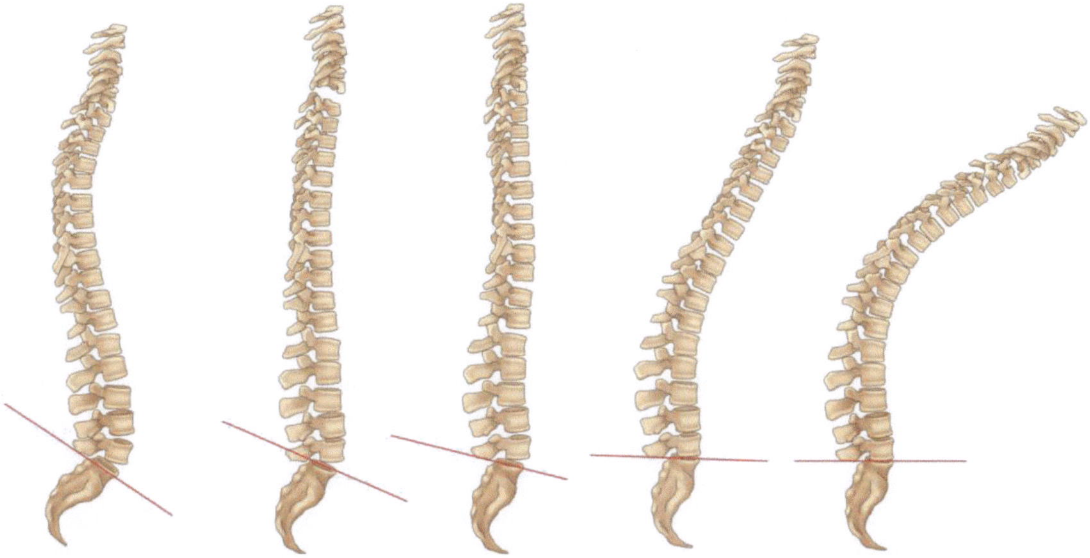

Fig. 13.10 The four types of lumbar degenerative kyphosis proposed by Takemitsu

walk from the initial standing position, the body bends forward over time. In order to maintain the center of gravity of the body, which is concentrated forward, even a little to the back, the hip and knee are bent. Second, they cannot lift heavy objects well. If you lift a slightly heavy object like a pot or flower pot, the body bends forward more, making it difficult to balance the body. It's tough. Third, when working in the kitchen, the body bends forward, so one has to support the body with one elbow to work. Therefore, there are calluses on one or both elbows. Fourth, uphill walking such as hills or stairs is particularly difficult. These four symptoms are referred to as the basic symptoms (cardinal symptom) of lumbar degenerative kyphosis.

13.3 Coronal Imbalance: Scoliosis

Scoliosis is a representative spinal arrangement disorder in the coronal plane. Scoliosis can be divided into pediatric scoliosis and adult scoliosis, and pediatric scoliosis can be further divided into congenital scoliosis, early onset scoliosis, and adolescent idiopathic scoliosis. In this chapter, we will only discuss degenerative lumbar scoliosis that occurs in adults.

13.3.1 Degenerative Lumbar Scoliosis

Adult scoliosis is defined as a coronal Cobb angle of 10 degrees or more in patients who have completed growth and is classified into two forms: adult idiopathic scoliosis and adult degenerative scoliosis [14].

Degenerative lumbar scoliosis begins to appear mainly after the age of 50 without previous spinal deformities and due to degenerative changes. As age increases, the frequency of scoliosis increases and the curvature progresses. This is thought to be due to asymmetric disc space collapse and facet degeneration accompanied by lateral and/or rotatory listhesis [15]. These degenerative changes cause loss of lumbar lordosis and sagittal plane malalignment. Compared to adult idiopathic scoliosis, degenerative lumbar scoliosis has a smaller curvature angle, involves fewer segments, and rotational deformity is concentrated at the apex of the lumbar curve (Table 13.1).

Table 13.1 Comparison of adult idiopathic scoliosis and adult degenerative scoliosis

	Adult idiopathic scoliosis	Adult degenerative scoliosis
Age	Younger	Older
Spinal stenosis	Rare	Common
Cobb angle	Large	Small
Rotatory deformity	At entire curve	At apex of curve
Lateral subluxation of vertebral body	Not common	Common
Coronal and sagittal imbalance	Rare	Common

13.3.1.1 Pathophysiology

Degenerative spinal disease in adults appears as gradual degenerative changes in soft tissues with age. As disc desiccation and proteoglycan loss progress with disc degeneration, asymmetric disc height loss and loss of shock absorption function occur. This causes erosion and contact of the adjacent endplate, leading to sclerosis and osteophyte formation. This disc collapse transfers the physiological load to the posterior column, increasing stress and abnormal motion in the facet joint. As a result, facet hypertrophy, capsule degeneration, and ligamentous hypertrophy, i.e., facet arthropathy, occur. Facet hypertrophy and osteophytes not only cause stenosis of the central canal and neural foramina but also cause abnormal motion and instability. Multiple spondylitic and arthropathic segments form biomechanical shifts such as spondylolisthesis and rotatory subluxation, creating degenerative deformity. Since degenerative scoliosis mainly starts to appear in postmenopausal women in their 50s, there is a theory that postmenopausal osteoporosis is involved as a cause. Early onset osteoporosis can exacerbate spinal deformity and instability [14, 15].

13.3.1.2 Anatomy

The progression of lumbar degenerative scoliosis involves structural changes in local anatomy. On the convex side of the curve in patients with lumbar degenerative scoliosis, hypertrophy of the psoas and paravertebral muscles is observed, while degeneration occurs on the concave side. In patients with lumbar degenerative scoliosis, the morphology of the pedicle changes, leading to a decrease in pedicle diameter on the concave side. Due to the anatomical change of the foramina, the foraminal height, the interval between the pedicle and the superior articular process, and the foraminal area decrease.

13.3.1.3 Clinical Symptoms

The most common symptom of lumbar degenerative scoliosis patients is pain. The frequency of pain varies according to reports, but it appears in approximately 90%. Approximately 60~80% of lumbar degenerative scoliosis patients who complain of symptoms report back pain. Patients complain of diffuse axial lower back pain, mainly on the convex side of the curve. Pain can occur due to muscle fatigue and spasm of the scoliotic curvature convexity, and it appears that facet degeneration also causes lower back pain as the pain decreases with fluoroscopically guided facet injection.

Asymmetric disc space collapse and facet degeneration cause nerve root compression according to the concavity of the degenerative curve, resulting in symptomatic radiculopathy. The frequency varies according to reports, but it appears in approximately 47~78% (Fig. 13.11). However, the main cause of radiculopathy is foraminal stenosis rather than central spinal stenosis. Foraminal stenosis, posterior joint hypertrophy, and vertebral rotation atrophy cause the intervertebral space to narrow at the concave part of the curve. Pedicular kinking, where the nerve root is compressed between the spinal canal and the intervertebral disc, also causes radiculopathy. On the convex side of the curve, the nerve root can be excessively stretched to cause nerve symptoms. Thus, in patients with lumbar degenerative scoliosis, the frequency of pain is high, and it is uncommon for patients to complain solely of clinical or cosmetic deformity.

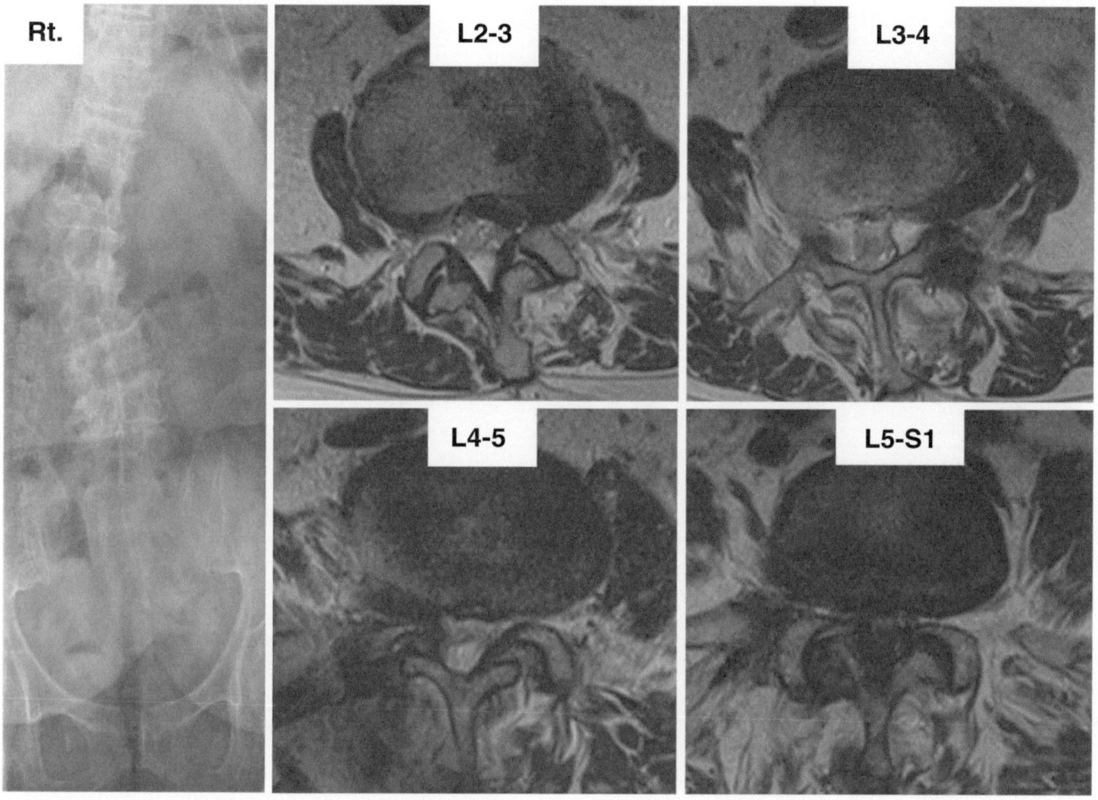

Fig. 13.11 In the case of degenerative lumbar scoliosis, various stenosis are accompanied

The primary focus of the clinical evaluation is to accurately identify the factors causing the symptoms. The cause of the pain can be a combination of deformity progression, deconditioning, neurological compromise, or it can be pain associated with degenerative arthritis of the sacroiliac, hip, knee joint. Through careful medical history taking, the location of the pain, the radiating area, and the aggravating/relieving factors should be accurately identified. Pain is mainly aggravated by standing for a certain period of time and is relieved by sitting or lying down.

In physical examination, a detailed neurological evaluation including motor strength, sensory function, and reflexes must be performed. It is also important to check for cervical and thoracic myelopathy/radiculopathy. Through visual inspection, hump, rib asymmetry, pelvic obliquity, shoulder asymmetry, overall spinal alignment in the coronal and sagittal plane should be checked. Leg length discrepancy or hip and/or knee flexion contracture should also be checked. The patient's standing posture and gait should be observed to evaluate the patient's sagittal and coronal balance, compensatory maneuver.

13.3.1.4 Radiological Examination

Standing anteroposterior and lateral 36-inch cassette spinal radiographs are important for patients with spinal deformities. This image should include not only the entire spine but also the base of the skull proximally and both femoral heads distally. The degree of deformation can be known by measuring the angle with the Cobb method, and the coronal, sagittal spinal alignment and balance can be evaluated by measuring the center sacral vertical line and sagittal vertical axis. Flexion, extension lateral radiographs are important for evaluating instability. EOS imaging is a new method that can obtain a perpendicular, whole body radiograph. With a method that uses 6–9 times less radiation than standard thoraco-

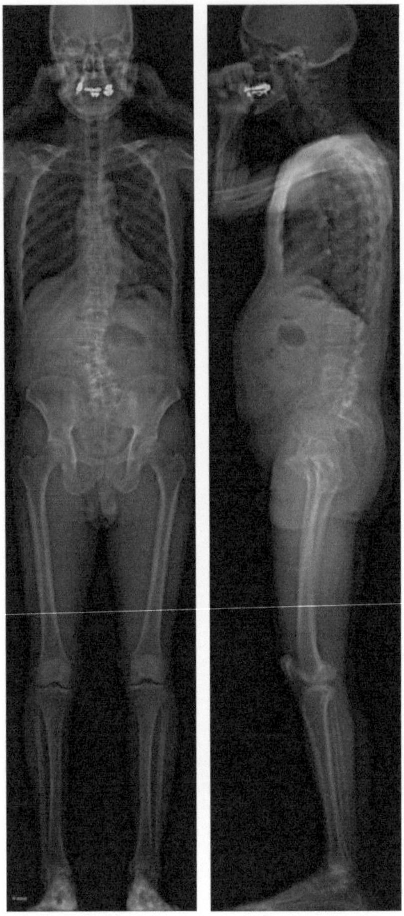

Fig. 13.12 EOS full body photo of a patient with degenerative lumbar scoliosis

lumbar radiographs, better quality images can be obtained. Through EOS imaging, information such as total body alignment, compensatory mechanisms, sagittal and coronal alignment can be obtained (Fig. 13.12).

In patients with neurological symptoms, MRI is a necessary test to evaluate central or foraminal stenosis. Through MRI, nerve root compression, disc degeneration, modic change (changes in signal intensity of the vertebral end plates and subchondral bone) can be evaluated. Noncontrast CT is essential for evaluating bony structures when planning surgery. CT can evaluate thoracolumbar anatomy, bridging osteophytes, autofused segments, etc. In patients who have had spinal surgery before, the degree of enhancing of scar tissue can be considered through postintravenous contrast images.

Bibliography

1. Schwab F, Patel A, Ungar B, Farcy JP, Lafage V. Adult spinal deformity-postoperative standing imbalance: how much can you tolerate? An overview of key parameters in assessing alignment and planning corrective surgery. Spine (Phila Pa 1976). 2010;35(25):2224–31. https://doi.org/10.1097/BRS.0b013e3181ee6bd4.
2. Dubousset J. Three-dimensional analysis of the scoliotic deformity. In: Pediatric spine: principles and practice. New York, NY: Raven Press; 1994.
3. Boulay C, Tardieu C, Hecquet J, et al. Sagittal alignment of spine and pelvis regulated by pelvic incidence: standard values and prediction of lordosis. Eur Spine J. 2006;15(4):415–22. https://doi.org/10.1007/s00586-005-0984-5.
4. Lafage V, Schwab F, Patel A, Hawkinson N, Farcy JP. Pelvic tilt and truncal inclination: two key radiographic parameters in the setting of adults with spinal deformity. Spine (Phila Pa 1976). 2009;34(17):E599–606. https://doi.org/10.1097/BRS.0b013e3181aad219.
5. Roussouly P, Nnadi C. Sagittal plane deformity: an overview of interpretation and management. Eur Spine J. 2010;19(11):1824–36. https://doi.org/10.1007/s00586-010-1476-9.
6. Roussouly P, Pinheiro-Franco JL. Biomechanical analysis of the spino-pelvic organization and adaptation in pathology. Eur Spine J. 2011;20(Suppl 5):609–18. https://doi.org/10.1007/s00586-011-1928-x.
7. Mendoza-Lattes S, Ries Z, Gao Y, Weinstein SL. Natural history of spinopelvic alignment differs from symptomatic deformity of the spine. Spine (Phila Pa 1976). 2010;35(16):E792–8. https://doi.org/10.1097/BRS.0b013e3181d35ca9.
8. Weinberg DS, Morris WZ, Gebhart JJ, Liu RW. Pelvic incidence: an anatomic investigation of 880 cadaveric specimens. Eur Spine J. 2016;25(11):3589–95. https://doi.org/10.1007/s00586-015-4317-z.
9. Schwab FJ, Blondel B, Bess S, et al. Radiographical spinopelvic parameters and disability in the setting of adult spinal deformity: a prospective multicenter analysis. Spine (Phila Pa 1976). 2013;38(13):E803–12. https://doi.org/10.1097/BRS.0b013e318292b7b9.
10. Terran J, Schwab F, Shaffrey CI, et al. The SRS-Schwab adult spinal deformity classification: assessment and clinical correlations based on a prospective operative and nonoperative cohort. Neurosurgery. 2013;73(4):559–68. https://doi.org/10.1227/NEU.0000000000000012.
11. Lafage R, Schwab F, Challier V, et al. Defining spino-pelvic alignment thresholds: should operative goals in adult spinal deformity surgery account for age? Spine (Phila Pa 1976). 2016;41(1):62–8. https://doi.org/10.1097/brs.0000000000001171.
12. Acaroglu E, European Spine Study Group. Decision-making in the treatment of adult spinal deformity. EFORT Open Rev. 2016;1(5):167–76. https://doi.org/10.1302/2058-5241.1.000013.

13. Takemitsu Y, Harada Y, Iwahara T, Miyamoto M, Miyatake Y. Lumbar degenerative kyphosis. Clinical, radiological and epidemiological studies. Spine (Phila Pa 1976). 1988;13(11):1317–26.
14. York PJ, Kim HJ. Degenerative scoliosis. Curr Rev Musculoskelet Med. 2017;10(4):547–58. https://doi.org/10.1007/s12178-017-9445-0.
15. Koerner JD, Reitman CA, Arnold PM, Rihn J. Degenerative Lumbar Scoliosis. JBJS Rev. 2015;3(4):e1. https://doi.org/10.2106/JBJS.RVW.N.00061.

14 Spinal Exercise Therapy

Ju Seok Ryu

14.1 Introduction

Back pain is one of the most common musculoskeletal pain disorders, with 80% of adults experiencing pain at least once [1]. Most patients recover within 6–12 weeks, but many experience recurrence or progress to chronic back pain [2]. Chronic back pain, which limits daily life and work performance, is very important in social and economic aspects, so appropriate treatment is needed.

Back pain is related to various structures that make up the lumbar spine, such as intervertebral discs, muscles, and ligaments. These structures affect each other organically to cause back pain. Chronic muscle weakness is known to cause back pain [3, 4], and the way to strengthen these muscles is exercise. In this chapter, we will look at various structures that can cause chronic back pain in the spine, point out the problems of various exercise methods currently being performed to treat chronic back pain and propose a new effective and convenient exercise method.

14.1.1 Structures that Can Cause Spinal Pain

Chronic back pain is caused by various structures of the spine, and there are many causative diseases. Chronic back pain is caused by various diseases such as fractures and array abnormalities of the spinal bones that make up the spine, stenosis where the spinal canal narrows, weakness of the muscles around the spine, herniated discs, and arthritis of the posterior joint.

The spinal stabilization system can be divided into the spinal column, spinal muscles, and neural control unit (Fig. 14.1) [5]. The minimum weight that bends the spine is called the critical load. The threshold of the lumbar spine is known to be about 20 lbs, and it is known to be over 1500 N when predicted in a biological model [5]. As shown in Fig. 14.2, weights exceeding the threshold bend the spine. Leaning, and preventing this, can be referred to as guy wires, and in the human body, muscles take on this role [5]. Therefore, the role of muscles is very important in stabilizing the spine.

J. S. Ryu (✉)
Department of Rehabilitation Medicine, Seoul National University College of Medicine, Seoul, Republic of Korea
e-mail: jseok337@snu.ac.kr

© The Author(s), under exclusive license to Springer Nature Singapore Pte Ltd. 2025
H. S. Kang, J. W. Lee (eds.), *Spinal Imaging*, https://doi.org/10.1007/978-981-95-1386-4_14

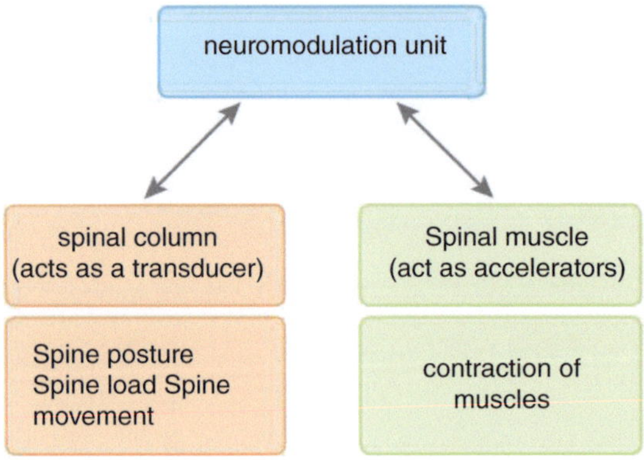

Fig. 14.1 This figure shows the stabilization system of the spine [5]

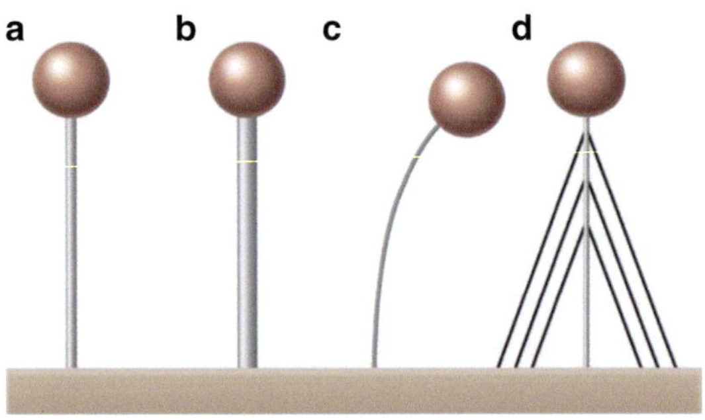

Fig. 14.2 The threshold of the spinal column refers to the minimum weight that makes the column tilt when placed on top of the spinal column. (**a**) Represents a state where a weight less than the threshold, just before the spinal column bends or shows instability, is placed, (**b**) represents a state where the spinal column is thickened and stabilized, (**c**) represents a state where the spinal column is thinned and destabilized by a weight exceeding the threshold, and (**d**) represents a state where the unstable column is stabilized by guy wires

The spinal muscles, which play an important role in stabilizing the spine, can be divided into the superficial muscle layer and the deep muscle layer (Fig. 14.3). The superficial muscles refer to the muscles located on the outside of the spinal muscles, which are generally composed of fast-twitch fibers and have a long lever arm, forming the global muscle system. Typically, this includes the erector spinae muscle, external oblique muscle, rectus abdominis muscle, quadratus lumborum muscle, etc. On the other hand, the deep muscles are composed of slow-twitch fibers and have a short lever arm, mainly controlling and stabilizing the movement of each segment, forming the local muscle system. These muscles include the transversus abdominis muscle, multifidus muscle, internal oblique muscle, deep transversospinalis muscle, pelvic floor muscle, etc.

14.1.2 The Importance of Exercise Therapy

The safety of the spine is absolutely necessary to prevent chronic lumbar pain. Instability refers to a state without mechanical stability, showing excessive and abnormal range of motion beyond the muscle's protective control. Generally, chronic pain occurs in the mid-range motion of the lumbar spine, so mid-range segmental motion abnormality would be more appropriate. In this way, stabilizing mechanical instability can improve pain and function, and exercise is responsible for this role. A strong core increases the protective ability of the trunk, supports the waist, induces regulated movement, and enhances safety and balance ability.

14.1.3 Types of Exercise Therapy

Current exercise therapies for chronic pain include flexibility exercises, core exercises, stabilization exercises, motor control exercises, Pilates, yoga, flexion exercises, extension exercises, bracing exercises, walking exercises, etc. The types of exercises are divided according to the purpose and main mechanism of exercise therapy, so most of the actual application methods of spinal exercises include similar postures, and there are quite a lot of overlapping elements between exercises.

Posture stabilization exercise is a term mixed with core exercise, and its purpose is to maintain intersegmental stability between spinal segments. Through this exercise, it enhances the neuromuscular control, strength, and endurance of various muscles in the trunk and pelvic floor, which play an important role in dynamic stability. On the other hand, motor control exercise has a conceptual difference from posture stabilization exercise.

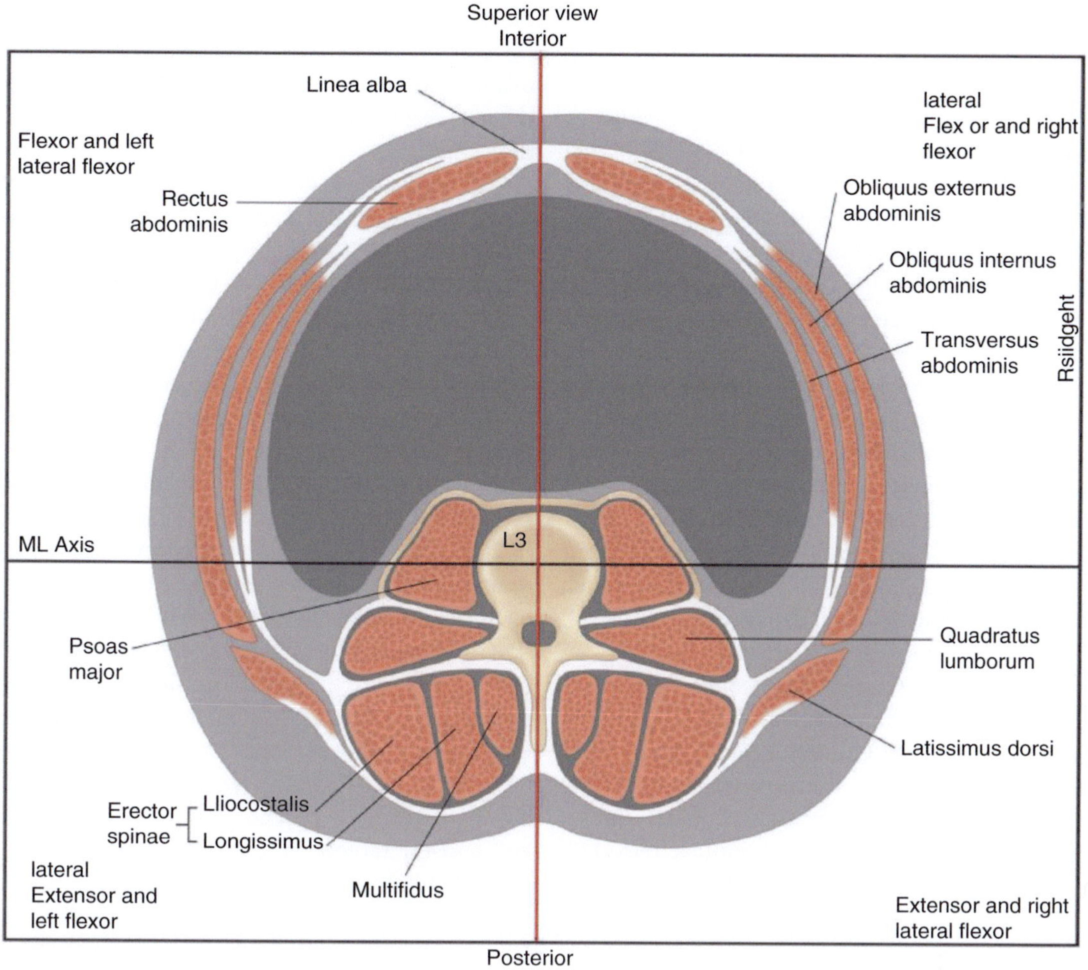

Fig. 14.3 This diagram illustrates the deep and superficial muscles surrounding the spine that make up the vertebral column

Motor control exercise is based on two hypotheses that the stability of the spine is important and that patients with chronic pain have abnormalities in muscle control when moving the spine. In a normal state, when the trunk muscles are moved, the deep muscles contract first, followed by the superficial muscles contracting [6, 7]. However, in patients with chronic low back pain, deep muscles contract later, which causes superficial muscles to contract excessively, increasing the stiffness of the spine and leading to the recurrence or progression of low back pain. This is the theoretical basis for performing motor function control exercises [6, 7]. There may be disagreements about this theory, which I will explain further later.

Flexion exercises are commonly known as Williams' flexion exercises, and they mainly use flexion movements to control lumbar pain [8]. On the other hand, extension exercises use extension movements as the main element of the exercise. According to this theory, a derangement syndrome occurs due to abnormalities in the intervertebral disc and adjacent tissues, causing pain of centralization or peripheralization. The aim is to reduce pain through one-directional movement. It is reported that 67~85% of patients with centralization improve their pain through extension movements, and due to this preferred direction, McKenzie exercise is used almost synonymously with extension exercise [9].

14.1.4 Evidence-Based Spinal Exercise Therapy

Evidence-based medicine narrows the scope of evidence more than traditional medicine and treats patients based on scientific evidence only. Therefore, randomized controlled trials are considered the highest level of evidence, and rather than relying on a single study, the aim is to raise the level of evidence by comprehensively judging the results of various studies. Since 2010, the author has been looking for effective exercise therapy methods for each disease to develop a standardized treatment program for chronic low back pain. Chronic low back pain is divided into non-specific chronic low back pain, spinal stenosis, spondylolisthesis, and disc herniation, and the author aimed to develop particularly effective exercise methods for each disease.

First, let's look at non-specific chronic low back pain. Many studies have been conducted on exercise therapy for non-specific chronic low back pain. Studies by Jordan K and Laurisen HH showed significant effects for both posture stabilization exercises and general exercises, with no difference between the two methods [10, 11]. Goldby LJ compared posture stabilization exercises with manual therapy, but again, there was no significant difference between the two groups [12]. Ferreira ML compared the effects between motor function control exercises, manual therapy, and general exercises, and after 8 weeks, motor function control exercises and manual therapy showed slightly superior effects, but after 6 and 12 months, there was no difference between the three exercise methods [13].

On the other hand, studies that showed outstanding effects of these specific exercise methods have common features. In 2009, Costa LOP found that motor function control exercises were superior to thermoelectric therapy. It showed significant effects, and Kim Tae-hoon and others also showed significant effects compared to thermoelectric therapy [14]. In other words, in studies where the control group was set to exercise therapy, there was no difference, but in studies where the control group was set to thermoelectric therapy or placebo, significant effects were observed. The recently published Cochrane review also concluded that the evidence that exercise function control exercise is superior to other exercises is very low, and it shows similar effects to physical therapy or other general exercise therapy, so the method of exercise therapy is based on the patient and therapist's preference, skills, and cost. It should be determined [15, 16].

For spondylolisthesis, two important research results can be found. Sinaki M and others compared flexion and extension exercises, and in the evaluation after 3 months, pain persisted in 67% of the extension exercises, but only 27% of the flexion exercises remained, so the flexion exercises were more effective. Also, this effect was reported to persist even after 3 years [17]. Later in 2005, Hicks GE and others reported that combining flexion exercises and posture stabilization exercises is more effective, and it is more effective in cases over 40 years old, 90 ° or more in the lower limb straight leg test, positive findings of the prone instability test, and the presence of aberrant motions [18].

For spinal stenosis, various results were shown depending on the exercise method and comparison target. In studies comparing non-surgical treatments for spinal stenosis, physical therapy and posture stabilization exercises showed superior results compared to group therapy, drug therapy, and self-treatment (home exercise) [19, 20], on the other hand, studies comparing exercise therapy and surgical treatment showed various results depending on the time. The results of studies before 2015 showed that surgical treatment was superior to exercise therapy, and it was recommended to perform conservative treatment first as the disease progresses slowly and then perform surgical treatment if it fails [21, 22]. However, after 2015, when abdominal exercises became popular, it was reported that there was no clear difference in effect between exercise therapy including abdominal exercises and surgical treatment [23]. According to the clinical practice guidelines announced in 2019, supervised exercise (exercise method under the guidance of a therapist, for example, a combination of posture stabilization exercise, walking exercise, etc. according to the patient's muscle strength and pain status) and postoperative supervised exercise are recommended for patients with spinal stenosis. On the other hand, physical therapy, drug therapy, and decompression surgery performed together with spinal fusion are not recommended [24]. However, as with most treatment methods, there are individual differences, so it is necessary to choose an appropriate treatment method according to the patient's condition.

The extension exercise known as the McKenzie exercise is also known to be effective, and the McKenzie directional preference-based exercise has been proposed to increase the treatment effect of patients who did not have an effect on this exercise [25]. However, in 2013 in a comparative study with posture stabilization exercises, posture stabilization exercises showed superior effects in muscle strengthening [26], and in a comparison with exercise function control exercises in 2018, there was no difference in effects between the two exercises [27].

Pilates and yoga are also commonly used exercise methods for chronic low back pain. However, the Cochrane review also found no evidence that Pilates and yoga are superior to other forms of exercise, and suggested that the exercise method should be determined considering the preferences of patients and therapists, cost, etc. [28, 29].

In summary, various exercise methods are used, but there is no significant difference between exercise methods, and it can be said that the general consensus is that they are more effective than thermoelectric treatment or placebo.

14.2 New Concept of Exercise Therapy

Logical approach to the movement of the spine: anatomy, physiology, movement-based approach

1. Which muscle should be strengthened? Generally, when back pain persists and movement decreases, muscle degeneration occurs. That is, it is a well-known fact that the muscle mass of the multifidus muscle and erector spinae muscle is reduced in patients with chronic low back pain. Then, what would the muscles be like before the onset of chronic pain? According to previous studies, patients with chronic pain after trauma had atrophy of the erector spinae muscle and multifidus muscle around the fifth lumbar vertebra from the time of the accident. Especially, this muscle atrophy was more prominent in the erector spinae muscle (Fig. 14.4) [3, 4]. These results imply two possibilities: patients with reduced muscle mass around the spine had weak resistance

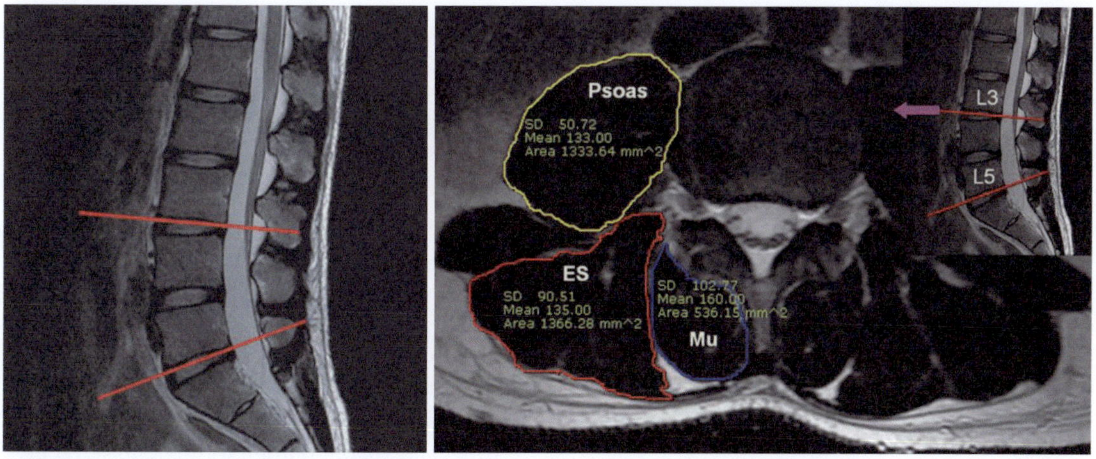

Fig. 14.4 This diagram shows a method of measuring the muscle mass of the spine using magnetic resonance imaging

to trauma, leading to chronic pain after trauma, or the muscle weakness was severe, and trauma at a stage with a high risk of chronic pain triggered chronic pain. If we apply these results to treatment, we can speculate that to prevent chronic pain after trauma, it is necessary to strengthen the muscles of the lower lumbar spine and increase muscle mass.

2. What exercise should be performed?
   When strengthening the muscles of the spine, it can be largely divided into methods that strengthen the deep muscles more and methods that strengthen both the deep and superficial muscles. Generally, posture stabilization exercises and core exercises strengthen both deep and superficial muscles, while exercise function control exercises target the deep muscles connecting the short vertebral bodies. Therefore, exercise function control exercises use various feedbacks such as ultrasound and electromyography to induce independent contraction and movement of the deep muscles and strengthen the muscles.

   However, the author would like to think differently about exercise function control exercises. The following picture shows that the intervertebral disc space has decreased due to a herniated disc of the spine. It is shown in Fig. 14.5. According to this figure, the length of the muscles between the third and fourth lumbar vertebrae decreased by about 20%, but the length of the second to fifth lumbar vertebrae decreased by about 10%. In other words, the deep muscles (e.g., multifidus muscle) connecting one segment had about 20% muscle laxity, but the laxity of the superficial muscles (e.g., erector spinae muscle) connecting four segments was only about 10%. This means that the deep muscles appear to contract later due to increased laxity, but this is not the cause of chronic back pain [30]. Also, as mentioned in the theoretical basis of spinal movement, there is no difference in the effects of focused exercises such as motor function control exercise and physiotherapy from general exercises, so there is a need to develop a simple and easily applicable new exercise.

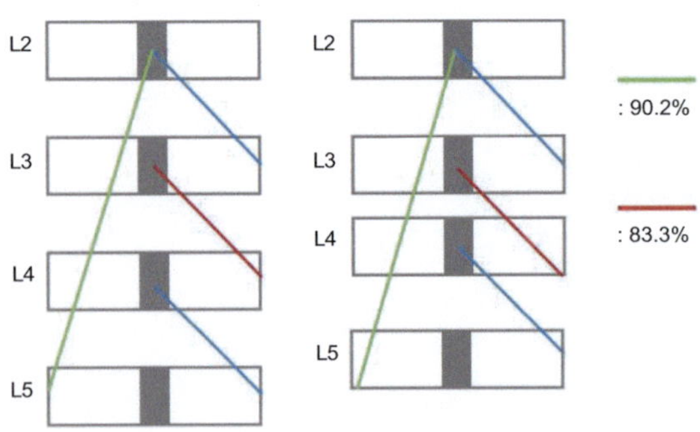

Fig. 14.5 This diagram shows that when a herniated disc occurs, the deep muscles of the spine increase in laxity relative to the superficial muscles

14.3 SNUBH Exercise Protocol for Back Pain

1. Background of introducing individualized graded stabilization exercise
   Several basic assumptions were made to develop a new exercise method. First, it is to develop a reasonable method in terms of cost. Physiotherapy that patients receive every day at the hospital is expensive, and there are many doubts about its effectiveness, so it is necessary to develop an exercise method that can be used at a low cost. The second is accessibility in terms of time and space. Patients should be able to get enough exercise effect within 30 min a day, and it should be possible to perform anywhere. If more than 30 min of exercise time is required, compliance decreases, leading to the problem of not continuing the exercise. Also, if you can only exercise at the hospital, it is difficult to apply in daily life because it takes a lot of time to move along with the cost. In previous studies, the exercise of distributing simple booklets had a weak effect, but the exercise method under the supervision of a therapist showed excellent effects [20]. However, it is thought that the method of supervised home exercise is reasonable because it is a great economic, time, and spatial burden for patients to receive supervision from a therapist every time.

Based on the above assumptions, we need an exercise method that can be performed within 30 min and can be performed independently at home after receiving education on the exercise method at the hospital several times by introducing the method of supervised home exercise. For this, the author developed an individualized graded stabilization exercise composed of five stages (Fig. 14.6) [31]. This exercise program has two features: safety and stages. From a safety perspective, posture stabilization exercise induces only isometric contraction of muscles without bending or straightening the waist, so the risk of side effects is very low and safe. And in terms of stages, this exercise program is divided into 1~5 stages depending on the difficulty and fatigue, and when the contraction strength of muscles was evaluated step by step using surface electromyography, it was proven that as the steps increased, the contraction movement of the muscles (integral, uA * second) increased (Fig. 14.7). This increase was also confirmed in the rectus abdominis and transversus abdominis muscles, along with the muscles around the lumbar spine [32]. If steps are set, a lower level can be applied to elderly patients with muscle weakness, and a higher level can be applied to young patients with good muscle strength. This allows for a customized exercise program according to the patient's condition, and if the patient's function improves, the intensity of the exercise can be increased to achieve a large exercise effect in a short time. Also, by using steps, exercise can be simplified, and it can be fully acquired with only 1–2 training sessions, which can be performed at home [31, 32]. And individualized step-by-step posture stabilization exercises, like other focused exercises, were able to confirm superior clinical effects compared to thermoelectric therapy [31]. In a prospective, randomized clinical study published in 2019, the effect of individualized step-by-step posture stabilization exercise showed significant effects [30].

2. Background of introducing walking exercise
   Walking exercise is included in the international clinical guidelines for chronic back pain [33–35], and its effectiveness as a treatment for chronic back pain has been proven [36]. According to a recent study, it shows excellent effects in both the effective aspect of exercise and the economic aspect, and it has a high compliance rate [37]. Therefore, walking should be actively performed for patients with

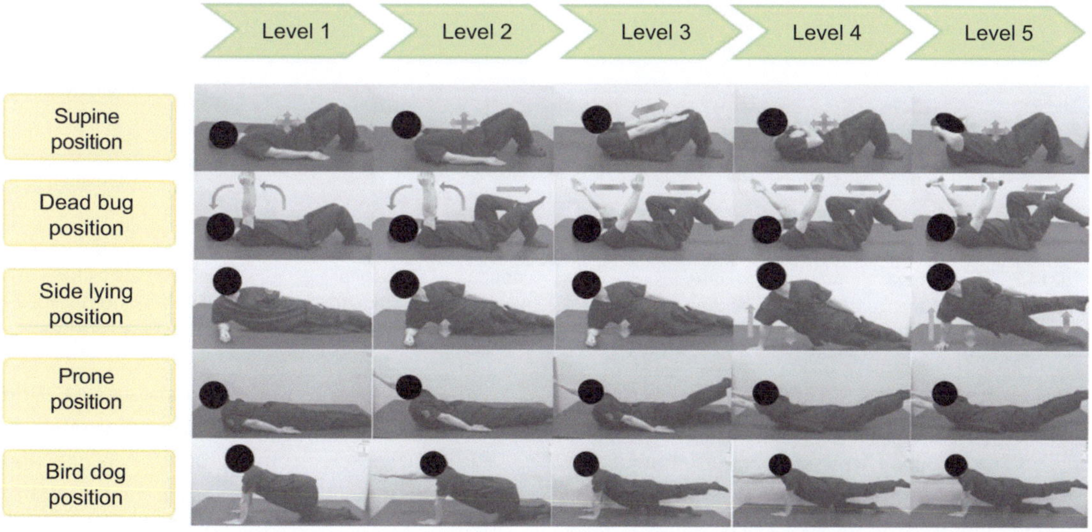

Fig. 14.6 This diagram shows the individualized graded stabilization exercise composed of five stages according to posture

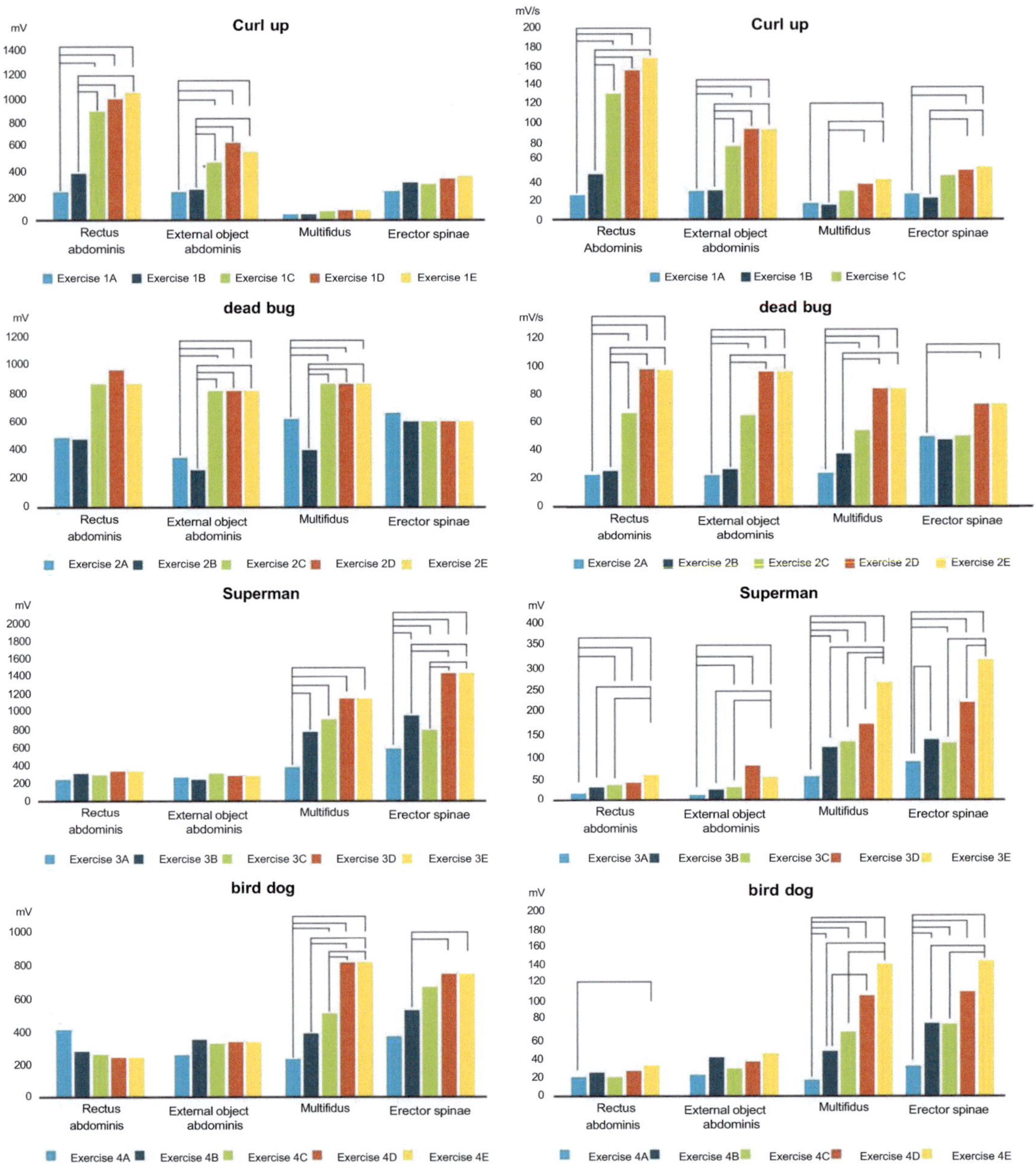

Fig. 14.7 This diagram shows that when muscles are evaluated using surface electromyography, the amount of muscle contraction movement increases proportionally as the stage increases in the individualized graded stabilization exercise

chronic back pain. Then, several questions may arise. How should I walk? Should I walk fast? Or should I walk slowly for a long time? Will hiking help? Can I go up and down the stairs? It is difficult to clearly answer these questions, but it is possible to infer an appropriate walking exercise method based on scientific evidence. When walking, if you analyze the movement of the lumbar muscles with surface electromyography, you can find something peculiar. As shown in the figure below, as the walking speed increases, the muscle contraction of the multifidus of the lumbar 3 and 5 and the erector spinae of the lumbar 5 increases (Fig. 14.8a) [38]. This result shows that fast walking is more effective for chronic back pain, as most back pain is related to muscle atrophy in the lower lumbar spine. On the other hand, when climbing uphill like a mountain trail, the muscle contraction of the lower lumbar spine no longer increases, and the muscle contraction of the upper lumbar spine rather increases (Fig. 14.8b). Also, when climbing uphill, the lumbar spine is flexed and force is applied, which can have a negative effect on the intervertebral disc. Therefore, it is better to educate to walk as fast as possible on flat ground for walking exercise. It is expected to be effective.

3. Background of the introduction of core exercises
   The importance of core exercises has been greatly emphasized since the announcement of a 10-year follow-up study in 2014 [39]. Especially after the publication of this paper,

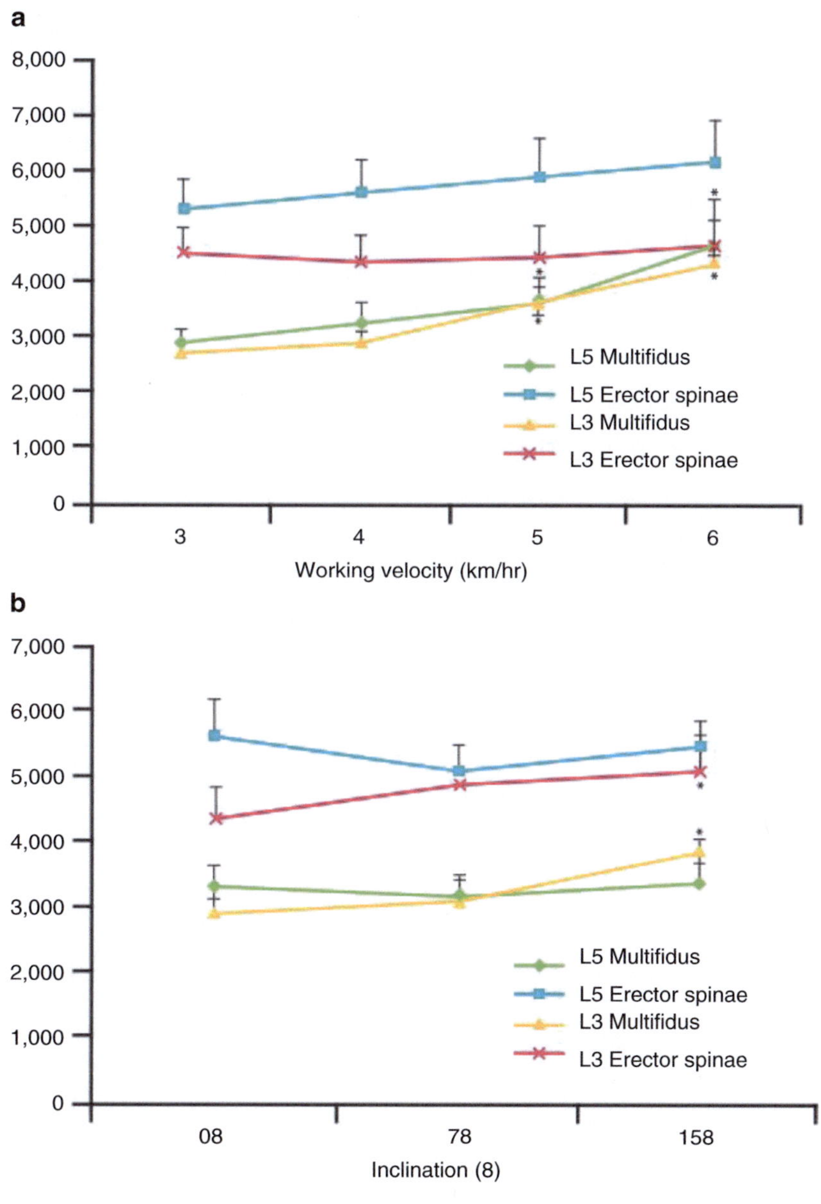

Fig. 14.8 (**a**) Shows that as the walking speed increases, the muscle contraction of the multifidus of the third and fif5th lumbar vertebrae and the erector spinae of the fifth lumbar vertebrae increases, and (**b**) shows that when climbing up a slope like a mountain trail, the muscle contraction of the lower lumbar does not increase any further, but the muscle contraction of the upper lumbar actually increases

it showed excellent results compared to previous studies for spinal stenosis, which had minimal effects from exercise therapy [23]. Core exercises consist of two main elements. First, sit in a chair, imagine your belly button touching your back, apply maximum force, hold for 5–7 s, then relax. Second, always apply 10–20% of your maximum force to your abdomen to maintain posture. This not only strengthens the muscles around the spine but also protects the spine, making it very useful. Core exercises can prevent the recurrence of back pain solely through core exercises, regardless of the presence or absence of strength training and flexibility exercises, as seen in research results [39].

4. Background of the introduction of posture correction

   A normal spine shows lordosis. Normally, the nucleus is located in the front of the intervertebral disc, forming lordosis with the back of the disc narrowed, and the muscles around the lumbar spine hold the back of the vertebral body strongly, maintaining lordosis. However, when a herniated disc occurs and the nucleus moves to the back or the muscles that fix the back of the spine weaken, the lordosis of the lumbar spine decreases, and the decreased lordosis promotes the posterior movement of the nucleus, causing a herniated disc and chronic back pain. Since the lordosis of the spine has the effect of preventing herniated discs by the lordosis itself, this posture should always be maintained (Fig. 14.9) [40]. For example, imagine sitting on the floor or on a sofa or chair. If the lordosis decreases or shows kyphosis at this time, a force that always pushes the nucleus of the intervertebral disc to the back is applied, so caution is required (Fig. 14.10). Therefore, it is necessary to always maintain a posture that maintains lordosis in daily life.

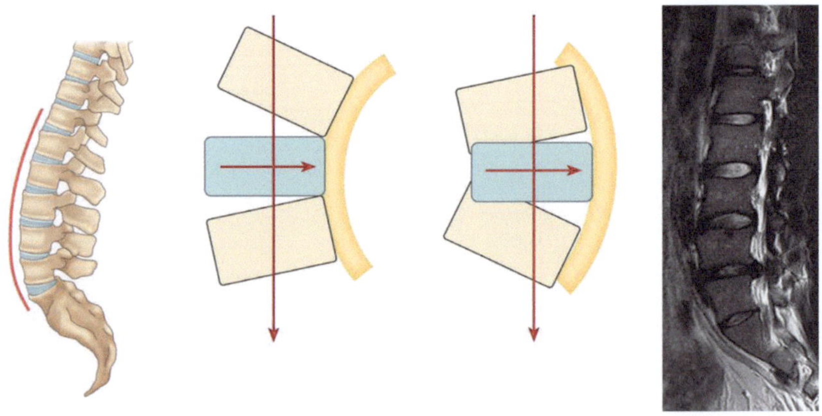

Fig. 14.9 This figure shows the impact of lumbar flexion on disc herniation

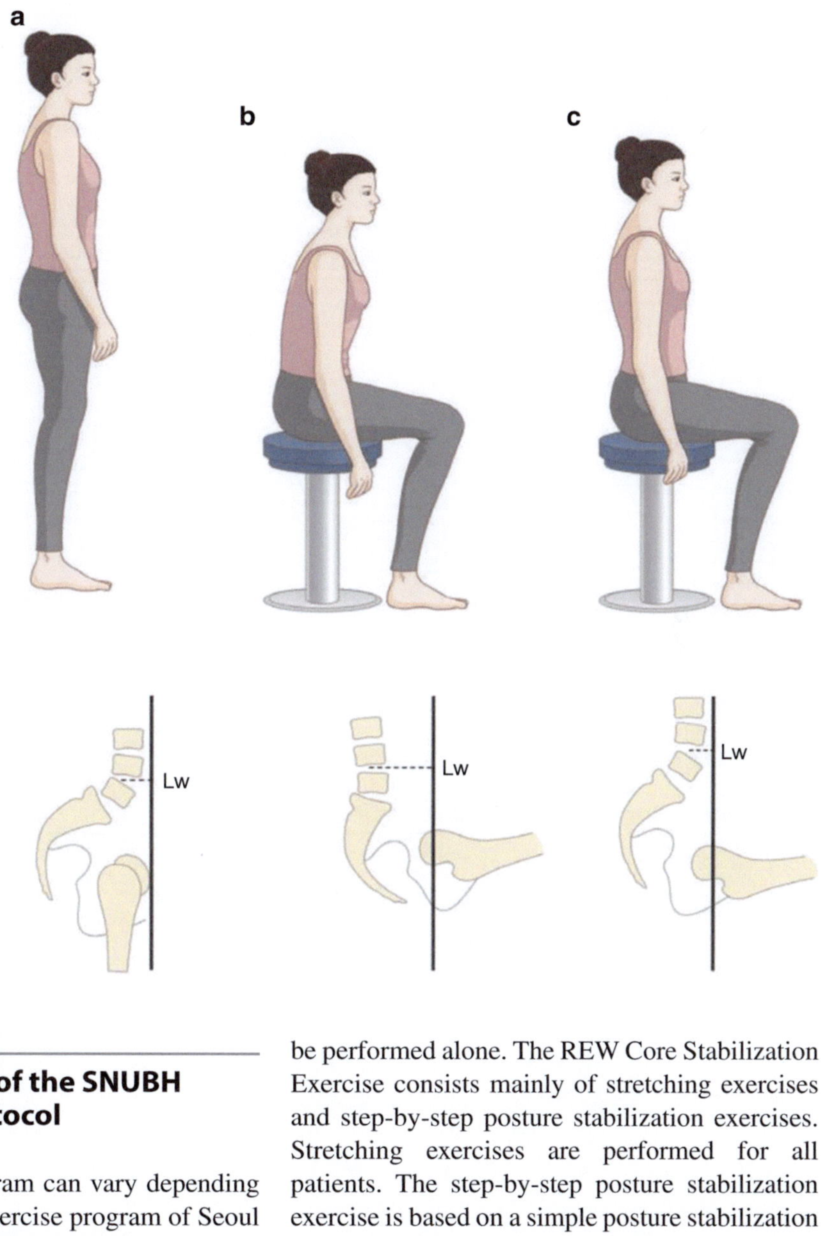

Fig. 14.10 This figure shows the difference in lumbar lordosis in standing (**a**) and sitting postures (**b**, **c**). In the sitting posture, the lumbar lordosis decreases (**b**), so it is especially necessary to straighten the back and maintain the lumbar lordosis (**c**)

14.4 Completion of the SNUBH Exercise Protocol

The spine exercise program can vary depending on the researcher. The exercise program of Seoul National University Bundang Hospital is characterized by being scientifically and systematically organized based on existing research results. The Seoul National University Bundang Hospital exercise program consists of exercise education materials (two pages) and the REW Core Stabilization Exercise (individualized graded stabilization exercise) program (one page).

The exercise education materials explain in detail how to perform posture education, core exercises, and walking exercises so that they can be performed alone. The REW Core Stabilization Exercise consists mainly of stretching exercises and step-by-step posture stabilization exercises. Stretching exercises are performed for all patients. The step-by-step posture stabilization exercise is based on a simple posture stabilization exercise, not a complex exercise like exercise function control, and consists of seven postures and each posture.

It consists of a five-step exercise. The patient visits the hospital and receives an evaluation of their muscle strength. They then receive training in stretching exercises and one of seven postures (a total of seven exercise methods). After about 2 weeks of exercising on their own, they revisit the hospital to relearn the exercise method or, if their muscle strength has improved, to learn a

1. Correct back posture

Ⓐ The lumbar spine is made up of five bones, with discs located between them, and the spinal nerves behind them. The normal lumbar spine has a C-shape that is curved forward, and if this is slightly exaggerated, it looks like below figures: If you maintain normal lumbar curvature (lordosis), you can prevent the herniation of nucleus pulposus of the disc, but if you do not maintain lordosis and apply a load, the space between the backs of the lumbar vertebrae will widen, making it easy for the nucleus pulposus of the disc to protrude. The protruded nucleus will induce pressure on the ligaments and nerves of the lumbar spine, causing pain.

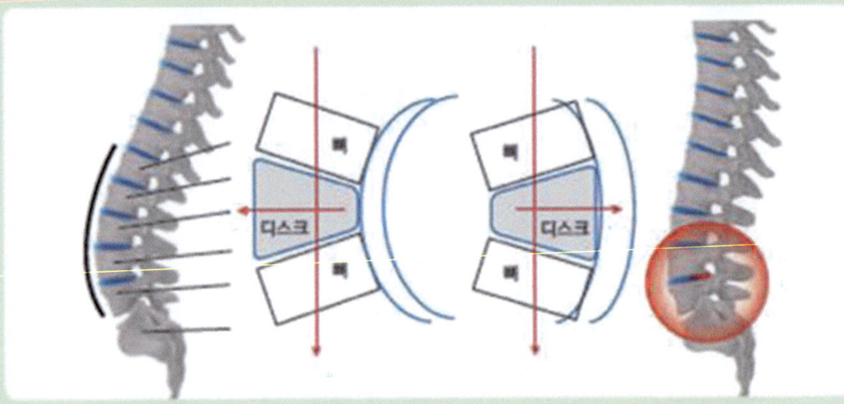

2. Important posture to keep in daily life

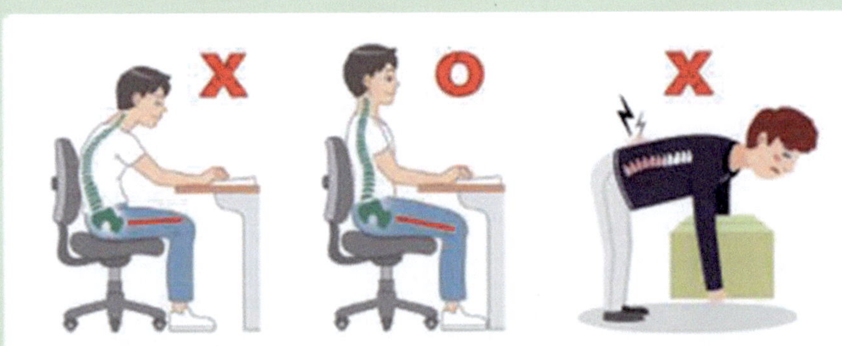

Ⓐ When performing various movements, it is important to maintain proper lumbar lordosis and avoid postures that involve bending the back.

Fig. 14.11 Educational material of the lumbar exercise program at Bundang Seoul National University Hospital

new exercise. They then continue to exercise at home. The following figure shows the exercise program, the exercise education material (Fig. 14.11), and the REW Core Stabilization Exercise program (Fig. 14.12).

- **B** When sitting on a chair or driving, keep your buttocks deep in the chair to maintain the correct extension angle (lordosis) of your back.
- **C** When sitting on the floor or sofa, your back tends to bend, so sit on a chair rather than on the floor or sofa, and if you must sit on a sofa, use a cushion to maintain the lordosis angle of your lumbar spine.
- **D** When lifting a heavy object, go close to the object and lift it with your back straight.
- **E** When washing your face or washing your hair, keep your back straight to avoid straining or herniated intervertebral disc of your back. When washing your hair, it is best to do it while standing while showering.

3. Bracing exercise

- **A** When someone hits your stomach with a fist, you will automatically tense your abdominal muscles to reduce the impact. You should tense your abdomen in the same way, as if you're contracting all the abdominal muscles along with the deep muscles of your back simultaneously.
- **B** While sitting on a chair, always engage about 10-20% of the maximum force you can exert with your abdomen to maintain good posture.
- **C** If you have been sitting for a long time, imagine that your belly button is touching your back, and then apply maximum force. Hold it for 5-7 seconds and then relax.

4. Walking exercise

- **A** Walk for at least 30 minutes, 5 times a week.
- **B** When walking, try to walk at a fast pace. Walking faster helps strengthen the back muscles and reduce lower back pain.
- **C** Walk on flat ground. Walking uphill or downhill can cause your back to bend, reducing the effectiveness of your back exercises.
- **D** While walking, also perform abdominal brace exercises. Apply 10-20% of the maximum strength you can exert on your abdomen while walking.

5. REW Core Stabilization Exercise

SNUH
분당서울대학교병원

Fig. 14.11 (continued)

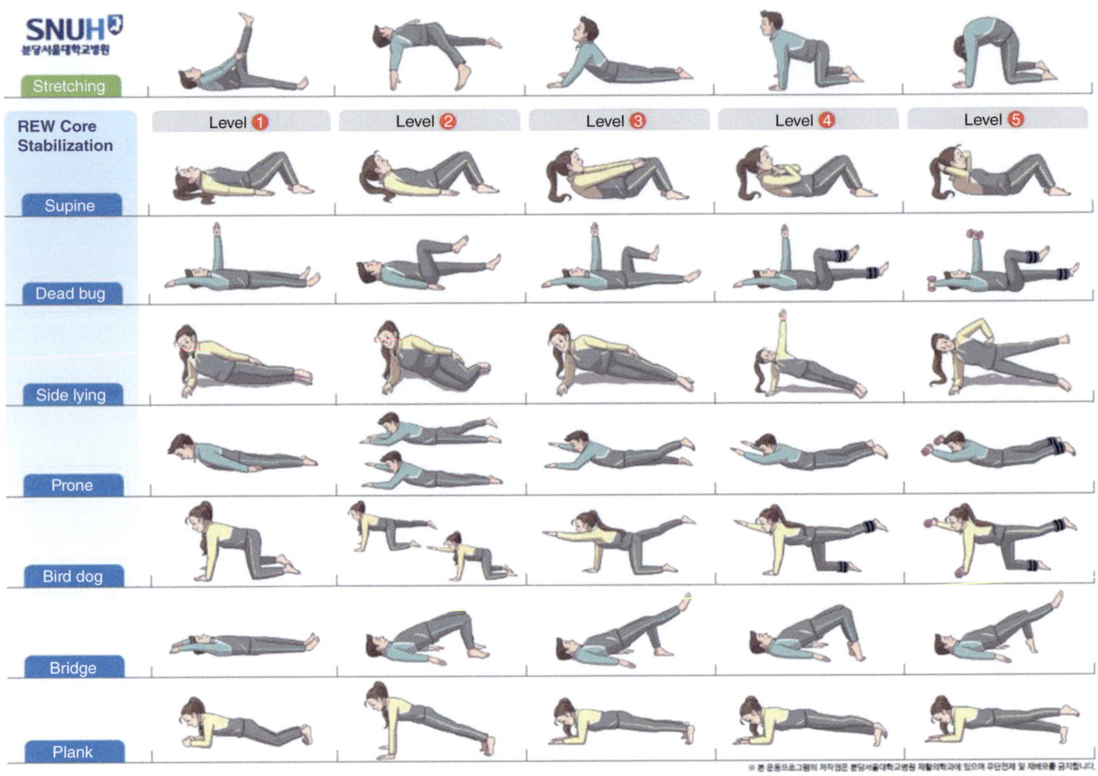

Fig. 14.12 REW core stabilization exercise of Seoul National University Bundang Hospital

14.5 Conclusion

Various exercise methods are used for spinal physiotherapy, but there is no significant difference between the methods. Therefore, an exercise that is easy to perform, economically feasible, and can be done at home in a short time is needed. The Seoul National University Bundang Hospital has developed a program where you can learn spinal exercises with one or two lessons and has proven its clinical effectiveness. It is currently being used in actual treatment. We hope that through this exercise program, patients with back pain can be free from back pain.

Bibliography

1. Waddell G. 1987 Volvo award in clinical sciences. A new clinical model for the treatment of low-back pain. Spine (Phila Pa 1976). 1987;12(7):632–44.
2. Kovacs FM, Seco J, Royuela A, Corcoll Reixach J, Abraira V. Predicting the evolution of low back pain patients in routine clinical practice: results from a registry within the Spanish National Health Service. Spine J. 2012;12(11):1008–20.
3. Lee HI, Lee ST, Kim M, Ryu JS. Sex differences in predicting chronicity of low-back pain after acute trauma using lumbar muscle area. Am J Phys Med Rehabil. 2015;94(2):123–30.
4. Lee HI, Song J, Lee HS, Kang JY, Kim M, Ryu JS. Association between cross-sectional areas of lumbar muscles on magnetic resonance imaging and chronicity of low back pain. Ann Rehabil Med. 2011;35(6):852–9.
5. Panjabi MM. The stabilizing system of the spine. Part I. Function, dysfunction, adaptation, and enhancement. J Spinal Disord. 1992;5(4):383–9; discussion 397.
6. Richardson CA, Jull GA. Muscle control-pain control. What exercises would you prescribe? Man Ther. 1995;1(1):2–10.
7. Jull GA, Richardson CA. Motor control problems in patients with spinal pain: a new direction for therapeutic exercise. J Manip Physiol Ther. 2000;23(2):115–7.
8. Blackburn SE, Portney LG. Electromyographic activity of back musculature during Williams' flexion exercises. Phys Ther. 1981;61(6):878–85.

9. Mann SJ, Lam JC, Singh P. McKenzie back exercises. In: StatPearls. Treasure Island (FL): StatPearls Publishing; 2019.
10. Jordan K, Dunn KM, Lewis M, Croft P. A minimal clinically important difference was derived for the Roland-Morris Disability Questionnaire for low back pain. J Clin Epidemiol. 2006;59(1):45–52.
11. Lauridsen HH, Hartvigsen J, Manniche C, Korsholm L, Grunnet-Nilsson N. Responsiveness and minimal clinically important difference for pain and disability instruments in low back pain patients. BMC Musculoskelet Disord. 2006;7:82.
12. Goldby LJ, Moore AP, Doust J, Trew ME. A randomized controlled stabilization and walking exercises on chronic low back pain: a randomized controlled trial. Medicine (Baltimore). 2019;98(26):e16173.
13. Ferreira ML, Ferreira PH, Latimer J, et al. Comparison of general exercise, motor control exercise and spinal manipulative therapy for chronic low back pain: a randomized trial. Pain. 2007;131(1–2):31–7.
14. Costa LO, Maher CG, Latimer J, et al. Motor control exercise for chronic low back pain: a randomized placebo-controlled trial. Phys Ther. 2009;89(12):1275–86.
15. Macedo LG, Saragiotto BT, Yamato TP, et al. Motor control exercise for acute non-specific low back pain. Cochrane Database Syst Rev. 2016;2:CD012085.
16. Saragiotto BT, Maher CG, Yamato TP, et al. Motor control exercise for nonspecific low back pain: a Cochrane review. Spine (Phila Pa 1976). 2016;41(16):1284–95.
17. Sinaki M, Lutness MP, Ilstrup DM, Chu CP, Gramse RR. Lumbar spondylolisthesis: retrospective comparison and three-year follow-up of two conservative treatment programs. Arch Phys Med Rehabil. 1989;70(8):594–8.
18. Hicks GE, Fritz JM, Delitto A, McGill SM. Preliminary development of a clinical prediction rule for determining which patients with low back pain will respond to a stabilization exercise program. Arch Phys Med Rehabil. 2005;86(9):1753–62.
19. Schneider MJ, Ammendolia C, Murphy DR, et al. Comparative clinical effectiveness of nonsurgical treatment methods in patients with lumbar spinal stenosis: a randomized clinical trial. JAMA Netw Open. 2019;2(1):e186828.
20. Minetama M, Kawakami M, Teraguchi M, et al. Supervised physical therapy vs. home exercise for patients with lumbar spinal stenosis: a randomized controlled trial. Spine J. 2019;19:1310–8.
21. Jarrett MS, Orlando JF, Grimmer-Somers K. The effectiveness of land based exercise compared to decompressive surgery in the management of lumbar spinal-canal stenosis: a systematic review. BMC Musculoskelet Disord. 2012;13:30.
22. Macedo LG, Hum A, Kuleba L, et al. Physical therapy interventions for degenerative lumbar spinal stenosis: a systematic review. Phys Ther. 2013;93(12):1646–60.
23. Zaina F, Tomkins-Lane C, Carragee E, Negrini S. Surgical versus non-surgical treatment for lumbar spinal stenosis. Cochrane Database Syst Rev. 2016;(1):CD010264.
24. Rousing R, Jensen RK, Fruensgaard S, et al. Danish national clinical guidelines for surgical and nonsurgical treatment of patients with lumbar spinal stenosis. Eur Spine J. 2019;28(6):1386–96.
25. Kent P, Mjosund HL, Petersen DH. Does targeting manual therapy and/or exercise improve patient outcomes in nonspecific low back pain? A systematic review. BMC Med. 2010;8:22.
26. Hosseinifar M, Akbari M, Behtash H, Amiri M, Sarrafzadeh J. The effects of stabilization and Mckenzie exercises on transverse abdominis and multifidus muscle thickness, pain, and disability: a randomized controlled trial in nonspecific chronic low back pain. J Phys Ther Sci. 2013;25(12):1541–5.
27. Halliday MH, Pappas E, Hancock MJ, et al. A randomized clinical trial comparing the McKenzie method and motor control exercises in people with chronic low back pain and a directional preference: 1-yearfollow-up. Physiotherapy. 2019;105:442–5.
28. Yamato TP, Maher CG, Saragiotto BT, et al. Pilates for low back pain: complete republication of a Cochrane review. Spine (Phila Pa 1976). 2016;41(12):1013–21.
29. Wieland LS, Skoetz N, Pilkington K, Vempati R, D'Adamo CR, Berman BM. Yoga treatment for chronic non-specific low back pain. Cochrane Database Syst Rev. 2017;1:CD010671.
30. Suh JH, Kim H, Jung GP, Ko JY, Ryu JS. The effect of lumbar stabilization and walking exercises on chronic low back pain: a randomized controlled trial. Medicine. 2019;98(26):e16173.
31. Lee HS, Kim DJ, Oh Y, Min K, Ryu JS. The effect of individualized gradable stabilization exercises in patients with chronic low back pain: case-control study. J Back Musculoskelet Rehabil. 2016;29(3):603–10.
32. Kim CR, Park DK, Lee ST, Ryu JS. Electromyographic changes in trunk muscles during graded lumbar stabilization exercises. PM R. 2016;8(10):979–89.
33. Airaksinen O, Brox JI, Cedraschi C, et al. Chapter 4. European guidelines for the management of chronic nonspecific low back pain. Eur Spine J. 2006;15(Suppl 2):S192–300.
34. Koes BW, van Tulder M, Lin CW, Macedo LG, McAuley J, Maher C. An updated overview of clinical guidelines for the management of nonspecific low back pain in primary care. Eur Spine J. 2010;19(12):2075–94.
35. Pillastrini P, Gardenghi I, Bonetti F, et al. An updated overview of clinical guidelines for chronic low back pain management in primary care. Joint Bone Spine. 2012;79(2):176–85.
36. O'Connor SR, Tully MA, Ryan B, et al. Walking exercise for chronic musculoskeletal pain: systematic review and meta-analysis. Arch Phys Med Rehabil. 2015;96(4):724–34.e3.

37. Hurley DA, Tully MA, Lonsdale C, et al. Supervised walking in comparison with fitness training for chronic back pain in physiotherapy: results of the SWIFT single-blinded randomized controlled trial (ISRCTN17592092). Pain. 2015;156(1):131–47.
38. Lee HS, Shim JS, Lee ST, Kim M, Ryu JS. Facilitating effects of fast and slope walking on paraspinal muscles. Ann Rehabil Med. 2014;38(4):514–22.
39. Aleksiev AR. Ten-year follow-up of strengthening versus flexibility exercises with or without abdominal bracing in recurrent low back pain. Spine (Phila Pa 1976). 2014;39(13):997–1003.
40. Been E, Kalichman L. Lumbar lordosis. Spine J. 2014;14(1):87–97.

Spinal Intervention

15

Jong Won Kwon and Eugene Lee

Spinal intervention refers to various procedures performed on spinal lesions through a percutaneous approach under the guidance of imaging equipment such as fluoroscopy and angiography, CT, etc. Its application areas are expanding. Fluoroscopy is most widely used in spinal intervention because it provides real-time imaging, clear bone contours, and allows procedures to be performed under guidance from various angles and directions. This chapter introduces epidural steroid injection, facet joint injection/sacroiliac joint injection, vertebroplasty, discography, and spinal biopsy, which are commonly performed in spinal intervention.

15.1 Epidural Steroid Injection

Back pain and radiating pain are conditions that most people can experience in their lifetime, and conservative treatments include rest, physical therapy, and oral intake of non-steroidal anti-inflammatory drugs (NSAIDs). If symptoms are severe or persistent, imaging tests are performed to find anatomical abnormalities such as herniated intervertebral disc (HIVD) or spinal stenosis, typically using plain radiography and MRI. Epidural steroid injection can be a very effective treatment method when there is little response to other conservative treatments or when severe pain is reported.

The first use of epidural steroid injection in common treatment was in 1952 [1], and Macnab et al. described selective nerve root block in 1971 [2]. Initially, these injection methods were performed without the help of imaging equipment, but with the introduction of fluoroscopy and CT equipment, procedures could be performed much more accurately and safely.

The purpose of the epidural steroid injection is not to treat anatomical abnormalities, but to improve the patient's symptoms [3]. It helps acute back pain patients to start rehabilitation treatment and return to daily life quickly. That is the purpose of the epidural steroid injection.

15.1.1 Anatomy

The epidural space is a potential space between the inner surface of the spinal canal and the outer surface of the dura, extending from the foramen magnum to the sacrococcygeal ligament. It connects to the space around the spine through the neural foramen, and the nerve root surrounded by the dura is located in the anterolateral epidural space. The nerve root has a dorsal root ganglion, which is generally located at the neural foramen. The dura surrounds the nerve root up to the dorsal

J. W. Kwon (✉)
Department of Radiology, Dongcheon Donggang Hospital, Ulsan, Republic of Korea

E. Lee (✉)
Department of Radiology, Seoul National University Bundang Hospital, Seongnam-si, Republic of Korea

© The Author(s), under exclusive license to Springer Nature Singapore Pte Ltd. 2025

H. S. Kang, J. W. Lee (eds.), *Spinal Imaging*, https://doi.org/10.1007/978-981-95-1386-4_15

root ganglion, and after that, it is called the peripheral nerve, and the dura merges with the epineurium. The posterior epidural space is most visible in the lumbar region, appearing as a triangle filled with fat in cross-sectional images (Fig. 15.1). In some patients, there is a structure called the plica mediana dorsalis (or epidural dorsomedian septum) in the center of the dura posterior, causing the drug injected into the spine to flow only to one side. In areas where posterior lumbar surgery has been performed previously, the posterior epidural space is not well visible, and if there is hypertrophy of the ligamentum flavum, it narrows. The posterior epidural space is hardly visible normally at the cervical or lumbar L5–S1 level.

There is a caudal approach to access the epidural space. The sacrum and coccyx are attached, and there is an area not covered by bone structures in the posterior at the fourth and fifth sacrum, which allows access to the spinal canal. This area is called the sacral hiatus and is covered by the sacrococcygeal ligament. The lateral side of the sacral hiatus is bordered by the sacral cornua, and the floor has the fifth sacral body. The dural sac is located up to the second sacral body on average in adults.

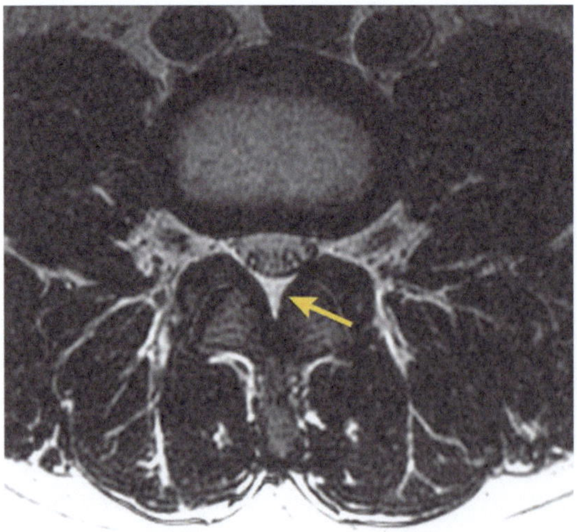

Fig. 15.1 Posterior epidural space. The epidural space refers to the outer space of the dura inside the spinal canal. In axial T2-weighted MR images, the posterior epidural space of the lumbar spine appears as a triangular space between the dura and the ligamentum flavum, normally containing adipose tissue (arrow)

15.1.2 Mechanism of Action and Effects

Pain caused by nerve compression occurs not only from simple physical pressure but also from the stimulation of chemicals. Green et al. reported inflammation around the nerve root in surgical findings [4], and in the early 1990s, it was reported that phospholipase A2 causes inflammation around the nerves. According to research so far, it has been reported that a large amount of chemical pain transmitters such as matrix metalloproteinases, phospholipase A2, nitric oxide, and cytokines like tumor necrosis factor-α are distributed around the disc that has escaped from HIVD [5], and in experiments related to spinal stenosis, chronic pressure caused venous congestion, edema in the nerve, conduction disorders, and leakage of neurotoxic substances. Epidural steroid injection is known to suppress the action of substances like phospholipase A2 and reduce inflammation. Also, corticosteroid is the signal transmission of unmyelinated C-fibers is reduced, decreasing the transmission of pain sensation [3]. The local anesthetic administered simultaneously reduces immediate pain and blocks the "pain-muscle spasm-ischemia-pain" cycle.

The effect of epidural steroid injection varies in different literature, but it is reported to have an effect in about 70~80% of cases, and it is reported to have a short-term effect (a few weeks to a few months) rather than a long-term effect (several years). It can be performed primarily before surgery in patients without neurological symptoms such as paralysis or nausea. However, it is difficult to clarify the exact degree of efficacy of epidural steroid injection due to the fact that most back pain naturally improves over time and it is difficult to study with a control group.

Generally, patients experience symptom improvement immediately after the procedure, which is due to the local anesthetic administered simultaneously. The effect of the steroid usually appears on the second to sixth day, and the degree of improvement varies from patient to patient. In some cases, the first injection may not have an effect, but the second or third injection may improve pain.

15.1.3 Indications and Contraindications

Radiating pain is the most effective and common indication. It is used in back pain, but back pain can be caused by various causes such as muscle or spinal joint problems, not just nerve stimulation, so the effect may not be significant. Indications for epidural steroid injection include acute or chronic radiating pain due to HIVD, back pain, or radiating pain due to spinal stenosis, post-spinal surgery pain, postherpetic neuralgia, and similar symptoms of idiopathic radiating pain. It can also be used for radiating pain in the cervical spine, degenerative spinal disease, cervical sprain, acute or chronic neck pain.

Blood coagulation disorders, pregnancy, systemic infection, or local skin infection at the puncture site, allergy to drugs, cases where the maximum allowable amount of steroid injection has already been received, uncontrolled diabetes, glaucoma, and pain due to psychological factors are contraindications.

15.1.4 Procedure

15.1.4.1 Preparation Before the Procedure

First, the pattern, degree, location, and duration of the patient's pain are identified. It is checked whether the patient has had surgery or spinal injections before, and diabetes or hypertension is also checked. After explaining the procedure method, risks, and effects to the patient, consent is obtained. If CT or MRI has been performed before the procedure, it is reviewed and the injection method and location are determined.

Epidural steroid injection is mostly performed under fluoroscopic guidance, and a contrast agent is used to confirm whether the tip of the spinal needle is properly located in the epidural space. If the injection is performed only by the operator's feeling without fluoroscopic equipment, the needle may be placed in the wrong position. White et al. reported that without using fluoroscopy, the needle was placed in the wrong place in 30% of cases with lumbar interlaminar approach and 25% of cases with caudal approach [6].

15.1.4.2 Lumbar Interlaminar Epidural Steroid Injection

This procedure is performed when the main symptoms are lumbar central canal stenosis at the L3–4 level or higher, or lower back pain. The patient lies face down on the procedure table with a pillow under their lower abdomen or pelvis to widen the interspinous space. There are two approaches to access the posterior epidural space through the center of the interspinous space: the midline approach and the slightly lateral paramidline (or paramedian) approach. Generally, the midline approach is used, but if the interspinous space is too narrow (example, in Baastrup's disease), the approach is made obliquely about 2~3 cm aside. If the patient's symptoms are located on one side, the paramidline approach on the symptomatic side may be more effective. The injection site is preferably at the lesion if the posterior epidural space is sufficient, but if the central canal stenosis at the lesion site is severe or if surgery has been performed before, access to the posterior epidural space at the lesion site may be difficult or impossible, so it is advisable to perform the procedure one or two levels below. A 22G spinal needle can be used, and the needle is advanced targeting the center of the interspinous space in the anteroposterior view (Fig. 15.2). Depending on the patient, if the spinous process is slightly posteriorly oriented, the anteroposterior view's angle is adjusted parallel to the spinous process, and the spinal needle is advanced slightly towards the head when accessing the posterior epidural space. There is a firm resistance when the needle passes through the ligament area, but when the ligamentum flavum is pierced and enters the posterior epidural space, the resistance disappears momentarily, which is called loss of resistance. The approach to the epidural space begins near the imaginary line connecting the central part of the facet joint in the lateral view, and the stylet of the spinal needle is removed and the contrast medium is connected to the cannula, and the needle is advanced slowly while testing the contrast medium. When the resistance disappears and the spread of the contrast medium along the epidural space is confirmed, the prepared injection drug is injected

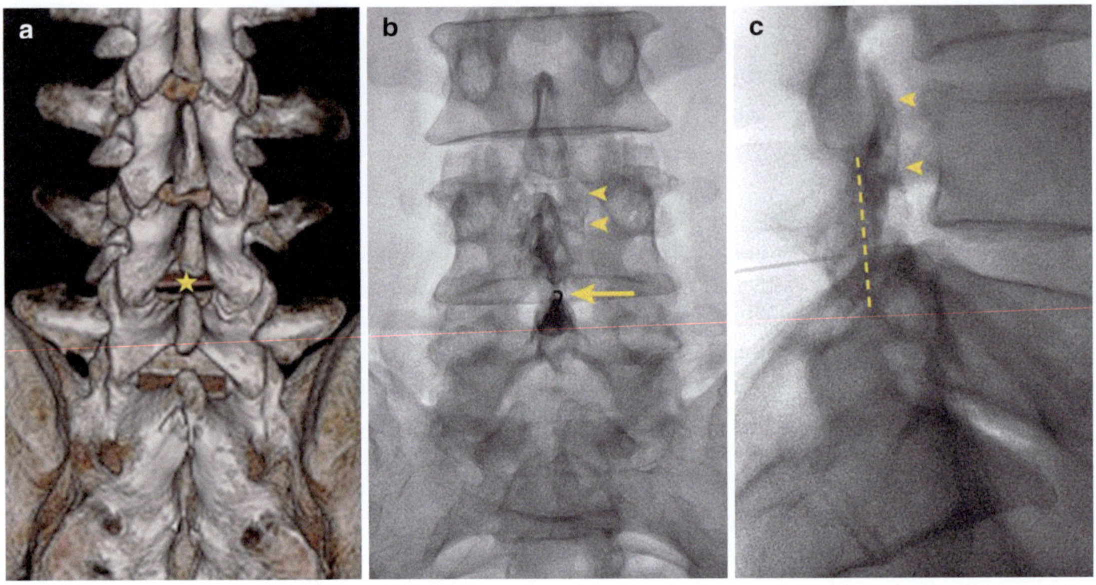

Fig. 15.2 Lumbar interlaminar epidural steroid injection. (**a**) The approach is to the central part (asterisk) between the lumbar L4–5 laminae, and the X-ray tube is rotated so that the interlaminar space can be visible. (**b**) In the anteroposterior fluoroscopic image, the spinal needle (arrow) is entering through the L4–5 interlaminar space, and the contrast medium (arrowhead) is spreading irregularly. (**c**) In the lateral fluoroscopic image, when the end of the spinal needle reaches near the imaginary line (dotted line) connecting the central part of the facet joint, the contrast medium is test injected to confirm the epidural space. The contrast medium (arrowhead) is spreading vertically

(Fig. 15.2). If a dural puncture occurs and the contrast medium is injected into the subarachnoid space, it quickly accumulates in the front part of the dural sac in the center because the patient is lying face down (Fig. 15.3). If a dural puncture occurs, the procedure is repeated after a week or attempted again at another site. If it is injected into the subdural space, the contrast medium spreads thinly along the dura in a tram-tract appearance. To confirm the epidural space, it must always be confirmed in both the anteroposterior and lateral views. If the contrast medium is correctly injected into the epidural space, the fluoroscopic findings in the case of the interlaminar approach show that the posterior epidural space is first filled linearly in the lateral view and then spreads around the dural sac to both sides.

15.1.4.3 Caudal Injection

This procedure is performed when there is radiating pain in both legs due to lumbar central canal stenosis, or when there are lesions in multiple areas and complex symptoms. Like the interlaminar approach, the patient is made to lie face down on the fluoroscopy table. The sacral hiatus at the bottom of the sacrum is identified in the anteroposterior fluoroscopic view (Fig. 15.4). This is an "inverted U-shape" hole surrounded by the bilateral sacral cornua, and it is confirmed by fluoroscopy. It is possible to confirm, but often it is not clearly visible due to overlapping with the air shadow in the rectum. In this case, the location of the sacral hiatus can be identified in the lateral radiographic image. A 22G spinal needle is advanced towards the apex of the sacral hiatus. The needle penetrates the sacrococcygeal ligament and the end of the needle is advanced to touch the posterior of the sacrum, while maintaining the needle's direction in the center in the anteroposterior radiographic image and advancing it towards the head. When advancing the needle, the bevel of the needle end is advanced while facing the dorsal aspect of the sacrum, as seen in the lateral radiographic image. When the end of

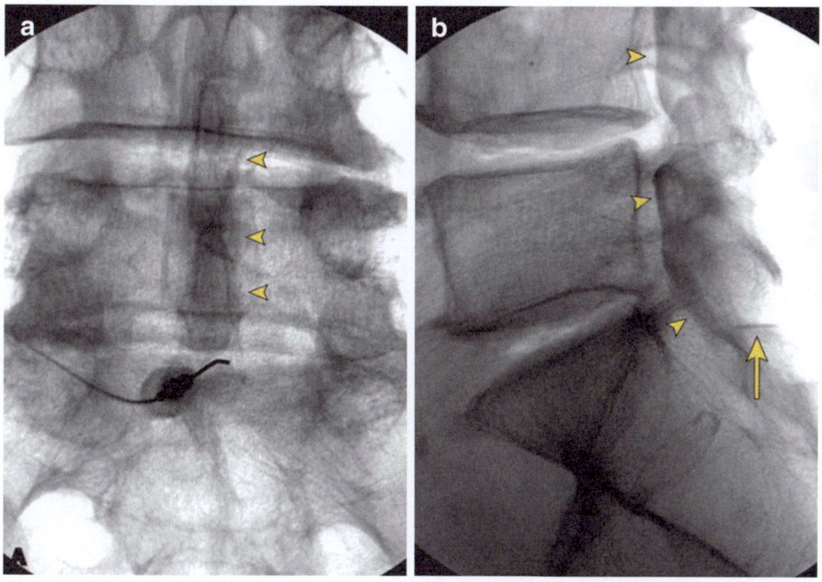

Fig. 15.3 Dural puncture occurring during lumbar interlaminar epidural steroid injection. (**a**) In the case of a dural puncture during an L5–S1 interlaminar epidural steroid injection, the contrast medium is pooled along the central part of the vertebral body (arrowhead) in the anterior and posterior images. (**b**) In the lateral fluoroscopic image, the spinal needle (arrow) is inserted into the L5–S1 interlaminar space. If the contrast medium quickly settles forward (arrowhead), a dural puncture can be confirmed

the needle advances to the height of the sacrum 2–3 times (since the dural sac of an adult is located up to the height of the sacrum 1–2 times on average, the end of the needle does not rise above the height of the sacrum two times to prevent the dura from being punctured), the stylet of the needle is removed and the contrast medium is connected to the cannula. If the contrast medium spreads towards the head when tested, the drug is injected. If the end of the needle is located on the ventral aspect of the sacrum, there may be cases where the needle scratches the periosteum, and in this case, the patient may complain of severe pain and the contrast medium and drug may be injected into the blood vessels, so the needle should be located on the dorsal aspect as much as possible and it should be confirmed that the contrast medium spreads softly into the epidural space. If the central canal stenosis is severe in the lower lumbar, the patient may complain of pain as the pressure in the spinal canal increases when injecting the drug, so the drug should be injected as softly and slowly as possible. Usually, when injecting with a caudal injection, the drug is diluted so that the total volume is about 7~10 mL.

After the caudal injection, the spread of the contrast medium appears as a Christmas tree shape in the anteroposterior radiographic image (Fig. 15.4). When the contrast medium fills around the dural sac, the dural sac appears as a filling defect in the lateral radiographic image and may appear as a railway track shape. If the dura is punctured and the contrast medium enters the intradural space, the contrast medium, which has a higher specific gravity than CSF, settles in the front part of the dural sac in a prone position, appearing as a fluid-fluid level with CSF. Also, it can be seen that the contrast medium is diluted and moved towards the head by CSF in real-time radiographic images.

15.1.4.4 Lumbar Transforaminal Epidural Steroid Injection

Transforaminal epidural steroid injection can be used to inject steroids for the treatment of unilateral radiating pain caused by HIVD or spinal stenosis, but it can also be used for diagnostic purposes by selectively blocking pain caused by nerve roots. When used for diagnostic purposes, local anesthetics that can only provide temporary

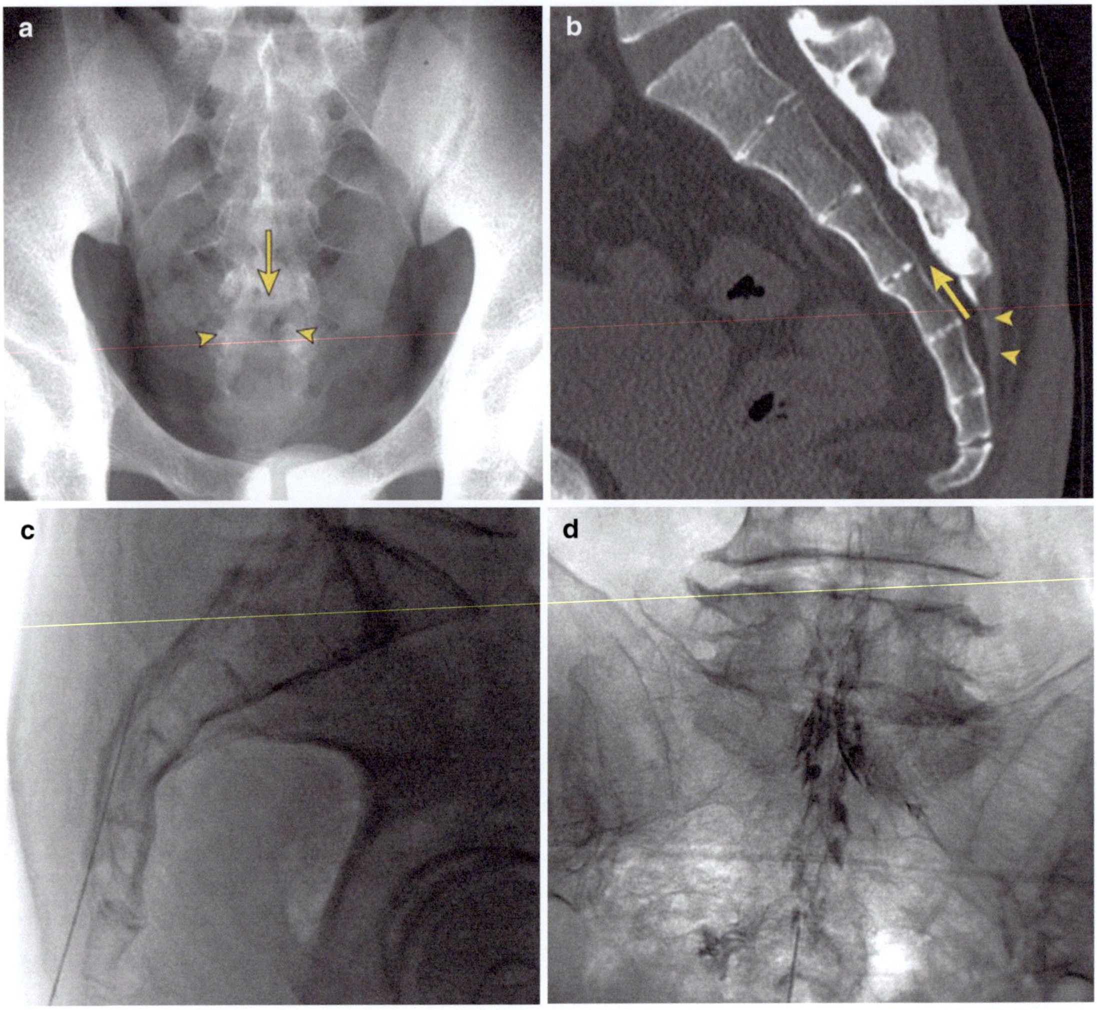

Fig. 15.4 Caudal injection. (**a**) In the plain radiography, the sacral hiatus (arrow) and sacral cornua (arrowhead) are visible. (**b**) In the sagittal reconstructed CT image, the needle is advanced through the sacrococcygeal ligament (arrowhead) (arrow). (**c**) This is a fluoroscopic image of another patient, and in the lateral image, the spinal needle is being advanced along the epidural space of the sacrum. To avoid dural puncture, it is advanced up to the height of the third sacrum. (**d**) In the anteroposterior fluoroscopic image, the needle is located in the center, and when the contrast medium and drug are injected, it spreads irregularly to both sides like a Christmas tree

effects, such as lidocaine, are mainly used. When the drug is distributed only around a single nerve root, the term selective nerve root block is sometimes used.

Unlike the caudal approach or interlaminar approach, the transforaminal approach can inject drugs into the anterior epidural space, making it more effective for nerve compression caused by a disc, and it can be used preferentially when symptoms are more severe on one side or nerve compression is confirmed by imaging.

To perform a lumbar transforaminal epidural steroid injection, first one must understand the anatomical relationships. To inject a steroid around the right L5 nerve root from the lumbar spine, it must be injected through the right L5–S1 neural foramen. Similarly, to inject around the left L4 nerve root, it must be injected through the left L4–5 neural foramen.

First, the patient is laid face down, and the X-ray tube is rotated towards the side to be injected to align with the oblique view of the

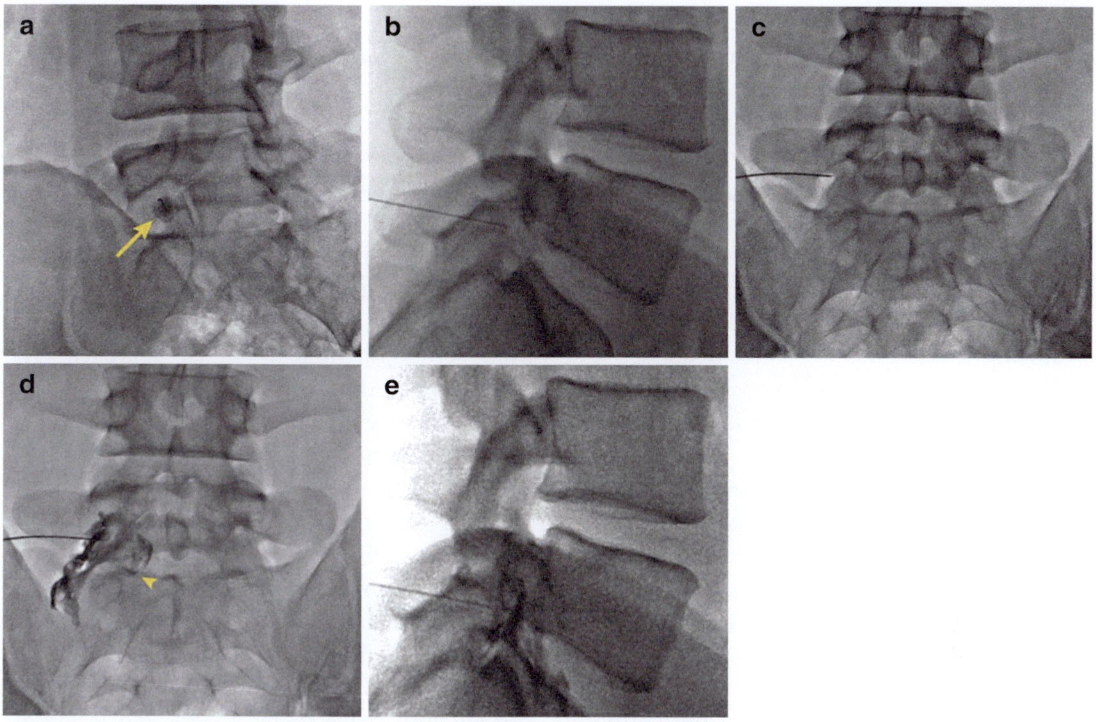

Fig. 15.5 Lumbar transforaminal epidural steroid injection. (**a**) In the left oblique view, the vertebral body shows a scotty dog appearance, and the spinal needle (arrow) is being advanced in a direction parallel to the X-ray tube below the target point, the pedicle. (**b**) In the lateral fluoroscopic image, the needle is advanced until the end reaches near the neural foramen. (**c**) After aligning the X-ray tube anteroposteriorly, when the end of the needle is near the outer boundary of the vertebral body, the contrast medium is test injected and the needle is carefully advanced. (**d**) When the contrast medium spreads around the nerve root and into the epidural space within the spinal canal (arrowhead), the drug is injected. (**e**) In the lateral fluoroscopic image, you can see the contrast medium spreading around the epidural space and nerve root

lumbar spine (Fig. 15.5). At this time, the vertebral body shows the so-called scotty dog shape, and the pedicle corresponding to the eye of the scotty dog is aligned with the superior articular process of the lower spine. In this oblique view, if you approach the 22G spinal needle aiming at the lower lateral part of the pedicle, you can access the safe triangle mentioned by Bogduk et al. [7]. This is a virtual triangular space with the pedicle as the upper boundary, the lateral surface of the vertebral body as the lateral boundary, and the spinal nerve as the lower inner boundary, which allows access to the anterior epidural space with a low risk of directly piercing the nerve, and is called a conventional approach. When the tip of the needle reaches near the neural foramen in the fluoroscopic lateral image, rotate the X-ray tube to inject a small amount of contrast medium from near the outer boundary of the vertebral body in the fluoroscopic anteroposterior image, slowly advancing the needle, and when the contrast medium spreads to the epidural space along the nerve and nerve root, inject local anesthetics and steroids. Another approach is the posterolateral approach, which can be used when the neural foramen is narrow and there is a risk of piercing the nerve root and it is difficult to access the safe triangle. In this case, you can approach along the lateral part of the superior articular process. The traditional method is to approach the needle to the front of the nerve root, but the posterolateral approach approaches the back of the nerve root by advancing towards a slightly lower point in the same oblique view. This method allows most of the drug to be injected into the epidural space without piercing the nerve root, and the probability of dural puncture is lower than the conventional approach [8]. When accessing the L5 nerve root, the needle may get caught on the iliac crest as it advances, so adjust the fluoroscopic angle to approach from above to below. In the case of the S1 nerve root, advance the needle aiming at the posterior sacral foramen, usually aiming at the superolateral of the foramen. During lumbar transforaminal epidural steroid injection, dilute the steroid and local anesthetic with saline to make a total volume of about 3 mL, and if the neural foramen is very narrow and the injection amount needs to be limited, inject without dilution.

During lumbar transforaminal epidural steroid injection, the needle should be able to go just below the pedicle to avoid the nerve root and access the anterior epidural space. If you go too far to the side of the pedicle, the contrast medium will not go enough towards the nerve root and will flow down the distal nerve. If the needle goes too far forward past the vertebral body, the contrast medium is injected into the psoas muscle. Depending on the position of the needle, it may get caught in the facet joint, or the contrast medium may leak towards the back muscles. During the progress of the needle, if the tip of the needle touches the nerve root, the patient complains of severe pain along the corresponding skin segment. In this case, pull the needle back a little so that the drug can be injected into the epineurium. Be careful not to inject into the inside. If it is injected into the epineurium, it is called an intra-epineural injection, and the pressure is high during the injection, causing the patient to complain of severe pain. In this case, the outer boundary is good when injecting the contrast agent, and the nerves appear as stripes on the inside [9]. To avoid this, if the needle touches the nerve root and the patient complains of severe radiating pain, do not test inject with a contrast agent, but slightly pull out the needle. Even during a transforaminal epidural steroid injection, the contrast agent can fill the subdural space, and the contrast agent spreads in the shape of a railway track.

15.1.4.5 Cervical Interlaminar Epidural Steroid Injection

In the cervical spine, interlaminar epidural steroid injection is safer than transforaminal epidural steroid injection, and both methods show similar effects, so the interlaminar approach is tried before the transforaminal approach. The patient is laid down in a prone position, and the neck is slightly flexed with a pillow on the chest so that the needle can pass through the interspinous space well. Adjust the posture so that the shoulder does not cover the injection site in the lateral image. The patient's hand is placed under the patient's thigh and pulled to fix it so that the shoulder can go down enough. Regardless of the location of the lesion, it is best to perform at the height of C5–6, C6–7, or C7–T1 where the posterior epidural space is the widest, and it is most commonly performed at C6–7. At this time, the midline approach, where the posterior epidural space is the widest, is safe. The epidural space of the cervical spine is a very narrow space, only 1–2 mm at the seventh cervical vertebra, and the upper part of the seventh cervical vertebra is <1 mm. Advance the needle while securing the center in the anterior and posterior images, and after advancing to some extent through the nuchal ligament and between the spinous processes, approach the spinolaminar line with a 22G spinal needle in the lateral image (Fig. 15.6). The spinolaminar line is a virtual line connecting the points where the spinous process and the lamina meet longitudinally, and it is the posterior boundary of the spinal canal, so care must be taken not to puncture the dura from this area [10]. When the end of the needle is located in the nuchal ligament or ligamentum flavum, a hard resistance is felt, and suddenly the resistance disappears when it enters the epidural space. At this time, a small amount of contrast agent is tested to confirm that

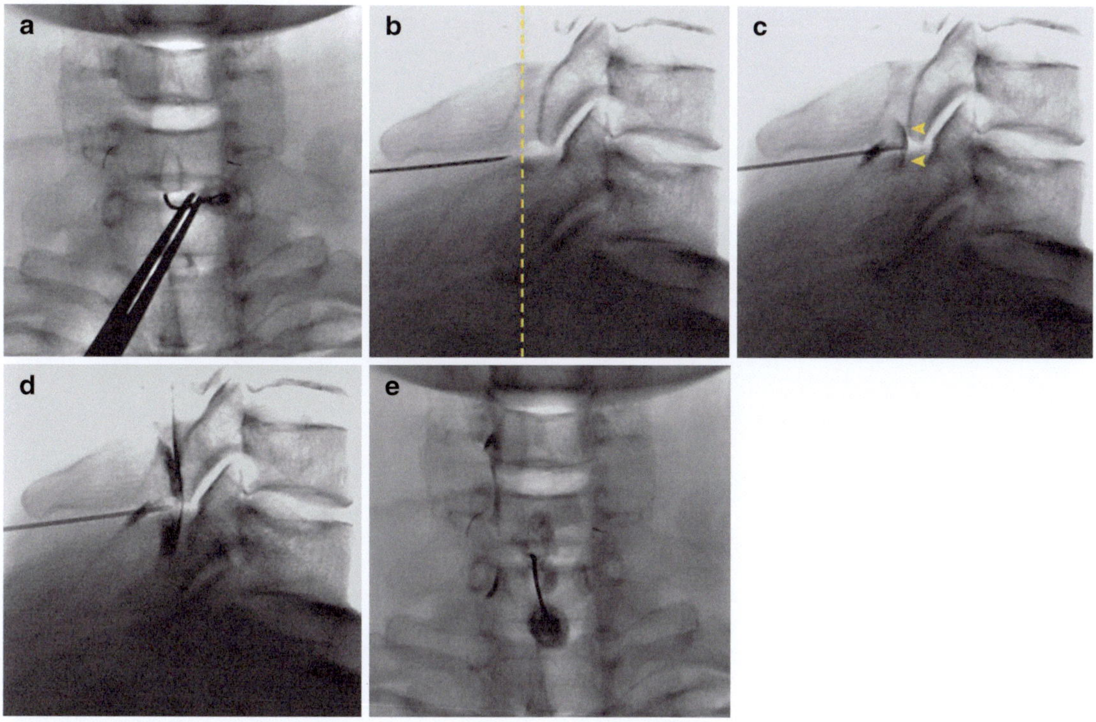

Fig. 15.6 Cervical interlaminar epidural steroid injection. (**a**) In the anteroposterior fluoroscopic image, the spinal needle is being inserted in the center of the interlaminar space. Forceps are used to prevent the operator's hand from being directly exposed to radiation. (**b**) In the lateral fluoroscopic image, the needle is advanced between the spinous processes and the spinal needle is advanced to near the spinolaminar line (dotted line). (**c**) The lateral fluoroscopic image is observed in real time, and the needle is carefully advanced while test injecting the contrast medium. When the contrast medium spreads vertically in a crescent shape (arrowhead), the epidural space can be confirmed. (**d**) The end of the needle is fixed in the epidural space and the drug is injected. It can be confirmed that the contrast medium is spreading vertically in a line in the posterior epidural space. (**e**) In the anteroposterior fluoroscopic image, you can see the contrast medium and drug spreading around the lateral epidural space and nerve root

it is the epidural space. Near the spinolaminar line, remove the stylet from the needle, connect a syringe containing the contrast agent to a preconnected short connector, and advance the needle while test injecting the contrast agent little by little. At some point, the resistance disappears and the contrast agent spreads smoothly up and down along the line (radiographic loss of resistance), and at this time, the drug is injected. The drug is usually diluted with a mixture of steroids and saline to make 2~3 mL. Although local anesthetics are sometimes mixed and injected, there is a risk of epidural anesthesia, and if local anesthetics are injected into the dura, a high level of spinal anesthesia can occur, so local anesthetics are generally not used. If a dural puncture occurs, the contrast agent disappears at a fast speed following the flow of CSF or accumulates in the front part, which is different from the shape of the blood vessels (Fig. 15.7).

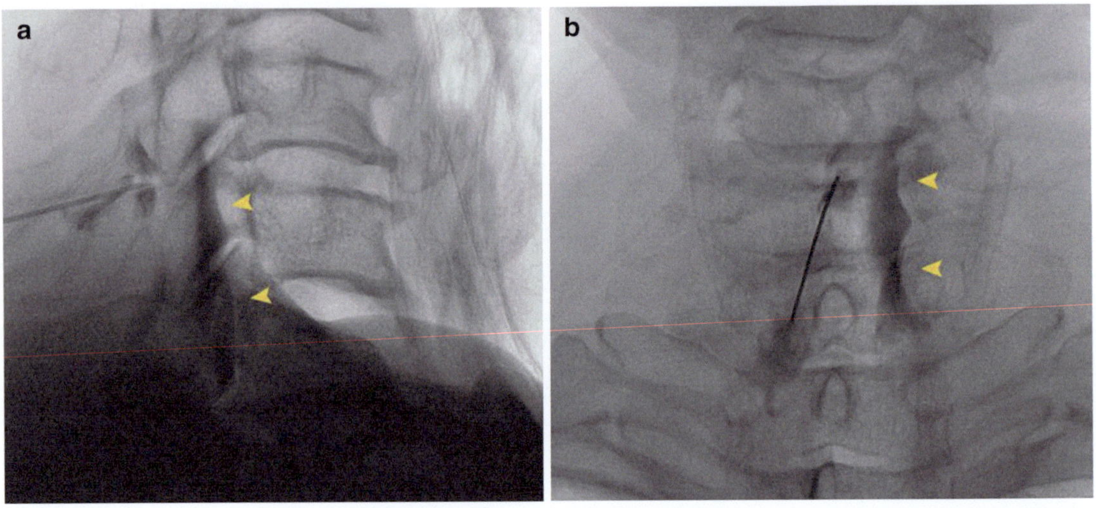

Fig. 15.7 Dural puncture occurred during cervical interlaminar epidural steroid injection. (**a**) After the dural puncture in the cervical spine, the contrast agent can be seen pooled in the front part of the dural sac (arrowhead) when injected. (**b**) When the contrast agent is injected into the dural sac, unlike when injected into the epidural space, it spreads inward (arrowhead) from the dura, showing a clear boundary on the lateral side in the pre- and post-fluoroscopic images. If a dural puncture occurs, the spinal needle should be removed and the injection should be attempted at a different level or a few days later

15.1.4.6 Cervical Transforaminal Epidural Steroid Injection

The effectiveness of cervical interlaminar epidural steroid injection is not significant and can be performed for the treatment of upper extremity radiating pain caused by the compression of a single nerve root or for diagnostic purposes before surgery. Cervical transforaminal epidural steroid injection is performed with the patient lying flat looking at the ceiling, and the X-ray tube is rotated to adjust the angle so that the neural foramen to be accessed is seen as widely as possible (Fig. 15.8). The cortical line of the lamina is made to overlap with the articular process to be clearly visible. Since the vertebral artery runs vertically right in front of the nerve root, the needle is aimed at the front wall of the superior articular process, the back part of the neural foramen, and is never directed towards the front of the neural foramen. Due to the risk of vertebral artery damage, CT-guided injection is sometimes recommended. A thin 25G spinal needle is used to minimize damage to important blood vessels. If the needle is thought to have touched the wall of the superior articular process, the angle of the X-ray tube is adjusted anteriorly and posteriorly to check the depth of the needle. If the tip of the needle enters the inside of the vertebral body, there is a risk of dural puncture, so a contrast agent is test injected from the outside of the vertebral body to confirm that the contrast agent spreads around the nerve root and into the epidural space, and then the steroid is injected. Anatomically, many blood vessels are distributed around the neural foramen (Fig. 15.9), and complications such as spinal cord infarction or cerebral infarction have been reported, so recent papers recommend a liquid form of preparation such as dexamethasone rather than a particle form of preparation such as triamcinolone [11].

15.1.5 Complications

Serious complications are very rare when the procedure is performed with accurate anatomical knowledge and the help of imaging equipment. The most common procedure-related complication is pain at the injection site, and nerve root injury, spinal cord injury (Fig. 15.10), epidural

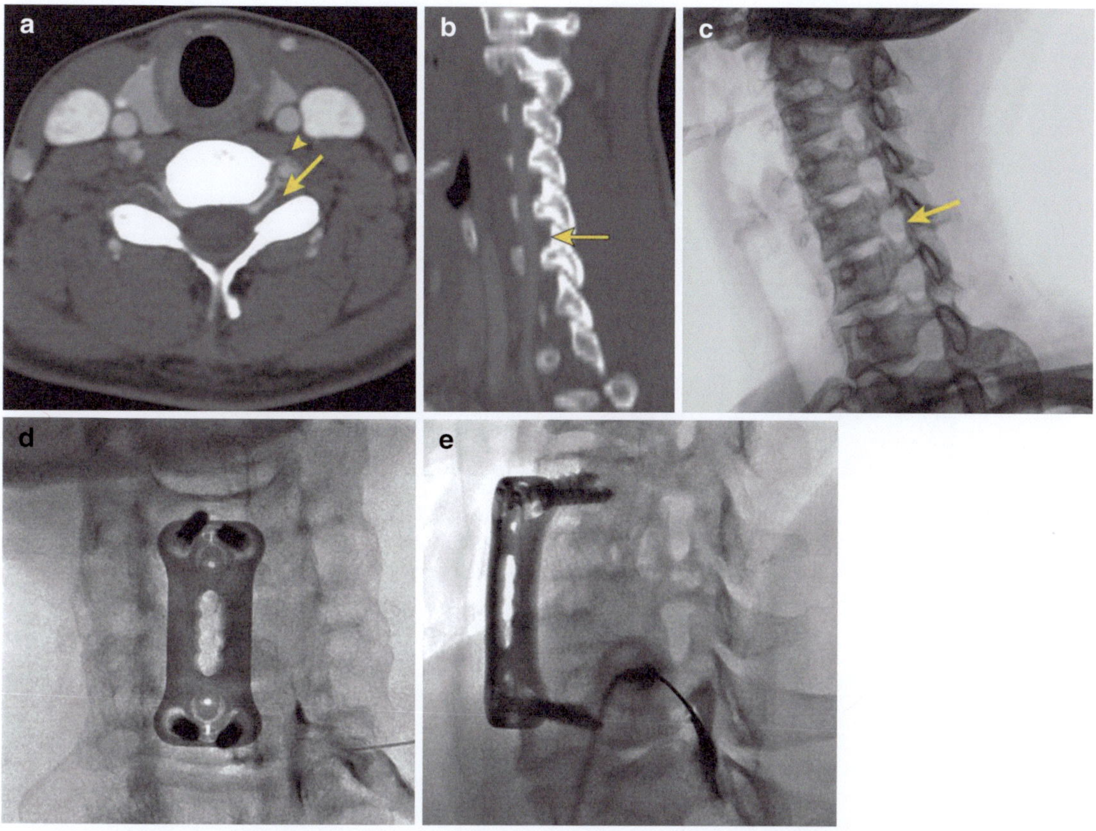

Fig. 15.8 Cervical transforaminal epidural steroid injection. (**a**) In the axial CT image, the vertebral artery (arrowhead) is located in the front part of the neural foramen, so to approach the neural foramen in the cervical spine, one must approach from the back (arrow). (**b**) In the sagittal reconstructed CT image, the vertebral artery is visible in front of the neural foramen. The spinal needle should be advanced targeting just in front of the superior articular process (arrow). (**c**) The X-ray tube is rotated to align the neural foramen to appear at its widest. The needle should be advanced targeting just in front of the superior articular process (arrow). (**d**) This is a pre- and post-fluoroscopic image of another patient, with the contrast agent spreading around the epidural space and the left C7 nerve root. (**e**) In the left oblique view of the fluoroscopy, the spinal needle is located at the back of the neural foramen, and the contrast agent is spreading along the back of the neural foramen

Fig. 15.9 Cervical transforaminal epidural steroid injection. In the cervical spine, there are many developed vessels around the neural foramen, so when injecting a contrast agent as a test, vessels often appear. In this case, the position of the spinal needle should be adjusted so that the vessels are not visible, and the drug should be injected. Since the drug can enter the artery, a liquid form of steroid preparation, not a particle preparation, is recommended

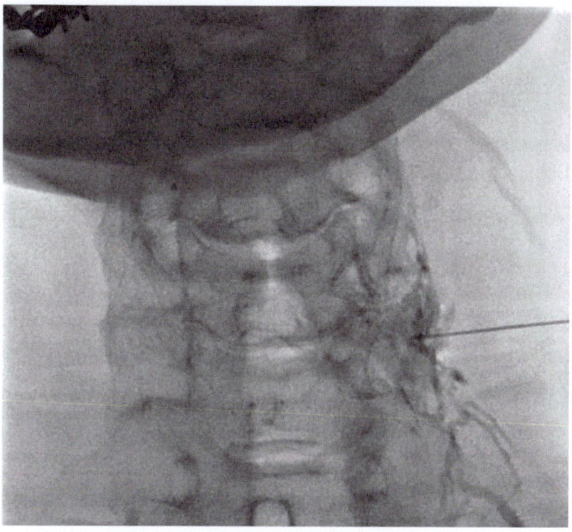

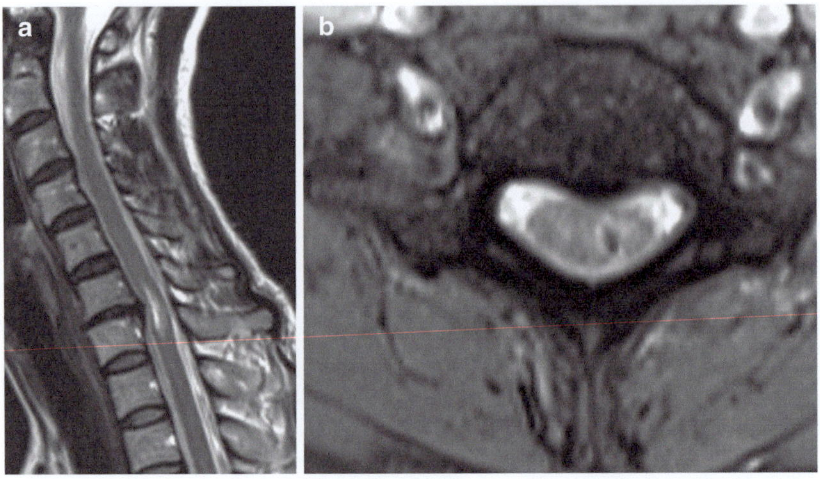

Fig. 15.10 Complications of epidural steroid injection—spinal cord injury. (**a**) This is an MR image of a 48-year-old female patient who suffered a spinal cord injury during a cervical epidural steroid injection a week ago. In the sagittal T2 weighted image, there is edema in the spinal cord at the C6–7 level. (**b**) In the axial gradient echo image, a punctate hemorrhage is visible at the same site

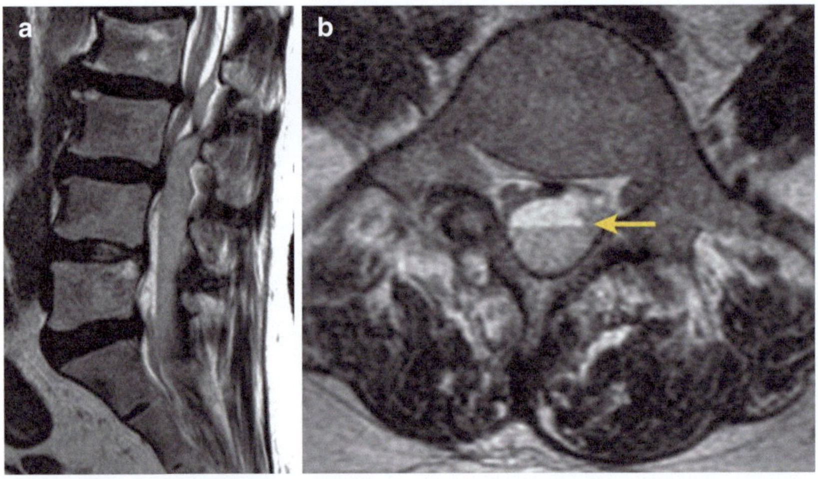

Fig. 15.11 Complications of epidural steroid injection—epidural hematoma. (**a**) This is an MR image of a 65-year-old female patient who complained of weakness in both legs after a lumbar interlaminar epidural steroid injection. In the sagittal T2 weighted image, there is a lesion of moderate signal intensity in the posterior epidural space from the L3 to S1 level. (**b**) This is an axial T2 weighted image at the L5 level, and there is a lesion with a fluid-fluid level (arrow) in the posterior epidural space. The acute epidural hematoma was surgically removed, and this patient had undergone an epidural steroid injection without stopping the use of Coumadin

hematoma (Fig. 15.11), epidural abscess, meningitis, osteomyelitis, headache due to dural puncture, temporary motor disorder, sensory paralysis, bowel disorder, hypotension or dizziness due to vasovagal reaction, and paralysis of the lower body due to Adamkiewicz artery puncture have been reported [3, 12]. Temporary weakness due to motor nerve block can commonly occur, and there have been cases of hypotension, deep vein thrombosis, and seizures. During cervical transforaminal injection, cerebral infarction or seizures can occur if local anesthetics or steroids are injected into the adjacent vertebral artery, and there have been case reports of cerebral infarction due to artery dissection and thrombus formation caused by damage to the vertebral artery itself.

Complications and side effects related to the drugs used include complaints of facial flushing, insomnia, and menstrual irregularities. However, most improve spontaneously without the need for special treatment. Possible allergic reactions can occur due to contrast agents, steroids, and local anesthetics. In diabetic patients, blood sugar levels can temporarily rise due to steroids, so it is advisable to consult with the attending physician about blood sugar checks and adjustments. Complications due to steroids can theoretically include pituitary function decline, Cushing's syndrome, osteoporosis, avascular osteonecrosis, systemic edema, and hypertension.

However, the possibility of such complications due to the therapeutic dose of steroids is very rare.

15.2 Facet Joint Injection/ Sacroiliac Joint Injection

The facet joint is a synovial joint covered with synovium, and pain associated with the facet joint (facet joint pain syndrome) is thought to occur when the sensory nerves that control the facet joint are stimulated by inflammation due to degenerative arthritis, sprains, segmental instability, etc. although the exact mechanism is unknown [13]. There are no specific findings on imaging that suggest facet joint pain syndrome, and it can be diagnosed as facet joint pain syndrome if symptoms disappear after injection. If facet joint pain syndrome is suspected, pain of nerve root origin such as HIVD or spinal stenosis should be ruled out first. It is when there is back pain and pain extends to the buttocks or back of the thigh, when pain is relieved by walking or exercising, when pain is complained of when getting up from a sitting position, when pain worsens during lumbar extension, when there is tenderness in the facet joint area (paramedian tenderness) and radiating pain extends below the knee but there are no neurological symptoms. If cervical facet joint pain syndrome is suspected, it is when there is neck pain slightly off the center of the spine, when there is localized tenderness, when the range of motion of the neck is reduced, when there is referred pain different from the dermatome distribution, and in the case of the upper cervical, it can also appear as a headache.

15.2.1 Lumbar Facet Joint Injection

If lumbar facet joint pain syndrome is suspected, the location of the injection is determined based on the location of the symptoms and the patient's existing images. A physical examination is performed under fluoroscopic guidance to find the joint that causes pain. The patient is made to lie face down on the procedure table, and if a pillow is placed under the patient's pelvis to reduce the lordosis of the waist, it is easier for the needle to access. First, the access angle of the facet joint is determined by checking the cross-sectional images such as CT or MR. In severe cases of bony spur, the needle often does not go in well even if the facet joint space is confirmed on the fluoroscopic image. The appropriate target point is just below the inferior articular process, which is the widest inferior recess in the facet joint [13]. Since the cross-sectional shape of the facet joint is curved inward, the angle of the X-ray tube is rotated to match the angle so that the back of the facet joint opens (Fig. 15.12). If the fluoroscopic angle is rotated a little more, the front of the facet joint opens, and if attempted in this state, access to the joint is not achieved. When the needle advances into the facet joint, it feels like the needle is stuck between some structures. Depending on the patient, when the needle enters the facet joint, the same pain as usual may be induced. The volume of a normal facet joint is only about 1.0~1.5 mL, so only a minimum amount of contrast medium is used. If the contrast medium is used as a test injection and the contrast medium spreads in the vertical direction, the needle is in the joint, and steroids and local anesthetics are injected.

In the lumbar region, a synovial cyst connected to the facet joint inside the spinal canal can cause severe. This can cause radiating pain and is usually associated with severe degenerative

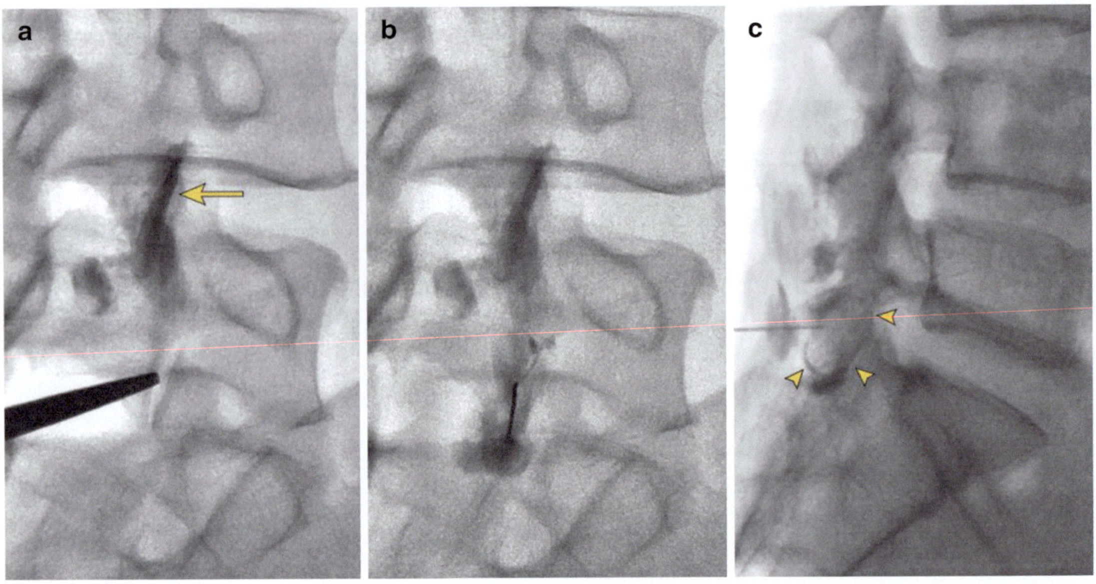

Fig. 15.12 Lumbar facet joint injection. (**a**) In the right oblique view, where the X-ray tube is rotated so that the facet joint space does not overlap and appears the widest, a small forceps was placed targeting the right L5–S1 facet joint. The right L4–5 facet joint already has contrast and medication injected (arrow). (**b**) After inserting a spinal needle into the right L5–S1 facet joint and performing a test injection of contrast, you can see the contrast spreading linearly inside the facet joint. (**c**) In the fluoroscopic lateral image, the contrast is spreading elliptically along the edge of the facet joint (arrowhead)

arthritis of the facet joint. Treatment of the synovial cyst is possible with a facet joint injection. Under CT or fluoroscopic guidance, a spinal needle is placed inside the facet joint, and a contrast agent is used to identify the synovial cyst connected to the facet joint. A mixture of steroids and local anesthetics is injected until the synovial cyst bursts [13]. This can temporarily cause severe pain, and the contrast agent and medication can leak into the epidural space.

15.2.2 Cervical Facet Joint Injection

Cervical facet joint injection can be approached from the back or the side. The lateral approach involves the patient lying face down and directly accessing the joint with a needle while viewing the lateral fluoroscopic image [13]. The posterior approach is similar to a cervical epidural injection, with the patient lying face down with a pillow under the chest. The cervical spine must be flexed for easy posterior access. The cervical facet joint is angled downward, so the injection starts from below the desired site. The needle should aim for the middle of the facet joint or slightly outside in the anteroposterior image for safety. The needle is approached while viewing the lateral fluoroscopic image, and the anteroposterior image is checked in the middle to ensure that the needle is not heading into the spinal canal (Fig. 15.13). Once the needle is determined to have entered the cervical facet joint, a contrast agent is used for a test injection. In the lateral fluoroscopic image, the contrast agent spreads linearly into the facet joint, and in the anteroposterior image, it spreads in a ring shape. In the case of cervical facet joint injection, only steroids are injected without using local anesthetics, like epidural injection. Since the volume of the facet joint is very small, a minimum amount of contrast agent is used, and steroids are injected undiluted. Complications related to facet joint injection are not common. Infections can occur related to the procedure, and complications related to steroid medication can occur.

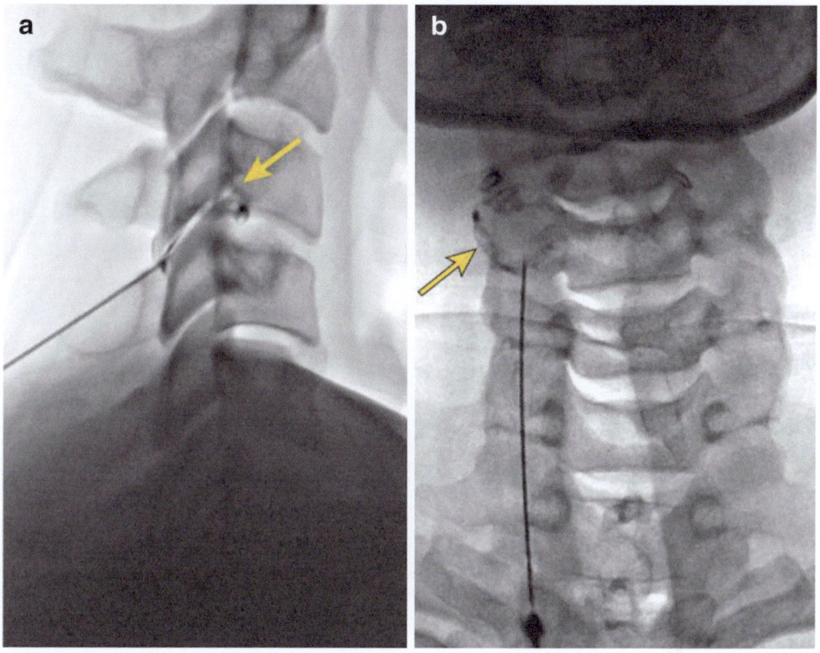

Fig. 15.13 Cervical facet joint injection. (**a**) In the fluoroscopic lateral image, when a test injection of contrast was performed after approaching the spinal needle to the posterior direction of the C3–4 facet joint, the contrast is spreading linearly inside the facet joint (arrow). (**b**) In the fluoroscopic anteroposterior image, the contrast is spreading in a ring shape in the right C3–4 facet joint (arrow)

15.2.3 Sacroiliac Joint Injection

The sacroiliac joint is a plane joint formed by the meeting of the sacrum and ilium, bearing vertical forces, and the normal volume of the sacroiliac joint is about 0.8~1.7 mL. Pain caused by the sacroiliac joint radiates from the medial side of the posterior superior iliac spine (PSIS) to the thigh, groin, and abdomen, and it is often difficult to distinguish from pain caused by the disc or facet joint [14]. Sacroiliac joint pain is thought to be due to stimulation of the synovium or chemical stimulation of the nerves branching into the synovium by the synovial fluid [13]. Indications for sacroiliac joint injection include pain due to arthritis and acute ankylosing spondylitis. The upper part of the sacroiliac joint is covered with synovium only in front, and the back is connected with strong ligaments. Therefore, to access the joint from the back, you need to approach from the bottom. It can be accessed under CT or fluoroscopic guidance in a prone position. If the sacroiliac joint is completely ankylosed, it may not be possible to access the joint. Once the needle enters the joint, a small amount of contrast agent is used for a test injection to confirm. Steroids and local anesthetics are injected (Fig. 15.14). If the needle is directed too far downward, it can touch the sciatic nerve that passes below the sacroiliac joint, and the local anesthetic can leak towards the sciatic nerve, causing temporary sensory loss in the sciatic nerve [13].

15.2.4 Spondylolysis Injection

In patients with spondylolysis, steroid injection at the site of the pars interarticularis defect is reported to be effective in controlling the pain of backache and radiculopathy and can reduce the frequency of surgical treatment [15]. In some cases, it is performed for diagnostic purposes to identify the cause of pain before performing fusion surgery, and there are reports that the therapeutic effect is good after fusion surgery if there is temporary pain relief after steroid injection at the site of spondylolysis. Spondylolysis injection is aimed at the pars interarticularis defect under fluoroscopic guidance (Fig. 15.15), and if this site is targeted, contrast medium can be seen filling the adjacent upper and lower facet joints through the pars interarticularis defect. In the case of L5 spondylolysis, the pars interarticularis defect is located directly below the inferior recess

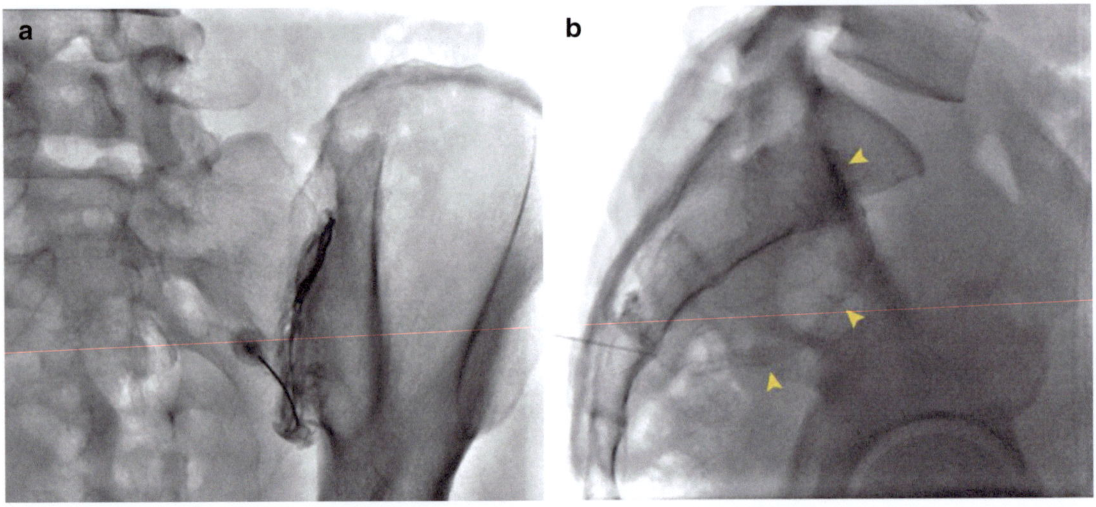

Fig. 15.14 Sacroiliac joint injection. (**a**) After inserting a spinal needle into the lower part of the right sacroiliac joint and performing a test injection of contrast, the contrast spreads linearly inside the joint in the fluoroscopic image. (**b**) In the fluoroscopic lateral image, the spinal needle is inserted in the posterior direction of the sacroiliac joint, and you can see the contrast spreading in a large ellipse (arrowhead)

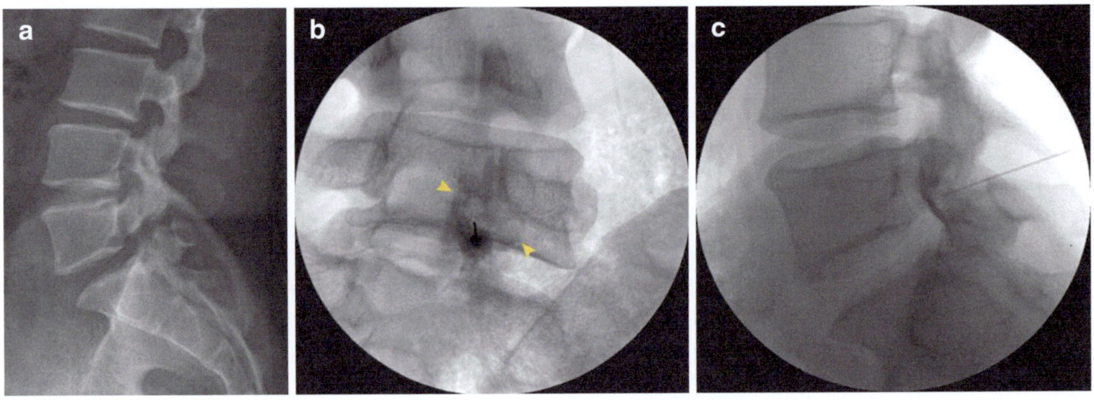

Fig. 15.15 Spondylolysis injection. (**a**) In the plain radiography lateral image, there is spondylolysis at L5. (**b**) In the right oblique view, after positioning the spinal needle at the site of spondylolysis (pars interarticularis defect), contrast is being injected. The contrast is spreading irregularly within a limited space (arrowhead). (**c**) In the fluoroscopic lateral image, you can see the contrast spreading at the site of spondylolysis

of the L4/5 facet joint, so the direction of needle advancement is usually similar to that of L4/5 facet joint injection.

15.3 Vertebroplasty

Vertebroplasty is a procedure in which an artificial cement called poly-methylmethacrylate (PMMA) is injected into the vertebral body where a compression fracture has occurred under imaging guidance, first reported in 1987 for a cervical hemangioma [16]. It is now performed worldwide as one of the important treatments for painful osteoporotic or malignant compression fractures. The therapeutic goal of vertebroplasty is to control pain and prevent the progression of existing compression fractures, i.e., additional collapse of the vertebral body. The mechanism of pain relief in vertebroplasty is not well known, but the most common hypothesis is that pain is relieved through mechanical stabilization, and there are hypotheses such as nerve terminal necrosis due to the heat generated when the cement hardens. Vertebroplasty is effective in treating back pain caused by vertebral compression fractures and is a relatively simple, safe, and economical procedure. Although vertebroplasty is a very useful treatment for rapid pain control, symptoms disappear in 66% of patients with compression fractures who have only received conservative treatment after several months, and after 6 weeks, the degree of pain relief is similar between vertebroplasty and conservative treatment [17]. There are also several complications associated with vertebroplasty, so it is thought that a more conservative approach should be taken.

15.3.1 Indications and Contraindications

The indications and contraindications are intended to introduce those presented in the "CIRSE (Cardiovascular and Interventional Radiological Society of Europe) guidelines, 2006" [18].

1. Indications
   (a) Osteoporotic vertebral compression fracture causing pain that does not respond to internal treatment.
   (b) Spinal pain caused by invasive primary bone tumors such as hemangioma or giant cell tumor.
   (c) Spinal pain associated with extensive osteolysis due to malignant invasion of multiple myeloma, lymphoma, metastasis.
   (d) Spinal pain associated with Kummell's disease.
   (e) Purpose of strengthening the vertebral body and pedicle before performing spinal posterior fixation surgery.
   (f) Chronic traumatic fracture related to nonunion of fractures or internal cystic changes.
2. Absolute contraindications
   (a) Asymptomatic vertebral compression fracture.
   (b) Cases showing improvement with internal medicine treatment.
   (c) Osteomyelitis, discitis, or active systemic infection.
   (d) Uncontrolled blood coagulation disorders.
   (e) Allergy to bone cement, etc.
   (f) Preventive treatment purpose for osteoporosis patients.
3. Relative contraindications
   (a) In case of radiating pain.
   (b) When a tumor invades into the spinal canal or there is spinal cord compression.
   (c) When there is a fracture in the posterior wall of the vertebral body: risk of cement leakage.
   (d) When the compression rate of the vertebral body is higher than 70%: difficulty in positioning the needle in the vertebral body.
   (e) In case of central canal stenosis: fractured fragments can move into the spinal canal and cause symptoms.
   (f) In case of more than five or diffuse bone metastases.
   (g) When surgery is not supported in case of emergency or when the devices to monitor the patient's condition are not equipped.

15.3.2 Considerations Before the Procedure

It is important to directly interview the patient and review the patient's clinical records and images in advance. In plain radiography, the level of compression fracture, the degree of compression of the vertebral body, the presence or absence of osteolytic lesions, the degree of pedicle invasion, fracture lines or cortex destruction are evaluated (Fig. 15.16). CT images are useful for evaluating the destruction of the posterior cortex of the vertebral body, the extent of bone tumor invasion, the posterior movement of bony fragments to the epidural space or neural foramen, etc. It is also performed to evaluate the shape of the vertebral body,

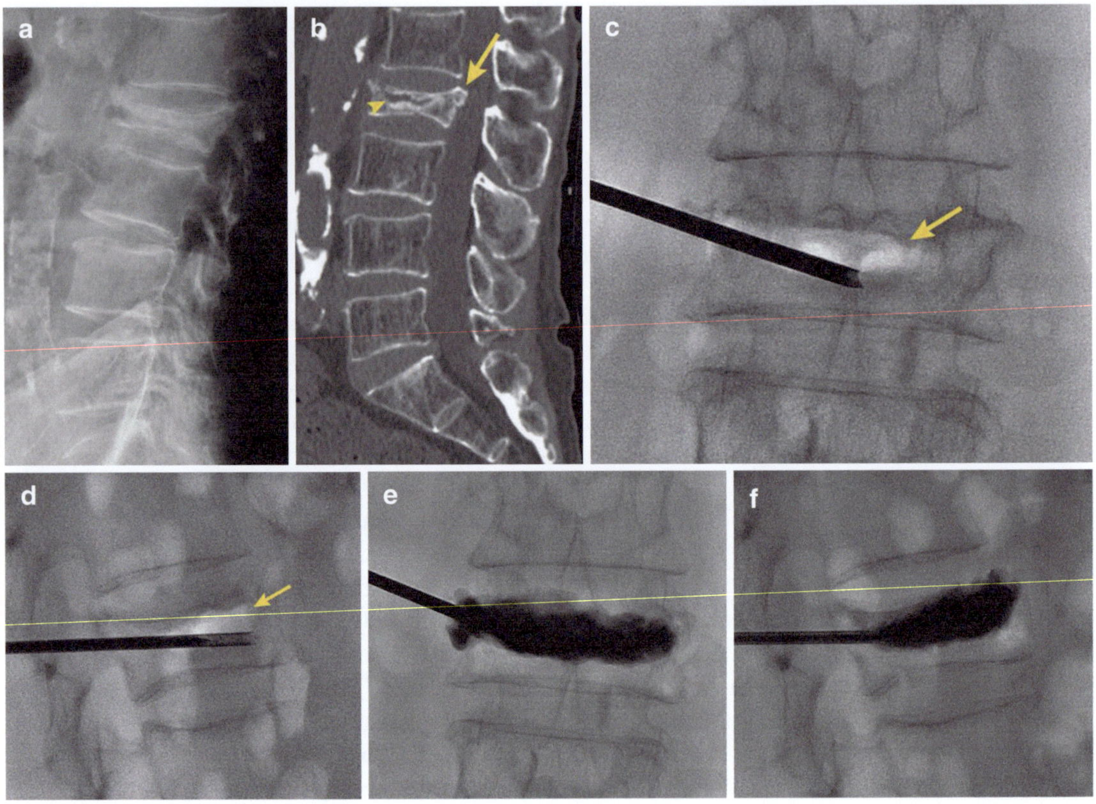

Fig. 15.16 Vertebroplasty for benign vertebral compression fracture with Kummell's disease. (**a**) In the plain radiography lateral image, there is a wedge deformity in the L2 vertebral body, and there is a linear osteosclerotic lesion inside. (**b**) In the sagittal reconstructed CT image, a cavity (arrowhead) is formed inside the L2 vertebral body with a wedge deformity, suggesting Kummell's disease. A small bone fragment moving into the spinal canal from the posterior of the vertebral body (arrow) is visible. (**c**, **d**) In the fluoroscopic image, the vertebroplasty needle is inserted and air is entering the vertebral body through the needle, clearly showing a vacuum shadow (arrow) inside the vertebral body. (**e**, **f**) The cement is densely filled in the area corresponding to the vacuum shadow, and there is no visible cement leakage outside the vertebral body. Compared to plain radiography, the height of the vertebral body has somewhat recovered

the width and shape of the pedicle, the invasion of posterior structures, and to plan the path of the vertebroplasty needle. Bone scans or MR images are useful for distinguishing acute fractures from healed fractures and are essential for selecting treatment targets in cases with multiple compression fractures [18]. In MR images, bone marrow edema in the fractured vertebral body and contrast enhancement suggest a pain-causing compression fracture (Fig. 15.17). MR images are also very useful for confirming the extent of bone tumor invasion. In a bone scan, the vertebral body with an acute compression fracture shows strong increased uptake.

15.3.3 Procedure Method

The methods for inserting the vertebroplasty needle into the vertebral body include the transpedicular, intercostovertebral, and anterolateral approaches. The most commonly performed transpedicular approach is used for the thoracolumbar vertebra. The patient lies face down on the procedure table. Most patients are elderly, so it is necessary to monitor vital signs such as blood pressure, pulse oximeter, and sometimes EKG during the procedure. If the patient's posture is not correct, do not force the patient's posture, but turn the X-ray tube to match the true anterior and lateral images of the target spine. After aligning the fluoroscopic anterior image so that the spinous process of the spine is in the center, determine the entry site where the needle will enter while turning the X-ray tube and looking at the lateral image together (Fig. 15.17). Infections after vertebroplasty can be difficult to treat and can leave serious sequelae, so the operator should wear sterile surgical gowns, hats, and masks, and use long tools such as sponge forceps to prevent the operator from being contaminated and disinfect the patient's skin with betadine. Initially in vertebroplasty, the needle was inserted through both pedicles and cement was injected (bipedicular approach), but nowadays, the needle is approached through one pedicle, the end of the needle is placed in the center of the vertebral body, and cement is injected (unipedicular approach). If the height of the vertebral body is very low due to severe spinal compression, or if there is endplate disruption due to fracture in the center, it is advantageous to insert the needle through both pedicles and inject cement rather than approaching from one side (Fig. 15.18). In such cases, if you approach from one pedicle, place the needle in the center of the vertebral body, and inject cement, there is a high risk of cement leakage into the disc space. If the cement is not sufficiently filled, you need to approach from the opposite side, so you need to disinfect the skin widely to the opposite side, and cover the disinfection cloth widely as in angiography. A sterilized vinyl is also put on the X-ray tube.

After anesthetizing the skin with lidocaine using a 25G needle, anesthetize up to the periosteum behind the pedicle using a spinal needle, and inject lidocaine into the soft tissue while removing the needle to prevent pain when approaching with a vertebroplasty needle. After making a small incision of about 0.5 cm at the entry site of the skin with a surgical knife, advance the vertebroplasty needle while looking at the fluoroscopic image, trying not to expose the operator's hand directly to radiation. The starting point is determined at the outermost part of the pedicle, and the end of the needle is positioned at the anterior 1/3~1/4, upper or lower 1/3 of the vertebral body in the lateral fluoroscopic image, and advances so that it passes through the center in the fluoroscopic anterior and posterior images. If the angle is wrong from the starting point where it first entered the bone, it cannot be corrected in the middle, so you should be careful about the progress angle from the beginning. What's important here is that in the fluoroscopic anterior and posterior images, when the needle is located inside the pedicle, it should approach inside the body after passing the posterior wall of the vertebral body in the lateral image. If the needle invades the medial wall of the pedicle before the needle passes the posterior wall of the vertebral body, the needle is located inside the spinal canal. If the needle damages the inner wall of the pedicle when passing the pedicle, it should be careful as it can cause dural injury, nerve compression due to cement leakage in the spinal canal, and spinal cord injury. In case of a vacuum cleft in the vertebral body, the bone cement should be filled into the vacuum cleft. The needle should be positioned at the end, and in this case, a significant height recovery can be expected (Fig. 15.16).

Afterward, using a ceramic or stainless container, adjust the PMMA powder (substrate):solvent (monomer) to 2:1 and mix in an appropriate amount of antibiotics to make a bone cement mixture with a pressurizer. If you are using a commercial vertebroplasty-specific cement, you can mix all the contents in the package and use it, and you need to add preventive antibiotics separately. If you are using cephalosporin antibiotics, you should have a skin sensitivity test before the procedure.

At the initial injection, do not inject all at once, but inject a drop as a test to check if it has not been injected into the blood vessel, then inject slowly. The injection speed should be adjusted considering the hardening speed of the cement, but if it is injected too quickly, it may be difficult to notice that the cement is leaking. Common areas of bone cement leakage are the basivertebral vein or azygos vein, and leakage often occurs through the gap in the posterior wall of the vertebral body. Cement leakage that should not be missed mainly occurs in front and behind the vertebral body, so when using a single X-ray tube, align it with the lateral image and perform cement injection, and occasionally turn it back and forth to check if both sides are evenly filled. If the bone cement fills up to the

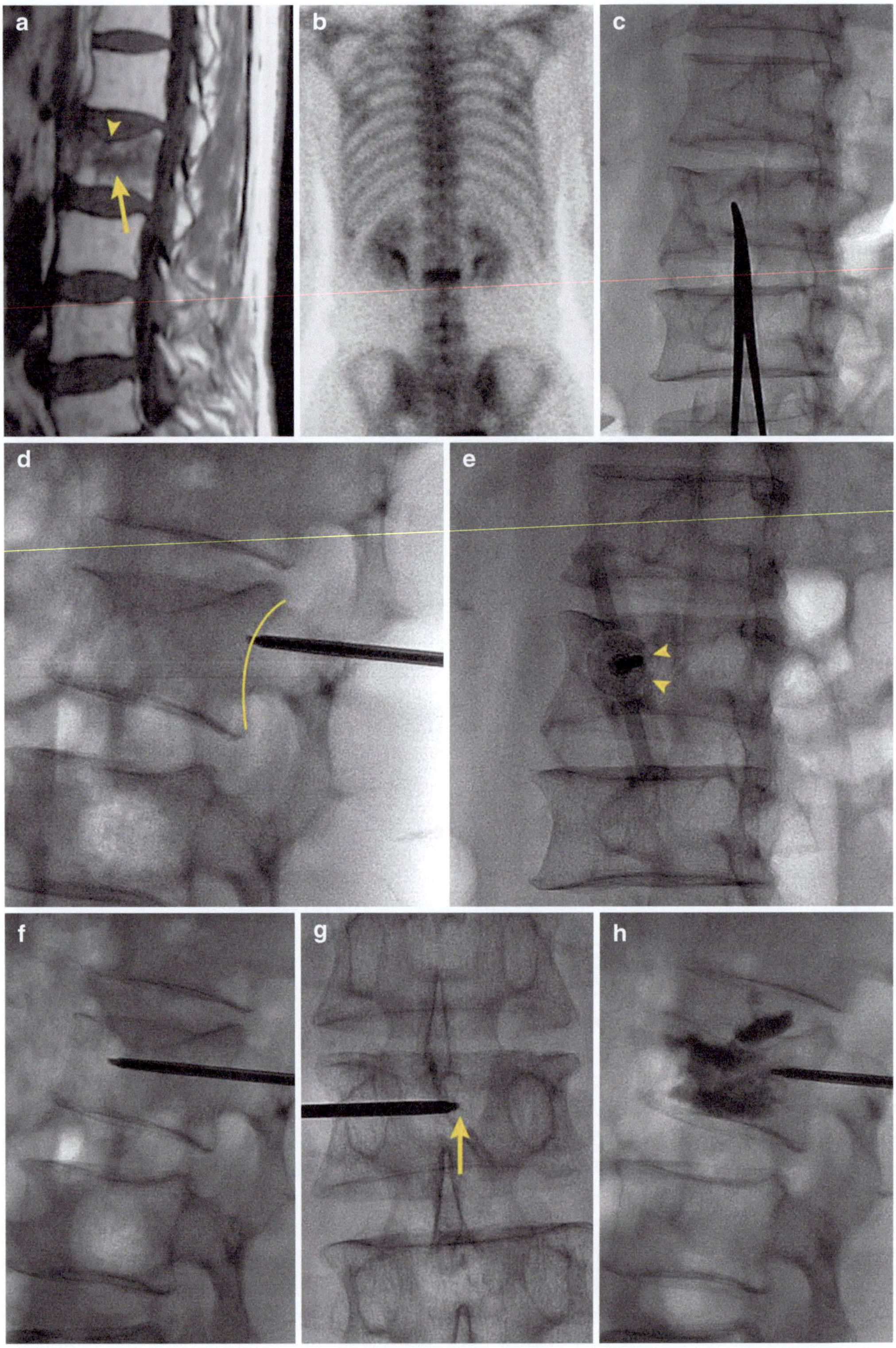
a
b
c
d
e
f
g
h

Fig. 15.17 Vertebroplasty for benign vertebral compression fracture. (**a**) In the sagittal T1-enhanced MR image, a fracture line (arrow) and surrounding bone marrow edema are visible within the L2 vertebral body. There is a defect (cortical defect, arrowhead) in the cortex of the upper vertebral endplate, and the vertebral body shows anterior wedging. (**b**) In the bone scan, there is a strong uptake increase in the L2 vertebral body, suggesting a painful compression fracture. (**c**) A clamp was placed on the left pedicle of L2 to mark the entry site for the needle in the left oblique view of L2. (**d, e**) In the lateral image, the vertebroplasty needle is inserted up to the pedicle, and the needle should not invade the inner boundary of the pedicle (arrowhead) in the oblique view until the end of the needle reaches the posterior of the vertebral body (solid line). (**f, g**) In the fluoroscopic lateral image, the needle is advanced to the anterior 1/4 point of the vertebral body, and in the anterior and posterior images, the end of the needle is slightly past the center point (arrow). (**h**) After filling up to the posterior 1/4 of the vertebral body with cement, the needle is slightly pulled back and waited until the cement hardens. Some of the cement leaked through the cortical defect of the vertebral endplate into the L2–3 disc space, but the patient's pain significantly improved and there were no other problems

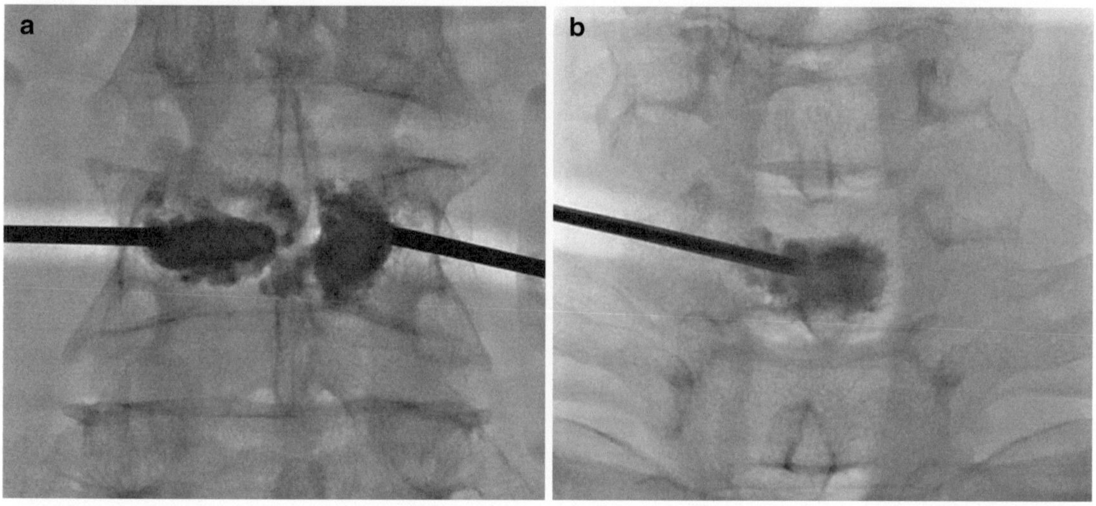

Fig. 15.18 Vertebroplasty for malignant compression fracture due to metastasis of renal cell carcinoma. (**a**) A 78-year-old male patient with a compression fracture in the L4 vertebral body on a sagittal T1-enhanced MR image. (**b**) After inserting the vertebroplasty needle through both pedicles, cement was injected. The cement was separately injected on both sides of the vertebral body

posterior 1/4 point of the vertebral body or leakage is observed, the injection should be stopped. If the injection is stopped early due to leakage, you can try injecting again after a while. After pulling the needle out to the back of the vertebral body and observing the remaining bone cement, remove the needle when it hardens and press the skin incision site to stop bleeding. If the cement is not completely hardened when removing the needle, the cement may leak along the route where the needle was inserted, so it should be removed after confirming that it is completely hardened.

If the pedicle is thin, or the direction of the pedicle does not point to the center of the vertebral body, making the transpedicular approach difficult, the intercostovertebral approach is used in the upper thoracic spine.

The cervical spine has the vertebral artery located next to the pedicle and the pedicle is small, making the transpedicular approach difficult, and the anterolateral approach is mainly used (Fig. 15.19). The patient is in the supine position, and the operator pushes the patient's carotid artery and jugular vein outward with one hand and pushes the trachea inward to palpate the vertebral body, then anesthetizes the skin and periosteum with the other hand. After making a skin incision, the vertebroplasty needle can be inserted directly into the vertebral body. Cement injection can be performed in a similar way to the lumbar spine while looking at the fluoroscopic image.

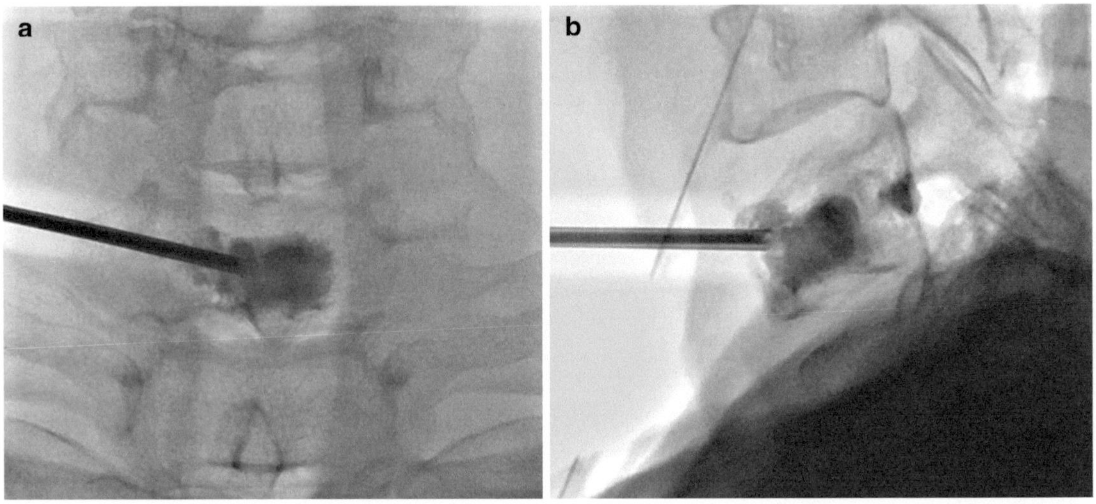

Fig. 15.19 Vertebroplasty for cervical malignant compression fracture due to metastasis of thyroid cancer. (**a**) The vertebroplasty needle is inserted from the anterolateral side of the C7 vertebral body and cement is injected. (**b**) In the fluoroscopic lateral image, the needle is inserted from the front of the vertebral body. There is no visible cement leakage outside the vertebral body

15.3.4 Complications

The incidence of complications after vertebroplasty is relatively higher in cases of malignant compression fracture than osteoporotic compression fracture. This is because if the tumor invades the cortical bone and pedicle, the cement is at high risk of leaking outside the vertebral body, and the tumor tissue can be pushed outwards by the cement injection, which can cause nerve compression. The most common complications are localized pain at the procedure site. During the procedure, cement leakage can occur in the epidural, vascular, and disc space. Cement leakage occurs frequently, found in about 30~72.5% of plain radiography and about 87.9~93% in CT, but actual symptoms occur in <1% of cases [19]. However, if a large amount of cement leakage occurs into the epidural space, it can cause persistent pain due to spinal or nerve root compression (Fig. 15.20). A small amount of vascular leakage does not cause a particular problem, but a large amount of leakage can cause a pulmonary embolism. To prevent a large amount of cement leakage, it is good to use high-resolution fluoroscopy equipment, use cement that is clearly visible in fluoroscopic images, and stop immediately when leakage is first detected. It is known that the incidence of new compression fractures in adjacent vertebral bodies is higher than in other areas due to the increased strength of the treated vertebral body and the effect of cement leaked into the disc in cases of vertebroplasty for osteoporotic compression fractures [20]. In rare cases, infection can occur at the procedure site (Fig. 15.21). Sometimes, performing vertebroplasty on a compression fracture accompanied by infectious spondylitis can worsen the spondylitis. It is important to carefully examine preoperative images and check the patient's blood test values. Other reported complications related to the procedure include fat embolism, pneumothorax, and rib fracture.

15.3.5 Kyphoplasty

Kyphoplasty is performed to correct kyphosis by restoring the height of the vertebral body compressed by a vertebral compression fracture, along with pain relief. The patient selection criteria are generally the same as for vertebroplasty, but it can be performed when the anterior compression deformation rate due to fracture is

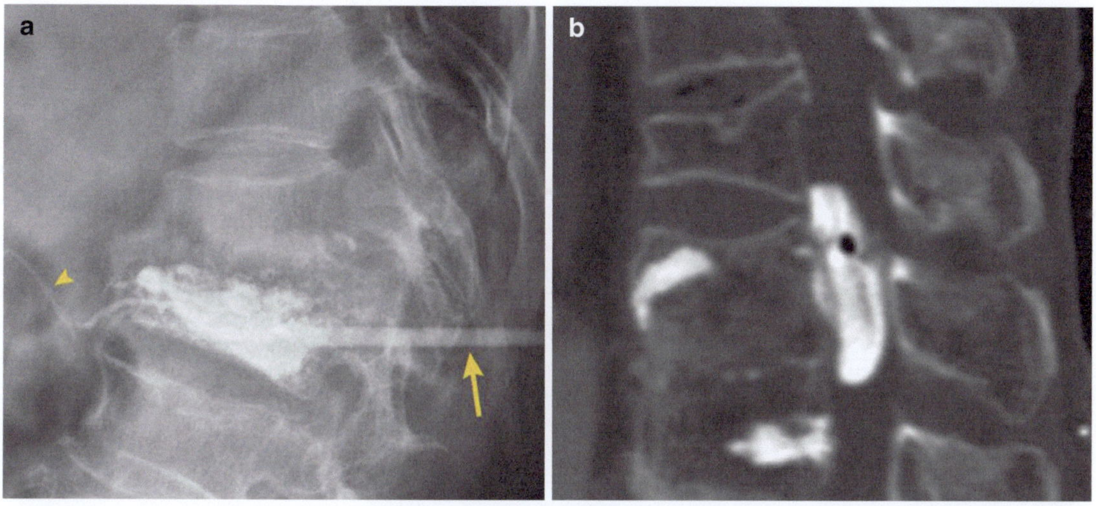

Fig. 15.20 Various cement leakages. (**a**) In the plain radiography performed after vertebroplasty, cement is leaking along the path where the vertebroplasty needle entered the anterior vessels (arrowhead) and the posterior of the vertebral body (arrow). Clinically, it did not cause symptoms. (**b**) This is a sagittal reconstructed CT image of a patient who developed lower limb paralysis after vertebroplasty, showing cement inside the dural sac. It is thought that the vertebroplasty needle passed into the spinal canal, and it was removed surgically

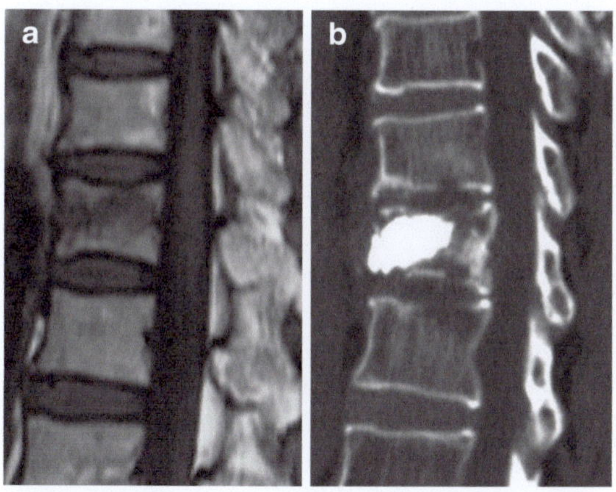

Fig. 15.21 Infectious spondylitis that occurred after vertebroplasty. (**a**) In the sagittal T1-enhanced MR image, a fracture line is visible within the T12 vertebral body along with bone marrow edema. No other accompanying findings are visible around the vertebral body. (**b**) A CT scan was performed due to persistent pain after vertebroplasty, and osteolytic lesions are visible around the injected cement and adjacent vertebral body in the sagittal reconstructed image. It was diagnosed as infectious spondylitis, and all the cement was removed by surgery and fusion surgery was performed

30~60%. Kyphoplasty involves inserting an 8G cannula into the vertebral body, creating a path for the balloon needle, and then inserting the balloon needle. After that, contrast medium is injected into the balloon to expand it (Fig. 15.22). The expanded balloon lifts the vertebral endplate to restore the height of the vertebral body, and when a cavity for the cement is formed, the balloon needle is removed and cement is injected into the newly formed cavity through the cannula. The advantage of kyphoplasty is that it restores the height of the vertebral body and injects cement into the newly formed cavity, reducing the possibility of cement leakage [21]. However, the procedure is expensive, the patient's pain during the procedure is more severe than with vertebroplasty, and due to the long procedure time, general anesthesia is sometimes required and there is a lot of fluoroscopic radiation exposure [21]. In reality, there is no difference in the long-term effects of vertebroplasty and kyphoplasty, and it is reported that the

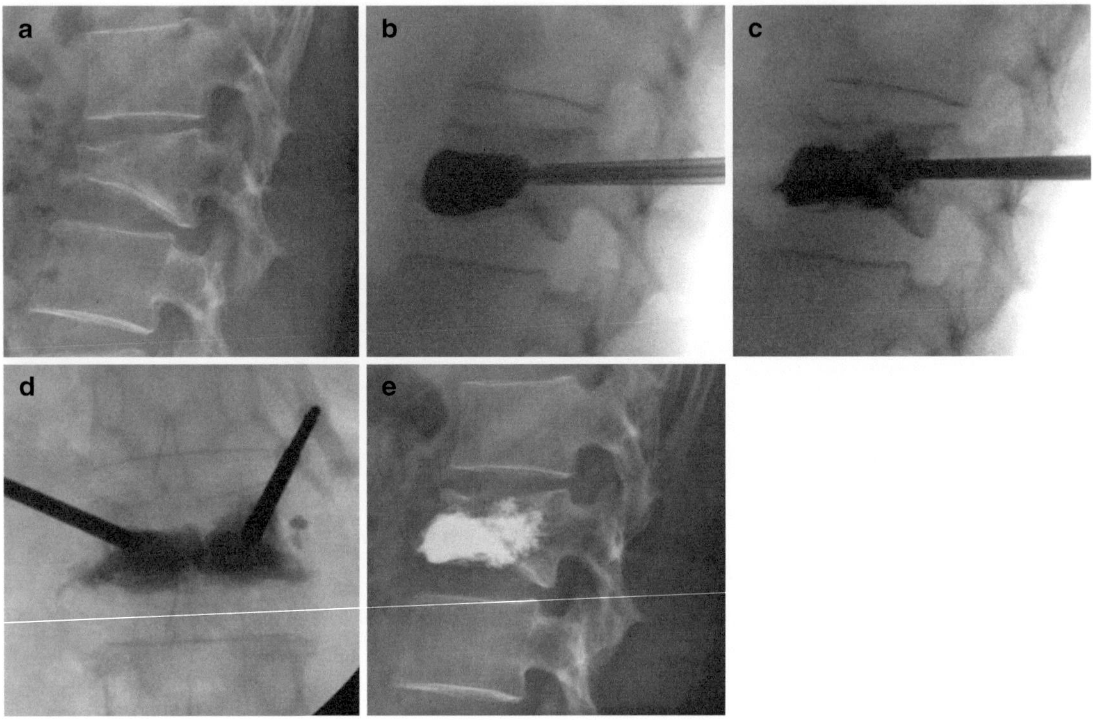

Fig. 15.22 Kyphoplasty. (**a**) Lateral plain radiography shows a wedge deformity caused by a compression fracture of the L2 vertebral body. (**b**) A needle is inserted into the fractured vertebral body, contrast medium is injected, the balloon is expanded to restore the height of the vertebral body, and a cavity is being created. (**c**, **d**) The needle was removed and cement was injected through the insertion tube. (**e**) Postoperative lateral plain radiography shows densely injected cement, almost no leakage of cement outside the vertebral body, and the height of the vertebral body has been restored

short-term effects of vertebroplasty and the medium-term effects of kyphoplasty are somewhat better.

15.3.6 Sacroplasty

Insufficiency fractures of the sacrum often occur in elderly patients or patients who have received radiation therapy and can sometimes cause disability due to severe pain. Recently, sacroplasty has been recognized as a useful and effective treatment for such fractures. It is being introduced. However, the sacrum is not anatomically simple, and there may be difficulties in simply confirming the sacral foramen by fluoroscopy. Before the procedure, using a three-dimensional reconstruction program, etc. to understand the anatomical structure of the sacrum, make sufficient plans, and if you use equipment that can do both fluoroscopy and CT, you can access it relatively easily (Fig. 15.23) [22].

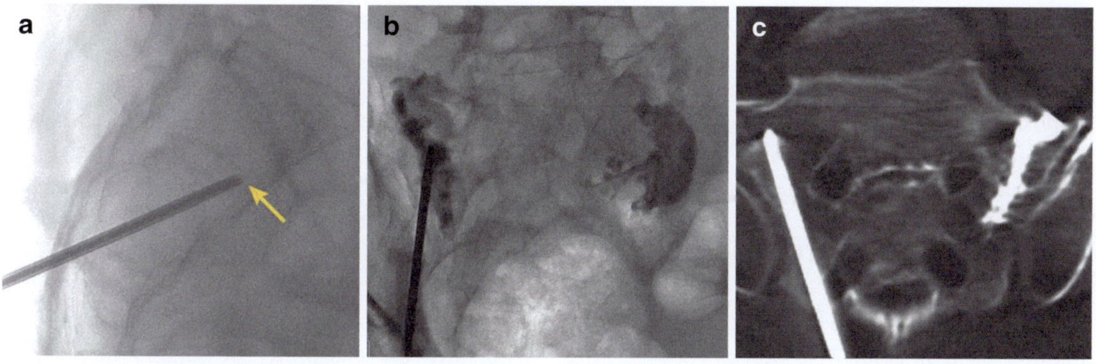

Fig. 15.23 Sacroplasty. (**a**) After laying a patient with an insufficiency fracture of the sacrum causing severe pain on the operating table, the vertebroplasty needle (arrow) is advanced while looking at the fluoroscopic image. (**b**) The X-ray tube is aligned in the right oblique view direction parallel to the left sacroiliac joint, and the vertebroplasty needle is inserted into the left sacral ala area and cement is being injected. The cement is being injected spreading in the vertical direction. Cement has already been injected into the right sacral ala area. (**c**) During sacroplasty, a CT scan was performed using fluoroscopic equipment to check the position of the needle. In the reconstructed CT image, the vertebroplasty needle is accurately located in the sacral ala area where the fracture is, and the path of the needle did not damage the sacral foramen. There is no sign of leakage of the cement injected on the other side

15.4 Discography

Discography was first attempted in 1948 for the purpose of diagnosing HIVD patients [23]. Before the introduction of MRI, discography was the only way to evaluate abnormal findings inside the disc that other imaging tests could not show. Now, simple, safe, and accurate test methods such as CT or MRI have been developed, so it is no longer used for the purpose of diagnosing HIVD or testing for abnormalities in the nerve root caused by it. However, it is mainly used for the purpose of diagnosing discogenic pain due to internal disc disruption (IDD), i.e., degeneration of the disc [24]. Discography, unlike other imaging diagnostic methods, can directly diagnose pathological causes and symptoms that the patient actually feels through not only the shape of the disc but also the presence or absence of pain induced during the test. However, there is still controversy over the diagnostic significance of discography and its usefulness for treatment, and there are objections to the term discogenic pain.

There is not much known about the imaging findings of internal disc disruption. Many studies report the high intensity zone (HIZ) of the degenerated disc in MRI T2 enhanced images as a pain indicator in patients with back pain [25]. It is known that the presence of HIZ in MRI has a significant correlation with pain induction and radial tear in discography.

Discography, which injects a contrast agent into the disc to induce pain for diagnosis, is also called provocative discography [26]. The pain-inducing mechanism of discography is not exactly known. The dominant hypothesis is that during discography, irritating substances such as neuropeptides or cytokines come out of the disc and stimulate the nerves in the outer annulus fibrosus to induce pain, and it is understood that pain occurs by the contrast agent contacting sensitized tissues and applying chemical stimulation or applying expansion pressure from the disc [27]. However, the debate over the diagnostic value of discography continues because the understanding of the onset mechanism of pain is still insufficient.

15.4.1 Discogenic Pain

The disc is composed of the nucleus pulposus, annulus fibrosus, and vertebral endplate. The disc is connected to the upper and lower vertebral bodies through the vertebral endplate in the center and the annulus fibrosus at the edge, functioning similar to a joint. The normal nucleus pulposus has no blood vessels, so it receives nutrient supply through diffusion from surrounding tissues such as the annulus fibrosus and vertebral endplate.

Until the 1940s and 1950s, it was thought that the disc, which is out of nerve control, could not cause pain. However, in reality, the annulus of a normal disc sensory nerves are connected up to the outer 1/3 of the fibrosus, and when degenerative changes occur, they progress further inward, with some nerves known to extend to the nucleus pulposus. Therefore, recently, the disc itself is being accepted as a factor in back pain.

In normal individuals, the disc develops abnormalities in weight load regulation as age increases. As early as the late teens, blood flow to the vertebral endplate can decrease, potentially causing nutritional supply issues. In such a state, if a force beyond the range that the disc can regulate is suddenly applied from the outside, or if low levels of stress are repeatedly and long-term applied, it can cause mechanical injury to the disc. Mechanical damage appears as annular tear (fissure) and cracks in the vertebral endplate, i.e., microfractures [28]. Compared to a normal disc evenly absorbing weight load, a damaged disc has more weight load applied to the damaged area, causing a vicious cycle of further rupture. Also, the nucleus pulposus is pushed out through the ruptured annulus fibrosus, resulting in findings of degenerative disc disease such as Modic change, endplate sclerosis, and bridging osteophyte [27]. If a microfracture occurs at the vertebral endplate site, inflammatory cytokines infiltrate the nucleus pulposus, leading to further disc degeneration. If the annulus fibrosus is ruptured, pain mediators can directly act on pain receptors, causing back pain. If sensory nerves grow to the nucleus pulposus due to degeneration, or if the nerve endings of the vertebral endplate are sensitized, the pain can be more severe [27].

15.4.2 Indications and Contraindications

Discography is used to distinguish between asymptomatic discs and symptomatic discs. Discography evaluates two elements: 1) Whether pain occurs when a contrast agent is injected into the disc and 2) the internal shape of the disc. Discography is an invasive test compared to other imaging tests, so it should be performed on patients who have the possibility of surgery after other imaging tests like MRI. In other words, it should be performed when the treatment direction is determined based on the results of discography.

The indications for discography are as follows [24, 28]:

1. When there is spinal pain that does not respond to conservative treatment for more than 4 months or when discogenic pain is suspected.
2. When there is severe spinal pain, but only disc degeneration, annular tears/fissures (high intensity zones), endplate changes (Modic changes), minor disc protrusions with questionable nerve root compromise are present on MRI.
3. When persistent pain after surgery is suspected to be due to disc degeneration or instability of adjacent level after spinal fusion surgery.
4. Before spinal fusion surgery, to determine which disc is the main area requiring surgery.

The purpose of discography is to obtain information about the type of pain induced. It is difficult to be sure that a specific disc is the cause of the patient's pain just by observing the shape of the disc. However, if morphological abnormalities are observed in disc where symptoms are caused in discography, the diagnosis of the cause of pain becomes clearer.

Congenital abnormalities in the spine and nerve root, hypersensitivity to contrast agents, local anesthetics, antibiotics, poor hemostasis, or use of anticoagulants are relative contraindications for the procedure. Inflammation at the procedure site, pregnancy, and difficulty for the patient to undergo the procedure are contraindications for discography.

15.4.3 Considerations Before the Procedure

Discography can be performed on an outpatient basis without the need for hospitalization. Prior to the procedure, the practitioners need to take a thorough medical history of the patients. They check the patient's overall medical condition, detailed medical history, and allergies. In particular, they need to confirm whether there is no suspicion of a systemic infection, whether there is an untreated infection around the procedure site, whether the patient has a problem with hemostasis, and whether there is a history of spinal surgery. Also, the procedure should be reconsidered for patients with neuropsychiatric problems and those who do not fully understand the purpose of the discography. It is also necessary to confirm whether there is a history of hypersensitivity to the local anesthetics and contrast agents used in the examination. Plain radiography, CT, MRI, and other imaging findings should be reviewed, and psychological testing may be needed if there is a somatization disorder or secondary gain, as these can increase the false-positive response of discography.

Before the procedure, the doctor explains the purpose, risks, and side effects of the procedure to the patient and obtains a consent form. It is very important for the patient to feel the same pain as usual during the procedure and to be able to distinguish it from other types of pain. The patient should be educated to express the intensity of the pain they feel using an appropriate pain scale. If the patient cannot express the pain induced during the procedure well, this test becomes meaningless.

15.4.4 Procedure Method

Discography should be performed by an experienced doctor who understands spinal diseases well. During the procedure, the patient should express their pain response through communication with the practitioner. However, a little sedation can be helpful in case of severe pain. Prophylactic antibiotics are needed to prevent infections that may occur due to the procedure. A part of the antibiotic is mixed with the contrast agent to be injected.

15.4.4.1 Lumbar Discography

The patient lies face down on the examination table for the procedure, and local anesthesia is applied to the procedure site after complete disinfection. In the case of lumbar discography, the posterolateral approach is generally preferred, and the double needle technique (using a 22G needle inside a short 18G needle, a coaxial technique) is sometimes recommended to reduce complications and increase success rates. This involves using a thick needle up to near the disc, and then a thin needle inside the thick needle. The method of injecting into the disc using a needle is claimed to have a lower risk of infection. The technique of using a single needle has the advantage of a short procedure time. If there is mainly pain on one side of the waist or buttocks, we approach the opposite side of the usual pain to distinguish between discogenic pain and phantom pain caused by inserting the needle.

In the anteroposterior image before and after fluoroscopy, the X-ray tube is aligned so that the target disc is parallel and the vertebral endplate is straight. Then, the X-ray tube is turned so that the lateral boundary of the superior articular process is located in the middle of the anterior and posterior diameter of the vertebral body (Fig. 15.24). At this angle, the needle must be inserted from the lateral point of the lateral boundary of the superior articular process so that the needle can pass through the center of the disc. The point

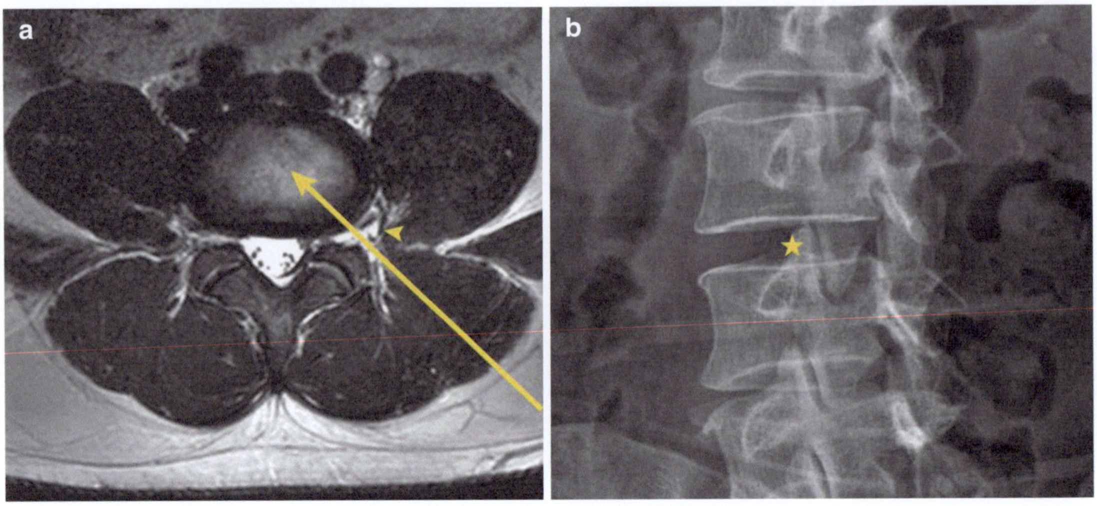

Fig. 15.24 Path of the needle in lumbar discography. (**a**) With the patient lying face down on the operating table, the needle is advanced following the direction of the arrow from the posterior lateral side. It should be careful not to damage the nerve (arrowhead) as it passes by the outside of the facet joint. (**b**) In the left oblique view, the X-ray tube is rotated to align the lateral surface of the L4 superior articular process with the center of the L3–4 disc. The lateral surface of the L4 superior articular process (asterisk) is the path where the needle will be inserted and pass

where the needle will be inserted is marked on the skin. At the L5–S1 level, there may be difficulty in the procedure due to the distance between the iliac crest and the widened facet joint. Before inserting the needle, local anesthesia is performed on the skin and subcutaneous and muscle tissues that become the path of the needle with 1% lidocaine. To avoid the risk of nerve damage, the direction of the needle should not deviate from the safety triangle. The boundaries of this safety triangle are the nerve root above, the endplate of the target disc below, and the lateral surface of the superior articular process inside. The needle approaches in the same direction as the fluoroscopic beam in the oblique view of the X-ray tube, and when the needle touches the annulus fibrosus of the disc, the X-ray tube is turned to see the lateral and anteroposterior images and the end of the needle is inserted so that it is located in the center of the disc. If necessary, the needle can be slightly pulled out to correct the path. When contacting the annulus fibrosus, a firm resistance is felt, and when passing through the outer boundary (Sharpey's fibers) of the annulus fibrosus, the patient may feel a sharp pain in the waist and buttocks momentarily.

After accurately positioning the end of the needle inside the nucleus pulposus, the contrast medium is slowly injected into the disc. The amount of injection should not exceed 2.5 mL, and if strong resistance is felt, the patient complains of severe pain, or if it is seen that the contrast medium leaks from the disc into the spinal canal, the injection should be stopped (Fig. 15.25).

In order for discography to have diagnostic significance when pain is induced in a specific disc, there must be a control disc around which symptoms are not induced. Therefore, at least one disc that looks normal should first be injected with a contrast medium to confirm that pain is not induced. If pain is induced from the disc where the contrast medium was injected, it may be difficult to confirm pain in the next disc. In this case, a small amount of lidocaine can be injected into the disc where pain was induced to confirm that the pain is relieved, and then the contrast medium can be injected into the next disc.

After confirming that the needle is in the correct position, the contrast medium is injected, but

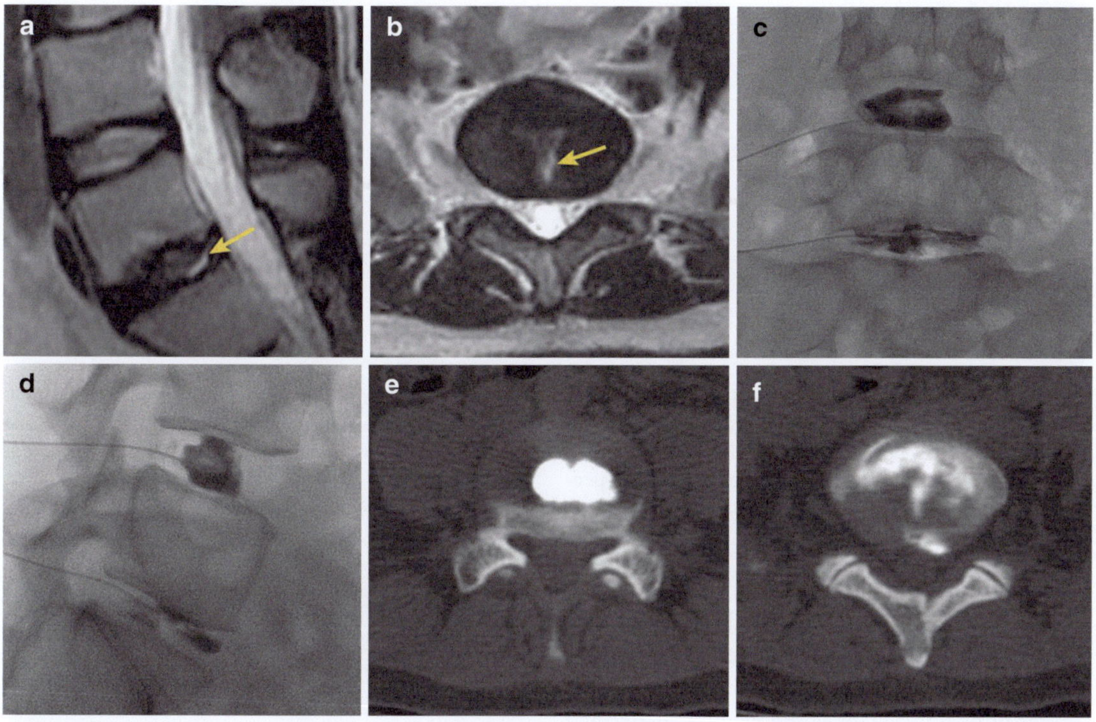

Fig. 15.25 Discography. (**a**, **b**) These are T2-weighted MR images of a 38-year-old female patient complaining of persistent low back pain. Degenerative changes in the L5–S1 disc, a high signal intensity area (HIZ, arrow) is seen in the center. (**c**, **d**) Needles are inserted into the L4–5 and L5–S1 discs, and pain provocation tests are performed by injecting contrast medium into each. The patient did not complain of pain in the L4–5 disc. However, when a small amount of contrast medium was injected into the L5–S1 disc, the patient complained of severe concordant pain. The contrast medium is spreading bilobularly in the central part of the L4–5 disc, and irregularly in the L5–S1 disc. (**e**) In the CT image examined immediately after discography, the contrast medium is confined to the nucleus pulposus area in the L4–5 disc. (**f**) In the L5–S1 disc, the contrast medium is spreading irregularly, and it is flowing out to the outer surface of the disc posteriorly, suggesting a radial tear. The patient's pain improved after disc replacement surgery at the L5–S1 level

in a normal disc, resistance is felt even before 1 mL of contrast medium is injected (high pressure endpoint), but in a degenerated disc, there is not much resistance even with a relatively large amount of injection (low pressure endpoint), and if the degree is severe, the annulus fibrosus of the disc is completely ruptured and the disc and epidural space are connected. In the case where the contrast agent can be injected almost without resistance, it becomes a state where the contrast agent can be infinitely injected (volume endpoint), and if severe pain occurs even when a small amount of contrast agent is injected, the injection should be stopped (pain endpoint). If the contrast agent is not properly injected from the beginning, there is a possibility that the end of the needle is located within the annulus fibrosus (intra-annular injection), and at this time, a positive reaction can be shown.

During the injection of the contrast agent, the patient is continuously asked to express the intensity of the pain, and the intensity of the pain is described in the following ways.

- No pain (no sensation)
- Heavy (pressure)
- Pain in a different area or of a different nature than usual (dissimilar pain)
- Pain similar to usual (similar pain)
- Severe pain that matches exactly as usual (exact pain reproduction)

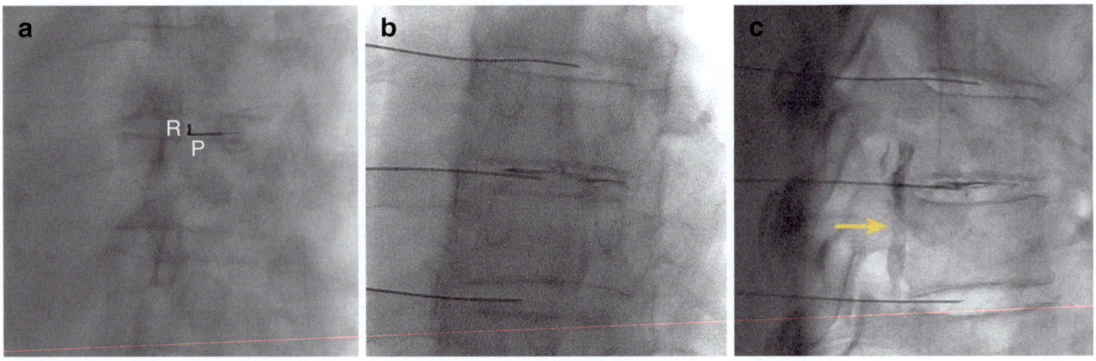

Fig. 15.26 Thoracic discography. (**a**) The needle is being inserted into the T7–8 disc while looking at the left oblique view. It advances towards the disc from the inside of the head of the left eighth rib (R = head of rib). P: pedicle. (**b**, **c**) In the anteroposterior and lateral fluoroscopic images, needles are inserted into the T7–8, T8–9, T9–10 discs. First, the contrast medium is being injected into the T8–9 disc, and the contrast medium is spreading irregularly and leaking into the epidural space (arrow). The patient complained of concordant pain

The most important finding in discography is whether the same pain as usual recurs in the patient. If pain is induced, its intensity, location, and nature are checked. If the induced pain is similar or exactly matches the usual, it is defined as concordant pain, and if not, it is defined as discordant pain. The intensity of pain is measured through the visual analog scale (VAS) and pain behavior.

15.4.4.2 Thoracic Discography

Thoracic discography is not commonly performed and can be performed under fluoroscopy or CT guidance. Thoracic discography can cause pneumothorax by piercing the pleura, so care should be taken. The procedure is similar to lumbar discography, using a 25G or 22G spinal needle, and the contrast agent is injected up to about 1.5 mL (Fig. 15.26).

15.4.4.3 Cervical Discography

Cervical discography is used to diagnose internal disc disruption (IDD) of the cervical spine, especially for persistent neck pain after cervical fusion surgery or neck pain that is difficult to confirm the exact cause on MRI after a traffic accident [29]. In the case of cervical discography, the patient lies flat with the neck slightly extended. After disinfecting the neck, a 25G spinal needle is approached anteromedially, inside the sternocleidomastoid muscle (Fig. 15.27). At this time, the trachea and esophagus are pushed medially by pressing the neck with the fingertips, and the carotid artery is pushed laterally while feeling the pulse, and the needle is inserted in between. The patient is made to hold a barium suspension in the mouth to check the pharynx and esophagus on the fluoroscope and is made to drink just before inserting the needle [29]. Under fluoroscopic guidance, the end of the needle is positioned in the central part of the disc. The amount of contrast agent is injected about 0.3~1.0 mL, and the pain response is evaluated in the same way as lumbar discography. Cervical

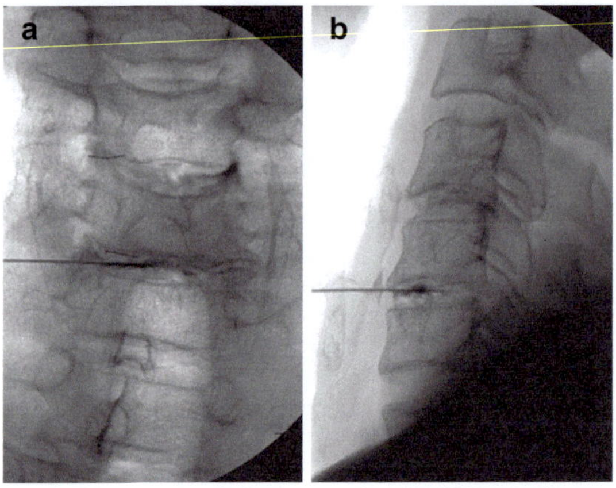

Fig. 15.27 Cervical discography. (**a**, **b**) The needle is inserted into the C5–6 disc from the anterolateral of the cervical spine. The contrast medium is spreading irregularly, but the patient did not complain of pain

discography requires the operator's attention as the risk of complications such as discitis or epidural abscess infection, hematoma, spinal cord injury is higher than lumbar discography.

15.4.5 Imaging Findings

In a normal disc, the contrast agent spreads in a lobular or bilobular pattern. In abnormal discs, various patterns are observed. The contrast agent spreads along the torn part of the annulus fibrosus within the disc. In the case of a completely torn annulus fibrosus, the contrast agent can flow into the epidural space, and in some cases, it can flow into the fracture site of the vertebral endplate. However, such forms alone cannot determine that the cause of the patient's pain is in the disc. The patient's subjective response to the contrast agent injection should be considered.

After discography, CT-discography is performed to clearly observe the fracture pattern of the annulus fibrosus.

The shape of the disc in discography is as follows [30]:

1. Cotton ball: Normal findings, the contrast agent is gathered in the middle of the disc.
2. Lobular, hamburger bun type: Normal shape, formation of intranuclear cleft within the nucleus pulposus.
3. Irregular: Initial degeneration, cracks or gaps are visible in the inner 2/3 of the annulus fibrosus.
4. Fissured: Advanced degenerative changes, radial tear or fissure.
5. Ruptured: Complete radial tear, contrast agent leakage into the epidural space.

It is known that radial tear is most closely related to discogenic pain, and based on this, the Modified Dallas Discogram Scale is the most commonly used CT classification method. Grade 0 is when the contrast agent is completely confined within the nucleus pulposus, and Grades 1, 2, 3 each mean that the contrast agent has spread to the inner 1/3, middle, and outer 1/3 of the annulus fibrosus. Aprill and Bogduk set Grade 4 as the case where the contrast agent spreads more than 308 concentrically along the outer boundary of the annulus fibrosus, and defined Grade 5 as the case where there is leakage into the epidural space [30].

15.4.6 Post-procedure Management

After the procedure, check the patient's vital signs and the presence of bleeding or hematoma. Explain to the patient that discomfort related to the procedure, such as some dysphagia after cervical discography or persistent back pain after lumbar discography, may occur. The patient is discharged on the same day after hearing about potential side effects that may occur over the next few days. The patient is educated to be able to contact immediately if symptoms suggesting infection, such as fever, occur.

15.4.7 Complications

Serious side effects related to discography are discitis and nerve damage. Like other intervention procedures, discography carries a risk of infection. Since the disc is a tissue with almost no blood supply, infection in this area is considered the most serious complication related to the procedure. The frequency of discitis after discography is reported to be about 0.1~0.2% [27]. There are cases where the original pain worsens after discography. However, the possibility of discography causing damage to the disc is almost none, and the pain returns to a similar level as before after a few days. Other complications may include nausea, convulsions, headaches, retroperitoneal hemorrhage, hives, subarachnoid hemorrhage, nerve root damage, and injection of contrast medium into the annulus fibrosus or vertebral endplate due to inappropriate needle positioning. The likelihood of HIVD occurring after discography is very low. However, some reports have pointed out the possibility of faster degeneration in the disc where discography was performed, especially in young adults.

15.5 Spinal Biopsy

A biopsy refers to the removal of tissue from a living body for accurate diagnosis, mainly for microscopic diagnosis, and can be performed through surgical open biopsy or percutaneous biopsy. Percutaneous bone biopsy is usually performed under the guidance of imaging equipment, with fluoroscopy and CT being mainly used, and occasionally ultrasound and MR can be used. Percutaneous spinal biopsy is not a new method, fluoroscopy-guided spinal biopsy has been performed since 1969, and CT-guided spinal biopsy has been performed since 1981 [31]. Percutaneous needle biopsy is superior to open biopsy in terms of speed and cost-effectiveness and has fewer complications. The diagnostic rate of percutaneous spinal biopsy is reported to be about 68~97% [32]. Osteolytic lesions have a high diagnostic rate, but osteoblastic lesions and infectious spondylitis have relatively low diagnostic rates [31]. The accuracy can vary depending on the appropriate patient selection, the choice of the appropriate biopsy site, and the experience of the operator. In particular, fluoroscopy equipment has the advantage of being able to perform the procedure while viewing the position of the biopsy needle in real time. For large lesions of the spine or lesions of the disc, biopsy is mainly performed under fluoroscopy guidance. CT-guided biopsy is performed for small bone lesions and paraspinal masses and is mainly performed for thoracic lesions to avoid puncturing the pleura.

15.5.1 Indications

Places where percutaneous biopsy or aspiration can be considered in the spine include paraspinal soft tissue, vertebral body, posterior arch of the spine, disc, and epidural space or neural foramen, etc.

The indications for spinal biopsy are as follows:

1. Confirmation of spine metastasis in patients with primary cancer.
2. Diagnosis of primary spinal bone tumor.
3. Evaluation of tumor recurrence.
4. Diagnosis of multiple myeloma.
5. Diagnosis of pathologic compression fracture.
6. Confirmation of benign lesions.
7. When diagnosis and culture test for the presence of infection are needed.

In the case of metastatic cancer, pathological diagnosis is possible with relatively small amounts of tissue, but in the case of benign tumors and especially infectious diseases, a large amount of tissue is needed [32]. For culture of the causative bacteria in infectious diseases, a thick needle should be used to collect tissue several times.

15.5.2 Contraindications

It is not performed in cases where diagnosis is possible only by imaging, such as bone island, degenerative spinal disease, bony sclerosis, insufficiency fracture, and hemangioma (do not touch lesions). Contraindications for percutaneous spinal biopsy include coagulopathy [International Normalized Ratio (INR) >1.5, or platelets < 50,000/mm^3], pregnancy, significant spinal cord compression due to a mass in the area to be examined, and epidural mass, etc. Also, locations that are difficult to reach with a percutaneous approach (C1 anterior arch, C2 odontoid process, sclerotic lesion near important arteries) can also be contraindications. In uncooperative patients such as children, general anesthesia may be required.

15.5.3 Considerations Before the Procedure

Before the procedure, check the test results related to blood coagulation. Anticoagulants such as aspirin or coumadin should be discontinued in advance. In a biopsy to determine the presence of infection, antibiotics should be discontinued at least 48 h before the biopsy, and if possible, antibiotics should not be used before the biopsy.

If a biopsy is to be performed, it must be decided where and how the biopsy will be performed, and what equipment will be used. Analyze pre-examined MRI or CT images and plain radiography, etc., and choose a method that is safe for the patient, convenient for the operator, and can increase the diagnostic accuracy. Biopsies are preferably performed on large lesions on the surface. When osteolytic lesions and sclerotic lesions are mixed, osteolytic lesions are collected first [31]. The soft tissue mass that comes out from the collected bone tissue should also be examined. If multiple lesions show different imaging findings, there may be times when tissue needs to be obtained separately. In the case of a mass, tissue is obtained from the contrast-enhanced area excluding the blood vessels, and necrotic tumors obtain tissue from the marginal area. If there is a PET image, it is performed in areas where isotope uptake is high.

For all spinal biopsies, the patient and guardian are explained about the procedure process, risks, and complications, and consent is obtained.

15.5.4 Imaging Equipment

The choice of imaging equipment usually depends on the operator's preference. Generally, fluoroscopy equipment that can track the needle in real time and adjust the angle in all directions is used for biopsies of bone lesions that occupy most of the vertebral body or discs, and CT is preferred for soft tissue masses or small bone lesions or precise needle positioning such as the spinal posterior arch or epidural space. Fluoroscopy has the advantage of being able to guide images in real time, short procedure time, and low cost, but the disadvantage is that the operator is exposed to radiation. And it is difficult to perform under fluoroscopy guidance for soft tissue next to the vertebral body that is not visible on plain radiography. Ultrasound can observe the needle in real time and has the advantage of no radiation exposure, but it can only be used for subcutaneous soft tissue mass or bone destructive lesion in the posterior spine, and it is difficult to use in the vertebral body. MRI can be used for lesions not visible on CT, but there is a problem that the interventional MR system is not widely distributed yet and the experience is not sufficient.

15.5.4.1 Fluoroscopy Guidance

When performing a biopsy under fluoroscopy guidance, it is important to match the beam projection angle of the fluoroscopy well. When performing a biopsy on the vertebral body through the pedicle, In the case of implementation (transpedicular approach), the angle of the fluoroscopic X-ray tube should be adjusted so that the pedicle is clearly visible, and when accessing between the rib and the spine in the thoracic spine (intercostovertebral approach), the beam projection angle should be adjusted so that the pedicle and the start of the rib are as separated as possible. After determining the biopsy path, disinfect the skin, and anesthetize the skin, subcutaneous tissue, and periosteum using lidocaine. First, advance the guiding needle to the area where you want to obtain tissue. In the case of a biopsy through the pedicle, advance the guiding needle to the pedicle. Remove the stylet of the guiding needle and insert the biopsy needle into the cannula to obtain tissue from the desired area (Fig. 15.28). If you want to obtain tissue several times, you need to slightly change the position and direction of the guiding needle, and at this time, you should insert the stylet, pull out the guiding needle to the bony cortex, then change the direction and advance again. If you try to change the direction too much when the end of the needle is in the cancellous bone, the guiding needle may bend or break.

15.5.4.2 CT-Guided

The patient is made to lie face down on the procedure table, and after attaching a marker to the patient's skin, the biopsy lesion is scanned with a thickness of 2~4 mm. Select the most appropriate section and determine the most appropriate path for the biopsy needle to enter, then mark the needle insertion point (needle entry site on the skin) on the patient's skin. When determining the approach path of the needle, nerves or the spinal canal should be avoided, and in the case of the thoracic spine, it should not pass through the pleura. Among the various parts of the lesion, the

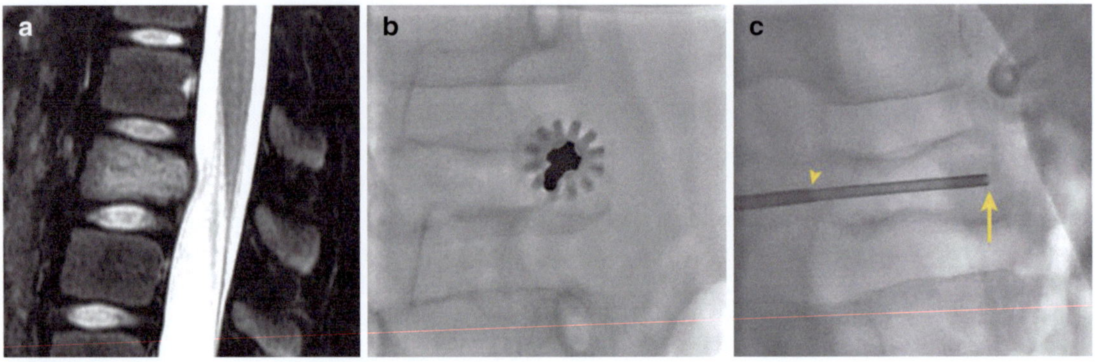

Fig. 15.28 Fluoroscopic-guided spinal biopsy. (**a**) In the sagittal T2-weighted MR image of a 5-year-old girl, the signal intensity of the L2 vertebral body is increased, and there is a wedge deformity. (**b**) The guiding needle is being inserted through the pedicel in the right oblique fluoroscopic view. (**c**) While looking at the lateral fluoroscopic image, the biopsy needle (arrow) is inserted into the guiding needle (arrowhead) and tissue is being collected from the vertebral body. Pathologically, it was diagnosed as Langerhans cell histiocytosis

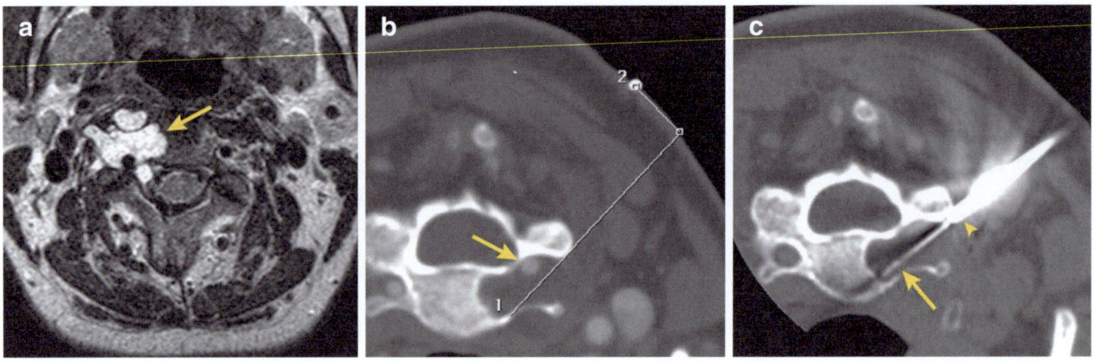

Fig. 15.29 CT-guided spinal biopsy. (**a**) In the axial T2-weighted MR image of a 59-year-old female patient who visited the hospital with a cervical mass found incidentally, there is a high signal intensity mass (arrow) in the right part of the C3 vertebral body. It invades the neural foramen and wraps around the right vertebral artery. (**b**) The patient was laid face down on the CT examination table, and contrast-enhanced CT was performed to check the blood vessels. The location of the vertebral artery (arrow) is confirmed, and the path of the biopsy needle is being planned using the mark (arrowhead) attached to the skin. (**c**) The guiding needle (arrowhead) is positioned near the mass, and tissue is being collected using a semi-automatic gun biopsy needle (arrow). Pathologically, it was diagnosed as chordoma

necrotic part should be avoided. Disinfect the skin with betadine, then first anesthetize the patient's skin with lidocaine using a thin needle. Then proceed to the biopsy site with a 22G spinal needle and perform local anesthesia. As with fluoroscopy-guided biopsy, advance the guiding needle to the desired area. Use CT to check the direction and position of the needle during the process. Once you have reached the desired area, remove the stylet of the guiding needle and insert the biopsy needle through the cannula to obtain tissue (Fig. 15.29).

15.5.5 Biopsy Path

Anterolateral approach is mainly performed for vertebral body lesions of the cervical spine (C4~7), and the biopsy needle can be inserted in a similar way to cervical vertebroplasty [31].

With one hand, push the sternocleidomastoid muscle, carotid artery, and jugular vein laterally and the trachea medially so that the anterior part of the vertebral body touches the fingertips. Anesthetize the skin and periosteum with the other hand, and approach the vertebral body with the biopsy needle to collect tissue. Since the needle needs to be observed in real time, it is mainly performed under fluoroscopic guidance. In the cervical spine, the posterior arch of the spine, soft tissue lesions behind the spine, or C1~3 vertebral body lesions can be performed with a posterolateral approach under CT guidance.

In the case of the thoracic spine, it is often difficult to find an access path due to obstacles such as the lungs and ribs. If there is a lesion in the vertebral body, there is an approach through the pedicle (transpedicular approach) and an approach between the vertebral body and the rib (posterolateral intercostovertebral groove approach), and sometimes through the joint between the rib and the thoracic transverse process. It is also possible to approach via the posterolateral costotransverse joint [33]. At this time, a biopsy should be performed after anesthetizing everything from the thoracic costotransverse joint to the vertebral body periosteum. If the mass is located large next to the vertebral body, it can also be approached posterolaterally through the ribs (posterolateral intercostal approach). At this time, it should be performed under CT guidance due to the possibility of pleural injury.

For the vertebral body of the lumbar spine, the transpedicular approach is safe in most cases [31]. It is performed under CT or fluoroscopic guidance, and it is very important that the needle does not invade the spinal canal. If the pedicle is very thin or the location of the lesion is difficult to approach through the pedicle, there is also a method of directly approaching the vertebral body from the posterolateral side of the spine under CT guidance (posterolateral extrapedicular approach). Soft tissue lesions next to the spine are approached posterolaterally, and lesions on the posterior arch of the spine are also directly approached under CT guidance. In the case of the sacrum, it is mainly performed under CT guidance and approached from the back (dorsal approach).

15.5.6 Biopsy Needle

It is important to choose the appropriate biopsy needle depending on the nature of the lesion. The ideal biopsy device is a device that can obtain as much tissue as possible while minimizing tissue damage and bleeding. Needles can be divided into central cutting and suction devices. The core biopsy needle cuts and collects tissue to see histological findings, and the aspiration needle is used for cell diagnosis. Recently, the Bonopty (RADI Medical system AB, Uppsala, Sweden) needle is widely used in the coaxial biopsy system. For osteolytic or osteodestructive lesions, a biopsy can be performed using a small size (18~22G) needle such as Chiba, E-Z-EM, spinal needle, and aspiration method, and an automatic biopsy device can also be used to biopsy soft tissue, osteolytic or bone marrow lesions.

An important consideration in choosing the appropriate biopsy device is the amount of tissue needed for accurate pathological diagnosis. The inner diameter size of the biopsy needle is inversely proportional to the gauge. That is, the smaller the gauge, the more tissue can be obtained. However, the smaller the gauge, the higher the possibility of local complications, so an appropriate size needle should be selected considering this.

15.5.7 Complications

In the case of skilled operators, complications are reported to be about 1~3%, and they mainly occur in the thoracic spine close to the lung or pleura [31]. Complications related to spinal biopsy include bleeding, infection, allergic reactions related to drugs, postdural puncture headache, pneumothorax related to thoracic spine biopsy, epidural abscess, vasovagal reaction, and rarely reported limb paralysis related to spinal cord puncture. If a hypervascular tumor invades the posterior wall of the vertebral body, cord compression can occur due to bleeding after biopsy. Rarely, the spread of tumors or infections through the biopsy path is also reported.

Bibliography

1. Robecchi A, Capra R. Hydrocortisone (compound F); first clinical experiments in the field of rheumatology. Minerva Med. 1952;43:1259–63.
2. Macnab I. Negative disc exploration. An analysis of the causes of nerve-root involvement in sixty-eight patients. J Bone Joint Surg Am. 1971;53:891–903.
3. Hession WG, Stanczak JD, Davis KW, Choi JJ. Epidural steroid injections. Semin Roentgenol. 2004;39:7–23.
4. Green PW, Burke AJ, Weiss CA, Langan P. The role of epidural cortisone injection in the treatment of diskogenic low back pain. Clin Orthop Relat Res. 1980;(153):121–5.
5. Biyani A, Andersson GB. Low back pain: pathophysiology and management. J Am Acad Orthop Surg. 2004;12:106–15.
6. White AH, Derby R, Wynne G. Epidural injections for the diagnosis and treatment of low-back pain. Spine (Phila Pa 1976). 1980;5:78–86.
7. Ghahreman A, Ferch R, Bogduk N. The efficacy of transforaminal injection of steroids for the treatment of lumbar radicular pain. Pain Med. 2010;11:1149–68.
8. Lee IS, Kim SH, Lee JW, et al. Comparison of the temporary diagnostic relief of transforaminal epidural steroid injection approaches: conventional versus posterolateral technique. AJNR Am J Neuroradiol. 2007;28:204–8.
9. Pfirrmann CW, Oberholzer PA, Zanetti M, et al. Selective nerve root blocks for the treatment of sciatica: evaluation of injection site and effectiveness--a study with patients and cadavers. Radiology. 2001;221:704–11.
10. Kwon JW, Lee JW, Kim SH, et al. Cervical interlaminar epidural steroid injection for neck pain and cervical radiculopathy: effect and prognostic factors. Skeletal Radiol. 2007;36:431–6.
11. Lee JW, Park KW, Chung SK, et al. Cervical transforaminal epidural steroid injection for the management of cervical radiculopathy: a comparative study of particulate versus non-particulate steroids. Skeletal Radiol. 2009;38:1077–82.
12. Abbasi A, Malhotra G, Malanga G, Elovic EP, Kahn S. Complications of interlaminar cervical epidural steroid injections: a review of the literature. Spine (Phila Pa 1976). 2007;32:2144–51.
13. Tuite MJ. Facet joint and sacroiliac joint injection. Semin Roentgenol. 2004;39:37–51.
14. Fortin JD, Dwyer AP, West S, Pier J. Sacroiliac joint: pain referral maps upon applying a new injection/arthrography technique. Part I: asymptomatic volunteers. Spine (Phila Pa 1976). 1994;19:1475–82.
15. Kang WY, Lee JW, Lee E, Kang Y, Ahn JM, Kang HS. Efficacy and outcome predictors of fluoroscopy-guided facet joint injection for spondylolysis. Skeletal Radiol. 2018;47:1137–44.
16. Galibert P, Deramond H, Rosat P, Le Gars D. Preliminary note on the treatment of vertebral angioma by percutaneous acrylic vertebroplasty. Neurochirurgie. 1987;33:166–8.
17. Diamond TH, Champion B, Clark WA. Management of acute osteoporotic vertebral fractures: a nonrandomized trial comparing percutaneous vertebroplasty with conservative therapy. Am J Med. 2003;114:257–65.
18. Gangi A, Sabharwal T, Irani FG, Buy X, Morales JP, Adam A. Quality assurance guidelines for percutaneous vertebroplasty. Cardiovasc Intervent Radiol. 2006;29:173–8.
19. Laredo JD, Hamze B. Complications of percutaneous vertebroplasty and their prevention. Skeletal Radiol. 2004;33:493–505.
20. Kim SH, Kang HS, Choi JA, Ahn JM. Risk factors of new compression fractures in adjacent vertebrae after percutaneous vertebroplasty. Acta Radiol. 2004;45:440–5.
21. Peh WC, Munk PL, Rashid F, Gilula LA. Percutaneous vertebral augmentation: vertebroplasty, kyphoplasty and skyphoplasty. Radiol Clin North Am. 2008;46:611–35, vii.
22. Kang SE, Lee JW, Kim JH, Park KW, Yeom JS, Kang HS. Percutaneous sacroplasty with the use of C-arm flat-panel detector CT: technical feasibility and clinical outcome. Skeletal Radiol. 2011;40:453–60.
23. Lindblom K. Diagnostic puncture of intervertebral disks in sciatica. Acta Orthop Scand. 1948;17:231–9.
24. Anderson MW. Lumbar discography: an update. Semin Roentgenol. 2004;39:52–67.
25. Won JH, Eun CJ, Hwan HS, et al. Internal disc disruption in patients with low back pain: correlation with magnetic resonance imaging and provoked discography and post-discography computed tomography. J Korean Radiol Soc. 2004;51:541–7.
26. Carragee EJ, Lincoln T, Parmar VS, Alamin T. A gold standard evaluation of the "discogenic pain" diagnosis as determined by provocative discography. Spine (Phila Pa 1976). 2006;31:2115–23.
27. Cohen SP, Larkin TM, Barna SA, Palmer WE, Hecht AC, Stojanovic MP. Lumbar discography: a comprehensive review of outcome studies, diagnostic accuracy, and principles. Reg Anesth Pain Med. 2005;30:163–83.
28. Saboeiro GR. Lumbar discography. Radiol Clin North Am. 2009;47:421–33.

29. Won KJ, Hyun KS, Woo LJ, et al. The significance of cervical discography before surgery. J Korean Radiol Soc. 2006;55:103–10.
30. Fenton DS, Czervionke LF. Discography. In: Fenton DS, Czervionke LF, editors. Image-guided spine intervention. Philadelphia: Saunders; 2003. p. 227–56.
31. Tehranzadeh J, Tao C, Browning CA. Percutaneous needle biopsy of the spine. Acta Radiol. 2007;48:860–8.
32. Gogna A, Peh WC, Munk PL. Image-guided musculoskeletal biopsy. Radiol Clin North Am. 2008;46:455–73.
33. Czervionke LF, Fenton DS. Percutaneous spine biopsy. In: Fenton DS, Czervionke LF, editors. Image-guided spine intervention. Philadelphia: Saunders; 2003. p. 141–80.

Postoperative Imaging Evaluation of the Spine

16

Suk-joo Hong

Spinal instrumentation was first performed in 1911 to treat Pott's disease, and since then, various devices and surgical techniques have been developed and used [1]. It is difficult to distinguish and understand all devices and surgical techniques in imaging, but it is necessary to know the basic surgical devices and methods to properly diagnose postoperative complications. This chapter aims to cover the general knowledge of spinal surgical techniques and devices necessary for postoperative imaging interpretation, postoperative imaging techniques and interpretation methods, and complications.

16.1 Spinal Surgery Techniques

16.1.1 Basic Principles and Devices of Spinal Surgery

Spinal surgery includes fusion, instrumentation, discectomy, decompression, and dynamic reconstruction, etc. [1, 2]. Spinal fusion is performed to treat spinal deformities, instability, and neurological dysfunction caused by scoliosis, kyphosis, spondylolisthesis, or fractures, and spinal instrumentation is often performed concurrently. It also becomes an indication for chronic intractable spinal pain caused by degenerative spinal diseases, infections, tumors, etc. It is a commonly performed surgery when decompression is needed for the treatment of discogenic neuropathy. Spinal instrumentation refers to internal fixation performed to promote fusion of the affected spinal area and prevent the occurrence of pseudoarthrosis [1]. The devices used in spinal fusion and concurrent instrumentation are not to replace the vertebral body or intervertebral disc, but to ensure stability until spinal fusion occurs, and generally, instrumentation that has not achieved complete bone fusion is considered a failure [3]. The basic metal devices used in spinal fusion and instrumentation include rods, plates, wires, cables, screws, hooks, cages, etc. [1, 3, 4]. Among them, rods and plates are mainly installed in the anterior column or posterior element of the spine to provide stabilization, traction, and compression in the longitudinal plane (Fig. 16.1). The rod is fixed to the spine with wires, cables, screws, hooks, etc. (Fig. 16.1b), and the plate has holes for screws. This is fixed to the bone (Fig. 16.1a). While a wire is a single line and comes in various thicknesses, a cable is made by twisting multiple wires and is used to fix bone fragments to the bone without using rods or plates (Fig. 16.2). A screw is partially or fully threaded, with closely spaced threads being a cortical screw and widely spaced threads being a cancellous screw. Cortical screws are mainly used in spinal surgery (Figs. 16.1 and 16.2). Screws can also be divided into unicortical and bicortical screws depending

S.-j. Hong (✉)
Department of Radiology, Korea University College of Medicine, Seoul, Republic of Korea
e-mail: hongsj@korea.ac.kr

© The Author(s), under exclusive license to Springer Nature Singapore Pte Ltd. 2025
H. S. Kang, J. W. Lee (eds.), *Spinal Imaging*, https://doi.org/10.1007/978-981-95-1386-4_16

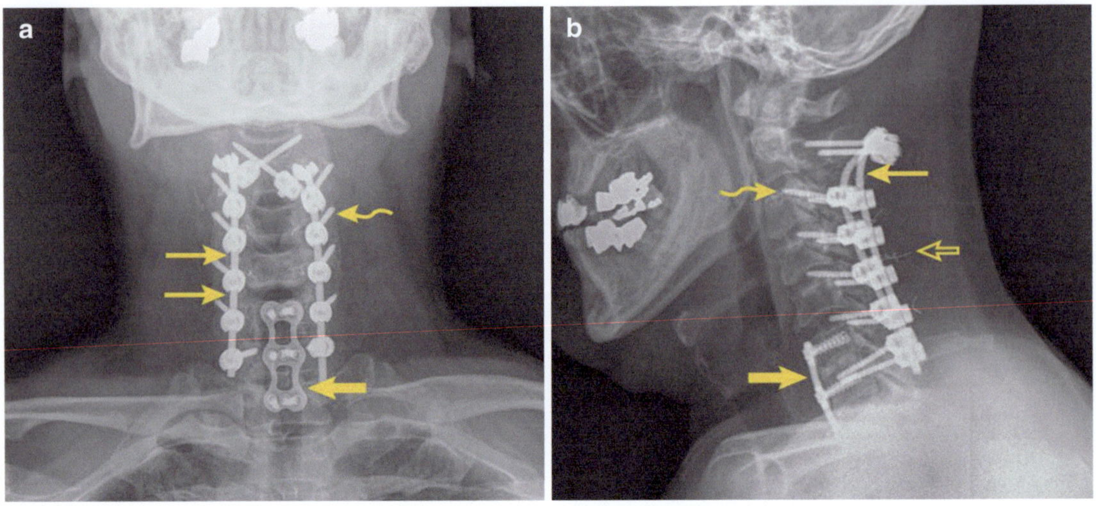

Fig. 16.1 Posterior and lateral images (**a**, **b**) of the cervical spine of a patient who underwent C2–C7 posterior instrumentation, C6–T1 anterior instrumentation, and interbody fusion. Various metal instruments used in spinal instrumentation—rod (arrow), plate (thick arrow), cortical screw (curved arrow), wire (empty arrow)—can be seen

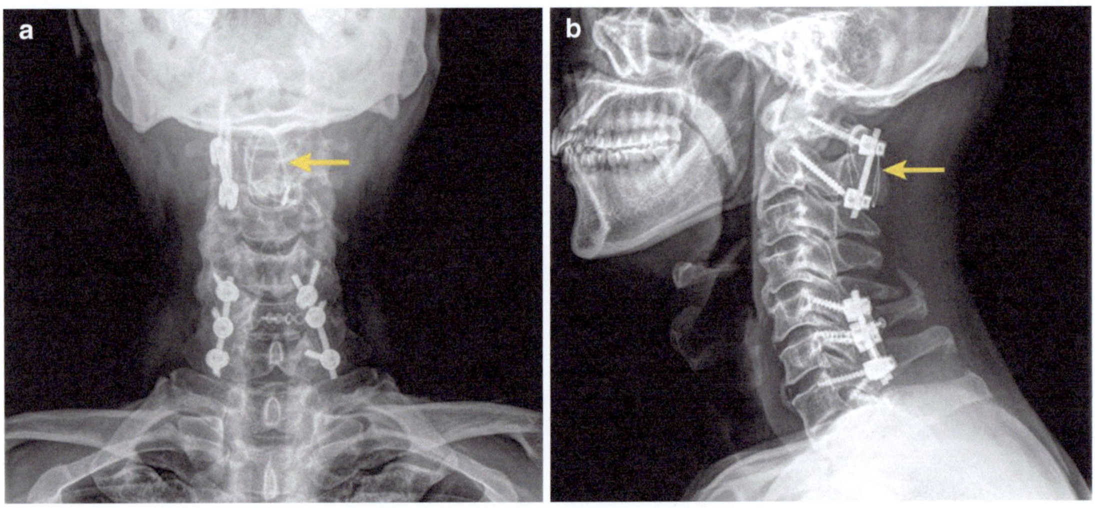

Fig. 16.2 Anterior and lateral images (**a**, **b**) of a patient who underwent C1–C2 sublaminar cable fixation. A thick cable can be seen compared to the wire, and usually a knot device is attached (arrow)

on the number of cortical bones they pass through. A hook is a metal attachment made to fit the shape of the posterior part of the spine, and it can be fixed to the posterior part of the spine without damaging the surrounding nerves and blood vessels. There are sublaminar hooks that can prevent dural damage with their blunt ends, and hooks that can be fixed to the pedicle or transverse process with their split ends. The shape of the spine is followed to fix rods or plates with screws or hooks. The defect of the vertebral body that occurs after corpectomy or vertebrectomy is replaced with allograft bone fragments or cages (Fig. 16.3). As mentioned earlier, spinal interbody fusion involves inserting an interbody spacer after partially or completely removing the intervertebral disc, and instrumentation is often used in conjunction to add fixation and stability.

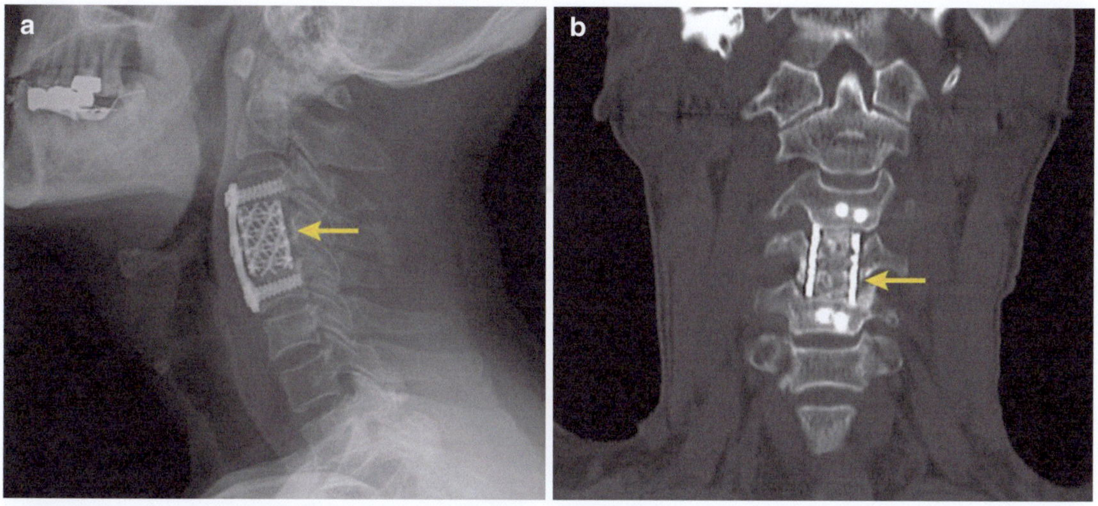

Fig. 16.3 Lateral image (**a**) and coronal CT image (**b**) of the cervical spine of a patient who underwent C4 corpectomy, cage insertion, C3–C5 anterior instrumentation and fusion. A metallic cage (arrow) is inserted to replace the removed C4 body, and the inside is filled with a bone graft

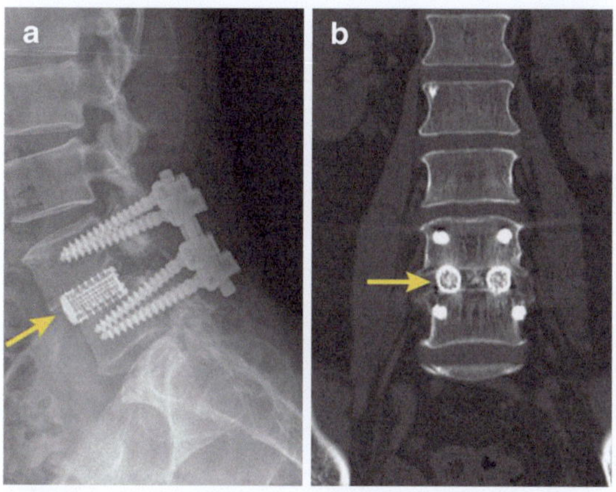

Fig. 16.4 Lateral image (**a**) and sagittal CT image (**b**) of the lumbar spine of a patient who underwent L4–L5 posterior lumbar interbody fusion (PLIF) and pedicle screw fixation. After the intervertebral discectomy, the area was filled with a titanium cage and bone graft (arrow), and interbody fusion was performed

The fusion materials commonly used between vertebral bodies are titanium cages, bone plugs, and radiolucent materials such as polyetheretherketone (PEEK) [3]. A cage is a hollow cylindrical metal device, which is filled with bone graft inside, making bone fusion easier between two vertebral bodies (Fig. 16.4). Bone graft is also usually filled around the cage to fill the remaining intervertebral disc space. Bone grafts use autografts, allografts, or a mixture of these bones, and autografts mostly use cortical cancellous bone blocks covered with cortical bone on two or three sides from the iliac bone [5]. Radiolucent fusion materials have radiopaque markers at both ends to indicate their location (Fig. 16.5).

Discectomy is mainly performed with laminectomy to treat symptomatic HIVD (herniated intervertebral disc) [6]. The approach for discectomy varies depending on the size and location of the herniated intervertebral disc. Small paracentral HIVD can be easily removed without laminectomy through partial or complete incision of the ligamentum flavum, which is called fenestration. When the herniated intervertebral disc is large, various degrees of laminectomy are required, and partial, complete laminectomy can be performed on one or both sides, and removal of the ligamentum flavum is also performed (Fig. 16.6). Recently, intervertebral discectomy is also performed using microscopic lumbar laminotomy, in which case the ligamentum flavum can be preserved [5]. When there is foraminal or extraforaminal HIVD, medial facetectomy is also performed [6]. In the cervical spine, discectomy and fusion are mainly performed through an anterior approach, which is called anterior cervical discectomy and fusion (ACDF) (Fig. 16.7),

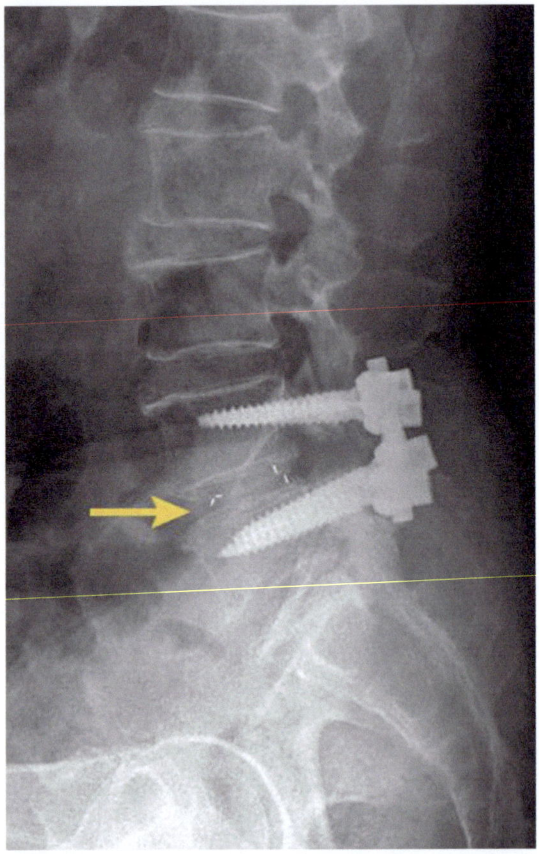

Fig. 16.5 Side view of a patient who underwent L4–L5 posterior lumbar interbody fusion (PLIF) and pedicle screw fixation. A radiopaque fusion material with metal markers at both ends was used (arrow)

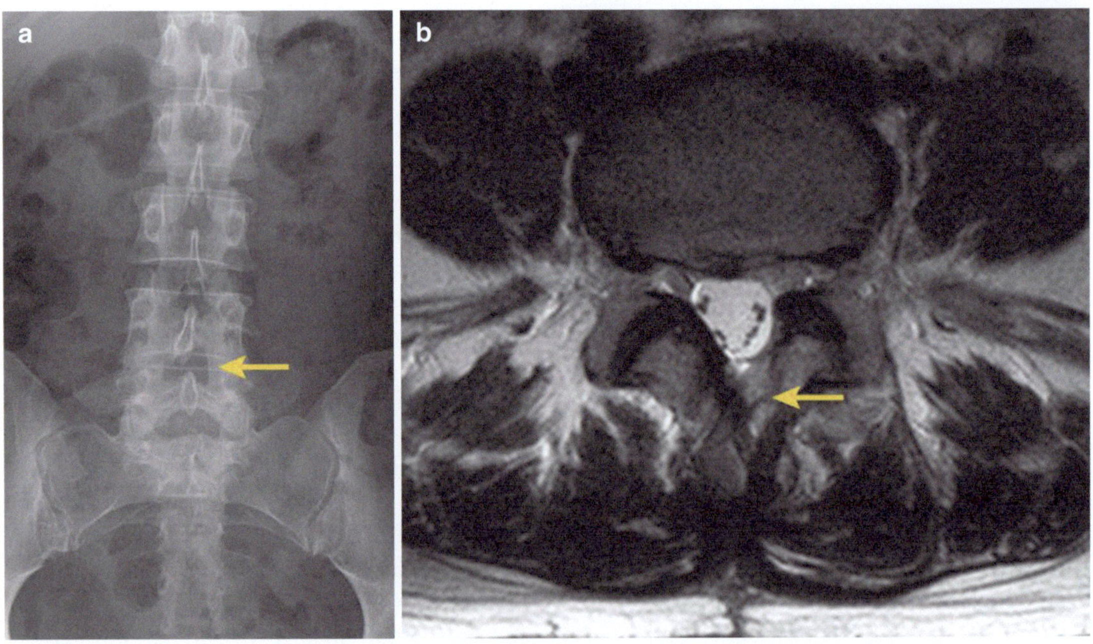

Fig. 16.6 Patient who underwent L4–L5 discectomy and left laminectomy. In the before and after photos (**a**), you can see that the left intervertebral foramen is asymmetrically widened (arrow), and in the axial T2-weighted image (**b**), you can see that the left lamina and ligamentum flavum have been partially resected (arrow)

and intervertebral discectomy is also performed through foraminotomy (Fig. 16.8). Various materials are inserted to prevent epidural fibrosis after laminectomy, including silastic sheet, Dacron, composite membrane, fat. There are grafts, methyl cellulose, etc. [6].

Decompression is performed to treat conditions such as spinal stenosis, and this includes

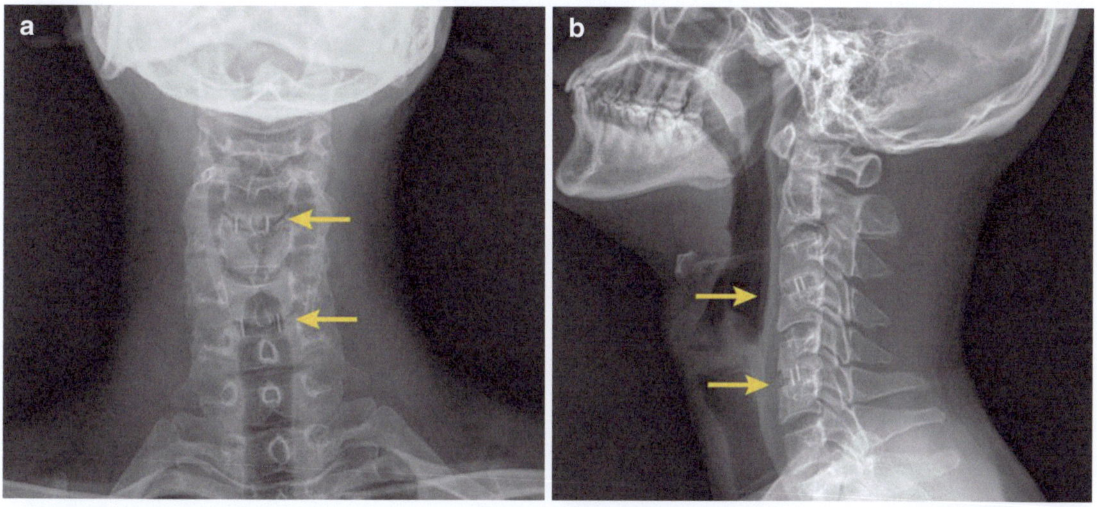

Fig. 16.7 Front (**a**) and side (**b**) photos of the cervical spine of a patient who underwent C3–4, C5–6 anterior cervical discectomy and fusion (ACDF) (arrow)

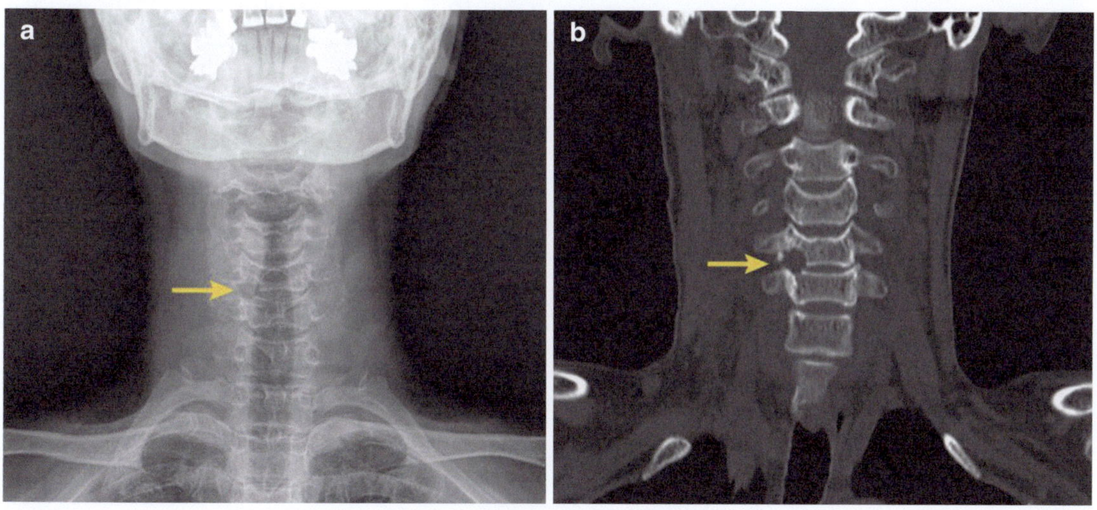

Fig. 16.8 Front view of the cervical spine (**a**) and sagittal CT image (**b**) of a patient who underwent C5–6 right foraminotomy. The right neural foramen of C5–6 where the foraminotomy was performed is widened (arrow)

procedures like laminectomy, laminoplasty, and foraminotomy [7, 8]. Laminectomy is mainly performed through a posterior approach in lumbar stenosis, and when instability is present or expected, spinal fusion is performed concurrently, which is called posterior lumbar interbody fusion (PLIF) (Fig. 16.9). Laminoplasty is performed through a posterior approach in the cervical spine when there is spinal compression due to OPLL (ossification of posterior longitudinal ligament). More details will be discussed in the next chapter.

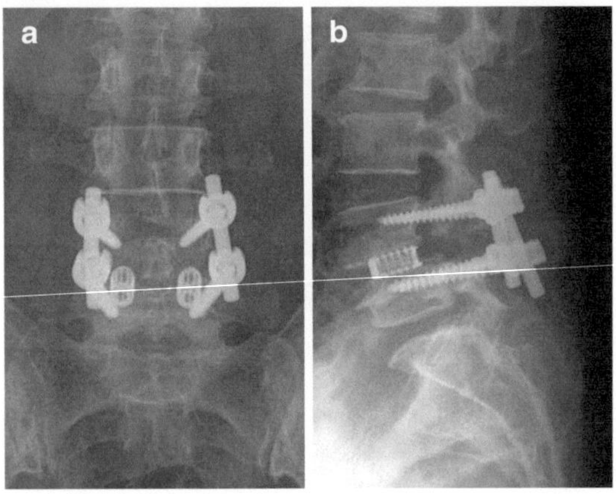

Fig. 16.9 Front (**a**) and side (**b**) photos of the lumbar spine after laminectomy, posterior lumbar interbody fusion (PLIF), and pedicle screw fixation in a patient with L4–5 lumbar spinal stenosis

Dynamic spinal reconstruction, unlike traditional spinal fusion, aims to preserve the mobility and function of the spine and eliminate pain caused by damaged intervertebral discs. It has been clinically used since the late 1980s [2]. Fusion, which was considered the standard for treating symptomatic segmental intervertebral disc disease, changes the biomechanical characteristics by eliminating spinal mobility and flexibility, leading to problems such as acceleration of adjacent segmental disease (ASD), collapse of the graft site, and pain at the graft site. Non-fusion spinal surgery or dynamic spinal reconstruction, which aims to overcome these problems, includes spinal arthroplasty or total disc replacement (TDR) and dynamic stabilization. TDR or ADR (artificial disc replacement) involves removing all or most of the intervertebral disc and inserting a completely new material between the vertebral bodies. The most common form involves fixing two metal plates to the top and bottom of the spine and filling the middle space with a compressible polyethylene material (Fig. 16.10) [2, 3]. Lumbar spine TDR was first attempted by Fernstrom in the late 1950s, and many studies were conducted in the 1980s. In

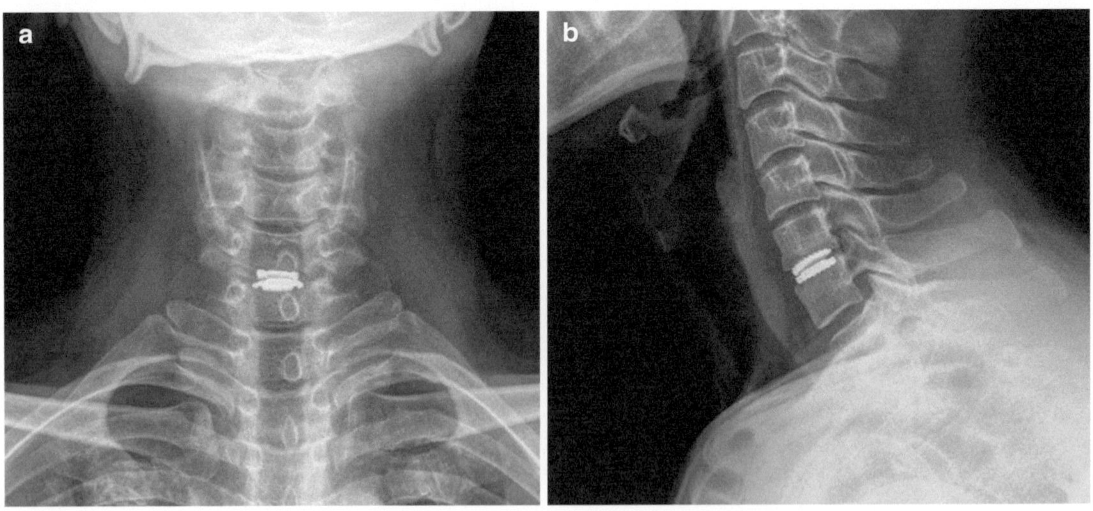

Fig. 16.10 Front (**a**) and side (**b**) photos of a patient who underwent total disc replacement (TDR) at C6–7

2004, the SB Charite III (Depuy Spine, Raynham, MA) was approved by the US FDA as the first lumbar spine arthroplasty device [2, 9]. Lumbar spine TDR is known to have similar short-term effects to spinal fusion, but research on long-term effects is still lacking [9]. The indications for lumbar spine TDR are patients with discogenic lumbar pain without facet arthrosis, but it is contraindicated in most patients with back pain [3, 9]. Cervical spine TDR is currently more widely performed clinically than lumbar spine, and many short-term studies report similar or superior results to ACDF (Fig. 16.10). There are also reports that it can potentially prevent the disadvantages of ACDF, such as ASD and graft site pain, but long-term follow-up is still needed [9]. Dynamic stabilization is a surgery that stabilizes the motion segment while preserving the intervertebral disc and spinal structures by attaching a device to the back of the spine. This includes interspinous process spacer, pedicle screw-based system, facet replacement, etc. (Fig. 16.11) [2, 3].

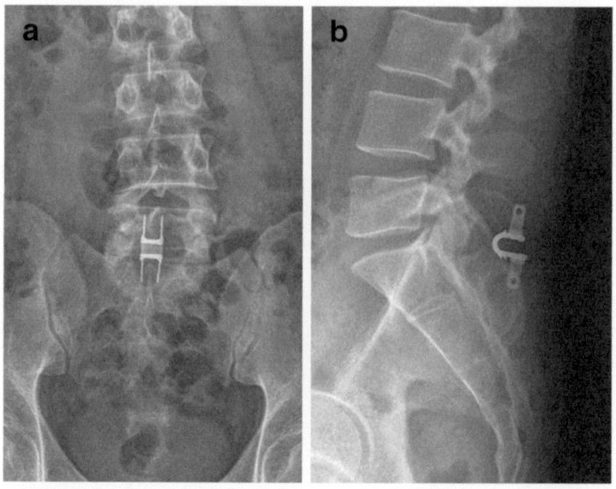

Fig. 16.11 Front (**a**) and side (**b**) photos of a patient who had an interspinous spacer, a type of dynamic stabilization, inserted at L5–S1

16.1.2 Surgical Approaches and General Surgical Techniques

16.1.2.1 Cervical Spine

The surgical approaches in the cervical spine can be broadly divided into anterior approach and posterior approach (Table 16.1) [1, 10]. The anterior approach can be divided into the craniovertebral junction and upper cervical spine, and mid to lower cervical spine. The anterior approach to the craniovertebral junction and upper cervical spine is used for tumors, infections, trauma, and spinal deformities. It is used when the main disease such as degenerative spinal disease is located in the vertebral body [10]. The surgical techniques commonly used include the transoral approach, high cervical retropharyngeal approach, anterior odontoid screw fixation (Fig. 16.12), anterior atlantoaxial facet screw fixation, etc. The transoral approach is a good indication for extradural lesions located relatively centrally in the lower clivus, atlas, and axis. It is mainly used for tumor or abscess excision and is also used for craniovertebral decompression such as odontoid process non-union and basilar invagination [10]. The anterior approach of the mid to lower cervical spine is the most commonly performed surgery in cervical spine surgery for degenerative disc disease, myelopathy, infection, trauma, tumor, etc., causing spinal deformity or instability to perform decompression or stabilization [1, 11]. Through the anterior approach, intervertebral discectomy, fusion, and instrumentation are mainly performed (Fig. 16.13), and foraminotomy is also performed through the anterolateral approach (Fig. 16.8). The posterior approach of the cervical spine can be divided into the upper cervical spine from the occiput to the axis and the lower cervical spine below C3 [12]. It can be applied to all diseases of the cervical spine such as fractures, dislocations, ligament injuries, cervical intervertebral disc her-

Table 16.1 Surgical approaches, techniques, and typical indications for the cervical spine

Approach	Location	Technique	Indication
Anterior approach	Upper cervical spine	Transoral approach	Lower clivus, anterior lesions of C1/C2
		High cervical retropharyngeal approach	C1–C3, Hangman fracture
		Anterior odontoid screw fixation	Type II Odontoid process fracture
		Anterior atlantoaxial facet screw fixation	Atlantoaxial instability
	Mid to lower cervical spine	Anterior cervical discectomy with fusion (ACDF)	Radiculopathy, myelopathy
		Anterolateral foraminotomy	Unilateral radiculopathy
Posterior approach	Upper cervical spine	Foramen magnum decompression	Chiari malformation, achondroplasia, syringomyelia
		Posterior occipitocervical fusion	Occipito-atlantal subluxation, Atlantoaxial instability
		C1–2 Sublaminar wire fixation	Atlantoaxial instability
		C1–2 Transarticular screw fixation	Atlantoaxial instability, odontoid process non-union
		C1 lateral mass-C2 pedicle screw fixation	Atlantoaxial instability
	Mid to lower cervical spine	Laminectomy	Cervical spinal stenosis
		Laminoplasty	Cervical spinal stenosis, OPLL
		Posterior cervical laminoforaminotomy	Unilateral radiculopathy
		Interspinous wire fixation	Anteroposterior instability
		Facet wire fixation	Cervical spinal instability
		Lateral mass screw fixation	Cervical spinal instability
		Pedicle screw fixation	Cervical spinal instability

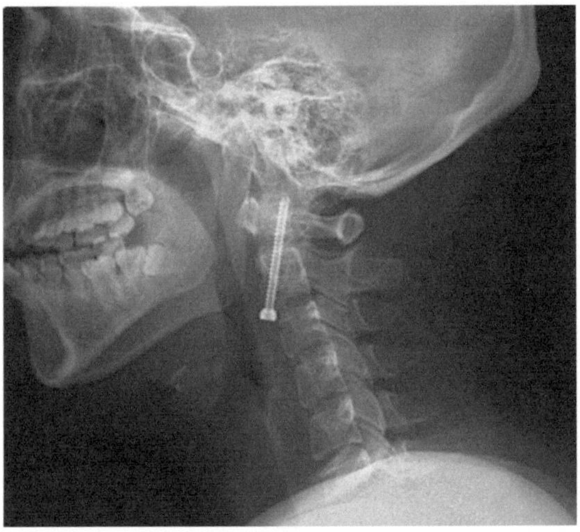

Fig. 16.12 In a patient with an odontoid process fracture, a lateral image of the cervical spine after performing an anterior odontoid screw fixation

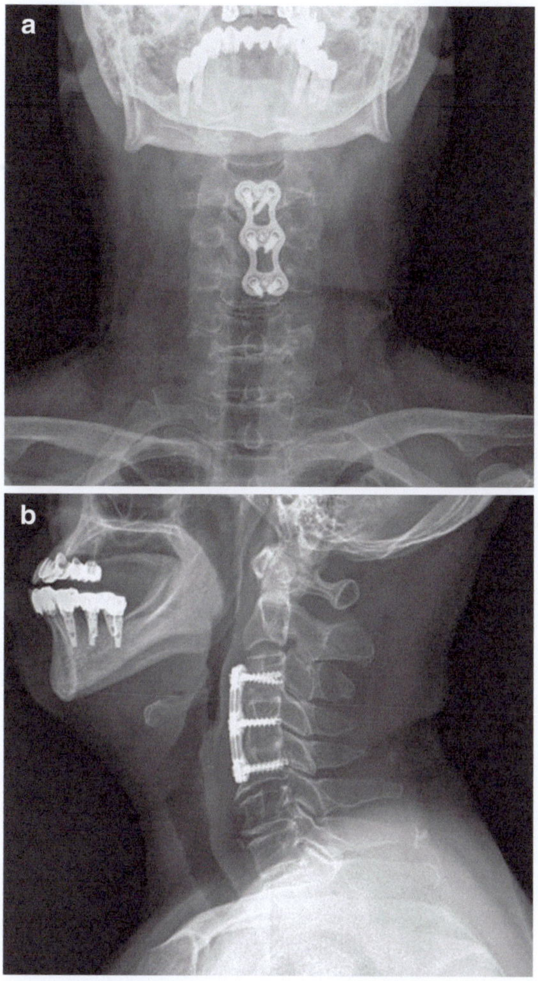

Fig. 16.13 A patient with C3–5 intervertebral disc herniation who underwent anterior cervical discectomy with fusion (ACDF) and concurrent anterior instrumentation (C-spine AP (**a**) and lateral (**b**) views)

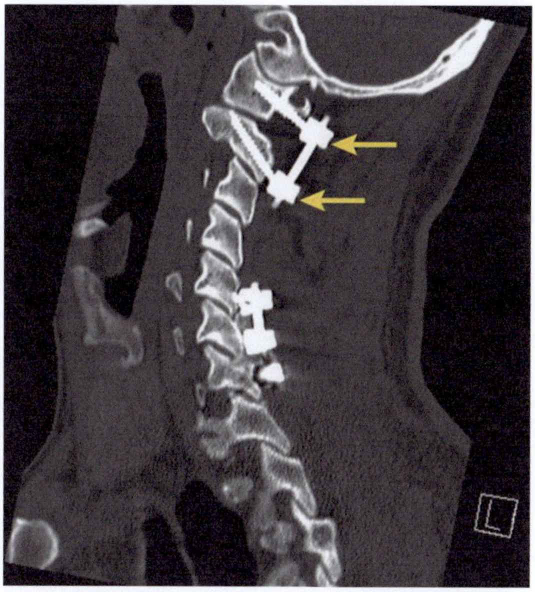

Fig. 16.14 Axial CT image after performing C1 lateral mass-C2 pedicle screw fixation (arrow) in a patient with C1–2 cervical spinal instability

niation, tumors, and stenosis caused by trauma. Surgeries performed through the posterior approach in the upper cervical spine include foramen magnum decompression performed in Chiari malformation, achondroplasia, etc. and posterior occipitocervical fusion, C1–2 sublaminar wire fixation, C1–2 transarticular screw fixation, C1 lateral mass-C2 pedicle screw fixation can be performed for atlantoaxial instability [1, 11]. Among them, sublaminar wire fixation can cause damage to the dura mater or spinal cord when the wire passes sublaminar (Fig. 16.2b) [1, 11]. C1 lateral mass-C2 pedicle screw fixation was introduced most recently and has become popular as a surgical method that can minimize neurovascular damage (Fig. 16.14), and posterior occipitocervical fusion is no longer performed for traumatic atlantoaxial instability without damage to the posterior arch of the atlas. The posterior approach of the lower cervical spine performs laminectomy or laminoplasty for cervical canal decompression, and fixation techniques include interspinous wire fixation, facet wire fixation, lateral mass screw fixation, pedicle screw fixation, etc. (Fig. 16.15). Laminectomy or laminoplasty can be performed through a posterior approach to treat cervical spinal stenosis caused by degenerative spondylosis or OPLL. Laminectomy has a high risk of nerve damage, and if performed extensively, it can

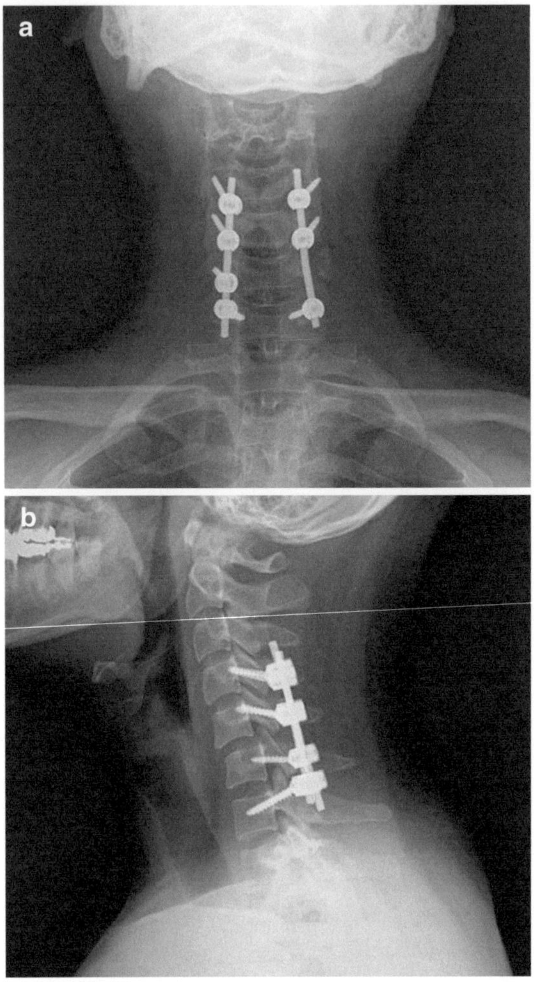

Fig. 16.15 Anterior and lateral (**a**, **b**) images of a patient who underwent C4–7 posterior instrumentation. Lateral mass screw fixation was performed at C4–6, and pedicle screw fixation was performed at C7

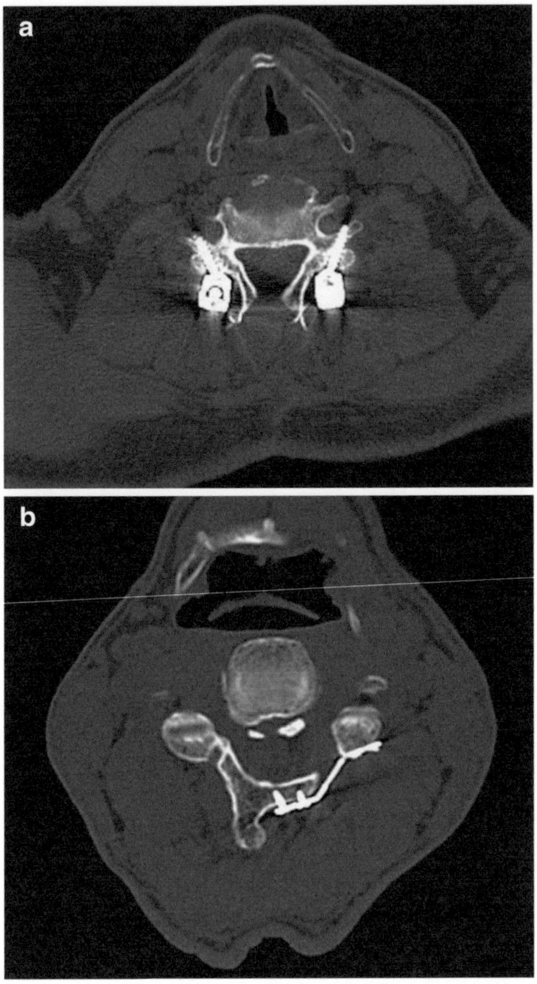

Fig. 16.16 (**a**) Axial CT image after performing midline expansive laminoplasty in a patient with cervical spinal stenosis. (**b**) Axial CT image after performing open door laminoplasty in a patient with cervical spine OPLL

exacerbate spinal instability, so laminoplasty is mainly chosen recently. Laminoplasty includes the Kurokawa method, which cuts the center to expand the spinal canal, and the expansive open door laminoplasty, which opens the spinal canal by cutting the lateral side of the posterior arch (Fig. 16.16) [1, 8, 12]. In addition, posterior cervical laminoforaminotomy can be performed in patients with soft HIVD with unilateral neuralgia [8, 12].

16.1.2.2 Thoracic Spine

The surgical approach to the thoracic spine can be divided into anterior and posterolateral approaches [13]. The anterior approach to the thoracic spine includes transthoracic, transsternal, and thoracoscopy methods. The transthoracic approach is performed in conjunction with thoracotomy, and access is possible from T2 to L2 (Fig. 16.17). Generally, the left transthoracic approach is performed, which is easier to handle the aorta and its branches than the

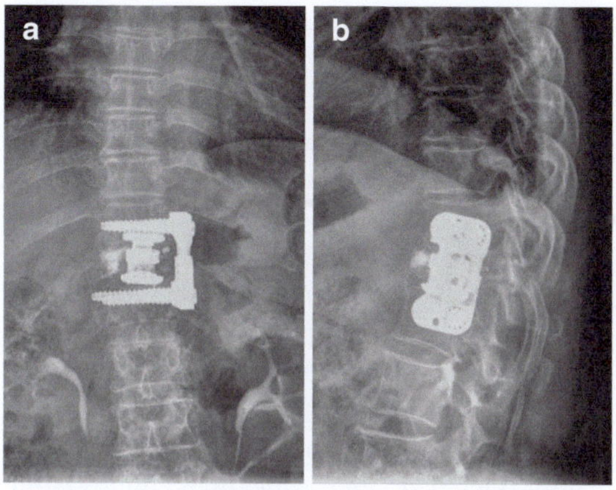

Fig. 16.17 This is a patient who underwent a left transthoracic partial corpectomy and instrumentation at T10–12 (T-L spine AP (**a**) and lateral (**b**) views)

right, but access becomes quite difficult above T4 due to the aortic arch. The posterior approach to the thoracic spine varies, including laminectomy, transpedicular, costotransversectomy, lateral extracavitary is present [13]. Laminectomy is generally performed for various diseases such as posterior decompression, thoracic discectomy, posterior fusion, tumor removal, and intradural tumors, but is not performed for anterior diseases of the spine. In the thoracic spine, spinal nerves are easily damaged by even minor stimuli, so many methods have been studied to reduce stimulation. To reach the vertebral body or intervertebral disc, a transpedicular approach is performed, and the vertebral body is removed by bilateral approach. Costotransversectomy is used for partial vertebrectomy, fusion, decompression, etc. with a posterolateral approach. It is accessed after medial rib resection and separation of costotransverse, cost-vertebral joint. The lateral extracavitary approach can perform both anterior and posterior approaches at the same time, but it is technically difficult and has the disadvantage of a long operation time. With this approach, the lateral dura can be directly confirmed and accessed to the disease.

16.1.2.3 Lumbar Spine

The anterior approach of the lumbar spine includes transperitoneal and retroperitoneal approaches, but about 6% can be accompanied by vascular complications, the overall complication rate is about 20%, and important complications account for 12% [13]. Spinal fusion performed in the lumbar spine includes posterior fusion (PF), posterior lateral fusion (PLF), anterior lumbar interbody fusion (ALIF), posterior lumbar interbody fusion (PLIF), and transforaminal lumbar interbody fusion (TLIF) [5, 13]. Among them, PLIF is mainly performed to treat spinal instability due to degenerative intervertebral disc disease or spondylolisthesis, and can correct all three columns of the spine with a single posterior approach through discectomy, fusion, and segmental fixation using screws and wires (Fig. 16.9). It also has the advantage of avoiding vascular or sympathetic nerve damage that often accompanies the anterior approach. In the classical PLIF, it consists of bilateral laminectomy, medial facetectomy, and preservation of midline structures such as the spinous process and interspinous ligament. More extended PLIF involves total facetectomy and extended laminectomy, which can be accompanied by instability, so instrumentation is needed (Fig. 16.18) [13]. TLIF is a modification of PLIF, completely removing one facet joint to expose the intervertebral space to the outside of the dura and minimizing nerve traction, so it can prevent nerve traction damage that can occur in PLIF (Fig. 16.19) [5]. Microscopic lumbar discectomy

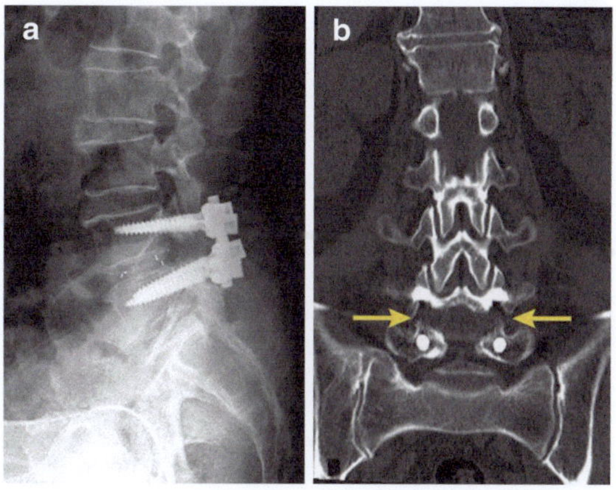

Fig. 16.18 In a patient with L4–5 lumbar spinal stenosis, an expanded PLIF was performed, which included discectomy, interbody fusion, total facetectomy (arrow), laminectomy, and pedicle screw fixation. (**a**) Lateral photo of the lumbar spine. (**b**) Sagittal CT image

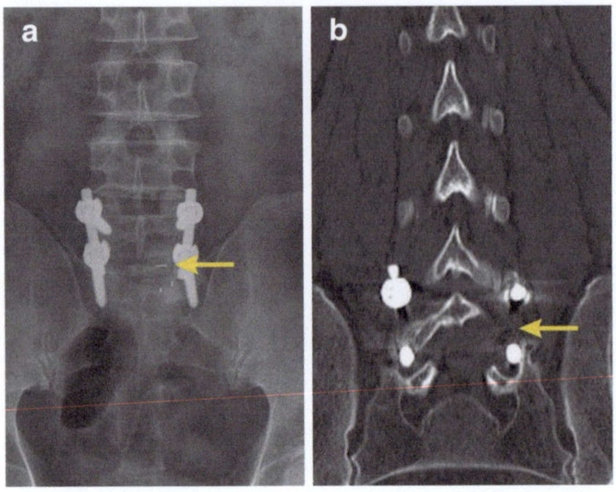

Fig. 16.19 Anterior and posterior photos of the lumbar spine (**a**) and sagittal CT image (**b**) of a patient who underwent transforaminal lumbar interbody fusion (TLIF) at L4–5. A partial discectomy and interbody fusion were performed on the left side through a left facetectomy and partial laminectomy (arrow)

using a microscope is also performed as a posterior approach to the lumbar spine, and depending on the location of the lesion, it is performed through one lamina, so all midline ligaments including the interspinous ligament are preserved to prevent postoperative instability and recovery is fast. With this approach, both sides of the central canal, lateral recess, and intervertebral foramen can be decompressed [5].

16.2 Postoperative Spinal Imaging

Postoperative spinal imaging is performed for the following purposes [3]. First, to determine the degree of bone fusion, second, to evaluate the position or condition of the inserted devices, third, to detect the occurrence of complications such as infection, bleeding, and fourth, to discover new diseases or evaluate the progress of existing diseases [3]. Choosing the appropriate imaging technique after surgery is an essential element in the evaluation of devices or bone grafts, and the assessment of complications [14].

16.2.1 Plain Radiography

Postoperative standard plain radiography is essential for tracking the position of devices and can be considered the starting point of all postoperative evaluations [14]. Changes in the position of the device or device failure can usually be easily detected in continuous plain radiography, and it is important to compare not only the most recent images but also several previous images [3]. Anteroposterior, lateral, oblique, dynamic views (flexion, extension, lateral flexion, etc.) are mainly included, and sometimes fluoroscopic images can be helpful. However, in plain radiography, it is impossible to evaluate lesions such as spinal metastasis or cauda equina compression, and in such cases, MRI should be performed.

16.2.2 CT

CT is the most suitable imaging technique for accurately evaluating bones such as bone fusion, and it is useful for evaluating the position of the device, spinal alignment, spinal canal, and complications such as pseudarthrosis [3, 14]. However, there is a disadvantage that the image quality is degraded by beam hardening artifact, streak artifact, or starburst-type, sunburst artifact caused by X-ray attenuation in metal devices (Fig. 16.20). Titanium devices produce less of these artifacts than stainless steel, and patient movement can exacerbate these artifacts. However, recently, with the spread of multidetector CT (MDCT), image acquisition time has been reduced and multiplanar reconstruction (MPR) has become possible, and the development of image reconstruction algorithms has minimized the degradation of image quality due to metal artifacts [3]. To minimize metal artifacts, it is necessary to apply imaging conditions and indicators optimized for this, such as placing the shortest part of the metal device perpendicular to the table to minimize the distance the X-ray passes through the metal, increasing the maximum voltage (kVp) and current (mAs), reducing

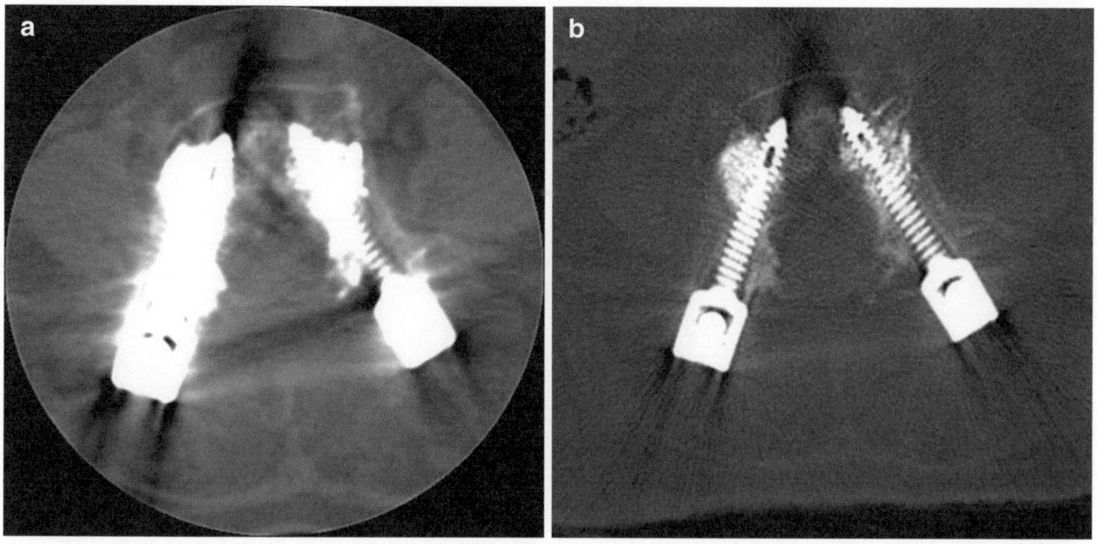

Fig. 16.20 (**a**) Streak artifact caused by metal device is seen in the axial CT image. (**b**) 16-channel CT image obtained as an imaging indicator to minimize metal artifacts

the detector collimation and pitch, acquiring with thin slice thickness, using a large focus, etc. (Fig. 16.20b) [15, 16]. The recommended maximum voltage is 140 kVp for the thoracolumbar spine and 120 kVp for the cervical spine, and recently, image processing technology that can effectively minimize metal artifacts with low tube voltage and current using the iterative reconstruction algorithm has been released [17]. Image reconstruction is recommended to be done with a soft tissue algorithm and thick slice thickness [15–17]. Also, acquiring images by expanding the CT's Hounsfield scale larger than the HU of the metal device (about 8000~20,000 HU) can minimize the degradation of image quality, and MPR, 3D volume rendering, etc. can contribute to artifact minimization [15, 16].

16.2.3 MR

MR imaging is most suitable for evaluating the inside of the spinal canal, especially for detecting postoperative infections, fluid retention, recurrence of intervertebral disc herniation, recurrence of tumors, etc. It is most useful for evaluation [3, 14]. However, the problem is the image distortion caused by the magnetic susceptibility artifact of the metal object, and this artifact also occurs more severely in stainless steel products than in titanium products. Most of the metal tools used recently are made of titanium, so the image distortion caused by artifacts is less than in the past, but it is still difficult to evaluate around the metal tool. Therefore, a separate imaging indicator is needed to minimize these artifacts. The gradient recalled echo (GRE) sequence is the most vulnerable to susceptibility artifacts, so it is an imaging sequence that must be avoided, and it is recommended to use the fast spin echo (FSE) image, which is less sensitive to magnetization [3, 14, 16]. Reducing TE, reducing voxel size, widening receiver bandwidth, and using low magnetic field strength are necessary to reduce metal artifacts (Fig. 16.21) [3, 14, 16]. Fat suppression images can minimize artifacts by using the short tau inversion recovery (STIR) sequence or the Dixon technique, which are less affected by the homogeneity of the main magnetic field [16]. Contrast-enhanced MR images are very useful for evaluating complications such as infection after surgery and are particularly useful for differential diagnosis of recurrent disc herniation

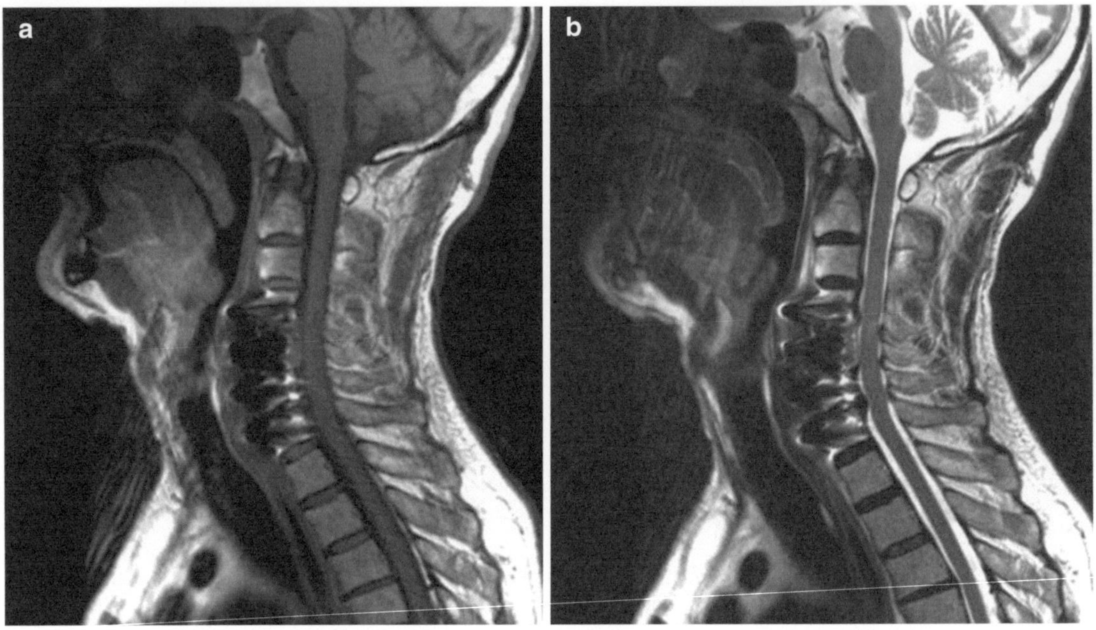

Fig. 16.21 T1 (**a**), T2 (**b**) enhanced images of the cervical spine obtained as imaging indicators to minimize metal artifacts. Although anterior cervical discectomy with fusion (ACDF) was performed at C4–7, it does not interfere with the evaluation of lesions within the spinal cord

and postoperative fibrosis after discectomy [6]. However, opinions are divided on the need for fat suppression images.

16.2.4 Others

Ultrasound is usually useful for evaluating fluid retention after surgery and aspirating fluid with a needle and is also used as a primary screening test for postoperative pain [3, 14]. Whole body bone scans are sometimes used to evaluate bone fusion, and the fused segment should be observed with cold sores after 6~12 months [3]. Technetium-leukocyte scans, gallium scans, or PET scans are also useful for evaluating infections around metal tools [14]. When the metal artifact is too severe and the MR image is not diagnostic, myelography is performed. However, lumbar spine puncture may be difficult due to postoperative soft tissue changes, and sometimes cervical spine puncture is needed [3]. Recently, by performing CT myelography along with conventional myelography using MDCT, MPR images can be obtained, which is very useful clinically (Fig. 16.22).

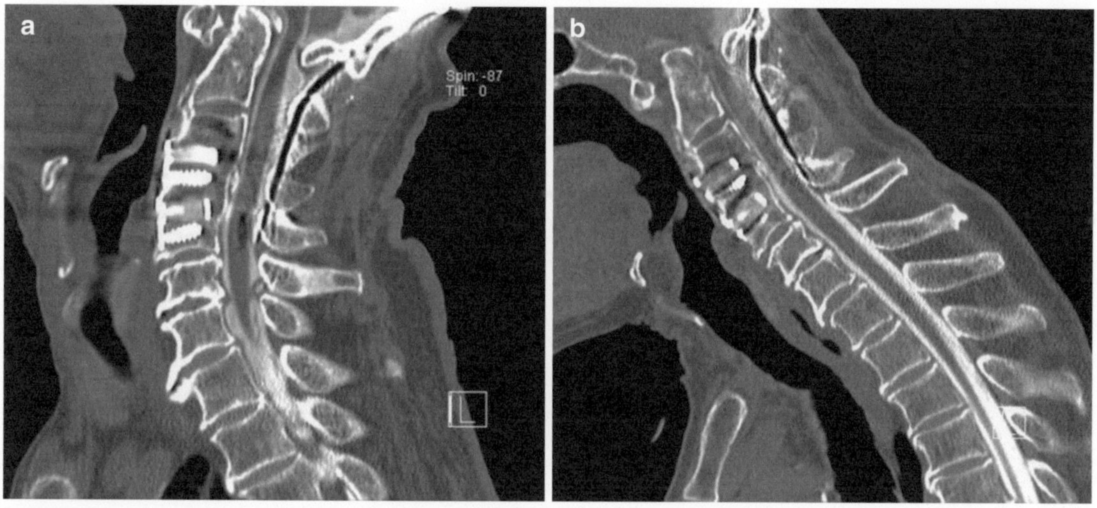

Fig. 16.22 CT myelography extension (**a**), flexion (**b**) sagittal reconstruction images of a patient who underwent C3–5 anterior cervical discectomy with fusion (ACDF) and posterior occipitocervical fusion. It is helping to diagnose spinal cord compression at the cranio-cervical junction by acquiring as an imaging indicator to minimize metal artifacts on MDCT devices

16.3 Post-spinal Surgery Imaging Findings and Complications

16.3.1 Postoperative Imaging Findings

Generally, it is evaluated by dividing it into about 6 months after intervertebral discectomy. Cases where early imaging is needed within about 2 weeks after surgery are cases where the sciatic nerve pain does not improve or recur early, cauda equina syndrome, and worsening of back pain [6]. The normal findings that can be seen within 6 months after intervertebral discectomy are as follows [6]. A high signal intensity band leading from the nucleus pulposus to the annulus fibrosus can be observed in the T2 enhanced image, and this finding can be found up to about 2 months. Contrast enhancement in the annulus fibrosus. This is also normal, and disc space enhancement can be seen in about 67% up to 6 weeks after surgery (Fig. 16.23a). The nucleus pulposus may appear as a low signal or weak high signal intensity, and the height of the intervertebral disc may decrease depending on the extent of the discectomy. The bone marrow around the endplate can show signal intensity similar to Modic type 1 (fibrovascular) endplate change, that is, T1 low signal, T2 high signal intensity. Immediately after surgery, the anterior epidural space may increase in soft tissue, and due to tissue cuts, swelling, bleeding, etc. the boundary of the annulus fibrosus may be unclear, showing findings similar to preoperative disc herniation (Fig. 16.23b). This tumor-like effect with increased epidural soft tissue is seen in about 80%, and it is said to be found in about 50% after 2 months of surgery, gradually reducing in volume as swelling and hematoma decrease and are replaced by fibrosis [6, 18]. Early after surgery, due to damage to the blood–nerve barrier, enhancement along the nerve root can occur and can be observed in about 20~62% within 3~6 weeks, but it is normal not to enhance after 6 months (Fig. 16.23d). It is also often observed that the nerve root is invaded by epidural soft tissue. At this time, adhesion of the cauda equina at the discectomy site can often be seen, which gradually normalizes. The thecal sac expands further up to 3 weeks and then gradually contracts [18]. The laminectomy site may be filled with medium signal intensity tissue, other than the partially resected ligamentum flavum. There are cases where a fat graft is filled to minimize epidural fibrosis, which should not be confused with post-operative bleeding. Enhancement of the facet joint can be observed normally up to 6 weeks, and the paraspinal muscle can appear as T1 low signal, T2

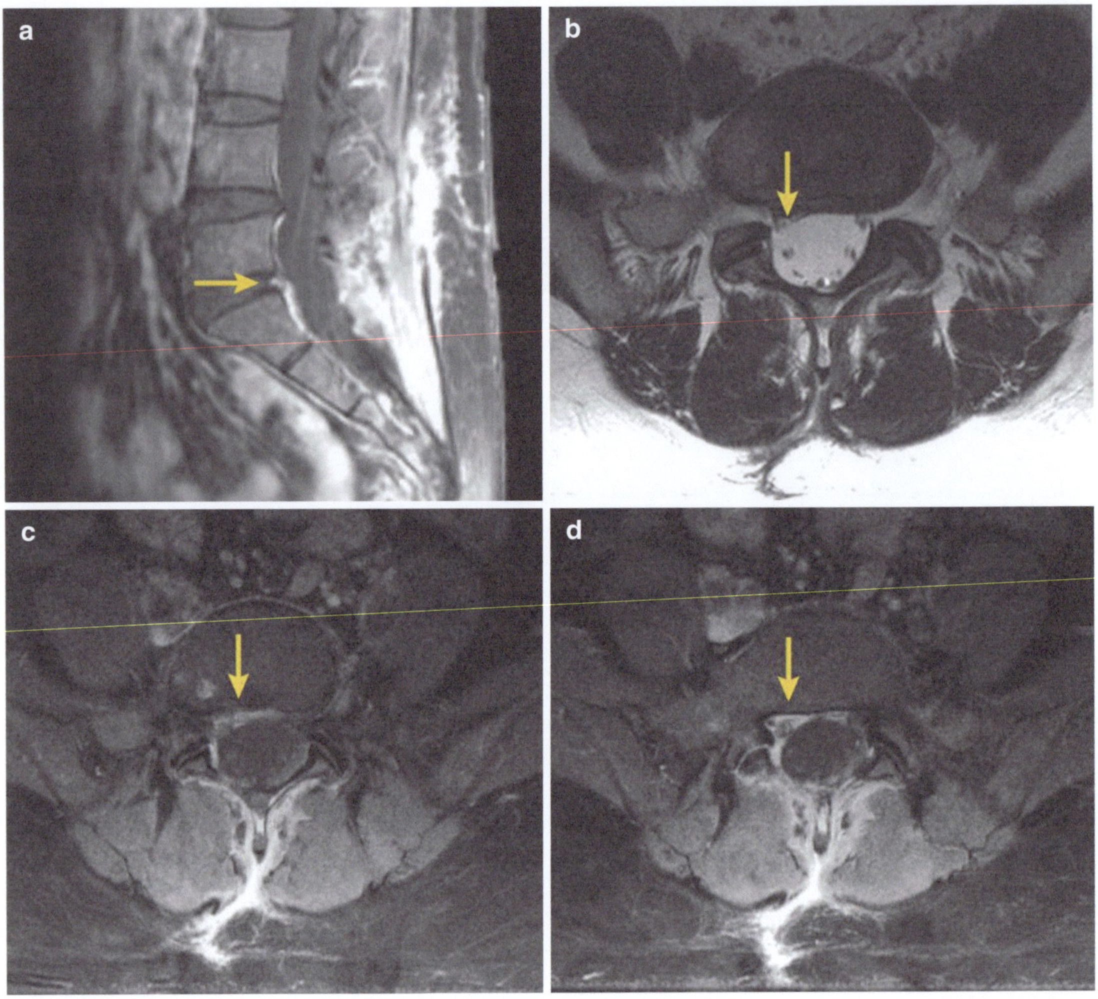

Fig. 16.23 MR image taken 3 months after performing right partial laminectomy and discectomy at L5–S1. (**a**) A small contrast enhancement is seen in the posterior disc on the fat-suppressed contrast-enhanced sagittal T1-weighted image (arrow). On the axial T2 (**b**), contrast-enhanced T1 (**c**) weighted images, unclear contrast enhancement findings due to edema, increased extradural connective tissue, etc. are seen in the right subarticular zone of the disc where discectomy was performed (arrow). On the axial contrast-enhanced T1 (**d**) weighted image, the soft tissue of the right anterior epidural space directly below the disc and the right L5 nerve root are being enhanced (arrow)

high signal intensity due to swelling. The incision path that enhances around the spinous process subcutaneous tissue layer can be observed, and this is almost seen in all patients up to about 3 weeks, and most of them do not enhance after about 3 months. Small fluid retention can be seen normally early after surgery, especially well observed where laminectomy was performed, and it is impossible to distinguish infected fluid retention only by MR imaging findings [6]. After discectomy, 6 months later, the defect site of the annulus fibrosus, which previously showed high signal intensity, gradually changes to low signal intensity on T2 enhanced images as it heals, and enhancement of the disc space can be seen in about 86% at 6 months after surgery (Fig. 16.24). There are reports that most epidural soft tissues are observed as scars that do not show a tumor-like effect after 6 months of surgery, but in other studies, it is said to persist as epidural fibrosis similar to a tumor-like shape in about 50% for 1 year after surgery [6]. The degree of enhancement of epidural fibrosis varies, and it is

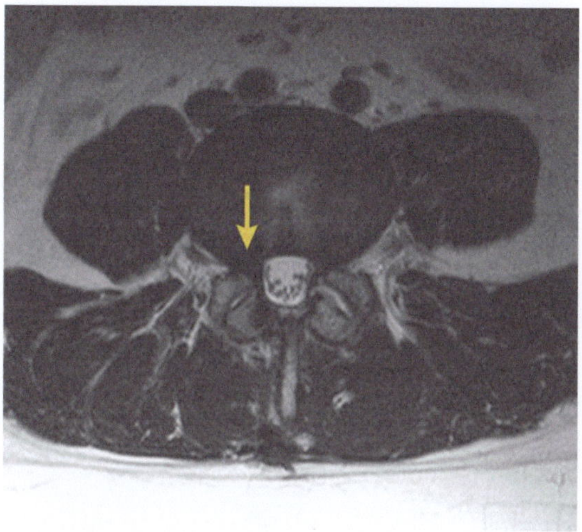

Fig. 16.24 On the axial T2-weighted image taken 24 months after performing L4–5 discectomy, the annulus fibrosus of the discectomy site appears as low signal intensity (arrow)

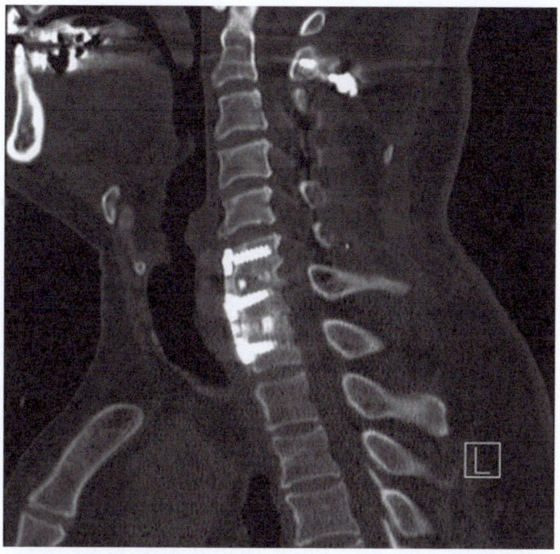

Fig. 16.25 Bone fusion is seen between the vertebral bodies in the sagittal reconstruction CT image of a patient who underwent C6–T1 ACDF

known to be most enhanced at 9 months after surgery [6]. At the laminectomy site, scarification progresses to appear as a T1 intermediate, T2 low signal intensity area with blurred boundaries, and enhancement remains at the boundary area with soft tissue. It can be. After 6 months of alcohol, facet joint enhancement can be seen in about 53%, and paraspinal muscle enhancement is observed in about 18% [6].

The primary purpose of using devices in spinal fusion is to stabilize the spine until fusion is complete [1]. The strictest definition of spinal fusion is the connection between two bone structures with trabecular bone, especially between the transverse processes in posterior fusion, between the two joint surfaces in facet fusion, and between the two adjacent vertebral bodies, which is referred to as bony fusion (Fig. 16.25). Pseudarthrosis is known to occur in about 5~34%, but there is still no non-invasive gold standard to check the status of fusion [1, 3]. Usually, movements within 2~5° in simple radiographic flexion/extension images are considered normal, but there are various variables such as limited movement when shooting in patients with back pain, so it is difficult to use flexion/extension images as a gold standard. Clinically, successful fusion is evaluated when pain is reduced and a definite range of motion restriction is confirmed, which is called functional arthrodesis. However, radiologically, immature bone grafts or incomplete bone connections may be seen, which is explained by the contribution of unmineralized osteoid to stability [1]. It is difficult to evaluate the fusion material covered by metal devices, especially it is difficult to evaluate the fusion of bone grafts filled inside the interbody cage, and it is known that bone fusion is complete by observing the bony connection formed in front and behind the cage (Fig. 16.3) [4]. The Brantigan cage made of carbon fiber is radiolucent, so the maturity of the bone graft can be well evaluated in simple radiographs [1, 3]. In studies compared with surgery, it is said that actual bone fusion is underestimated in simple radiographs, and CT is reported to be more accurate, but in CT, it is said that about 22% shows inconsistency with surgical findings [1]. CT is most useful for evaluating bone fusion, especially useful for evaluating fusion between facet joints, and MR imaging has limitations in evaluating bone fusion. Immediately after surgery, basic anteroposterior and lateral simple radiographs are performed, and if there are no major problems, start shooting flexion/extension images around 6~8 weeks after surgery and it is good to perform continuous examinations until fusion is completed around 9~14 months [1].

16.3.2 Complications Related to Surgery Such as Spinal Fusion, Instrumentation

The incidence of all complications occurring after spinal surgery is reported to be about 16.4% [19]. Complications occur more frequently after thoracolumbar spine surgery than after cervical spine surgery, with about 8.9% after cervical spine surgery and about 17.8% after thoracolumbar spine surgery [19].

Spinal fusion has been widely performed to date, but there are still unresolved issues. These include adjacent segmental disease (ASD), pseudoarthrosis, and donor site morbidity [9]. The rigidity caused by spinal fusion affects adjacent abnormal stress can be provided to the segment, which can induce the acceleration of degenerative changes in adjacent segments (ASD) (Fig. 16.26) [9]. Symptomatic ASD requiring additional decompression or fusion after lumbar spine fusion is known to occur in about 17% within 5 years and about 36% within 10 years [20]. After cervical spine fusion, symptomatic ASD is said to occur in about 25% within 10 years [8]. However, reports continue to suggest that ASD is a continuum of natural degenerative changes [8, 9]. The incidence of pseudarthrosis or non-union has been reported variably, and it is said to occur in about 2.3~83.3% after lumbar spine fusion (Fig. 16.27) [9]. Fractures or dislocations of

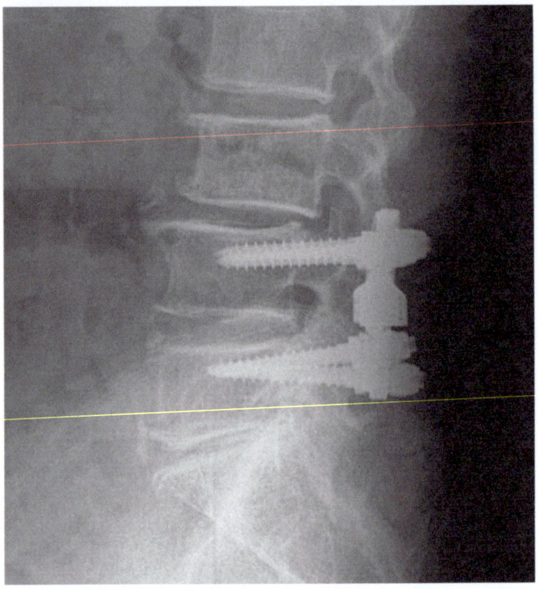

Fig. 16.26 Lateral photo of a patient who underwent L4–5 pedicle screw fixation. More severe degenerative changes and retrolisthesis are seen in the adjacent L3–4 disc than in other areas

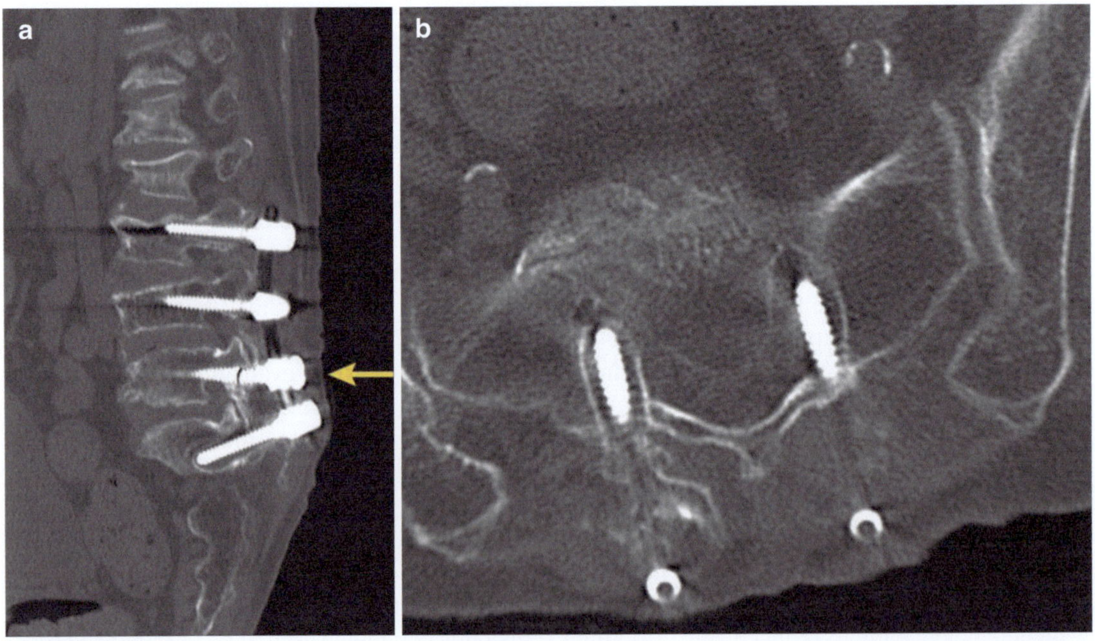

Fig. 16.27 Sagittal (**a**), axial (**b**) reconstruction CT images of a patient who underwent L3–S1 pedicle screw fixation. Osteolysis is seen around the screws on both sides of S1, and a fracture is seen on the right screw of L5 (arrow)

metallic rods, plates, screws, etc. are strong indicators of pseudarthrosis (Fig. 16.27), and the more segments that undergo fusion, the higher the probability of union failure [1]. After anterior instrumentation of the cervical spine, device fractures or loosening occur in about 35%, and screws not fixed to the metal plate fail more frequently [8]. In the cervical spine, if only laminectomy is performed without instrumentation, it can lead to postoperative instability, kyphosis, or worsening of nerve damage [8]. Especially in children or young people, it is severe in cases where there was pre-existing kyphosis or segmental instability, and it is a method to maintain preoperative lordosis by performing laminectomy and instrumentation together [8]. Kyphosis can also occur after laminoplasty, especially when C2 is included or the preoperative lordotic angle is <10° [8].

16.3.3 Arachnoiditis

Postoperative arachnoiditis can be divided into three forms, the first of which is the formation of a central connective tissue mass in the dural sac where the nerve roots adhere (Fig. 16.28a) [6, 18]. Instead of the normal feather shape, the nerve roots are tangled together, and it is well observed in CT myelography or MR T1, T2 enhanced axial images. The second form is when the nerve roots adhere to the dura, showing an "empty thecal sac sign," and in MR images, only the CSF signal intensity in the dural sac is found, and the nerve roots can be seen adhered to the dura at the edge (Fig. 16.28b). The third form is when inflammatory nodules, which appear to be the final stage of the inflammatory response, fill the inside of the dural sac, and in myelography, you can see the contrast medium filling in a candle-dripping shape along with the blockage of the contrast medium column, and in MR and CT myelography, it appears like a nonspecific connective tissue nodule. These three forms can be mixed, especially central adhesion and peripheral adhesion often occur together [18]. In most cases, contrast enhancement is not well done, and even when it appears in the form of inflammatory nodules, contrast enhancement is much less than in tumorous arachnoiditis. After surgery, cauda equina adhesion usually occurs early, which is known to naturally disappear within 1~6 weeks [18].

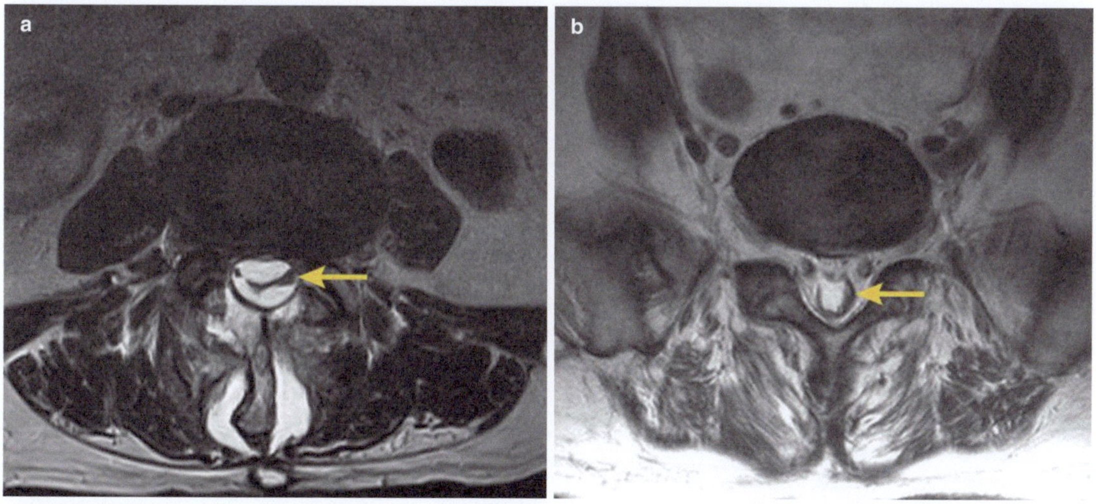

Fig. 16.28 Arachnoiditis that occurred after lumbar spine surgery. (**a**) Bilateral laminectomy was performed and the nerve rootlets inside the dural sac are adhered in the center (arrow). (**b**) The nerve rootlets inside the dural sac are adhered along the periphery of the dural sac (arrow)

16.3.4 Spinal Stenosis

Bony stenosis accounts for about 60% of the causes of failed back surgery syndrome (FBSS). It is known to account for a certain degree. Various mechanisms can cause bony spinal stenosis, including lateral recess stenosis due to bone hyperplasia after facetectomy (Fig. 16.29a,

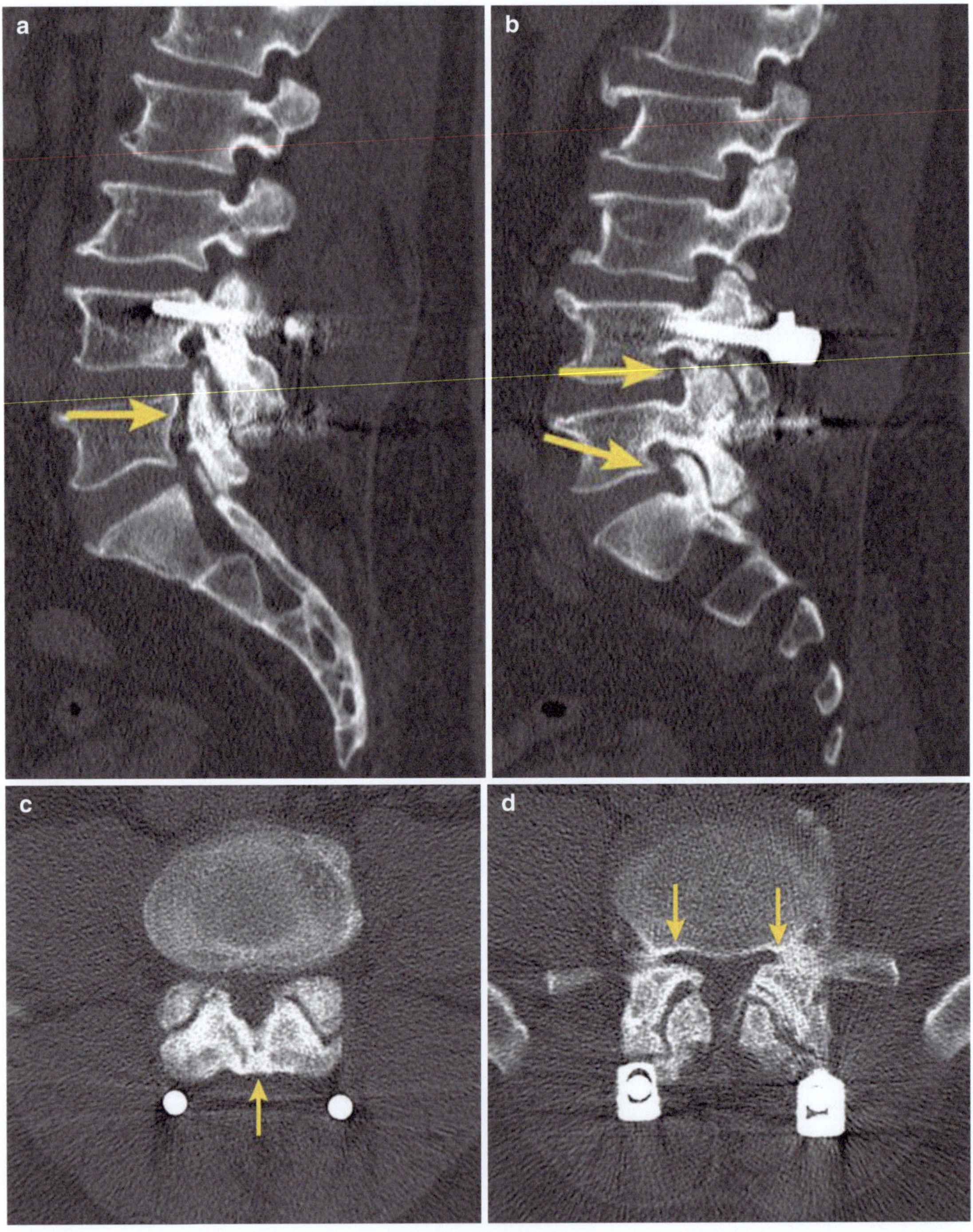

Fig. 16.29 CT images of a patient who underwent L4–5 interfacet fusion and pedicle screw fixation. Lateral recess stenosis due to bony hypertrophy (**a**, **d**), neural foraminal stenosis (**b**), and central canal stenosis (**c**) are seen (arrow)

d), posterior central canal, or lateral recess stenosis due to bone hyperplasia after posterior fusion (Fig. 16.29c), cases where the bone hyperplasias into the spinal canal or nerve foramen after anterior fusion, osteophyte that occurs as degenerative changes in the intervertebral disc continue, nerve foramen or lateral recess stenosis due to the facet joint that sinks together as the height of the intervertebral disc space decreases after discectomy, and spinal canal stenosis due to postoperative spondylolisthesis [18]. Bony stenosis appears variously on MR depending on the degree of bone marrow formation and hardening inside, with the hardened part showing low signal intensity in both T1 and T2 enhanced images, eroding the epidural or nerve foramen and eliminating fat. Osteophytes containing fatty bone marrow can confirm the high signal intensity of fat in T1 enhanced images. It is useful to evaluate bony nerve foramen stenosis in the coronal plane, which mainly occurs due to osteophytes or downward movement and dislocation of the facet joint due to degenerative changes in the intervertebral disc (Fig. 16.29b) [18].

16.3.5 Epidural Fibrosis and Recurrent Disc Herniation

In the lumbar region, the formation of an epidural scar occurs when normal epidural fat tissue is replaced with fibrous tissue after discectomy and laminectomy. Such epidural fibrosis causes recurrent radiculopathy after surgery by adhering the dura mater and nerve roots to surrounding structures and is known to account for about 8~14% of FBSS [6, 18]. Many studies report that excessive fibrous tissue around the nerve root can cause various symptoms, as nerve roots surrounded by collagen scar are damaged by increased tension, axoplasmic transport disorders, and restricted blood circulation [18]. Therefore, epidural fibrosis after discectomy is known to have a negative impact on long-term surgical outcomes. In a double-blind randomized controlled trial involving 197 patients who underwent unilateral lumbar spine discectomy, the degree of radiculopathy was proportional to the degree of epidural fibrosis observed in MR findings obtained 6 months after surgery, and patients with excessive epidural fibrosis had a 3.2 times higher recurrence rate of radiculopathy than those without [21]. Numerous attempts and studies have been conducted to minimize such epidural fibrosis and various potential substances (silastic, Dacron, methacrylate, bone graft, synthetic membrane or foam, fat graft, carboxymethylcellulose, elastase, sodium hyaluronate) have been used and evaluated in surgery [6, 18].

Recurrent disc herniation is defined as disc herniation that occurs on the same or opposite side of the same level after a pain-free period of 6 months or more [6]. The incidence is about 5~11%, and symptoms can improve by removing the escaped intervertebral disc through reoperation. On the other hand, reoperation is contraindicated for epidural fibrosis, so it is important to distinguish these two complications, especially in the anterior epidural space [6]. Recurrent/residual disc herniation appears as a polyp-shaped T1, T2 low signal intensity in the anterior epidural. It appears as a structure connected to the mother disc in space (if not sequestration) (Fig. 16.30). However, when it is large, it can show a T2 high signal intensity in the center. The margin of the herniated disc usually shows a low signal intensity border, which is due to the surrounding posterior longitudinal ligament or annulus fibrosus. Epidural fibrosis generally shows a medium signal intensity and changes to a low signal intensity about 2 years after surgery (Fig. 16.31). Intervertebral disc fragments also have smoother boundaries than fibrosis. The mass effect can occur in both diseases, so it is not very helpful in differentiation, but dural retraction towards soft tissue suggests fibrosis (Fig. 16.31) [6]. Contrast-enhanced MR imaging is most useful for distinguishing between epi-

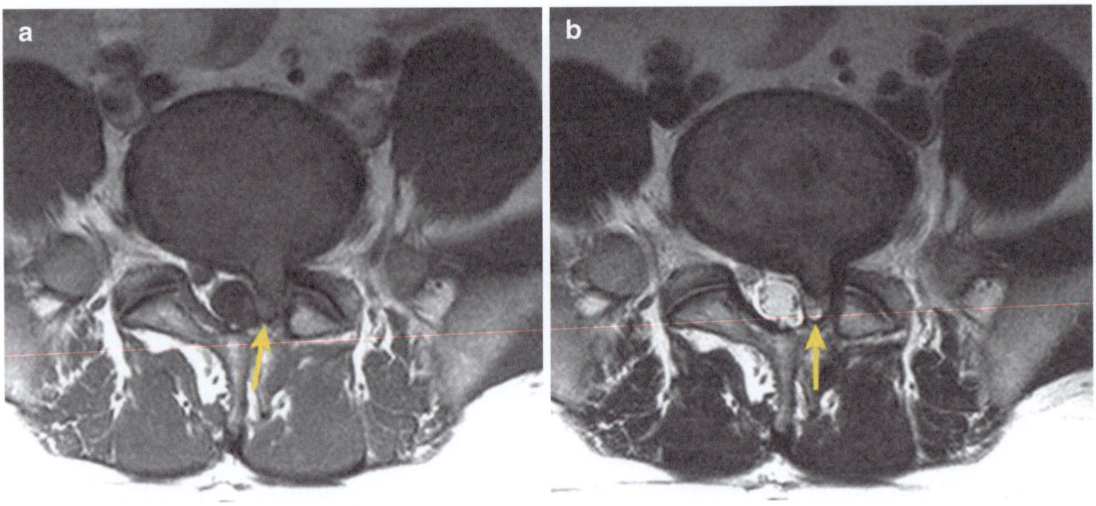

Fig. 16.30 Recurrent/residual intervertebral disc herniation that occurred after left L4–5 laminectomy and discectomy is seen on axial T1 (**a**), T2 (**b**) images. The left L5 nerve root is compressed (arrow)

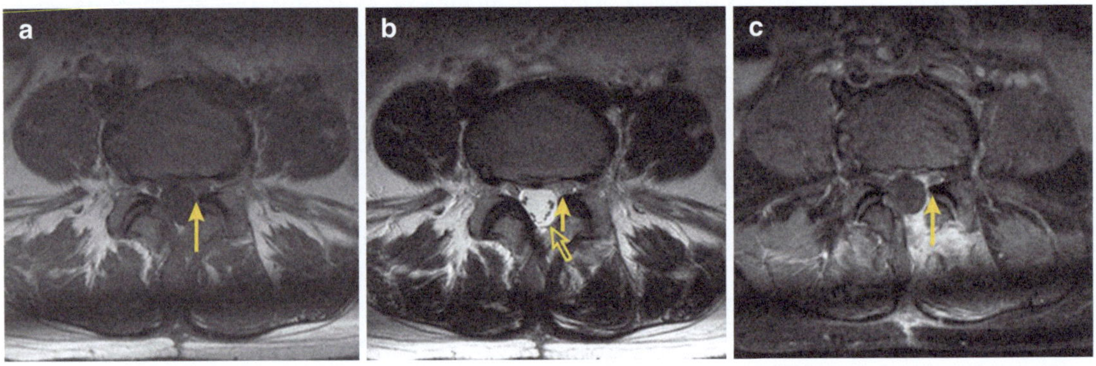

Fig. 16.31 Axial T1 (**a**), T2 (**b**), fat-suppressed contrast-enhanced T1 (**c**) images of a patient who underwent left L4–5 laminectomy and discectomy. Epidural fibrosis, which shows low signal intensity on T1, intermediate or slightly high signal intensity on T2, and is well enhanced, is seen around the left L5 nerve root, along with dural retraction to the left posterior (empty arrow)

dural fibrosis and recurrent disc herniation, with reported accuracy of 96~100%. Epidural fibrosis is well contrast-enhanced regardless of the post-operative period, but the escaped intervertebral disc is a non-vascular structure, so immediate contrast enhancement does not occur (Fig. 16.31). These findings can be divided into three categories: (1) only fibrosis, (2) only disc herniation, (3) fibrosis and disc herniation together [18]. However, the escaped intervertebral disc can also be contrast-enhanced in delayed images due to diffusion, can be contrast-enhanced at the border by granulation tissue, and if the fibrous tissue invades the escaped intervertebral disc or the escaped intervertebral disc is too small, the intervertebral disc can be contrast-enhanced (Fig. 16.32). It has also been reported that using fat-suppressed T1-weighted images when obtaining contrast-enhanced images is more useful for diagnosing epidural fibrosis [18]. It has also been reported that excessive epidural fibrosis or recurrent/residual intervertebral disc hernia-

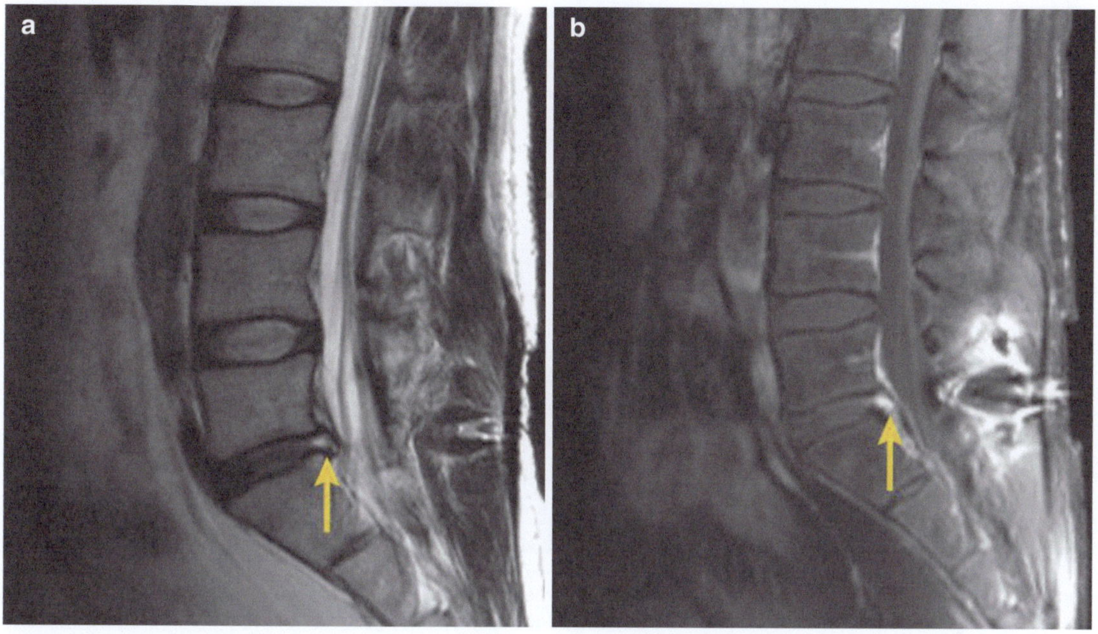

Fig. 16.32 Recurrent/residual intervertebral disc herniation is partially enhanced inside on coronal T2 (**a**), fat-suppressed contrast-enhanced T1 (**b**) images after L5–S1 discectomy (arrow)

tion can be seen even in asymptomatic patients after surgery [6]. Changes also occur in the affected nerve root, and generally, the finding of a thickened nerve root has no diagnostic meaning, and the position change of the nerve root or contrast enhancement findings seen after 6 months postoperatively are known to be related to clinical symptoms [6].

16.3.6 Pseudomeningocele

Pseudomeningocele occurs when cerebrospinal fluid leaks through the dura mater damaged during surgery. Pseudomeningocele can also be a potential cause of FBSS, can cause back pain, and radicular pain caused by trapped nerve roots has been reported [6]. On MR images, a round structure with cerebrospinal fluid signal intensity is seen at the location where laminectomy was performed behind the dura mater (Fig. 16.33) [18]. It can be contrast-enhanced and a fibrous capsule with medium signal intensity may exist, and a fluid-fluid level due to debris or blood components may be seen inside. However, it is often difficult to accurately identify the location of dural damage [6, 18].

16.3.7 Infection

Postoperative intervertebral discitis can be divided into aseptic and infectious, and generally, infectious intervertebral discitis is accompanied by back pain and fever within 8 weeks after surgery, and blood inflammatory markers such as CRP or ESR increase. Contrast-enhanced MR imaging is the most suitable imaging technique for diagnosing intervertebral discitis, osteomyelitis, soft tissue abscess, etc. [6, 18]. MR images show a decrease or loss of disc space, high signal intensity within the intervertebral disc on T2-weighted images, loss of intra-nuclear cleft, loss of endplate boundaries and erosion, and

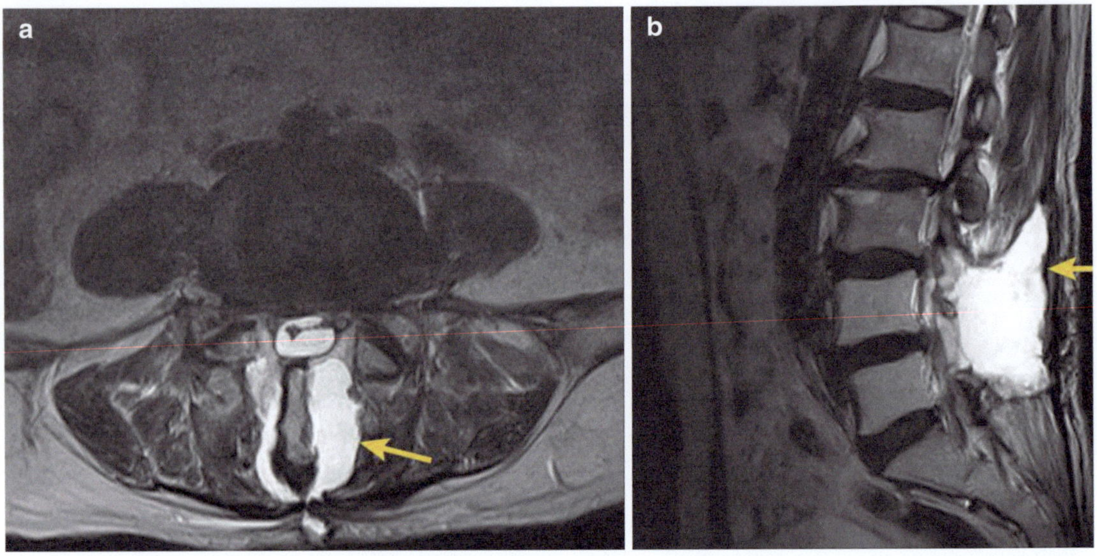

Fig. 16.33 Axial (**a**), coronal (**b**) T2 images of a patient who underwent laminectomy and discectomy between L3–5 show a high signal intensity pseudomeningocele at the laminectomy site and posterior paraspinal muscle (arrow)

bone marrow edema of the vertebral body (Fig. 16.34). After surgery, degenerative disc changes can also show similar findings, especially in Modic type 1 (fibrovascular) endplate marrow changes. However, the biggest difference is that the degenerative disc shows low signal intensity on T2-weighted images (Fig. 16.34b) [6]. More definitive differentiation is possible with contrast-enhanced images, with the most reliable contrast enhancement pattern suggesting infection being the overall, irregular enhancement of the intervertebral disc, annulus fibrosus, and bone marrow of the vertebral body [6, 18]. Postoperative degenerative intervertebral discs can also be enhanced, but they are mainly linear enhancements parallel to the endplate. Phlegmon appears as a finding of chronic enhancement in the soft tissue without abscess formation in the center, and it is well distinguished from an abscess accompanied by non-enhancing pus inside (Fig. 16.34e). MR imaging can accurately understand the relationship with surrounding soft tissues and neural structures, and it is much more accurate than gallium scans in differentiating from other tumors or degenerative changes. Gallium scans have the advantage of being able to detect intervertebral discitis earlier than MR imaging and more sensitively detect changes in treatment [18].

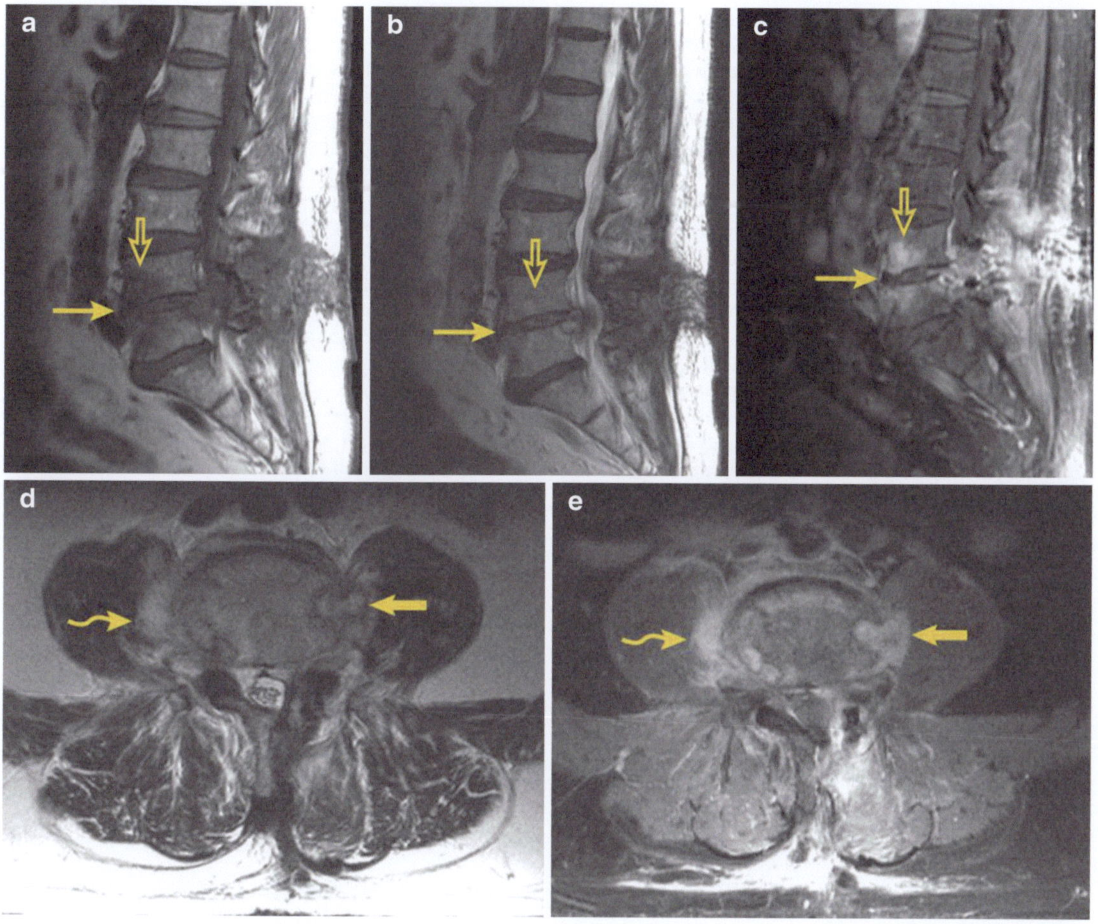

Fig. 16.34 Coronal T1 (**a**), T2 (**b**), fat-suppressed contrast-enhanced T1 (**c**) images, axial T2 (**d**), fat-suppressed contrast-enhanced T1 (**e**) images of a patient who developed infectious spondylitis after L4–5 laminectomy and discectomy. The intervertebral disc shows low signal intensity on T1, high signal intensity on T2, and some enhancement (arrow), and erosion of low signal intensity on T1 and bone marrow edema of low signal intensity on T1, high signal intensity on T2, and well-enhanced on the adjacent endplate (empty arrow) are seen. A poorly defined paravertebral phlegmon shows high signal intensity on T2, diffuse enhancement (curved arrow), and is accompanied by a small abscess that does not enhance in the center (thick arrow)

Bibliography

1. Andrews CL. Evaluation of the postoperative spine: spinal instrumentation and fusion. Semin Musculoskelet Radiol. 2000;4(3):259–79.
2. Ho-yeol J, Young-soo K. Dynamic spine reconstruction. I. Introduction. In: Korean spine neurosurgery society. Spine study the textbook of spine. 1st ed. Gunja Publishing Company; 2008. p. 1239–64.
3. Rutherford EE, Tarplett LJ, Davis EM, Harley JM, King LJ. Lumbar spinal fusion and stabilization: hardware, techniques, and imaging appearances. Radiographics. 2007;27:1737–49.
4. Shah LM. Hardware. Spine postprocedural imaging. In: Ross JS, et al., editors. Diagnostic imaging spine. 2nd ed. Amirsys; 2010. VII-2-2~41.
5. Seok-won K, Ho S. Lumbar spine posterior approach. In: Korean Spine Neurosurgery Society, editor. Spine study the textbook of spine. 1st ed. Gunja Publishing Company; 2008. p. 451–70.
6. Saifuddin SBA. MRI of the post-discectomy lumbar spine. Clin Radiol. 2002;57:969–81.
7. Djurasovic M, Glassman SD, Carreon LY, Dimar JR. Contemporary management of symptomatic lumbar spinal stenosis. Orthop Clin N Am. 2010;41:183–91.

8. Rao RD, Currier BL, Albert TJ, et al. Degenerative cervical spondylosis: clinical syndromes, pathogenesis, and management. J Bone Joint Surg Am. 2007;89:1360–78.
9. Kishen TJ, Diwan AD. Fusion versus disc replacement for degenerative conditions of the lumbar and cervical spine: quid est testimonium? Orthop Clin N Am. 2010;41:167–81.
10. Dae-cheol C, Ju-kyung S. Dual vertebral joint and upper cervical spine anterior approach. In: Korean Spinal Neurosurgery Society, editor. Spine study the textbook of spine. 1st ed. Gunja Publishing Company; 2008. p. 369–76.
11. Woo-kyung K. Middle-lower cervical spine anterior approach. In: Korean Spinal Neurosurgery Society, editor. Spine study the textbook of spine. 1st ed. Gunja Publishing Company; 2008. p. 377–91.
12. Yong-jae C, Sang-jin K. Cervical spine posterior approach. In: Korean spinal neurosurgery society. Spine study the textbook of spine. 1st ed. Gunja Publishing Company; 2008. p. 392–403.
13. Ross JS. Surgical approaches. Section 1. Postoperative imaging and complications. Part VII. Spine postprocedural imaging. In: Ross JS, Moore KR, Shah LM, Borg B, Crim J, editors. Diagnostic imaging spine. 2nd ed. Amirsys; 2010. VII-1-2.
14. Berquist TH. Imaging of the postoperative spine. Radiol Clin North Am. 2006;44:407–18.
15. Ohashi K, El-Khoury GY. Musculoskeletal CT: recent advantages and current clinical applications. Radiol Clin North Am. 2009;47:387–409.
16. Lee M, Kim S, Lee S, et al. Overcoming artifacts from metallic orthopedic implants at high field-strength MR imaging and multidetector CT. Radiographics. 2007;27:791–803.
17. Douglas-Akinwande AC, Buckwalter KA, Rydberg J, Rankin JL, Choplin RH. Multichannel CT: evaluating the spine in postoperative patients with orthopedic hardware. Radiographics. 2006;26:S97–S110.
18. Ross JS. Magnetic resonance imaging of the postoperative spine. Semin Musculoskelet Radiol. 2000;4(3):281–91.
19. Nasser R, Yadla S, Maltenfort MG, et al. Complications in spine surgery. J Neurosurg Spine. 2010;13:144–57.
20. Ghiselli G, Wang JC, Bhatia NN, et al. Adjacent segment degeneration in the lumbar spine. J Bone Joint Surg Am. 2004;86(7):1497–503.
21. Ross JS, Robertson JT, Fredrickson RA, et al. Association between peridural scar and recurrent radicular pain after lumbar discectomy: magnetic resonance evaluation. Neurosurgery. 2006;38:855–63.

17 Brachial Plexus Disorders

In Sook Lee

17.1 Overview

The brachial plexus is a network of nerves that supply motor and sensory nerve branches to the upper limbs, including the shoulder, chest, arm, and hand. It is quite difficult to clinically distinguish brachial plexopathy and other spinal-related abnormalities, and electrophysiological diagnostic methods are often difficult to perform due to the deep location of the brachial plexus, often resulting in intermediate results [1]. Moreover, due to ambiguous clinical symptoms, uncommon characteristics, and complex anatomical structure, diagnosing pathological conditions of the brachial plexus is difficult both clinically and radiologically, and there is a tendency to evaluate it necessarily through magnetic resonance imaging (MRI) [2–4]. Recently, the use of MR neurography (MRN) for more detailed evaluation in cases where brachial plexopathy or peripheral neuropathy is suspected or diagnosed has increased, and the results are also excellent [4–6].

I. S. Lee (✉)
Department of Radiology, Pusan National University College of Medicine, Yangsan-si, Republic of Korea
e-mail: lis@pusan.ac.kr

17.2 Anatomical Considerations of the Brachial Plexus

17.2.1 Root, Trunk, Division, and Cord

The brachial plexus is formed by the C5–8 and T1 spinal nerves and includes anterior (motor) and posterior (sensory) nerve rootlet fibers. The roots, the first part of the plexus, are named according to their origin. The axial plane best shows the anterior and posterior nerve rootlets, and each root exits the corresponding neural foramen. Each root is divided into pre-ganglionic and post-ganglionic parts based on the dorsal root ganglion (DRG). The pre-ganglionic area includes the ventral and dorsal nerve rootlet's spinal root entry zone, their intradural course, and their course within the neural foramen to their dorsal root ganglion. The anterior branches (rami) of the post-ganglionic part connect to the plexus (Fig. 17.1) [7, 8].

The brachial plexus includes roots, trunks, divisions, cords, and branches (Fig. 17.2) [9]. Occasionally, the brachial plexus receives additional distribution from the C4 and T2 roots as a variant [1]. The roots that have exited the nerve holes travel into the interscalene space. The interscalene space is bounded by the anterior scalene muscle in front, the middle/posterior scalene

© The Author(s), under exclusive license to Springer Nature Singapore Pte Ltd. 2025

H. S. Kang, J. W. Lee (eds.), *Spinal Imaging*, https://doi.org/10.1007/978-981-95-1386-4_17

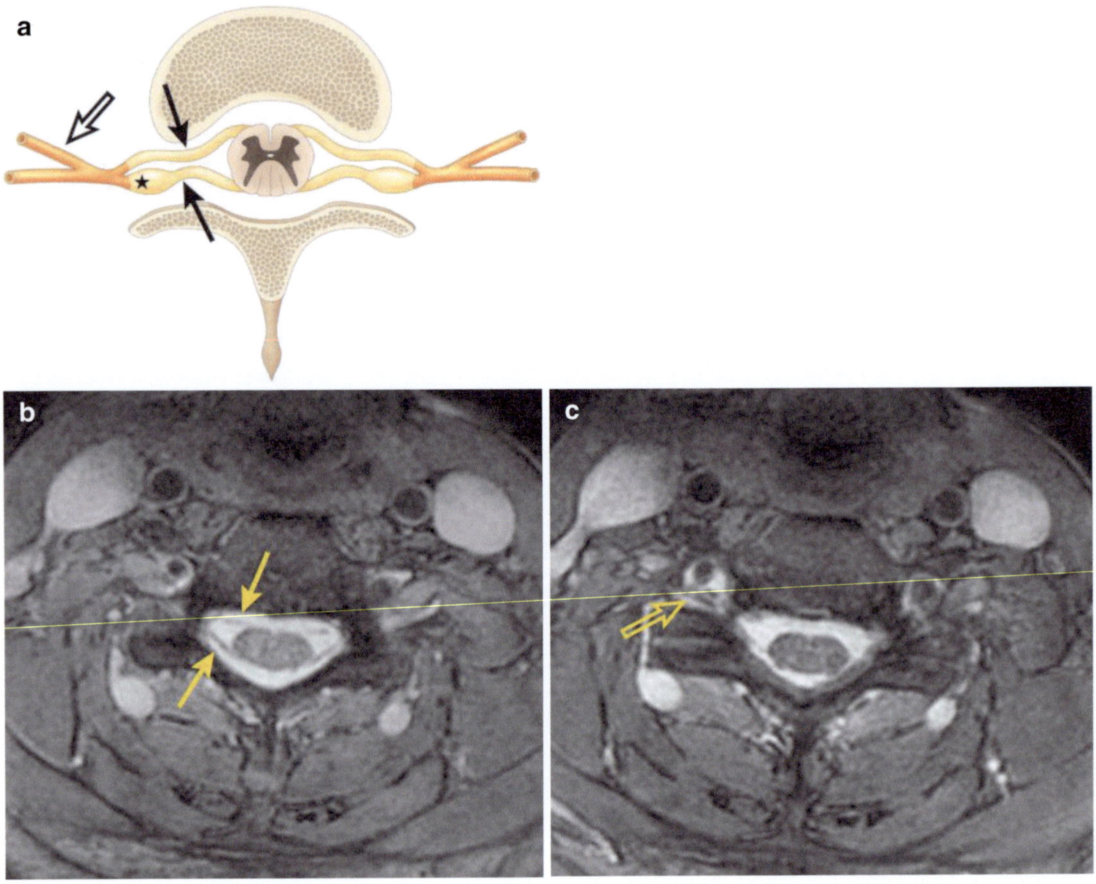

Fig. 17.1 Anatomical structure of the brachial plexus before and after the ganglion. (**a**) The nerve root is divided into pre-ganglionic (light yellow) and post-ganglionic (orange) around the dorsal root ganglion (asterisk). The anterior and posterior nerve rootlets (arrows) head towards the anterior ramus (empty arrow) through the neural foramen, which is connected to the brachial plexus. (**b**, **c**) In the continuous axial gradient echo images at the C5–6 position, the anterior and posterior nerve rootlets (arrows) merge to form the nerve root (empty arrow) and exit through the neural foramen

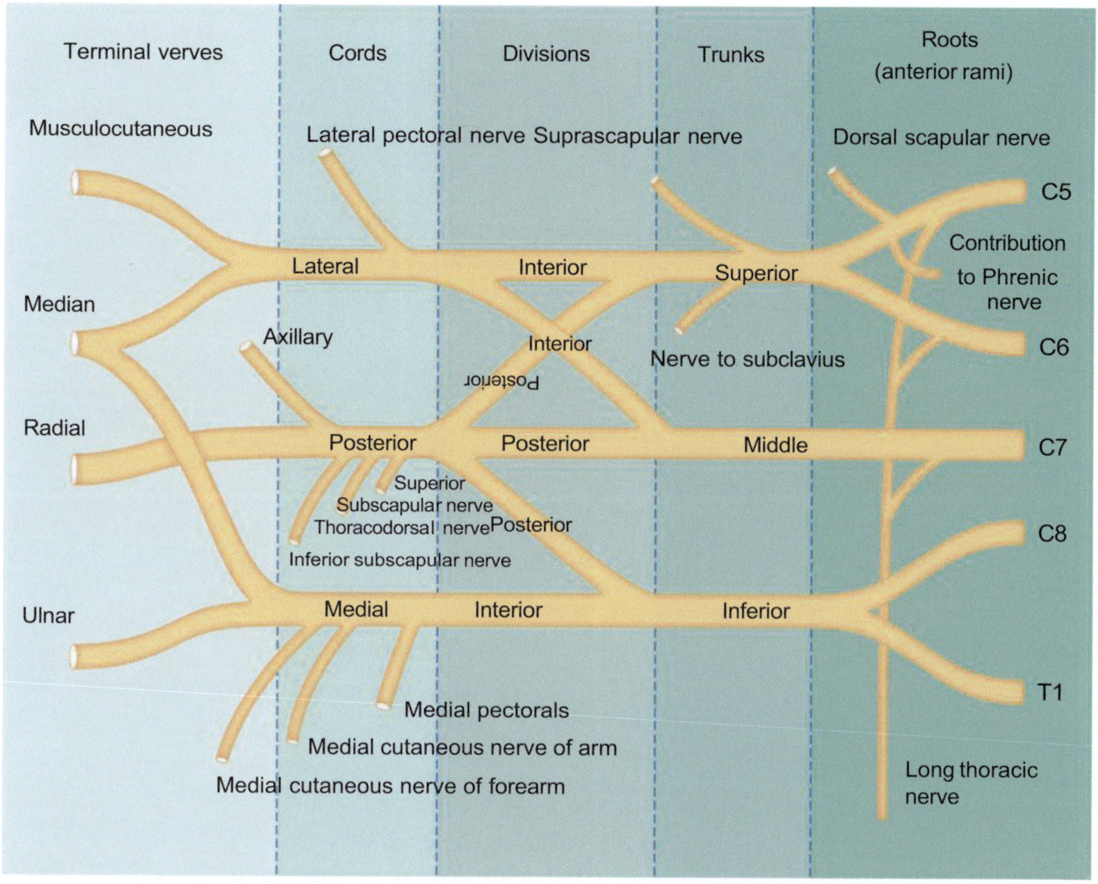

Fig. 17.2 Schematic of the entire brachial plexus. The brachial plexus is formed by the C5–8 and T1 spinal nerves and is divided into roots, trunks, divisions, and cords. It consists of five roots, three trunks, six divisions, three cords, and five terminal branches

muscles behind, and the subclavian artery and first rib below [2, 4]. A total of three trunks are located in this interscalene space (Fig. 17.3a, b) [1].

On the lateral side of the middle scalene muscle, the upper two nerve roots (C5 & C6) merge to form the upper trunk, the middle nerve root (C7) connects to the middle trunk, and the lower two nerve roots (C8 & T1) merge to form the lower trunk [2, 4]. These three trunks travel posterosuperior to the subclavian artery, divide into anterior and posterior divisions in the costoclavicular triangle, becoming a total of six divisions, which are located laterally to the scalene muscles and superior to the clavicle [9, 10]. The costoclavicular triangle is bounded by the clavicle superiorly, the subclavius muscle anteriorly, and the first rib and middle scalene muscle posteriorly (Fig. 17.3c) [2, 4]. On the lateral side of the first rib, the divisions merge to form medial, lateral, and posterior cords, depending on their relationship with the ipsilateral subclavian/axillary artery [2, 3]. The three cords are located medially to the lateral border of the pectoralis minor muscle. Another landmark for the cords in the coronal plane is the subclavian artery, which is used to distinguish the medial, lateral, and posterior components (Fig. 17.3d, e) [9].

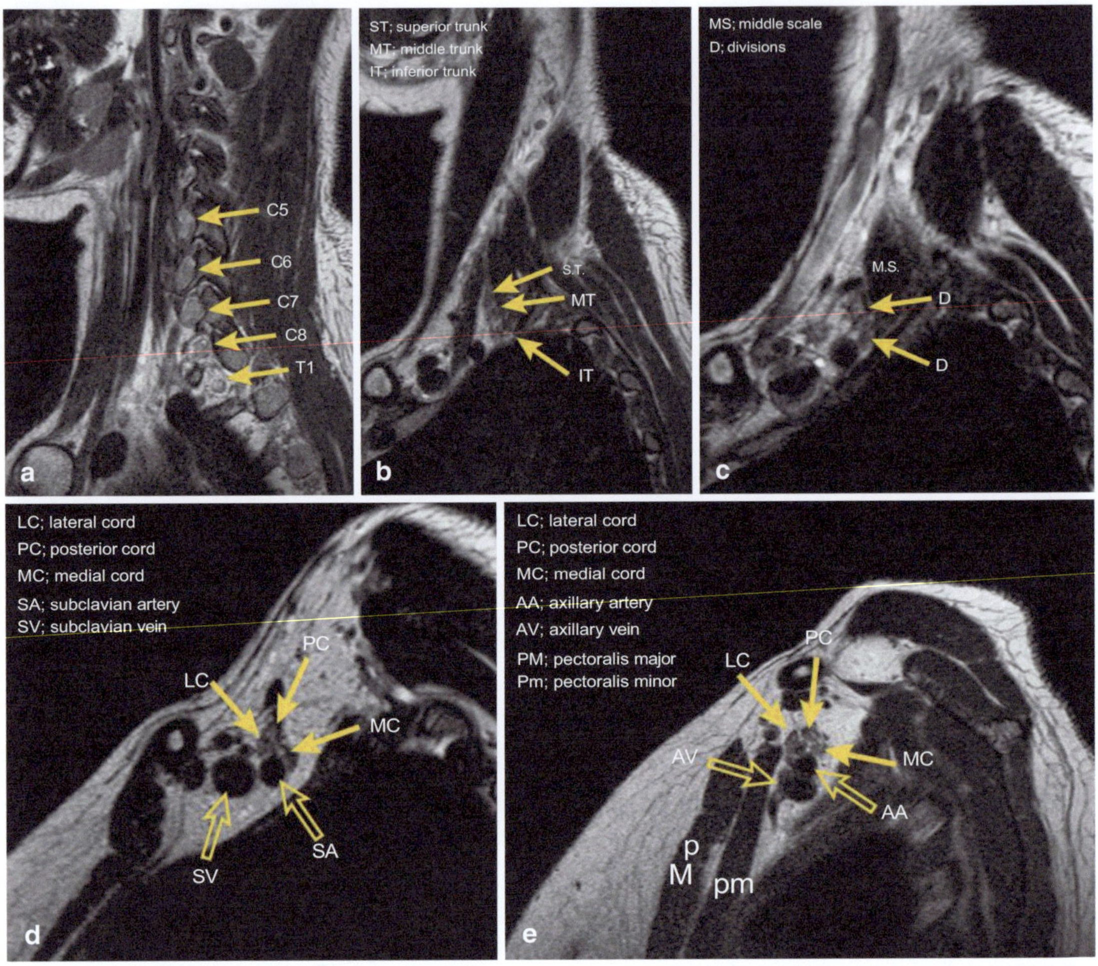

Fig. 17.3 Normal anatomy of the brachial plexus in a coronal T2-weighted MRI. (**a**) The nerve roots from C5 to T1 protrude through their respective foramina. (**b**) In the interscalene space, there are a total of three trunks (superior, middle, inferior). (**c**) In the costoclavicular triangle, there are six divisions, which are difficult to distinguish from each other in normal conditions. (**d**, **e**) On the lateral side of the first rib, and the medial posterior side of the pectoralis minor, the three cords are distinguished as medial, lateral, and posterior based on the subclavian/axillary artery

17.2.2 Terminal Branches and Innervation of the Brachial Plexus

The cords divide into five terminal nerves, the ulnar (medial cord), median (medial and lateral cords), musculocutaneous (lateral cord), radial (posterior cord), and axillary (posterior cord) nerves, slightly laterally to the lateral border of the pectoralis minor muscle [2, 4].

It is important to know the muscles innervated by the nerves that originate directly from the brachial plexus before the terminal branches are formed. The pattern of muscle atrophy caused by nerve block provides clues to the lesion site [9].

The long thoracic nerve, which branches off immediately after the C5–7 roots exit the nerve hole, innervates the serratus anterior muscle. A little further laterally, the C5 root branches off the dorsal scapular nerve and distributes to the levator scapulae and rhomboid major and minor muscles [9].

The posterior cords branch into the upper and lower subscapular nerves (distributed to the teres major and subscapular muscles), thoracodorsal nerve (distributed to the latissimus dorsi muscle), and axillary nerve (distributed to the teres minor and deltoid muscles). It innervates the distribution. The lateral cord innervates the biceps and coracobrachialis muscles through the musculocutaneous nerve. The medial cord branches the cutaneous nerves and the ulnar nerve to innervate the upper arm and forearm. The medial and lateral pectoral nerves originate from the medial and lateral cords, respectively, and they form a connection to distribute to the pectoralis major and pectoralis minor [9].

If you trace the peripheral nerves back to the spinal area, the C5 root innervates the supraspinatus, infraspinatus, and deltoid muscles, C6 innervates the biceps, C7 innervates the extensor muscles of the forearm and triceps, and C8 and T1 distribute to the flexor muscles of the fingers and the intrinsic muscles of the hand [10].

17.2.2.1 Suprascapular Nerve (C5, 6)

The suprascapular nerve is a motor-sensory nerve that supplies the shoulder joint and the supraspinatus and infraspinatus muscles. It originates from the upper trunk of the brachial plexus and travels laterally in the posterior triangle of the neck, entering the supraspinatus fossa covered by the transverse scapular ligament through the suprascapular notch of the scapula. This fibro-osseous tunnel is prone to nerve entrapment due to mass lesions such as joint periarticular cysts, varicosities, ligament or muscle attachment variants, rotator cuff tears, and tumors. The suprascapular nerve travels posteriorly to reach the infraspinatus fossa passing the spinoglenoid notch. This nerve distributes to the supraspinatus at the suprascapular notch, and further proximally to the infraspinatus. Therefore, if a lesion compressing this nerve is located around the suprascapular notch, both the supraspinatus and infraspinatus become denervated areas, and if it is located around the spinoglenoid notch, only the infraspinatus becomes a denervated area (Fig. 17.4). Patients may present with shoulder pain and weakness during abduction (supraspinatus) and external rotation (infraspinatus) [1, 11].

Electromyography can confirm abnormalities of the above nerves. In magnetic resonance neurography, the normal suprascapular nerve is usually not well seen, but in cases of abnormalities, it can be seen along the nerve path. Nerve entrapment by mass lesions and changes in denervated muscles are clearly visible [1, 11].

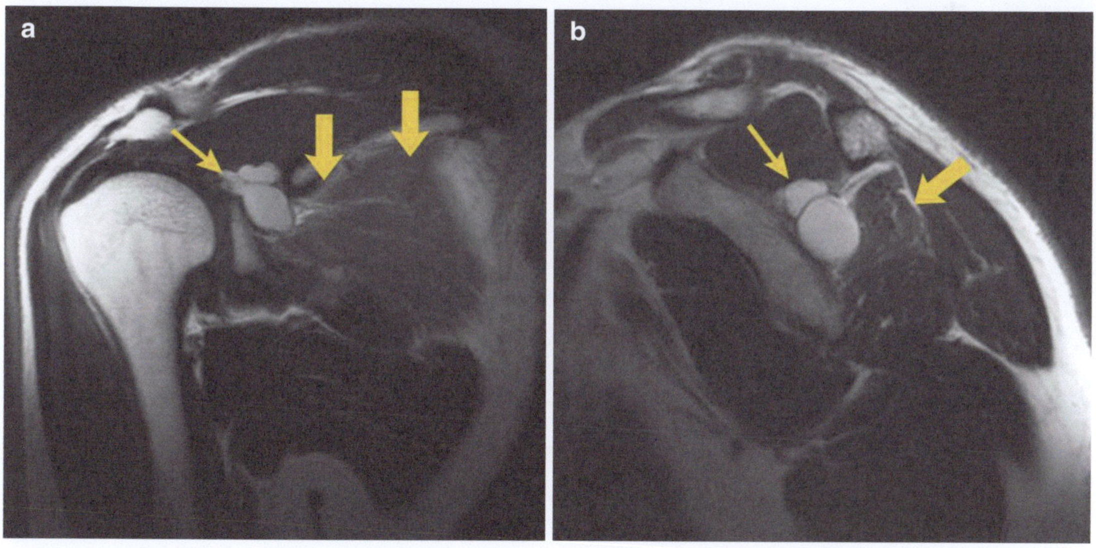

Fig. 17.4 Ganglion cyst compressing the suprascapular nerve. On the coronal (**a**) and sagittal (**b**) T2-weighted images, the ganglion cyst (arrow) is located in the spinoglenoid notch, showing high signal intensity swelling due to denervation changes only in the infraspinatus muscle (thick arrow) (acute and subacute phase)

17.2.2.2 Axillary Nerve (C5, 6)

The axillary nerve is a motor-sensory nerve originating from the posterior cord of the brachial plexus in the armpit. The nerve fibers originate from the C5, 6 nerve roots, the middle trunk, and its posterior division. The axillary nerve travels through the armpit, passing in front of the subscapularis muscle and behind the axillary artery, following the circumflex humeral vessels downward to the shoulder joint, and terminates in the quadrilateral space. After exiting the quadrilateral space, the axillary nerve finally ends in the anterior, posterior, and lateral branches that branch into the long head of the triceps muscle. It wraps around the surgical neck of the humerus in the anterior or superior branch and ends after distributing to the deltoid muscle and adjacent skin. The posterior or inferior branch is distributed to the teres minor muscle, the posterior belly of the deltoid, and adjacent skin [1, 12].

The axillary nerve can be compromised by inflammation or injury to the brachial plexus, and can also be damaged alone during shoulder dislocation, humeral fracture, penetrating injury, rotator cuff surgery, or improper use of crutches. Patients may feel weakness during flexion, abduction, and external rotation of the shoulder and may complain of sensory abnormalities in the lateral shoulder [1, 12].

In magnetic resonance neurography, the axillary nerve is often well seen, surrounded by normal fat without local expansion or mass. Abnormal nerve signal intensity, size, and associated brachial plexopathy can be clearly seen on high-resolution images. Denervation changes in the teres minor or deltoid muscle confirm the pathological condition of the nerve (Fig. 17.5). Isolated denervation changes in the teres minor are often seen as a single finding in patients with a frozen shoulder [12].

17.2.2.3 Musculocutaneous Nerve (C5–7)

The musculocutaneous nerve is a motor-sensory nerve originating from the lateral cord of the brachial plexus at the lower border of the pectoralis major muscle. Its nerve fibers originate from the C5–7 roots. This nerve passes through the armpit, pierces the coracobrachialis muscle, and passes between the biceps and brachialis muscles. In the

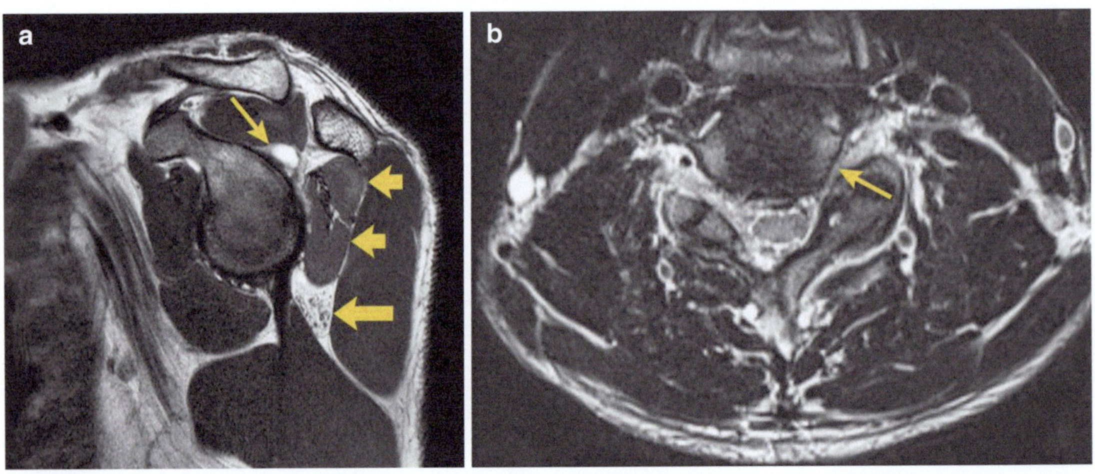

Fig. 17.5 Isolated atrophy of the teres minor muscle due to compression of the C6 nerve root. (**a**) On the sagittal T2-weighted image, there is a ganglion cyst (arrow) in the spinoglenoid notch, and due to this, denervation changes of the infraspinatus muscle (high signal intensity swelling, short thick arrow) are seen. Regardless of this, characteristically, severe fatty infiltration and atrophy (long thick arrow) of the teres minor muscle are seen. (**b**) Compression of the left C6 nerve root is seen at the C5–6 level on the cervical axial T2-weighted image

anterosuperior position of the main joint, the musculocutaneous nerve pierces the deep fascia from the lateral side of the biceps tendon and connects to the lateral cutaneous nerve of the forearm. The musculocutaneous nerve controls the coracobrachialis, biceps, and brachialis muscles.

This nerve is rarely damaged, but it can be compressed between the aponeurosis of the biceps and the fascia of the brachialis, dislocation of the shoulder joint, proximal fracture of the humerus, weightlifting injury, and sometimes traction injury during anesthesia.

Normal nerves are isointense and barely visible, but when the lateral cord and C5–7 nerve roots are compromised, regardless of the presence or absence of associated brachial plexopathy, MRN can show abnormal nerves with T2 high signal intensity or edema. Denervation changes in muscles can be observed in the coracobrachialis, biceps, and brachialis muscles [1, 2, 13].

17.2.2.4 Long Thoracic Nerve (C5–7)

The long thoracic nerve is a motor nerve that distributes to a single muscle and is a proximal branch of the brachial plexus formed by the C5–7 nerve roots. It originates from the posterior side of the plexus, passes through the middle scalene muscle, and runs along the thoracic wall on the outer surface of the serratus anterior muscle, distributing to the muscles along its path.

This nerve can be damaged by traction injuries due to falls, traffic accidents, axillary and lymph node dissection, mastectomy, or sports injuries, or it can be entrapped within the middle scalene muscle or entrapped by a thoracic mass. This nerve is also the most commonly affected by brachial neuritis.

Patients show a laterally winged scapula accompanied by dull shoulder joint pain and weakness when lifting their arms. The diagnosis can be confirmed by electromyography of the serratus anterior muscle. Because the nerve itself is too small to be detected in magnetic resonance neurography, the role of imaging is to confirm the denervation changes of each muscle in clinically confusing cases. Sometimes, abnormal nerves in MRN may follow denervation changes in the serratus anterior muscle. Imaging also excludes tumors in patients without trauma or brachial neuritis [1, 4].

17.2.3 Anatomy of the Thoracic Outlet

From medial to lateral, it can be divided into three anatomical spaces: the interscalene triangle, the costoclavicular space, and the retropectoralis minor space (subcoracoid tunnel) (Fig. 17.6). These are best seen in the sagittal and coronal planes.

The interscalene triangle is bounded anteriorly by the anterior scalene, posteriorly by the middle/posterior scalene, and inferiorly by the first rib. This space contains the subclavian vessels, and the roots and trunks of the brachial plexus. The costoclavicular space is bounded anteriorly by the subclavius muscle, anterosuperiorly by the clavicle, and posteriorly by the first rib and middle scalene. This space contains the subclavian vessels and the divisions and cords of the brachial plexus. The most lateral space of the thoracic outlet, the retropectoralis minor space, is bounded anteriorly by the pectoralis minor, posterosuperiorly by the subscapularis, and posteroinferiorly by the anterior chest wall. This space contains the proximal cords and terminal branches of the brachial plexus. These cords are adjacent to the axillary artery and vein at the following locations (clockwise): anterosuperior (lateral cord), posterosuperior (posterior cord), posteroinferior (medial cord). Denervation muscle changes can be observed in the coracobrachialis, biceps, and brachialis [1, 14].

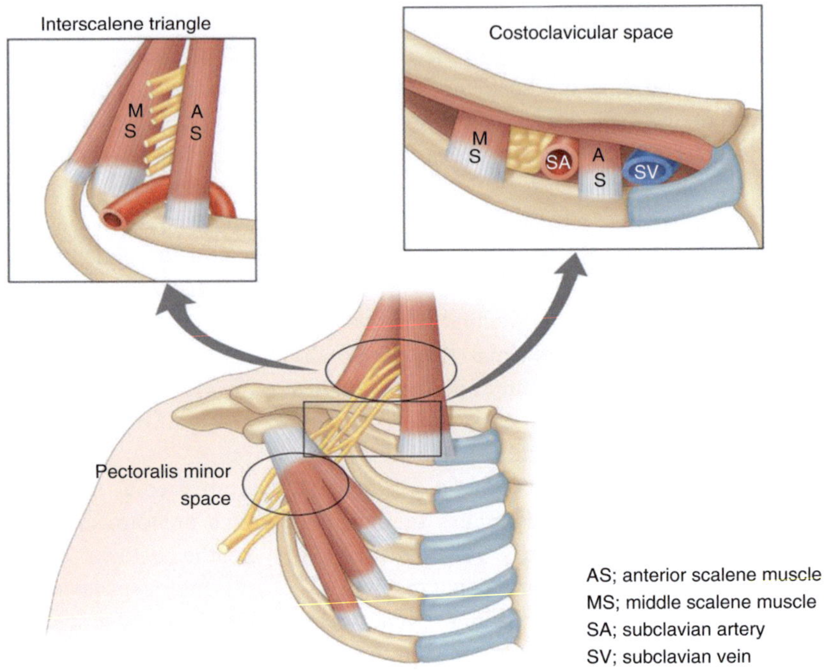

Fig. 17.6 Anatomy of the thoracic outlet. It can be divided into three anatomical spaces from medial to lateral, the interscalene triangle, costoclavicular space, and retropectoralis minor space (or subcoracoid tunnel)

17.3 Practical MR Imaging Protocol

17.3.1 General MR Protocol

The purpose of brachial plexus imaging is to show the entire course of the neural network from the pre-ganglionic segments (e.g., rootlets and intradural nerve segments) and the dorsal root ganglion (DRG) to the post-ganglionic branches. To obtain good images of the brachial plexus, a field strength of at least 1.5 T is required, and 3 T further enhances the signal-to-noise ratio (SNR) and contrast-to-noise ratio (CNR) [1, 2]. A neurovascular coil, such as a surface coil with a multichannel phased array structure, is needed. Or a body surface coil with a curved end improves the signal-to-noise ratio [4, 5].

Because the normal course of the brachial plexus runs from the medial to the lateral direction, it can be difficult to interpret with conventional coronal, axial, and sagittal images. In other words, oblique sagittal and coronal images are preferred techniques for clearly defining the anatomical structure of the brachial plexus and its relationship with important surrounding structures [15]. Oblique axial images tilted 5~10° downward from the medial to the lateral direction are obtained from C4 to T1 vertebrae. The vertebrae are placed not in the middle of the image range (field-of-view, FOV), but at the edge, to clearly show the plexus from the proximal branch to the distal. Oblique sagittal images tilted about 15° on the vertical axis are obtained from the neural foramen on the east side to the shoulder joint. Oblique coronal images are tilted about 5~7° forward from the horizontal plane (the axis connecting the middle part of the transverse process and the humeral head), and scans are obtained from the sternum to the spinous process of the spine [9].

In the case of unilateral damage, bilateral coronal T2-weighted images help effectively compare the injured side with the normal opposite side. A sagittal technique with a narrow scan area that only includes one side is better for evaluating swelling, hypertrophy, or contrast enhancement patterns of brachial plexus segments [2, 16].

To fully image the brachial plexus, a focused multiplanar, multisequence MRI is required, which provides higher contrast images than CT. The scan area should include the position from C4 to T2 due to anatomical variations of the pre-fixed (C4–8) and post-fixed (C6–T2) brachial plexus [4, 5].

The sequences used can be selected according to each patient's situation and suspected pathological conditions [2]. Also, various sequences are being used depending on the needs of radiologists or clinicians in each hospital (Table 17.1).

T1-weighted images are most useful for evaluating nerves, fat surrounding nerves, scalene and regional muscles, and the structure of the thoracic outlet. T2-weighted images are obtained with various contrasts (fat suppression technique/STIR) for an appropriate evaluation of the brachial plexus. Sagittal STIR images are useful for evaluating each segment of the plexus. Also, STIR images have various advantages, such as clearly showing the symmetrical normal high signal intensity and size of the posterior root ganglion. If a lateral abnormality is suspected in the proximal segments (cords) of the brachial plexus, focused 3D imaging of the east side should be performed at that site [1].

Gadolinium-based intravenous contrast enhancement is not essential for routine brachial plexus evaluation. However, if infection, trauma, or tumor is primarily considered, it is necessary to clarify the extent of invasion and evaluate potential collections for discharge. Contrast enhancement is essential [2, 16]. Fat-suppressed contrast-enhanced T1-weighted imaging is performed when a local tumor or edema is seen in the nerve in the first image, or when neuritis is clinically suspected, especially in patients with a history of trauma, for the evaluation of subtle nerve root damage [5–7, 11, 15, 17]. Contrast enhancement of the intradural nerve root suggests functional impairment despite the clear persistence of the morphological form, due to damage to the damaged vascular-nerve barrier. However, this is a very rare finding [1].

In many cases, cervical MRI is additionally examined in addition to the brachial plexus. The additional cervical MRI enables the evaluation of fractures, ligament damage in trauma patients, evaluation of degenerative diseases of the upper cervical spine, or evaluation of other related abnormalities in non-traumatic cases [9].

Table 17.1 Various recommended brachial plexus MRI protocols on 3 T MRI

Type I
Coronal T1 TSE & T2 FSE Sagittal T1 SE (each side) and sagittal T2 FSE (affected side or each side) Axial T1WI & T2WI Axial and sagittal (affected side) T1 fs contrast enhancement
Type II
Axial (5~10° off axis) • T2-weighted SPACE, T2-weighted with fat saturation or STIR, T1-weighted contrast-enhanced with fat suppression Coronal (5~7° off axis) • T2-weighted with fat saturation or STIR, T1-weighted or proton density-weighted, contrast-enhanced with fat suppression Sagittal (15° off axis) • T2-weighted with fat saturation or STIR, T1-weighted contrast-enhanced with fat suppression
Type III
3 T MRN examination protocol for evaluation of the brachial plexus (FOVs from C2 to T2) • T1 coronal (T1 axial), 3D coronal STIR SPACE, 3D sagittal T2 SPACE • STIR sagittal, bilateral, affected side Additional arm examination if desired • Axial T1WI, Axial T2 SPAIR (spectral-attenuated inversion recovery)

On the other hand, since spinal lesions can be a major disturbance similar to brachial plexopathy, 3D T2 SPACE imaging focused on the cervical spine is needed. The intradural nerve segments before the ganglion are best seen in this sequence [1].

17.3.2 Advanced MRI

Three-dimensional T2-weighted techniques using steady-state-free procession (SSFP) can help visualize segments within the dura mater and within the neural foramen with high contrast and resolution. To see the intradural nerve root, or if myelographic imaging is needed, in addition to basic T1-weighted and T2-weighted imaging, 3D SSFP or heavily T2-weighted 3D imaging suppressing fat and flow can be performed [7].

MR myelography is a superior examination method as it is non-invasive compared to CT myelography, has no radiation exposure, and can detect pseudomeningocele regardless of the connection with the thecal sac [7].

Three-dimensional imaging and multiplanar postprocessing techniques show the nerve rootlets in the subarachnoid space, posterior root ganglion, and neural foramen structures much better. The 3D STIR SPACE sequence enables excellent background fat suppression and isotropic multiplanar and curved planar reconstructions. The reconstructed images can be observed along the longitudinal plane of the nerve, and can be further enhanced by constructing 3D maximum intensity projection (MIP) images that emphasize abnormalities more [4]. MIP images are useful for evaluating asymmetry of bilateral nerve plexus with high-resolution near-isotropic fat-suppressed T2-weighted imaging that better shows the brachial plexus (Fig. 17.7) [1].

DTI (diffusion tensor image) reconstructs the DTI parameter map, evaluating the ratio and direction of water diffusion in tightly bound nerves. This technique can provide a quantitative analysis of anisotropic (directional) diffusion representing microstructure in axons [1].

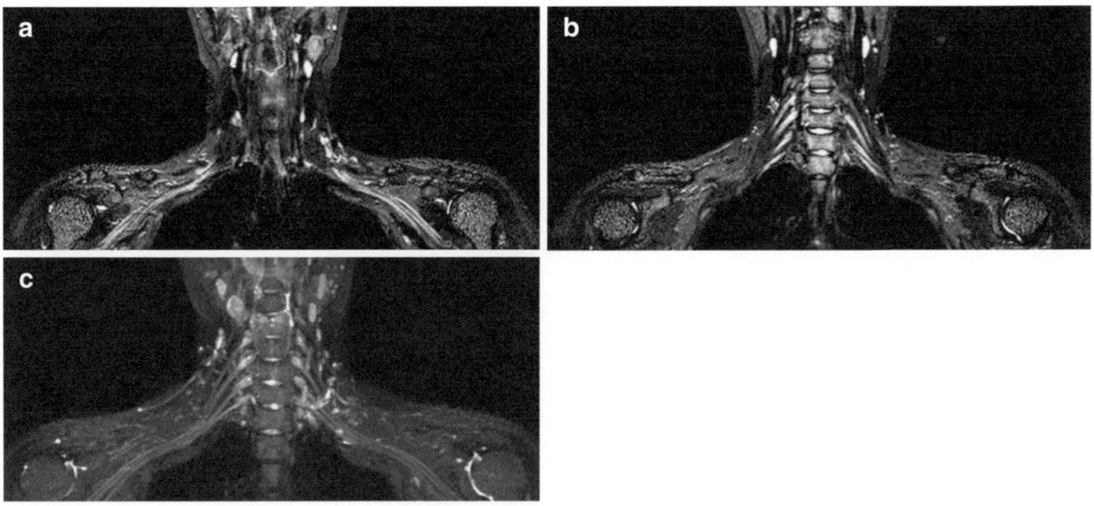

Fig. 17.7 3D STIR SPACE sequence of the brachial plexus (**a**, **b**) and 3D maximum intensity projection (MIP) (**c**) image. With excellent background fat suppression, the contrast is high, showing the brachial plexus better, and especially the MIP image, which is reconstructed isotropically, allows observation along the longitudinal plane of the plexus, useful for evaluating the presence or absence of asymmetry in both plexuses

17.4 Evaluation Form of Brachial Plexus MRI and Judgment of Abnormalities

17.4.1 Evaluation Form for Brachial Plexus MRI

The basic evaluation form recommended for the evaluation of the brachial plexus MRI starts from the axial T2-weighted images. The spinal cord should be centrally located within the dural sac without contour deformation, and the nerve rootlets are evaluated for their connectivity with the spinal cord [3]. The spinal cord, nerve rootlets, pre-ganglionic, and post-ganglionic nerve roots should normally have a homogeneous low signal intensity on T2-weighted images [3]. Abnormal signal intensity or fluid accumulation in the extradural space, neural foramen, or perispinal space may suggest hemorrhage or pseudomeningocele, and should be reviewed in comparison with the signal intensity on T1-weighted images. The post-ganglionic nerve roots and proximal trunks are well seen in the axial sequence because they run between the anterior and middle scalene muscles. These surrounding muscles and fat should be evaluated for edema, hemorrhage, and mass [9].

The coronal plane provides the longest in-plane images of the brachial plexus and is used to evaluate the trunks through the branches. In the absence of pathological conditions, nerves surrounded by fat and muscle should show homogeneous signal intensity. The clavicle, ribs, and muscles that have the nerve distribution of the brachial plexus should be evaluated in this coronal plane [9].

The sagittal plane is useful for evaluating the cords. These nerves are adjacent to the subclavian artery, making it difficult to distinguish from the subclavian artery in other directional planes. Any changes in the fat surrounding the vessels or nerves can be abnormal. Vascular abnormalities (e.g., subclavian artery aneurysm) or mass effects from displaced clavicle fractures can be found. Care should be taken to distinguish and confirm other causes of neuropathy, including secondary signs of brachial plexus abnormalities, nerve block, intervertebral disc abnormalities, muscle swelling, and atrophy caused by vertebral body or rib fractures [9].

17.4.2 Abnormal Findings of Nerves in MRI

Abnormal findings of nerves in magnetic resonance neurography include asymmetric T2 high signal intensity, enlargement, kinking of the nerve due to fibrosis/compression due to intramuscular course/entrapment due to mass lesions, discontinuity due to injury/local formation of neuroma [1]. Sometimes, it may be difficult to distinguish the size abnormality of the nerve root due to old cervical degenerative changes in middle-aged or elderly people and the T2 signal intensity associated with hyperextension injury/brachial plexitis. Generally, asymmetric T2 high signal intensity in the scalene triangle while preserving the most proximal part of the nerve root and the posterior root ganglion distinguishes plexopathy from nerve impingement/irritation associated with cervical degenerative disease (involvement of the most proximal part of the nerve located in the neural foramen or immediately adjacent to it, abnormality confined to the nerve corresponding to the narrowest neural foramen) [1].

3D imaging shows the full range of nerves and local signal intensity changes. Deviations and size changes in the neural pathway can be easily evaluated by the isotropic reconstruction of the image along the longitudinal plane of the nerve. However, this 3D image is not very helpful in detecting abnormalities in nerve fiber bundles. The total or partial loss of the adipose plane around the brachial plexus reflects fibrosis, tumors, or hemorrhage. Changes in the local nerve-blocking muscles of the neck and shoulder are very helpful in suggesting nerve damage/inflammation. These changes can range from swelling and similar T2 signal intensity abnormalities in the early stages of nerve blockage to fat replacement and atrophy in the subacute and chronic stages. The degree of muscle fat replacement and atrophy can help determine surgical treatment for nerve restoration or tendon grafting [3, 4, 6, 18].

17.5 Common Clinical Symptoms

Brachial plexopathy is a neurological disease that causes pain or functional disability in the ipsilateral upper limb. It can be caused by internal disease, excessive extension, penetrating wound, or direct trauma [9]. Symptoms associated with the brachial plexus range from vague and nonspecific symptoms such as local shoulder pain, upper limb weakness, and sensory changes in the upper limb or shoulder to symptoms according to specific nerve distribution such as pain or motor/sensory deficits. They may also complain of more specific symptoms such as scapular winging due to long thoracic nerve damage, diaphragmatic dysfunction due to the phrenic nerve of C3–5, and Horner's syndrome due to C8–T1 after the ganglion [2].

17.6 Pathological Situations

17.6.1 Classification by Location Centered on the Clavicle

17.6.1.1 Lesions Above the Clavicle

It includes roots and trunks in the scalene triangle, generally occurring more frequently and in more severe forms than lesions in other areas. Erb-Duchenne paralysis is caused by damage to the C5, 6 nerve roots or upper trunk, accounting for about 90% of obstetric brachial plexus injuries. Less commonly, there may be Dejerine-Klumpke paralysis caused by damage to the C8, T1 roots or lower trunk. Common pathological conditions above the clavicle include brachial plexitis (Parsonage-Turner syndrome), traumatic injury, tumors (metastasis, neurofibroma, neurofibromatosis, pancoast tumor), and thoracic outlet syndrome (TOS) [3, 17, 18].

Involvement of C5, 6 (upper plexus) results in adduction and internal rotation of the arm, accompanied by not only weakness of the flexor muscles in the shoulder and arm, but also sensory loss in the lateral arm and thumb. Involvement of C7 (middle trunk) results in sensory loss in the middle finger and arm. It causes weakness in the extension of the forearm and wrist in the internal rotation of the forearm and wrist. C8, T1 (lower nerve plexus) infringement results in weakness of the intrinsic muscles of the hand, along with sensory loss on the ulnar side of the forearm and hand [3, 17, 18].

17.6.1.2 Posterior Clavicular Lesions

Lesions behind the clavicle include the divisions of the brachial plexus. Generally, lesions of the anterior division cause lesions of the flexor compartment, and lesions of the posterior division cause lesions of the extensor compartment [1].

17.6.1.3 Subclavicular Lesions

Lesions below the clavicle affect the cords and terminal branches of the nerves, and occur about three times less frequently than lesions above the clavicle. Lesions in this area generally have a better prognosis and recover earlier than those above the clavicle. Common causes include radiation neuropathy, humeral fractures with displacement, gunshot wounds, and iatrogenic injuries.

Lateral cord lesions cause weakness in elbow/wrist flexion and forearm pronation, along with sensory loss in the anterolateral forearm and hand. Medial cord lesions show similar symptoms to lateral cord lesions while relatively preserving finger extension. Posterior cord lesions affect the radial and axillary nerves, causing weakness in arm, wrist, and finger extension and sensory loss in the shoulder and back of the arm [1].

17.6.2 Classification According to Each Clinical Setting

17.6.2.1 Traumatic Plexopathy

Trauma is the most common cause of pathological conditions of the brachial plexus. Traumatic brachial plexus injuries have two distinct patient groups. The first is newborns with persistent extension injuries due to shoulder dystocia during labor. Such trauma can result in flaccidity of the ipsilateral arm. In most obstetric trauma cases, the brachial plexus nerves are more stretched than dislocated, so signs of injury improve within a few weeks to months. If a dislocation injury occurs, the C5, 6 nerve roots are often damaged, resulting in Erb palsy (arm adduction and internal rotation, wrist flexion). Imaging often shows sequelae of Erb palsy rather than the dislocation injury itself that causes Erb palsy. Secondary progressive shoulder joint deformities due to muscle imbalance can be seen as early as age 2 [7, 8, 19]. The second patient group is young men in their 10s and 20s. They can fall from high places, suffer blunt force injuries after motorcycle or car accidents, or suffer penetrating injuries from gunshot wounds. These injuries can delay diagnosis because they often accompany head or spinal injuries that are somewhat distant from the brachial plexus [7, 19]. Brachial plexus injuries can cause neurological sequelae and inhibit use of upper limb in young patients [7]. In addition, brachial plexus injuries can be caused by sports injuries, rucksack (backpack for climbing) injuries, and iatrogenic traction injuries during anesthesia.

The usefulness of brachial plexus MRI in trauma situations is to distinguish between pre-ganglionic and post-ganglionic injuries, and this distinction is very important for prognosis and future management [7]. The overall spectrum of nerve injuries ranges from neuropraxia/nerve stretch injuries (most common), axonotmesis, partial nerve lacerations with continuous neuromas (neurotmesis) to complete nerve lacerations/nerve root avulsions (most severe injuries). These injuries can also affect various nerves in the upper limb (e.g., suprascapular, musculocutaneous, axillary nerves).

The detection of pre-ganglionic injuries can be difficult, and avulsion injuries of the nerve root require major surgery and neurotization, so it is very important to carefully observe the nerve roots from the spinal cord. It is often necessary to make a judgment by combining direct images such as high-resolution 3D MRI or CT myelography and indirect radiological features. Pre-ganglionic injuries do not usually restore well directly, so there are many limitations in treatment. In order to recover some function in denervated muscles, surgery to transplant an intact nerve to the proximal cut end (stump) is sometimes performed. The primary goal is to recover the biceps function (C6) and subsequently recover shoulder mobility [3, 4, 7, 20].

Post-ganglionic injuries have better prognosis and treatment options. Many of these will undergo clinical and radiological follow-up examinations. In cases where surgery is indicated, if direct restoration is impossible, autologous nerve transplantation may be considered. To prevent irreversible atrophy of denervated muscles, the neurotraumatic effect on muscles should be confirmed acutely for early surgical intervention. If there is no significant denervation effect or if the denervation effect progresses slowly, the continuity of the nerve fascicles is considered. For intact nerve fascicles (continuity maintained), conservative treatment (rehabilitation/neurolysis) is recommended. If the nerve fascicles are damaged (discontinuity of the nerve), nerve restoration and nerve transplantation are considered [3, 7, 20].

Direct Signs

High-resolution 3D T2-weighted images and CT myelography can show the anatomical continuity or discontinuity of the nerve roots within the dura. The course of the nerve root should be traced from the root entry zone to the posterior root ganglion in the foramen [3, 4, 7]. High-resolution heavily T2-weighted sequences such as SSFP or CISS (3D constructive interference in steady-state) should be used with conventional images to track the nerve roots within the dura. It is a very useful test method that helps to see the anatomical continuity of nerves [21]. MRN can show the continuity of nerves regardless of the location of nerve damage and the formation of neuroma, or it can show nerves that are completely ruptured or peeled off.

In the case of damaged nerves, but structurally intact (metabolic/functional disorder), contrast-enhanced sequences can show abnormal contrast enhancement of damaged nerves compared to the normal side. The expected mechanisms include the collapse of the vascular–nerve barrier or the expansion of the radicular vein [3, 7].

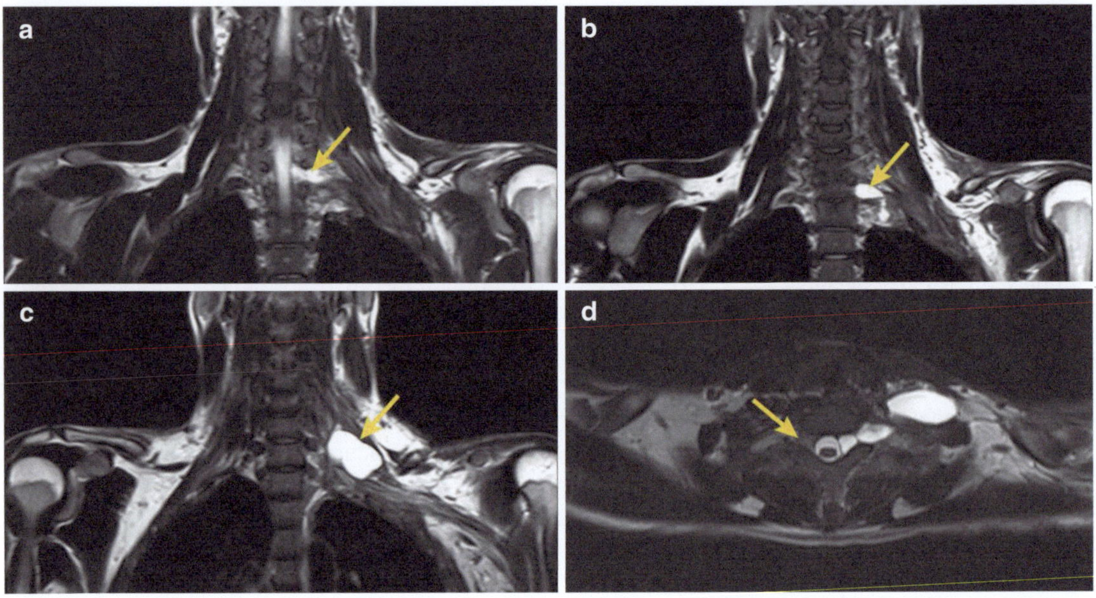

Fig. 17.8 Traumatic pseudomeningocele (pre-ganglionic brachial plexus injury). Continuous coronal T2 enhanced images (**a–c**) show a meningocele (arrow) associated with the C8 nerve root around the left neural foramen and the corresponding space between C7–T1. On the axial T2 enhanced image at the corresponding location (**d**), the right nerve root (arrow) appears normal, but a pseudomeningocele is seen in the left neural foramen instead of the normal nerve root, suggesting avulsion injury of the nerve root

Indirect Signs

In pre-ganglionic damage, pseudomeningocele can be seen in T2 enhanced images, which is common enough to be seen in about 80% of avulsion injuries, but it is not highly specific in diagnosing root avulsion [3]. This will usually show a form that has been invaded into the affected nerve hole, and there may or may not be a peeled nerve inside, and it is often difficult to judge (Fig. 17.8). If you consider indirect signs where the affected side's nerve is not visible or there is no traction due to peeled nerves, and the spine is displaced to the opposite side, you can diagnose it. Normally, the nerve root fixes the spinal cord in the middle of the dural space. The peeling of the nerve root results in unresisted traction by the intact nerve root on the opposite side [3, 4, 7, 10, 17, 22]. MRI findings for penetrating injuries and traction injuries without root avulsion include hematoma or soft tissue swelling depending on the vector of force at the nerve plexus site [3]. The T2 high signal intensity and contrast enhancement of the intact nerve with maintained connectivity suggest damage or disability despite the maintenance of connectivity [7, 8, 19].

In MRN, in addition to pseudomeningocele, another important imaging finding can show local denervation changes in muscles. Abnormal muscles show contrast enhancement within 24 h after injury, and T2 high signal intensity like swelling can be seen within a few days. Abnormal contrast enhancement of muscles around the spine (especially multifidus) can be a more accurate indirect sign suggesting root avulsion injury [1, 6].

Post-ganglionic traumatic nerve damage can show local swelling (high signal intensity in T2 enhanced images) (Fig. 17.9), clumping (Fig. 17.10), or retraction accompanied or unaccompanied nerve discontinuity, or hematoma or swelling around the nerve plexus anywhere in the proximal part of the nerve plexus than the dorsal root ganglion (DRG) [4, 7, 16].

MRI is an essential test method for identifying damage to the spinal cord itself, showing local spinal cord swelling, or bleeding in the acute phase, and myelomalacia in the chronic phase [3, 7, 17].

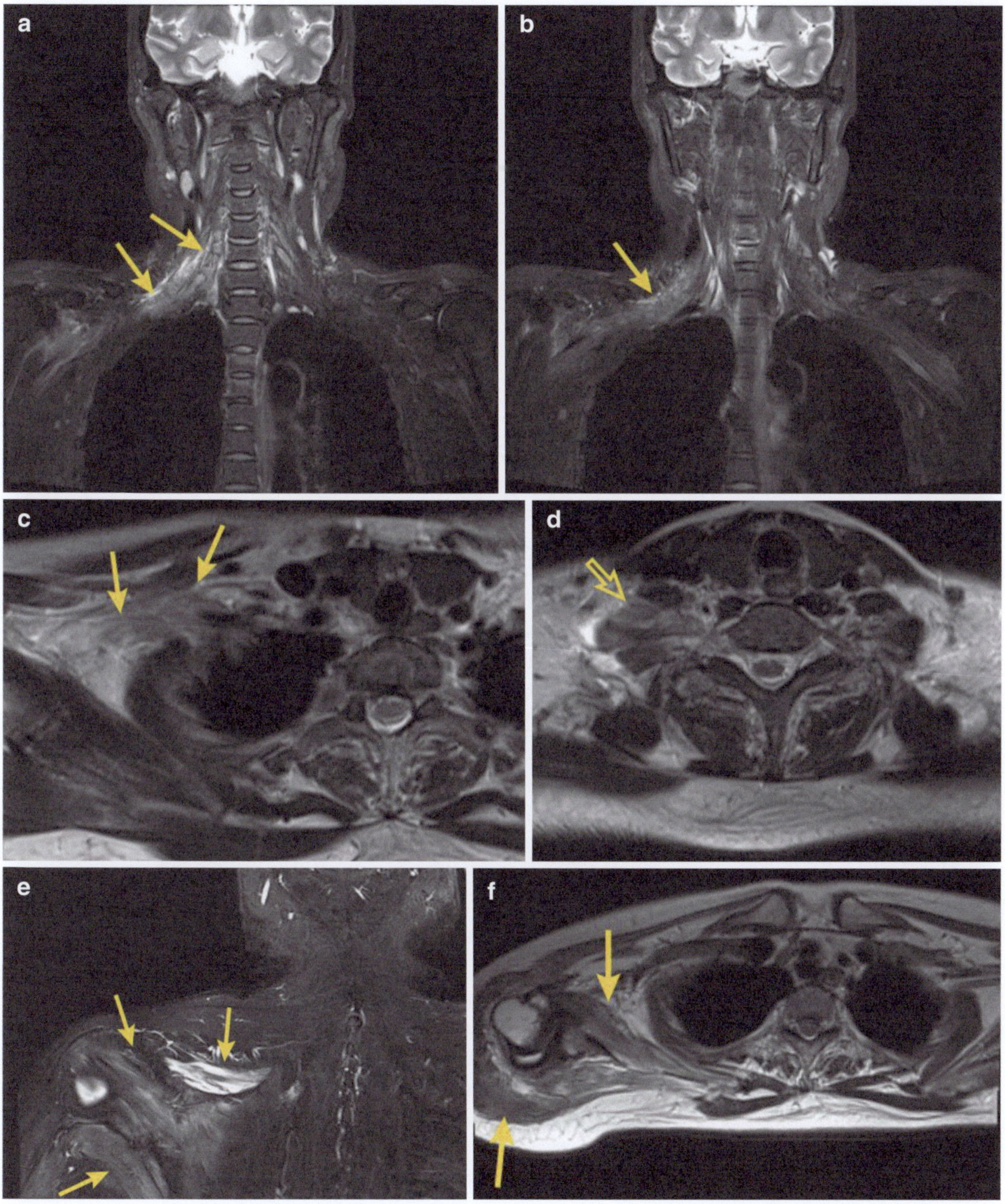

Fig. 17.9 Traumatic post-ganglionic plexus injury. On the fat-suppressed coronal T2 enhanced images (**a**, **b**), abnormal high signal intensity swelling is seen in the nerve and surrounding soft tissue throughout the right post-ganglionic plexus (roots, trunk, divisions, cords), and the nerves constituting the plexus are not distinguishable from each other. On the axial T2-weighted images (**c**, **d**), the normal adipose tissue surrounding the brachial plexus is lost (arrows), and the entire brachial plexus beyond the ganglion level shows overall swelling (empty arrow). In the follow-up MRI examination 6 months later (coronal fat-suppressed T2-weighted image **e**, axial T2-weighted image **f**), the right rotator cuff, teres major muscle, and deltoid muscle show denervation changes (arrows)

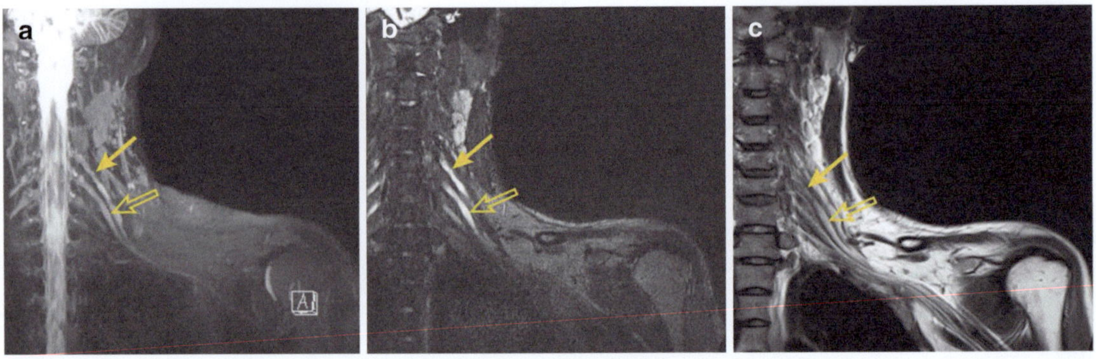

Fig. 17.10 Traumatic post-ganglionic brachial plexus injury. In the coronal MIP (**a**), STIR (**b**), T2-weighted images (**c**), the left C5 (arrow), C6 nerves (empty arrow) mainly show abnormal clumping at the trunk, division locations, and the nerves proximal to this are not well seen, suggesting avulsion injury. The patient complained of motor weakness in the upper extremity after a motorcycle accident, and electromyography showed damage to the axillary nerve and cutaneous nerve of the arm

CT myelography is used when MRI cannot be used or is contraindicated, or when it is ambiguous. It is a video technique that can be substituted when showing results. The most notable abnormal finding is the movement of the contrast medium injected into the epidural space through the torn dura of the meningocele or detached nerve root to the extradural space. Asymmetry of the nerve root can suggest signs of damage, but it is somewhat less clear [9].

17.6.2.2 Radiation Plexopathy

Patients complaining of recurrent symptoms after radiation therapy for malignant tumors consider both recurrence of the tumor and radiation plexopathy. In particular, atrophy and fibrosis of the brachial plexus due to radiation therapy can cause confusion in diagnosis, and often appear as nonspecific findings on MRI [1].

The time elapsed after radiation therapy is an important factor. Recurrence of the tumor usually occurs within 1 year after radiation therapy, and radiation plexopathy can occur from several months to 20 years after treatment (5~10% frequency), with the highest incidence occurring at 10~20 months. In other words, suspicious changes in imaging within 1 year after radiation therapy are more likely to be a recurrence of the tumor than fibrosis after radiation therapy. The average onset of fibrosis after radiation therapy is 5.5 years after treatment [4, 17, 23]. Radiation fibrosis can occur when the total radiation dose exceeds 6000 cGy in the treatment of breast cancer and lung cancer [8, 19, 23].

Radiation-associated plexopathy often involves the upper brachial plexus (C5, 6), while the lower brachial plexus (C8, T1, lower trunk) is a common site of direct tumor invasion from the lung apex or axillary malignant lesions. These findings can help predict radiation-associated fibrosis and recurrence, but the diagnosis is often unclear due to overlapping clinical or radiological findings [3, 4, 17].

The presence or absence of mass lesions is very important in radiological evaluation; contrast enhancement of mass-like features can indicate tumor recurrence or metastasis, but it can also be local atrophy associated with radiation therapy [2, 3, 23]. Fibrosis shows low signal intensity in both T1 and T2 enhanced images, while tumors generally have high signal intensity in T2 enhanced images [3, 17, 23].

Magnetic resonance neurography shows mass lesions with localized or diffuse contrast enhancement in cases of tumor recurrence, accompanied by asymmetric atrophy of the plexus (Fig. 17.11) [24]. Abnormal findings associated with radiation therapy show clear boundaries along the radiation area, diffuse symmetric contrast enhancement without localized mass-like con-

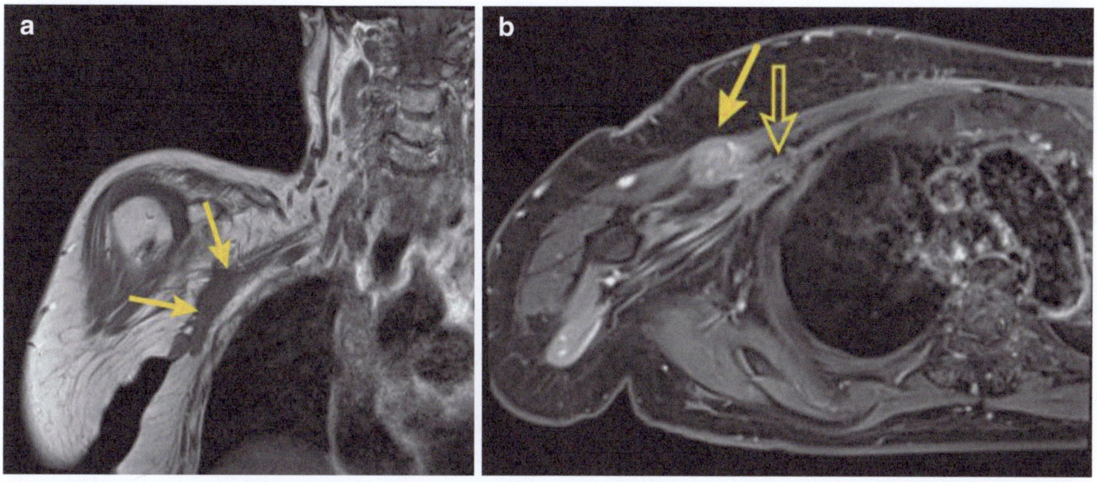

Fig. 17.11 Involvement of the brachial plexus by metastatic breast cancer. In the coronal T1-weighted image (**a**), an irregularly shaped mass lesion is located in the axillary skin and subcutaneous fat tissue, and this lesion is invading the cords of the brachial plexus. In the fat-suppressed contrast-enhanced axial T1-weighted image (**b**), a mass lesion showing enhancement in the pectoralis major muscle (arrow) and in the brachial plexus passing behind the minor pectoral muscle is seen

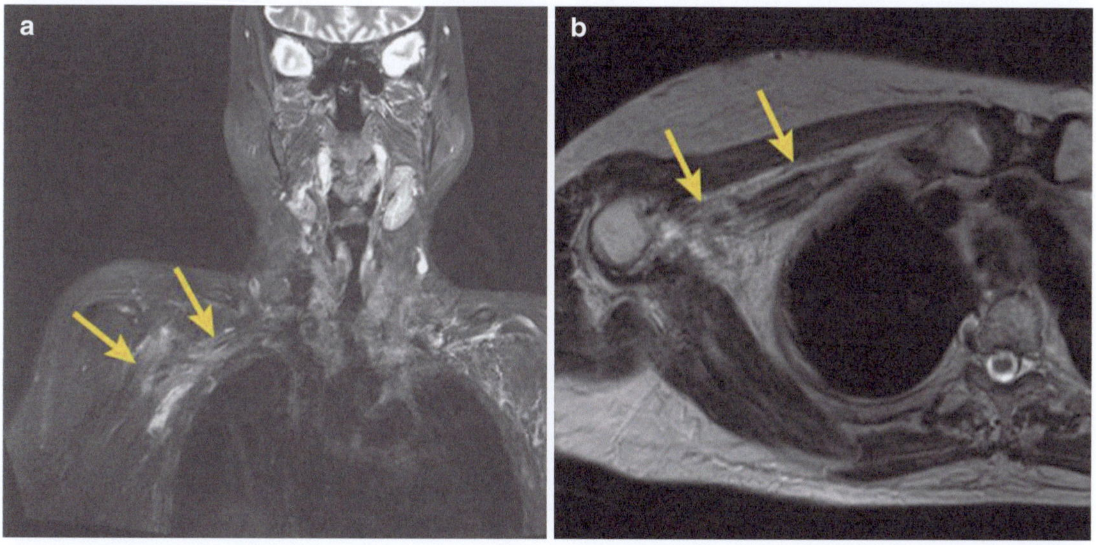

Fig. 17.12 Fibrosis of the brachial plexus after radiation therapy for breast cancer. In the coronal fat-suppressed T2-weighted image (**a**) and axial T2-weighted image (**b**), the right brachial plexus, especially at the divisions, cords locations, shows underdevelopment and high signal intensity of the nerve fibers, and the fat surrounding the plexus also shows underdevelopment invasion (arrow). There is no clear mass in that area

trast enhancement. Also, fibrosis after radiation therapy can show T1, T2 low signal intensity fat stranding accompanied by distortion and kinking of the nerve ganglion (Fig. 17.12) [1].

If an MRI cannot distinguish between radiation-related fibrosis and malignant lesions, some patients may undergo PET-CT or biopsy. PET-CT has been studied to evaluate radiation-related neuropathy in small-scale breast cancer patients and has shown positive results, but large-scale studies need to be conducted to clearly prove these findings [25].

Both tumor recurrence and radiation neuropathy can show symptoms of pain, sensory abnormalities, and motor weakness, but about 30% of radiation neuropathy shows characteristic myokymic discharge in electromyography [1]. On the other hand, radiation neuropathy often shows sensory symptoms associated with edema, while metastatic lesions have severe pain early on. Horner's syndrome can also be seen in metastatic lesions [4].

17.6.2.3 Infection

Infections of the brachial plexus can occur for various reasons, but are usually directly transmitted through the extension of spinal infections, empyema or lung parenchymal infections, septic arthritis of the shoulder, adjacent soft tissue infections, or iatrogenic entry of pathogens [2, 26].

Radiological features are similar to infections in other areas, showing edema with high signal on T2-weighted images, various forms of contrast enhancement, inflammation of surrounding soft tissues, and a clear source of infection may or may not be visible [4, 10].

17.6.2.4 Inflammation

Primary inflammatory processes invading the brachial plexus are rare and can secondarily invade the brachial plexus due to infections/inflammations of adjacent structures, i.e., the supraclavicular fossa or axilla. The upper part of the brachial plexus is more commonly invaded and is mostly associated with sensory symptoms. It is more common in men, with sporadic forms occurring around the age of 40, and hereditary forms around the age of 28. Diagnosis is usually based on clinical symptoms, with acute pain (severe burning pain in the shoulder) starting suddenly along the radicular distribution, followed by sensory abnormalities, and delayed associated shoulder weakness and atrophy being characteristic clinical symptoms [16]. Clinical symptoms can occur bilaterally, but about 29% show an asymmetrical pattern, and about 60% start with symptoms appearing at night. Many reports suggest that these symptoms most commonly improve without sequelae within 3–4 months, but some reports suggest that symptoms disappear in only about 25% of patients, and can persist for up to 3 years after symptom onset in about 75%. The clinical symptoms of inflammation are similar to those of cervical spondylitis, radiculitis, rotator cuff tear, shoulder impingement, and calcific tendinitis. Multiple dermatomal, myotomal location involvement, and pain relief before the onset of motor deficits can be somewhat differentiated, but imaging and nerve conduction studies are needed for definitive diagnosis and exclusion of other causes [2].

Brachial plexus neuritis can have various causes (vaccination, immune, toxin, rarely heredofamilial plexopathies (e.g., Charcot-Marie-Tooth disease)), but all show similar MRI findings [8]. That is, the radiological findings of inflammation are nonspecific, but the same as the inflammation situation that occurred in other parts of our body. MRI images range from the brachial plexus appearing normal to local edema and swelling of the brachial plexus structures accompanied by T2 high signal intensity and various contrast enhancements. Most of the involved shoulder and chest muscles show denervation changes, i.e., in the acute and subacute stages, the muscles show T2 high signal intensity and contrast enhancement with swelling and edema, and in the chronic stage, these muscles show atrophy and fat replacement (Fig. 17.13). The most commonly involved muscles are the serratus anterior, supraspinatus, and infraspinatus. The exact cause is not well known, but while nerves are involved in multiple, the spinal nerves are hardly affected. Most commonly, it invades along the distribution of the suprascapular nerve, less commonly along the distribution of the axillary nerve or the long thoracic nerve [2, 4, 11, 16, 17, 27].

Parsonage-Turner syndrome is more common in young or middle-aged patients and more common in men than women, and about 30% of patients are bilateral [4]. It presents with sudden onset of persistent severe pain in the neck, shoulder, and upper arm, followed by significant weakness and local muscle atrophy within a few weeks. The onset of symptoms is acute and

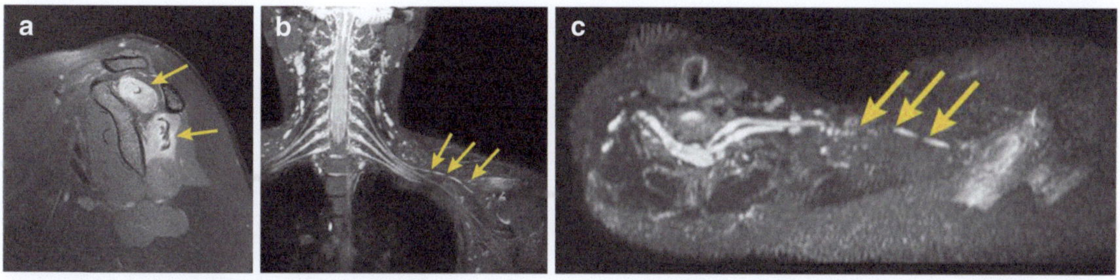

Fig. 17.13 Parsonage-Turner syndrome due to multiple stenosis of the C5 nerve. A 26-year-old female patient complained of rapidly progressing left shoulder, neck pain for 2 weeks, and motor weakness in the upper extremity after 1 week. In the coronal fat-suppressed contrast-enhanced image (**a**), underdevelopment enhancement of the supraspinatus and infraspinatus muscles is seen (arrow), suggesting muscle changes due to denervation. In the coronal (**b**) and oblique axial (**c**) MIP images, multiple stenosis (arrows) is seen at the cords of the C5 nerve, and the supraspinatus and infraspinatus muscles, which receive its distribution, show underdevelopment high signal intensity

subsides after 4–12 weeks [1, 8]. MRI findings are nonspecific and can show T2 high signal intensity in the brachial plexus with edema (acute phase) and later progress to muscle atrophy (chronic phase) [4, 17, 28].

17.6.2.5 Brachial Plexopathy Due to Tumors

Tumors include primary and secondary tumors. Primary tumors originating from nerves are more common in younger patients, are sporadic and benign (e.g., schwannoma), or can occur in conditions with a genetic predisposition (e.g., neurofibromatosis type 1) with both benign and malignant lesions (e.g., neurofibroma and malignant neuroblastoma) [8, 23]. Secondary tumors seen in older patients can cause brachial plexopathy from direct extension or metastasis [19]. Secondary involvement is more common than primary tumors [2].

Tumorous plexopathy, which often presents with vague symptoms, shows various MRI findings. It can be possessed. Although MRI shows high specificity and sensitivity for tumors occurring in the brachial plexus, false positives can also occur. Therefore, clinical information including clinical symptoms, underlying systemic diseases (e.g., neurofibromatosis type 1), and the course of the tumor (time course of chemotherapy/radiation therapy) is important in the complete imaging evaluation of the brachial plexus [29].

Benign Tumors

Various benign diseases such as fibromatosis, proliferative fasciitis, lipoma, hemangioma, brachial cleft cyst, lymphangioma, benign nerve tumors, or neuroblastoma can invade the brachial plexus [2].

Fibromatosis (abdominal desmoid) (Fig. 17.14) and proliferative fasciitis can both appear as large masses invading the brachial plexus. Fibromatosis is usually painless, while proliferative fasciitis can present with sharp tenderness. Both of these lesions show isointensity with adjacent muscles/soft tissues on T1-weighted images and heterogeneous high signal intensity on T2-weighted images. Fibromatosis shows strong contrast enhancement (Fig. 17.14), while proliferative fasciitis shows mild contrast enhancement [10, 29].

Lymphangioma, lipoma, brachial cleft cyst, and hemangioma are rare in the brachial plexus and show similar imaging features to those originating in other parts of our body [23].

Lipomas typically show high signal intensity on both T1- and T2-weighted images, and signal attenuation on fat suppression sequences, making it easy to distinguish from lesions without fat. An important pitfall is the differentiation between low-grade liposarcoma and benign lipoma. In the presence of large lesions over 10 cm, significant non-fat components, numerous septa, or heterogeneous contrast enhancement, PET-CT can be performed for better differentiation [10, 30].

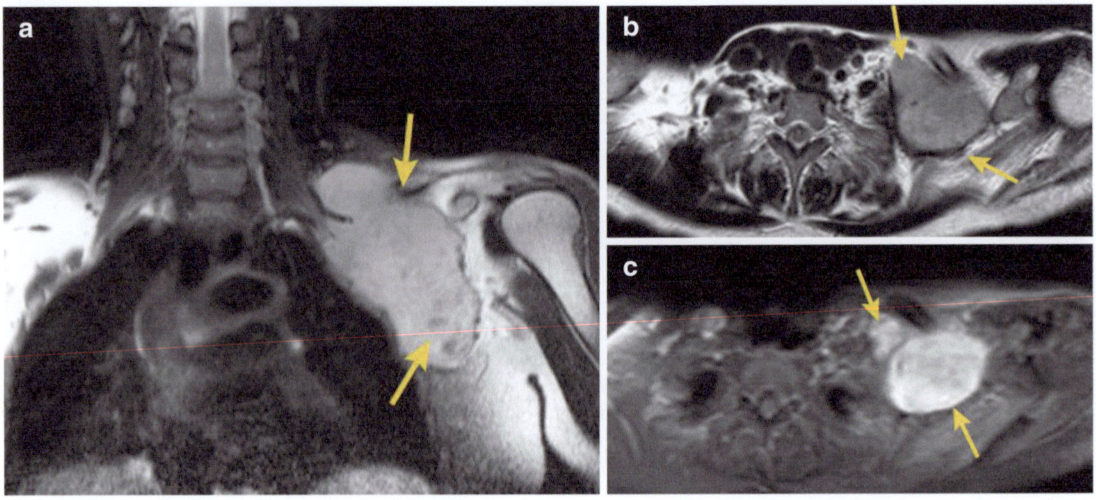

Fig. 17.14 Fibroma invading the left brachial plexus. On the coronal (**a**) and axial (**b**) T2-weighted images, a dumbbell-shaped mass (arrow) invading the trunk and cords of the left brachial plexus shows higher moderate signal intensity than the adjacent muscle. On the axial fat-suppressed contrast-enhanced image (**c**), the mass shows significant contrast enhancement (arrow)

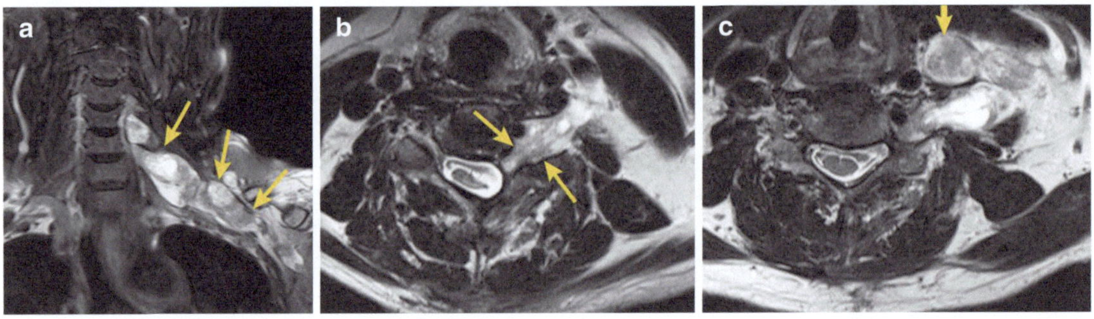

Fig. 17.15 Schwannoma invading the left brachial plexus. On the coronal T2-weighted image (**a**), the mass (arrows) is located along the root, trunk, division, and cord, and on the axial T2-weighted images (**b**, **c**) at the C5–6 level, the mass extends into the left neural foramen, showing a tail sign, and the normal root in the neural foramen is not visible due to the mass. The mass shows heterogeneous high signal intensity, and a target sign is seen in some areas (short arrow). Adjacent cortical bone shows mild erosion due to the expansion of the mass (arrows)

Benign nerve sheath tumors are the most common primary tumors invading the brachial plexus. They are commonly located in the nerve sheath, have well-defined ovoid shapes, high signal intensity on T2, and sometimes cause bone remodeling due to tumor expansion (Fig. 17.15) [3, 16, 23]. Neuroblastomas such as Schwannoma and neurofibroma are the most common benign tumors of the brachial plexus. The imaging features overlap, and solitary neurofibromas may not be distinguishable from schwannomas (Fig. 17.16). Both tumors are elliptical and are located parallel to the long axis of the invaded nerve. Schwannomas are eccentrically located relative to the associated nerve, pushing or compressing adjacent nerve bundles, while plexiform neurofibromas invade the nerve [17, 29]. Plexiform neurofibromas can be seen in cases of neurofibromatosis type 1 (Fig. 17.17) [16].

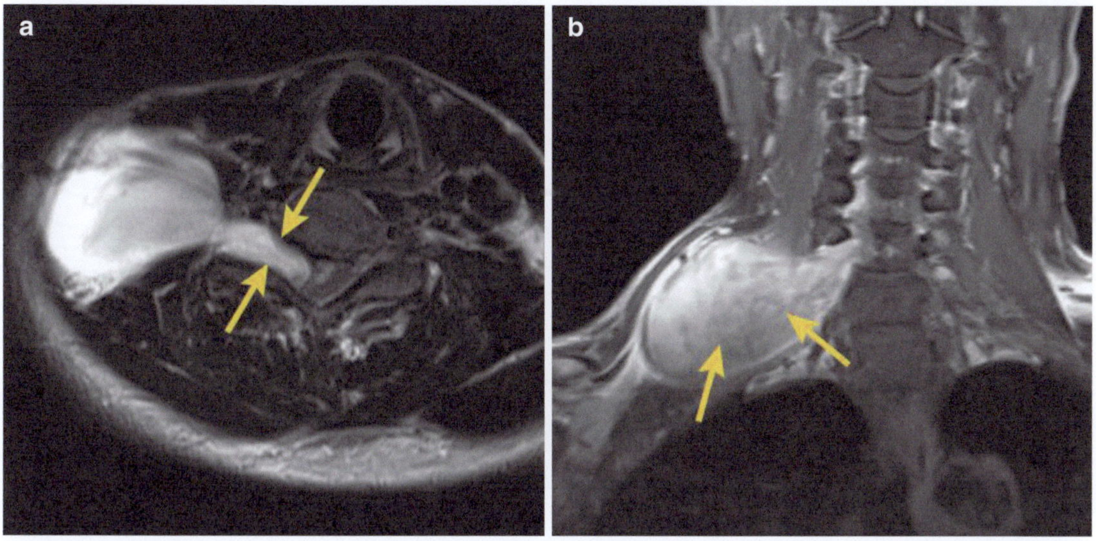

Fig. 17.16 Neurofibroma of the right brachial plexus. On the axial T2-weighted image (**a**) and coronal fat-suppressed contrast-enhanced image (**b**), the mass protruding through the right neural foramen at C6–7 widens the neural foramen mildly (arrow) due to its expanding nature and is located across the root, trunk, division, and cord of the brachial plexus. The mass shows heterogeneous high signal intensity on the T2-weighted image and strong contrast enhancement throughout the mass on the contrast-enhanced image, with a fascicular sign inside (arrows)

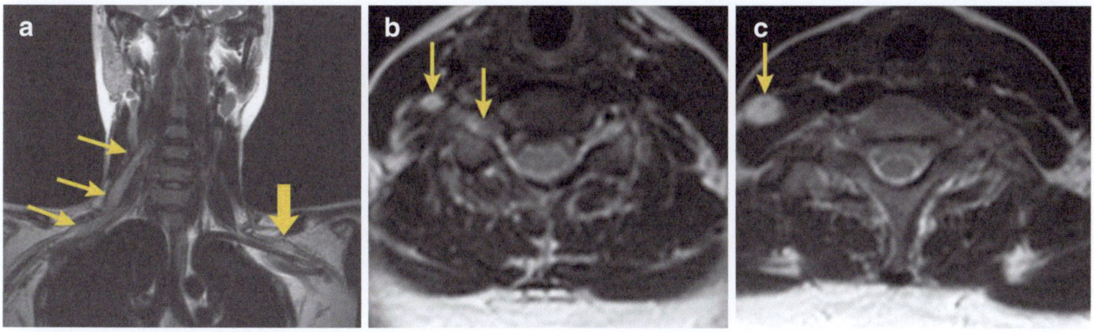

Fig. 17.17 Multiple neurofibromas in neurofibromatosis type I. On the coronal T2-weighted image (**a**), the right brachial plexus mainly shows tubular hypertrophy in a chronic manner (arrows), and on the left, a fusiform mass (thick arrow) is seen at the cord level. On the axial T2-weighted images (**b**, **c**), multiple nodular masses (arrows) are seen at various locations of the brachial plexus

Benign schwannomas typically show high signal intensity on T2-weighted images, with a central low signal intensity target sign (Fig. 17.18). They can also show split fat sign, fascicular sign, and tail sign (entering or exiting nerve sign). Homogeneous marked enhancement is most common. It is often difficult to distinguish schwannomas and neurofibromas based on imaging findings alone; features that may help differentiate these two include the orientation of the lesion to the originating nerve, multiplicity, history of neurofibromatosis type 1, and associated signs such as dural expansion. The ancient form, which shows cystic changes within the tumor, is difficult to diagnose on MRI and is often difficult to distinguish from malignant tumors [3, 15, 17, 23, 29].

Perineuromas are benign tumors that occur in the perineurium of the peripheral nerve sheath and can occur in the brachial plexus, presenting

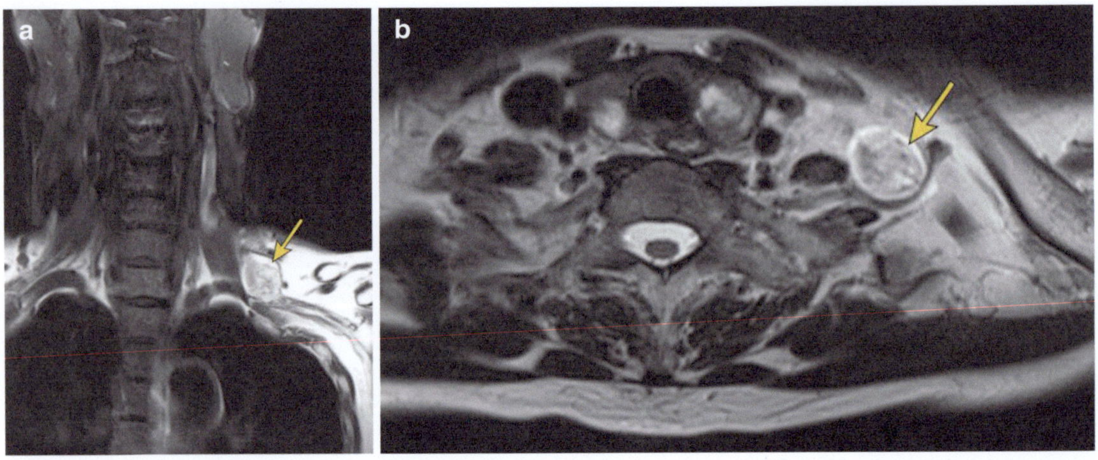

Fig. 17.18 A typical target sign of schwannoma. On the coronal (**a**) and axial (**b**) T2-weighted images, a nodular mass located at the division of the left nerve ganglion shows a typical "target sign" (arrow) with low signal intensity in the center and high signal intensity at the edges

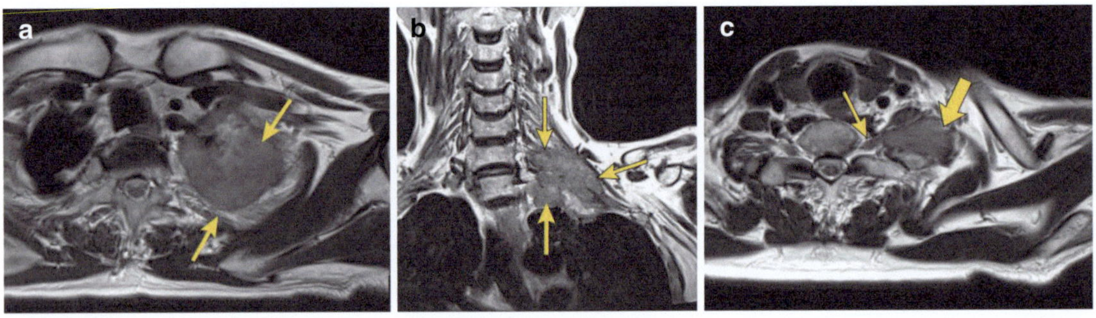

Fig. 17.19 Pancoast tumor invading the left brachial plexus. On the axial T2-weighted image (**a**), an irregularly bordered mass lesion (arrow) is seen in the left lung apex. On the coronal T2-weighted image (**b**), the mass (arrow) at the lung apex extends to the trunk, division of the left brachial plexus, invading several levels of nerves (mainly C8, T1). On the axial T2-weighted image (**c**) at the C7–T1 level, a mass lesion (thick arrow) connected to the C8 nerve root (arrow) is located between the quadrangular muscles

with distinct motor symptoms. The imaging findings are similar to other local lesions invading the brachial plexus [16].

Malignant Tumors

Malignant lesions can originate within the brachial plexus or spread secondarily to the brachial plexus [10]. Secondary invasion of the brachial plexus is more common than primary, with the most common primary cancers being breast cancer, lung cancer, and melanoma [4, 16, 23]. Breast cancer can invade the plexus either by direct extension or by metastasis to other adjacent structures such as the spine. Breast cancer metastasis most commonly takes the form of lymphadenopathy, surrounding, compressing, or occasionally invading the plexus. The signal intensity is similar to that of the primary cancer. Lung cancer often invades the plexus directly in the form of a Pancoast tumor (superior sulcus tumor) (Fig. 17.19), but like breast cancer, it can also invade in the form of lymph node metastasis. It typically invades the lower spinal nerves and the lower trunk of the plexus, causing clinical

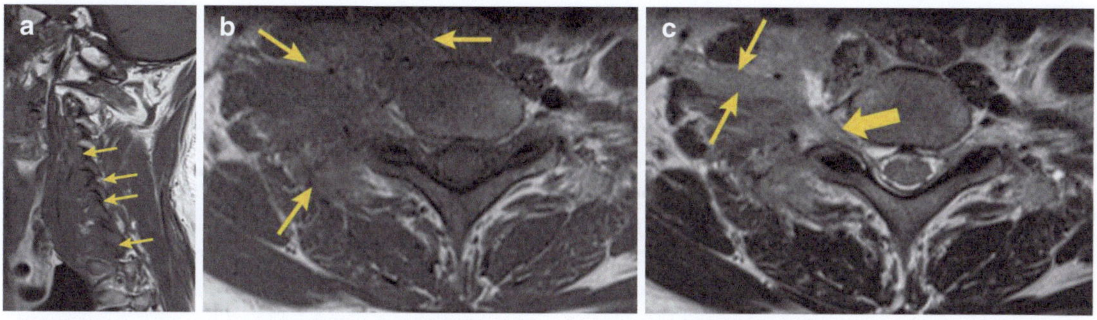

Fig. 17.20 Involvement of the brachial plexus in Non-Hodgkin's lymphoma. On the sagittal T1-weighted image (**a**), normal roots are not visible from several levels of the neural foramen, and the surrounding fat plane is lost (arrows). On the axial T1-weighted image (**b**), the nerve located in the space between the quadrangular muscles on the right side is not distinguishable compared to the left side, and a low signal intensity lesion with irregular boundaries around it and adjacent muscles is visible (arrows). On the axial T2-weighted image at the C7–T1 level (**c**), the root (thick arrow) and trunk (arrow) of the nerve ganglion located in the space between the right quadrangular muscles show atrophy and a higher medium signal intensity than the muscles

symptoms such as pain, sensory abnormalities, and weakness. In about 20% of cases, it invades the sympathetic chain, causing Horner's syndrome. Head and neck cancer can compress or invade the plexus through cervical or lymph node metastasis. Blood cancers such as leukemia and multiple myeloma can invade the brachial plexus due to the mass effect of enlarged lymph nodes [2].

The brachial plexus can also be invaded by lymphomatous nodular tissue in the spinal or intrathecal fluid spaces, or more rarely, by neurolymphomatosis (Fig. 17.20). Neurolymphomatosis or perineural lymphomatosis is a primary central nervous system lymphoma. It can also occur due to the expansion of a primary lymphoma of the peripheral nerves. On MRI, there may be subacute edema of the brachial plexus, distortion of fascicular morphology, and various contrast enhancements [17, 22, 23, 29, 31].

Primary malignant lesions invading the brachial plexus are mostly sarcomatous lesions (low-grade sarcoma, radiation-induced sarcoma, osteosarcoma, Ewing sarcoma, leiomyosarcoma, liposarcoma) [2, 29].

Malignant peripheral nerve sheath tumors are rare and are commonly seen after radiation therapy or in type 1 neurofibromatosis. In patients with type 1 neurofibromatosis, the presence of a plexiform neurofibroma increases the likelihood of developing a malignant peripheral nerve sheath tumor. This does not show any characteristic imaging findings. However, some findings can help in differential diagnosis: (1) rapid increase in size and large masses over 5 cm, (2) loss of target sign on T2-weighted images, (3) indistinct borders, (4) heterogeneous contrast enhancement associated with cystic/necrotic areas within the mass, (5) invasion into adjacent tissues, (6) edema around the lesion [3, 4, 23, 29, 32].

It is difficult to accurately distinguish between benign and malignant tumors based solely on imaging findings. It is expected that DTI (diffusion tensor imaging), a functional evaluation of MRI, can help distinguish tumors in addition to conventional MRI. In addition, high [18F] FDG PET uptake, especially when it shows delayed and persistent glucose uptake, suggests more aggressive or malignant lesions, but not always [1].

17.6.2.6 Thoracic Outlet Syndrome (TOS)

In 1900, Kinner Wilson first described it as a syndrome that compresses the neurovascular bundle passing between the anterior and posterior scalene muscles. Typically, thoracic outlet syndrome is diagnosed based on the results of clinical evaluations, including various dynamic tests such as raising the arm, and symptoms are caused by dynamic compression of the nerve/artery structures passing through the cervicothoracic junction. However, it is often difficult to diagnose with clinical examination alone. Especially in the early stages of the disease, electromyography has limitations in detecting mild symptoms [1]. Depending on the damaged component of the neurovascular bundle, it can be divided into arterial, venous, neurogenic, or a mixed form of TOS. Neurogenic TOS is the most common (over about 95% of all cases). Causes of TOS include impingement of the middle trunk by a fibrous band, kinking of the nerve root, flattening of the nerve due to intramuscular course of the nerve root, impingement by abnormal vessels, narrowing of the space between the scalene muscles due to atrophied muscles, and abnormalities of the bones impinging on the nerve (cervical rib, long transverse process of C7, callus or osteochondroma of the clavicle or first rib, costocostal pseudoarthrosis). Neurogenic TOS can be seen when the nerve is compressed in the interscalene. It is common in the triangle and costoclavicular space, and arterial TOS is most common in the costoclavicular space, followed by the interscalene triangle. The retropectoralis minor space rarely experiences nerve/vessel compression [6, 14, 33–35].

Other types can include disputed (most common), vascular (arterial, venous, or arteriovenous), true neurogenic (nerve), combined (nerve and vessel), droopy shoulder syndrome, etc. [14] The disputed type only presents sensory symptoms and is considered controversial. Vascular thoracic outlet syndrome is most common in young athletes who excessively abduct or raise their heads, caused by compression of the axillary or subclavian vessels. This compression can be static or dynamic (posture change) and can lead to stenosis, thrombosis, or aneurysm formation (known as Paget-von Schroetter syndrome). Possible symptoms include pain in the shoulder and arm accompanied by swelling, and color/temperature changes in the affected hand [1]. The true neurogenic type (Gilliatt-Sumner hand; a minority of TOS cases) is mainly caused by compression of the lower trunk of the brachial plexus due to anatomical variations. It is more common in women and presents with pain in the medial arm and sensory dysfunction (numbness) and weakness in the hand and forearm on the scapular side [1]. Droopy shoulder syndrome is common in young women and presents with shoulder pain and sensory abnormalities. It is usually bilateral and can lead to extension of the brachial plexus segment [1]. In addition, neck injuries from traffic accidents, or long-term non-ergonomic postures when using a computer, can also progress to thoracic outlet syndrome.

MRI plays an important role in identifying the compression of nerves/vessels, the structures causing the compression, and their location. Mild T2 high signal intensity of the C8 and T1 nerve roots is common but nonspecific. Changes in T2 signal intensity leading to the lower trunk or findings of associated nerve expansion are related to the clinical symptoms of thoracic outlet syndrome (Figs. 17.21).

Thoracic outlet syndrome can be treated with rehabilitation therapy or surgical treatments such as anterior scalene muscle resection or resection of abnormal ribs [1].

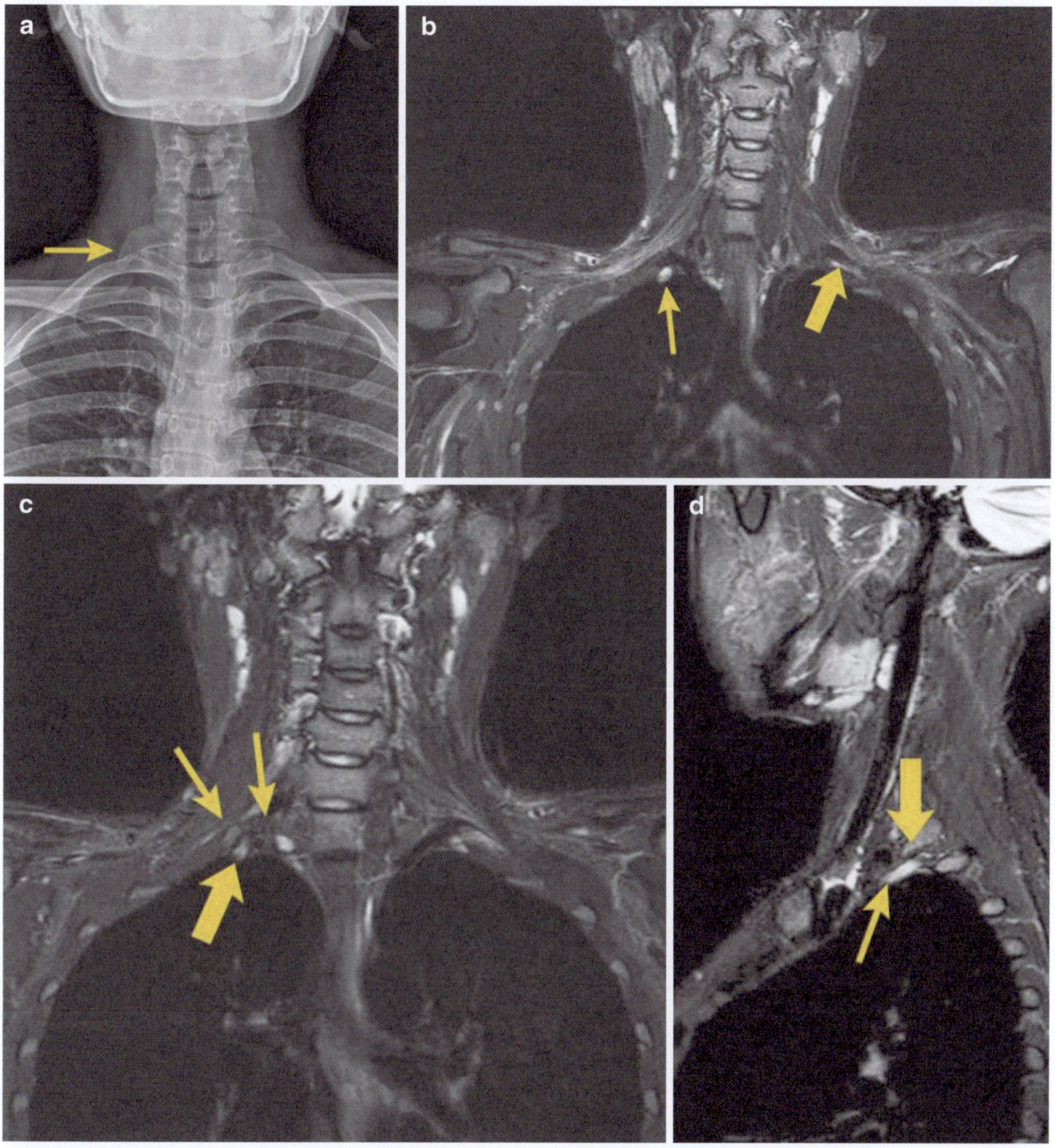

Fig. 17.21 Thoracic outlet syndrome complaining of numbness in the right hand. On the anteroposterior radiograph of the thoracic spine (**a**), the right transverse process of C7 (arrow) appears longer and more curved downward than the left. On the coronal STIR image (**b**), the T1 nerve at the trunk level shows asymmetry. That is, the right T1 nerve (arrow) shows atrophy compared to the left (thick arrow). On the consecutive coronal STIR images (**c**), the T1 nerve (thick arrow) located just below the right transverse process of C7 (arrows) shows slight compression. On the sagittal STIR image (**d**), the atrophy of the T1 nerve (arrow) passing below the right transverse process (thick arrow) is remarkable

17.7 Summary

The brachial plexus is anatomically complex and can be compromised in various pathological situations. Magnetic resonance imaging plays an important role in diagnosing these pathological conditions of the plexus, especially in early diagnosis.

Bibliography

1. Chhabra A, Thawait GK, Soldatos T, et al. High-resolution 3T MR neurography of the brachial plexus and its branches, with emphasis on 3D imaging. AJNR Am J Neuroradiol. 2013;34(3):486–97.
2. Mikityansky I, Zager EL, Yousem DM, Loevner LA. MR imaging of the brachial plexus. Magn Reson Imaging Clin N Am. 2012;20:791–826.
3. van Es HW, Bollen TL, van Heesewijk HP. MRI of the brachial plexus: a pictorial review. Eur J Radiol. 2010;74:391–402.
4. Martinoli C, Gandolfo N, Perez MM, et al. Brachial plexus and nerves about the shoulder. Semin Musculoskeletal Radiol. 2010;14:523–46.
5. Tagliafico A, Succio G, Emanuele Neumaier C, et al. MR imaging of the brachial plexus: comparison between 1.5-T and 3-T MR imaging: preliminary experience. Skeletal Radiol. 2011;40:717–24.
6. Chhabra A, Lee PP, Bizzell C, Soldatos T. 3 Tesla MR neurography: technique, interpretation, and pitfalls. Skeletal Radiol. 2011;40:1249–60.
7. Yoshikawa T, Hayashi N, Yamamoto S, et al. Brachial plexus injury: clinical manifestations, conventional imaging, findings, and the latest imaging technique. Radiographics. 2006;26:S133–43.
8. Castillo M. Imaging of the anatomy of the brachial plexus: review and self-assessment module. AJR Am J Roentgenol. 2005;185:S196–204.
9. Tharin BD, Kini JA, York GE, Ritter JL. Brachial plexopathy: a review of traumatic and nontraumatic causes. AJR Am J Roentgenol. 2014;202:W67–75.
10. Vijayasarathi A, Chokshi FH. MRI of the brachial plexus: a pictorial review. Appl Radiol. 2016;45:9–18.
11. Chalian M, Faridian-Aragh N, Soldatos T, et al. High-resolution 3T MRN of suprascapular neuropathy. Acad Radiol. 2011;18:1049–59.
12. Melis B, Defranco MJ, Ladermann A, Barthelemy R, Walch G. The teres minor muscle in rotator cuff tendon tears. Skeletal Radiol. 2011;40:1335–44.
13. Chhabra A, Lee P, Bizzell C, et al. High resolution 3-Tesla magnetic resonance neurography of musculocutaneous neuropathy. J Shoulder Elb Surg. 2012;21:e1–6.
14. Demondion X, Herbinet P, Van Sint JS, Boutry N, Chantelot C, Cotton A. Imaging assessment of thoracic outlet syndrome. Radiographics. 2006;26:1735–50.
15. Tagliafico A, Succio G, Neumaier CE, et al. Brachial plexus assessment with three-dimensional isotropic resolution fast spin echo MRI: comparison with conventional MRI at 3.0 T. Br J Radiol. 2012;85:e110–6.
16. Rehman I, Chokshi FH, Khosa F. MR imaging of the brachial plexus. Clin Neuroradiol. 2014;24:207–16.
17. Sureka J, Cherian RA, Alexander M, Thomas BP. MRI of brachial plexopathies. Clin Radiol. 2009;64:208–18.
18. Iyer VR, Sanghvi DA, Merchant N. Malignant brachial plexopathy: a pictorial essay of MRI findings. Indian J Radiol Imaging. 2010;20:274–8.
19. Lury K, Castillo M. Imaging of the brachial plexus. Appl Radiol. 2004;4:28–32.
20. Abul-Kasim K, Backman C, Bjorkman A, Dahlin LB. Advanced radiological work-up as an adjunct to decision in early reconstructive surgery in brachial plexus injuries. J Brachial Plex Peripher Nerve Inj. 2010;5:1–7.
21. Vargas MI, Viallon M, Nguyen D, Delavelle J, Becker M. Diffusion tensor imaging (DTI) and tractography of the brachial plexus: feasibility and initial experience in neoplastic conditions. Neuroradiology. 2010;52:237–45.
22. Gerevini S, Mandelli C, Cadioli M, Scotti G. Diagnostic value and surgical implications of the magnetic resonance imaging in the management of adult patients with brachial plexus pathologies. Surg Radiol Anat. 2008;30:91–101.
23. Wittenberg K, Adkins M. MR imaging of nontraumatic brachial plexopathies: frequency and spectrum of findings. Radiographics. 2000;20:1023–32.
24. Thawait SK, Chaudhry V, Thawait GK, et al. High-resolution MRN of diffuse peripheral nerve lesions. AJNR Am J Neuroradiol. 2011;32:1365–72.
25. Ahmad A, Barrington S, Maisey M, Rubens RD. Use of positron emission tomography in evaluation of brachial plexopathy in breast cancer patients. Br J Cancer. 1999;79:478–82.
26. White HD, White BA, Boethel C, Arroliga AC. Pancoast's syndrome secondary to infectious etiologies: a not so uncommon occurrence. Am J Med Sci. 2011;341:333–6.
27. Ryan M, Twair A, Nelson E, Brennan D, Eustace S. Whole body magnetic resonance imaging in the diagnosis of Parsonage Turner syndrome. Acta Radiol. 2004;45:534–9.
28. Linda DD, Harish S, Stewart BG, Finlay K, Parasu N, Rebello RP. Multimodality imaging of peripheral neuropathies of the upper limb and brachial plexus. Radiographics. 2010;30:1373–400.
29. Saifuddin A. Imaging of tumours of the brachial plexus. Skeletal Radiol. 2003;32:375–87.

30. Kransdorf MJ, Bancroft LW, Peterson JJ, Murphey MD, Foster WC, Temple HT. Imaging of fatty tumors: distinction of lipoma and well-differentiated liposarcoma. Radiology. 2002;224:99–104.
31. Bowen BC, Pattany PM, Saraf-Lavi E, Maravilla KR. The brachial plexus: normal anatomy, pathology, and MR imaging. Neuroimaging Clin N Am. 2004;14:59–85.
32. Wasa J, Nishida Y, Tsukushi S, et al. MRI features in the differentiation of malignant peripheral nerve sheath tumors and neurofibromas. Am J Roentgenol. 2010;194:1568–74.
33. Sabapathy SR, Venkatramani H, Bhardwaj P. Pseudoarthrosis of cervical rib: an unusual cause of thoracic outlet syndrome. J Hand Surg Am. 2010;35:2018–21.
34. Aralasmak A, Karaali K, Cevikol C, Uysal H, Senol U. MR imaging findings in brachial plexopathy with thoracic outlet syndrome. AJNR Am J Neuroradiol. 2010;31:410–7.
35. Parker EE, Glastonbury CM. MR imaging of the thoracic inlet. Magn Reson Imaging Clin N Am. 2008;16:341–53. https://doi.org/10.1016/j.mric.2008.02.018.

18 Imaging Diagnosis Tips for Major Spinal Diseases

Joon Woo Lee

18.1 Question 1

A patient came in with severe radiating pain in the lower extremities, suspecting disc herniation, so we took a lumbar MR, but the lesion is not clearly visible. What part should we pay close attention to in this case?

18.1.1 Answer 1 (Fig. 18.1)

Small disc herniations that cause severe pain are often overlooked in MR, such as cases where they have migrated inferiorly in the subarticular zone or superiorly in the foraminal zone. If disc herniation is not observed at the disc level in the axial T2 enhanced image, carefully observe the subarticular zone at one level below to check for small disc herniation around the nerve root, and at one level above the disc level, carefully observe the foraminal zone.

Also, if the disc herniation is small and round, pressing on the nerve root, the herniated disc can be mistaken for the nerve root. On the axial image, trace above and below the nerve root to check for signal changes. In T2 enhanced images, herniated discs usually have lower signals than nerve roots. Of course, in the case of acute disc herniation, the T2 signal is higher than the nerve root. In ambiguous cases, contrast-enhanced MR can be helpful. Herniated discs do not enhance or only the transitional part enhances, but the dorsal root ganglion uniformly enhances.

Acute disc herniation can show high signal shadows in T2 enhanced images, and in this case, it can be somewhat difficult to distinguish from epidural fat tissue. In this case, you can observe the disc herniation distinguished from the surrounding tissue in the T1 enhanced image. Therefore, it is important to carefully observe the posterior of the disc in the T1 enhanced axial image.

18.1.2 Tip 1

Commonly overlooked lumbar disc herniation

- Subarticular zone and inferior migration
- Foraminal zone and superior migration
- Nodular herniated disc with nerve root compression
- Acute disc herniation with T2-hyperintensity

J. W. Lee (✉)
Department of Radiology, Seoul National University College of Medicine, Seoul National University Bundang Hospital, Seongnam, Korea (Republic of)

© The Author(s), under exclusive license to Springer Nature Singapore Pte Ltd. 2025
H. S. Kang, J. W. Lee (eds.), *Spinal Imaging*, https://doi.org/10.1007/978-981-95-1386-4_18

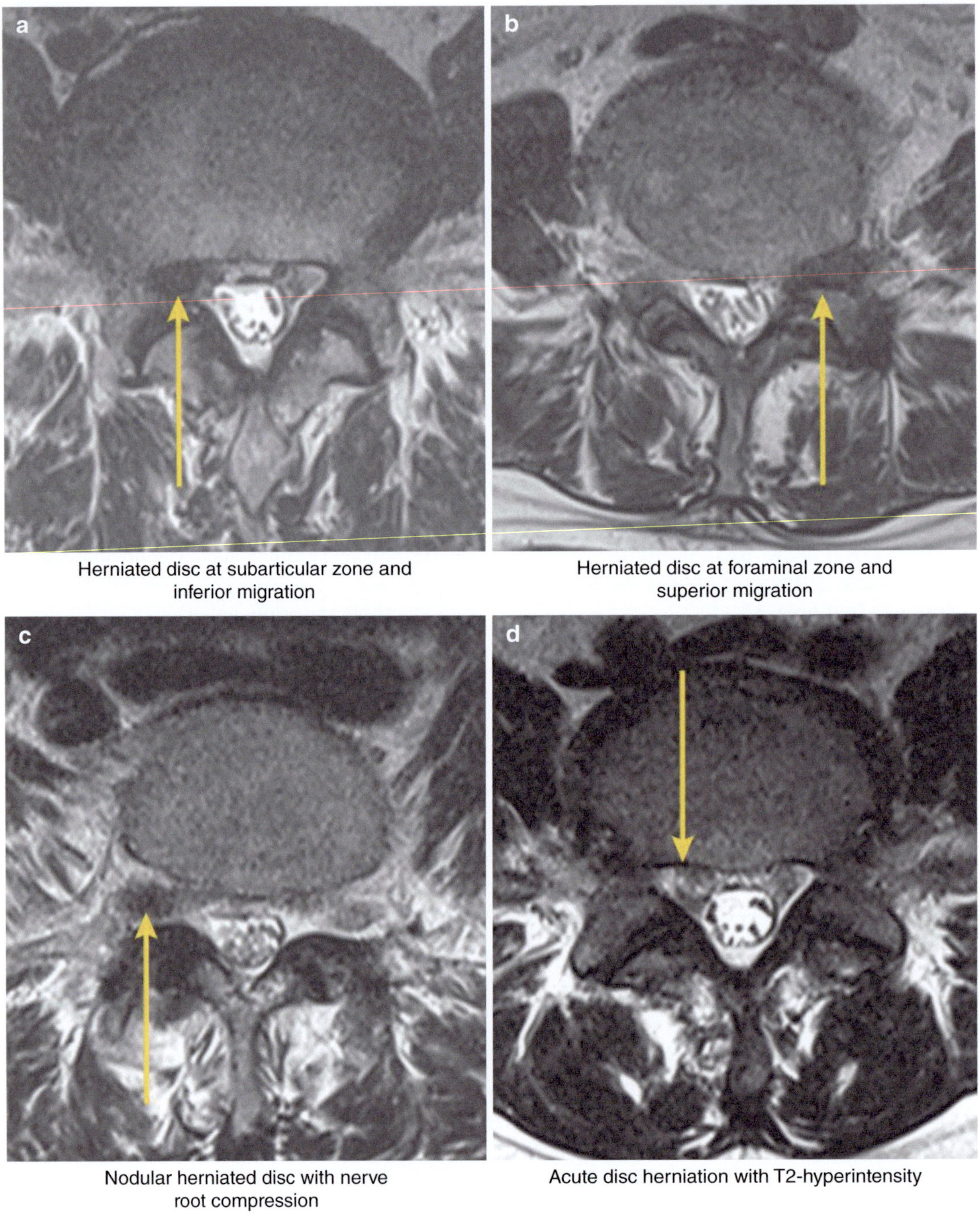

Fig. 18.1 Commonly overlooked lumbar disc herniation. (**a**) Herniated disc at subarticular zone and inferior migration. (**b**) Herniated disc at foraminal zone and superior migration. (**c**) Nodular herniated disc with nerve root compression. (**d**) Acute disc herniation with T2-hyperintensity

18.2 Question 2

An 80-year-old grandmother came to the emergency room with severe back pain after falling on her buttocks, but no signs of acute compression fractures are observed on the lumbar MR. What part should we pay close attention to in this case?

18.2.1 Answer 2 (Fig. 18.2)

In elderly patients suspected of compression fractures, the possibility of sacral insufficiency fractures should always be considered. Sacral insufficiency fractures are fractures that invade the sacral body and both sacral alae, and often the lesions are not scanned in routine L-spine MR axial images. Therefore, you should carefully look at the sacral body and both sacral alae in the sagittal T1 enhanced image. Check if there is buckling of the anterior cortex of the sacral body or signal changes within the sacral body in the sagittal T1 enhanced image. Also, both sacral alae are observed in the first and last images of the sagittal image, so check for linear fracture lines or signal changes within the sacral alae in these images. Usually, in the elderly, the sacral ala is replaced with fatty marrow, so it is common for the sacral ala to show high signal intensity in T1 enhanced images. If a T1 low-signal shadow is observed in the sacral ala, the possibility of sacral fracture, infection, or tumor must be confirmed. In this case, additional axial images should be taken up to the sacrum level to check for linear fracture lines and signal changes in both sacral alae. You should check. Also, in this

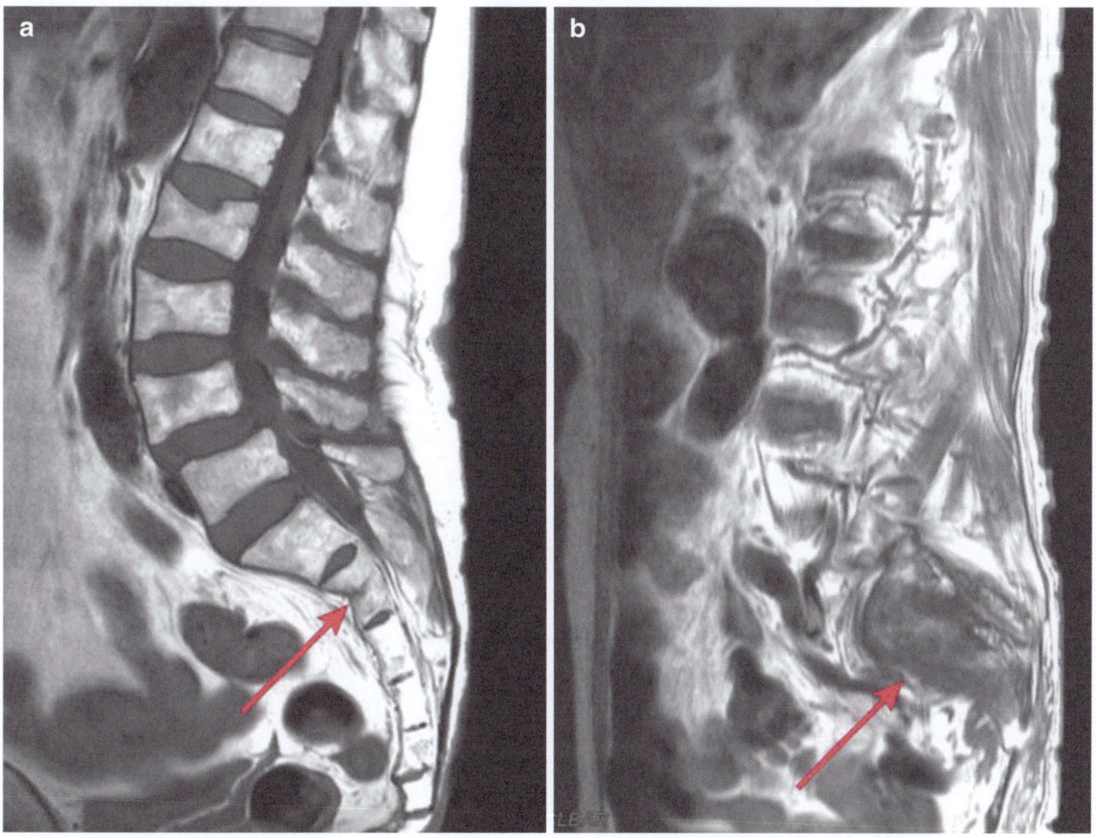

Buckling of the sacral body anterior cortex　　linear fracture line in sacral ala

Fig. 18.2 Sacral insufficiency fracture. (**a**) Buckling of the sacral body anterior cortex. (**b**) Linear fracture line in sacral ala case, if you take additional shots of the lesion in the axial and coronal plane with contrast enhancement, you can clearly identify the lesion and easily understand the extent of the lesion.

18.2.2 Tip 2

Reading tips for sacral insufficiency fracture

- Observe the sacrum in sagittal T1-weighted images
- Midline sagittal image: buckling of the sacral body anterior cortex
- First and last sagittal images: check for linear fracture line or signal change within the sacral ala

18.3 Question 3

A 65-year-old lung cancer patient had severe back pain and took an X-ray, which showed a compression fracture in the lumbar spine, so an MR was taken. In this case, is there a way to distinguish whether the compression fracture is a benign osteoporotic compression fracture or a malignant pathological fracture caused by metastatic cancer with MR?

18.3.1 Answer 3 (Fig. 18.3)

In the case of malignant compression fractures, the internal low-signal intensity is very low on T1-weighted images, and the T1 low-signal intensity is often distributed throughout the fractured vertebral body. During contrast enhancement, there are few or irregular areas that are not enhanced within the fracture, and the grid shadow caused by internal trabeculation is lost. Also, the posterior of the vertebral body often shows a curved surface. If a mass shadow is observed around the vertebral body, it can be more clearly considered as a malignant pathological fracture. Also, findings of metastatic cancer in other vertebral bodies are sometimes observed. The most important of these is that the signal intensity is very low on T1-weighted images, and the grid structure inside is lost.

In the case of benign osteoporotic compression fractures, normal bone marrow shadows are often observed somewhere in the fractured vertebral body on T1-weighted images. Also, the low-signal intensity due to bone marrow edema on T1-weighted images is not very low, and the grid shadow caused by internal trabeculation is reflected during contrast enhancement ("see-through appearance"). Also, during contrast enhancement, areas that are not enhanced along the fracture surface are observed in a linear or box shape. Also, in the case of benign osteoporotic compression fractures, a vacuum cavity can be seen inside, and water can enter here. Therefore, fractures in which air or fluid is observed inside suggest benign compression fractures. Even in the case of benign osteoporotic compression fractures, there can be edema around the cross-section of the spine, so the presence of signal changes around the spine cannot be definitively considered as a finding suggesting malignant compression fractures or infectious spondylitis. In the case of benign osteoporotic compression fractures, changes around the spine appear as relatively thin edema. However, in the case of an unstable unhealed compression fracture, a mass shadow can be observed around it, so be careful. In this case, other findings suggesting an unhealed fracture, such as increased bone shadow around the spinal fracture surface, should be carefully observed. Seeing old compression fracture findings in other vertebral bodies is also a finding that suggests a benign osteoporotic compression fracture.

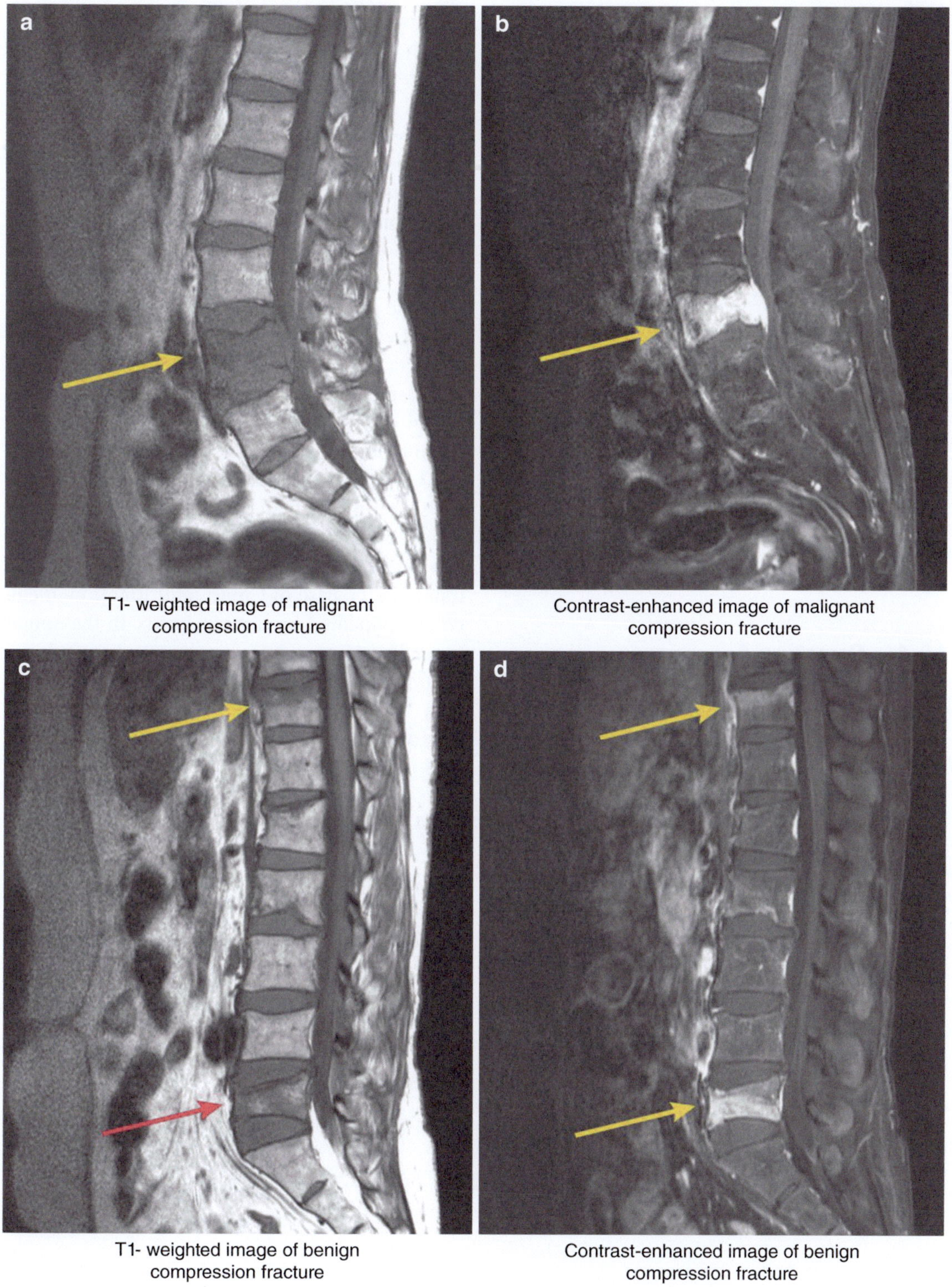

Fig. 18.3 Malignant compression fracture (**a**, **b**) vs benign compression fracture (C, D). (**a**) T1-weighted image of malignant compression fracture. (**b**) Contrast-enhanced image of malignant compression fracture. (**c**) T1-weighted image of benign compression fracture. (**d**) Contrast-enhanced image of benign compression fracture

18.3.2 Tip 3

	Malignant compression fracture	Benign compression fracture
Signal intensity on T1-weighted images	Very low signal	Slightly low signal
Normal marrow signal within the vertebral body on T1-weighted images	Loss	Preservation
Contrast enhancement signal intensity	Strong contrast enhancement	Weak contrast enhancement
Internal trabecular pattern	Loss	Preservation
Perivertebral tissues	Mass-like signal	Band-like edema
Other vertebral bodies	Metastatic findings	Old compression fractures

18.4 Question 4

A syrinx is observed within the spinal cord. What should you pay attention to in this case when interpreting?

18.4.1 Answer 4 (Fig. 18.4)

A syrinx is a case where fluid is filled in the spinal cord, showing a high signal shadow similar to cerebrospinal fluid in MR T2 enhanced images, and a low signal shadow similar to cerebrospinal fluid in T1 enhanced images. The causes of syrinx are very diverse.

When a syrinx is seen, it is very important to check the possibility of a syrinx caused by a tumor, so contrast-enhanced imaging must be taken. If a tumor that enhances contrast is observed in the center of the syrinx in the contrast-enhanced image, the possibility of ependymoma is high, and if a tumor located in the posterior subpial location behind the syrinx is observed, the possibility of hemangioblastoma is high.

If the syrinx is large, a flow artifact can occur inside, which can be mistaken for a tumor. Flow artifacts are unclear signals and do not enhance contrast, looking like they were drawn with a brush.

Another thing to check when a syrinx is seen is Chiari malformation. Chiari malformation is a disease in which an obstruction of the outflow of cerebrospinal fluid in the spinal cord occurs due to the downward herniation of the cerebellar tonsil. In the case of Chiari malformation, it can be accompanied by a wide syrinx in the spinal cord. Therefore, when a syrinx is observed, the foramen magnum area must be checked to confirm the presence or absence of chiari malformation.

18.4.2 Tip 4

Reading tips for Syrinx

- Contrast enhancement—ependymoma, hemangioblastoma
- Check the foramen magnum—Chiari malformation

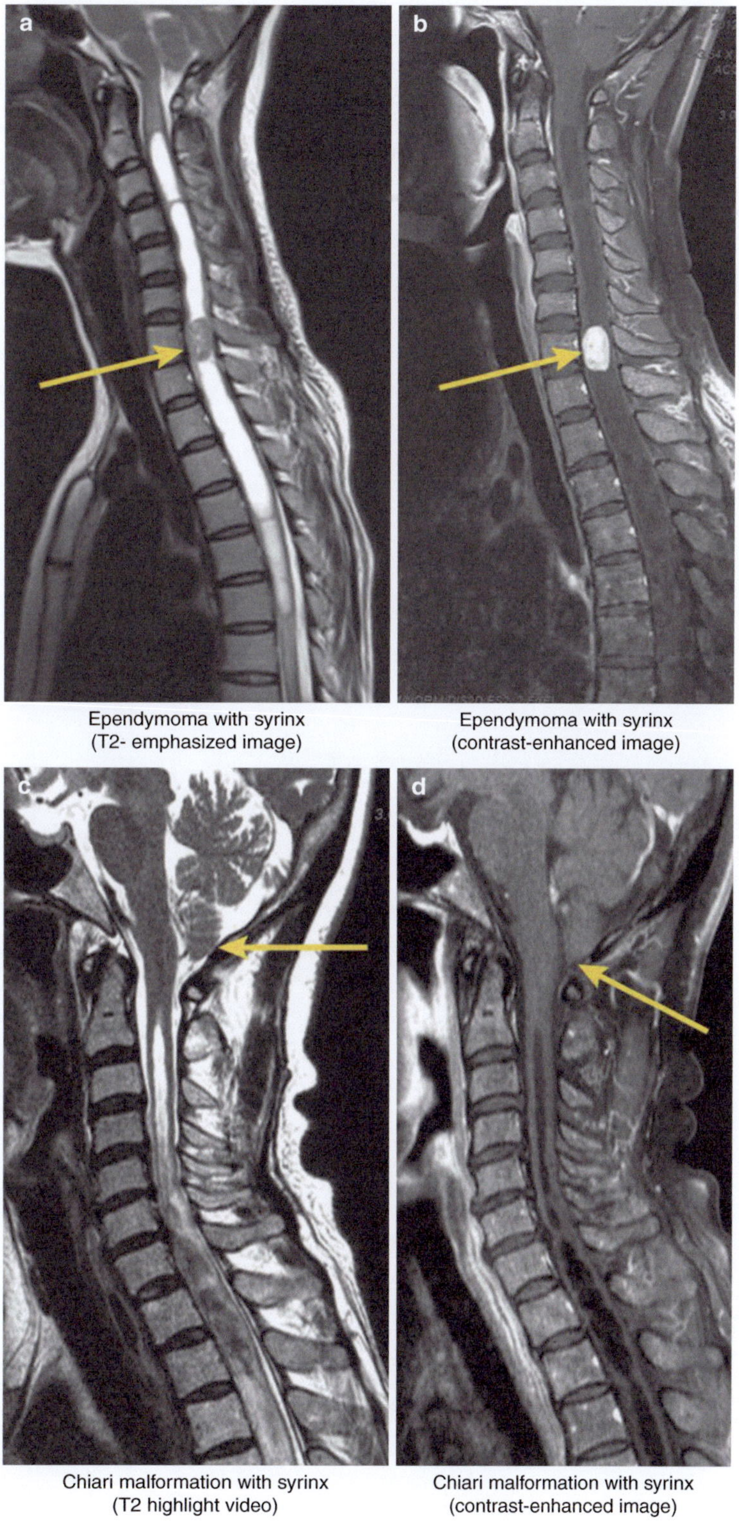

Fig. 18.4 Syrinx. (**a**) Ependymoma with syrinx (T2 enhanced image). (**b**) Ependymoma with syrinx (contrast-enhanced image). (**c**) Chiari malformation with syrinx (T2 enhanced image). (**d**) Chiari malformation with syrinx (contrast-enhanced image)

18.5 Question 5

No peculiarities were observed in the lumbar MR image of a patient with lower limb weakness. What should I pay special attention to in this case?

18.5.1 Answer 5 (Fig. 18.5)

If the lower limb weakness is acute and the timing is clear, you should consider the possibility of a cord infarct and observe the cornus medullaris area. Spinal cord infarcts most commonly occur in the cornus medullaris. Therefore, when taking a lumbar spine MR, it is best to include the lower portion of the spinal cord in the sagittal image to cover the lower thoracic spine. Spinal cord infarcts initially appear as pencil-like linear high signals in the anterior portion of the cord on T2 sagittal images, and it is difficult to distinguish them from artifacts, so axial images should be taken to confirm whether the lesion is a true lesion. Unlike the brain, diffusion-weighted images are not very helpful in the spinal cord when the lesion is small. Instead, if the lesion is ambiguous, it is useful to retake T2-weighted images within a day to confirm a spinal cord infarct. In the case of spinal cord infarcts, the lesion becomes more clear or pro-

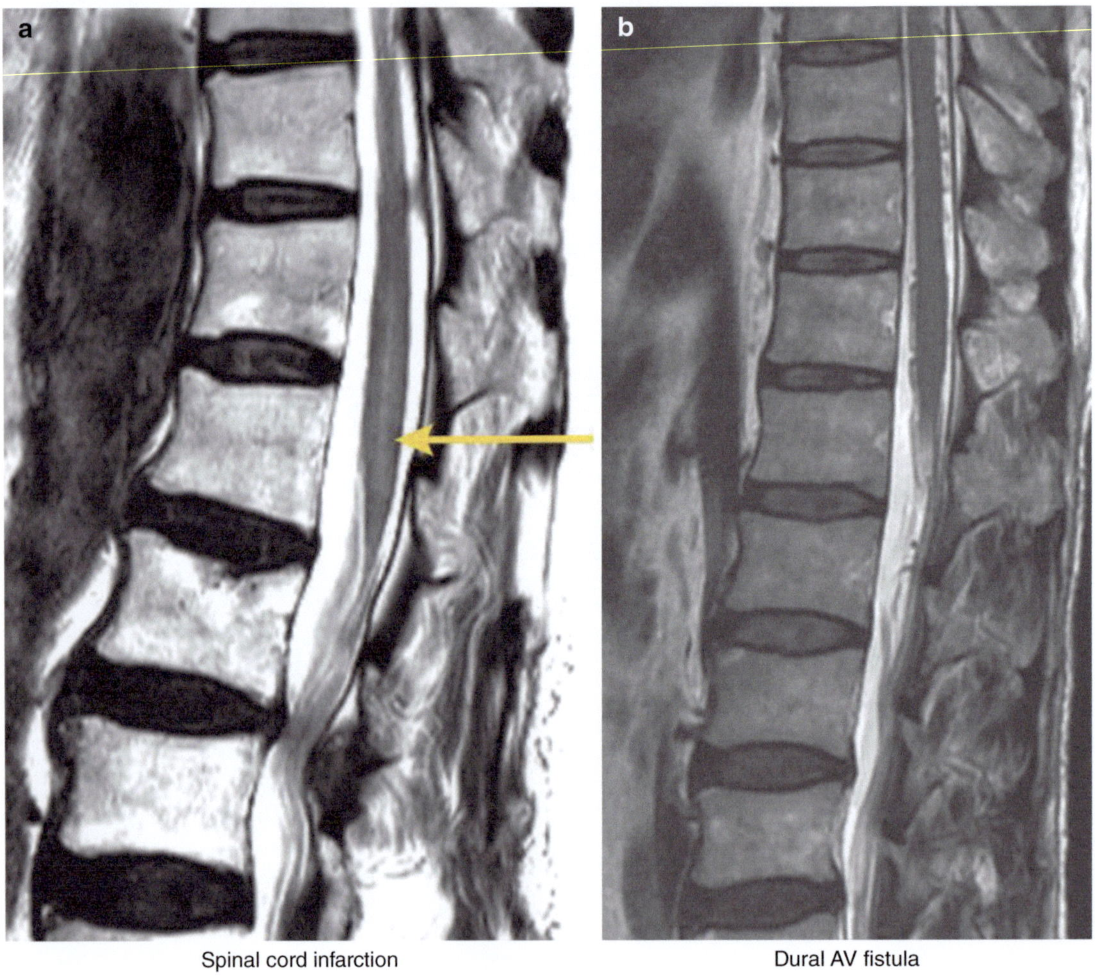

Fig. 18.5 Patient with lower limb weakness. (**a**) Spinal cord infarct. (**b**) Dural AV fistula. (**c**) Ossified ligamentum flavum with cord compression. (**d**) Guillain-Barre syndrome

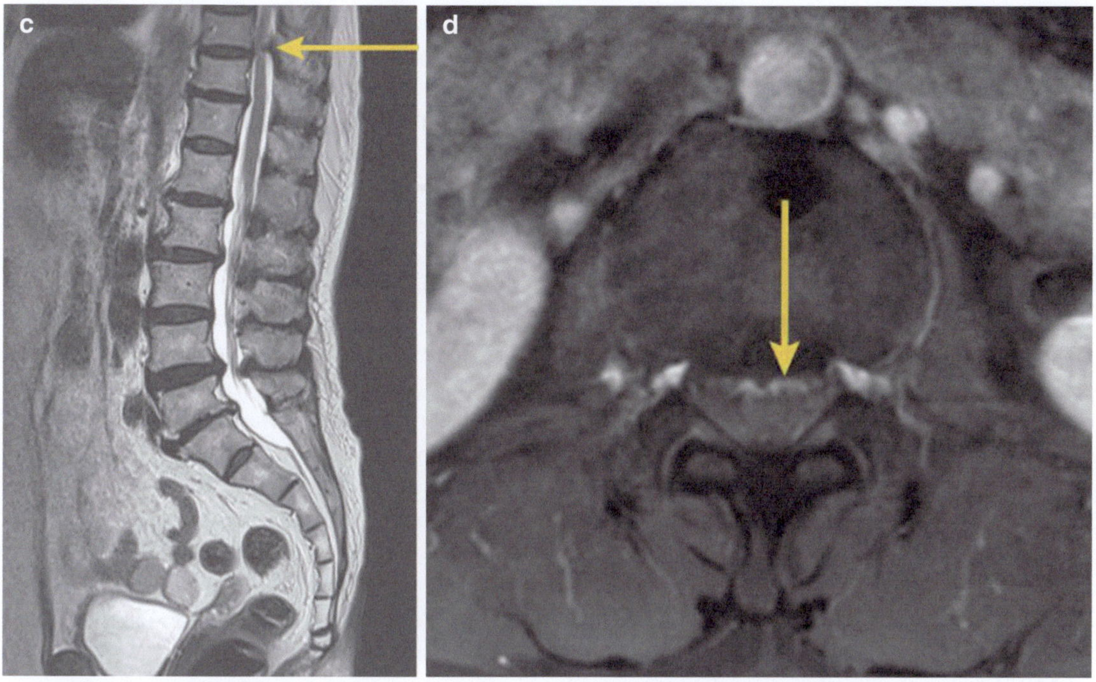

Ossified ligamentum flavum with cord compression

Guillain-Barre syndrome

Fig. 18.5 (continued)

gresses in a short time initially. Cord infarcts have less cord swelling compared to acute transverse myelitis or tumors, and initially do not enhance, but start to enhance after a few days. In conclusion, if a T2-high signal shadow is observed in the cornus medullaris in a patient with a clear onset of symptoms, progresses rapidly within the initial 1–2 days, and has little cord swelling, the possibility of a cord infarct is high. However, if the lower limb weakness is subacute or chronic, it is important to consider the possibility of vascular malformations such as dural AV fistula or perimedullary AF fistula, and to carefully observe whether there are tortuous flow voids caused by engorged perimedullary veins around the cord or cauda equina. In cases where the spinal cord is compressed at the cervical or thoracic level, lower limb weakness can occur, so it is necessary to definitely take images of the cervical and thoracic level. In the case of Guillain-Barre syndrome, the lesion is not observed unless it is enhanced. If selective enhancement is observed in the ventral rootlet of the cauda equina on the contrast-enhanced axial image, and there is no particular abnormality in the spinal cord on the T2-weighted image, the possibility of Guillain-Barre syndrome is high. If there is an abnormality in the spinal cord, the ventral root of the cauda equina may be enhanced due to Wallerian degeneration, so caution is needed. In the case of leptomeningeal metastasis, the lesion is not well observed unless it is enhanced.

18.5.2 Tip 5

Points to note in MR images of patients with lower limb weakness

- Possibility of spinal cord infarct
  - Conus medullaris
  - Pencil-like appearance, serial follow-up
- Possibility of dural AV fistula
  - Perimedullary flow voids (venous engorgement)

Spinal cord compression at cervical or thoracic level

- Guillain-Barre syndrome
  - Selective enhancement in the ventral rootlets

18.6 Question 6

A spine MR was taken to confirm infectious spondylitis as an infection was suspected clinically with fever and back pain. What should be noted in interpreting this case?

18.6.1 Answer 6 (Fig. 18.6)

In the early stages of infectious spondylitis, bone marrow edema is not severe, so it is easy to miss on MR. Check whether there is a T2-high signal shadow or enhancement along the ALL or PLL, and if there is a T2-high signal shadow or enhancement, check whether there is a signal change in the adjacent vertebral body corner. On the axial, check if there is a T2-high signal part inside the psoas muscle or in the paravertebral area, and confirm whether this part is enhanced. At this time, the part with fatty degeneration in the psoas muscle can appear as a T2-high signal shadow, so it is good to match the T1-weighted image together to confirm that it is not a fat signal. In the vertebral body, there is no signal change and the epidural abscess is mainly present. In cases where an abscess appears as a high signal shadow on T2-weighted images, care should be taken not to mistake it for cerebrospinal fluid. It is necessary to trace the dural interface and confirm the presence of fluid outside the dura. In contrast-enhanced images, initial abscesses may not enhance well and may appear as low signal shadows, so when a fluid signal is observed along the epidural space, the possibility of an epidural abscess should always be considered.

Also, depending on the case, infectious spondylitis may be confined to a single vertebral body, causing a bone marrow signal change, so such cases should be noted. If there is no depression of the cortex suggesting a compression fracture, no internal linear fracture line, and no clear solid portion suggesting a tumor, the possibility of infectious spondylitis should be considered even in cases of bone marrow edema of a single vertebral body.

If there is a compression fracture in the vertebral body and bone marrow edema is observed in the adjacent segment, it may be thought that there is also a compression fracture in the adjacent segment and it may be overlooked. If there are no findings suggesting a fracture in the adjacent segment, it may be accompanied by infectious spondylitis in the compression fracture, or compression may have occurred in infectious spondylitis such as tuberculous spondylitis. In this case, the presence or absence of a paravertebral phlegmon or abscess extending subligamentously should be carefully observed. In the case of osteoporotic compression fractures, the non-enhancing part inside is band-like or box-shaped. In the case of infection, the non-enhancing part inside is dot-like or irregular.

18.6.2 Tip 6

Findings to note in infectious spondylitis

- Initial infectious spondylitis
  - T2-hyperintensity in the psoas muscle
  - Paravertebral enhancement around ALL or PLL with focal bone marrow edema
- Be careful of epidural abscesses that appear as fluid signals without bone marrow edema and peripheral enhancement
- Infectious spondylitis can also involve a single vertebral body

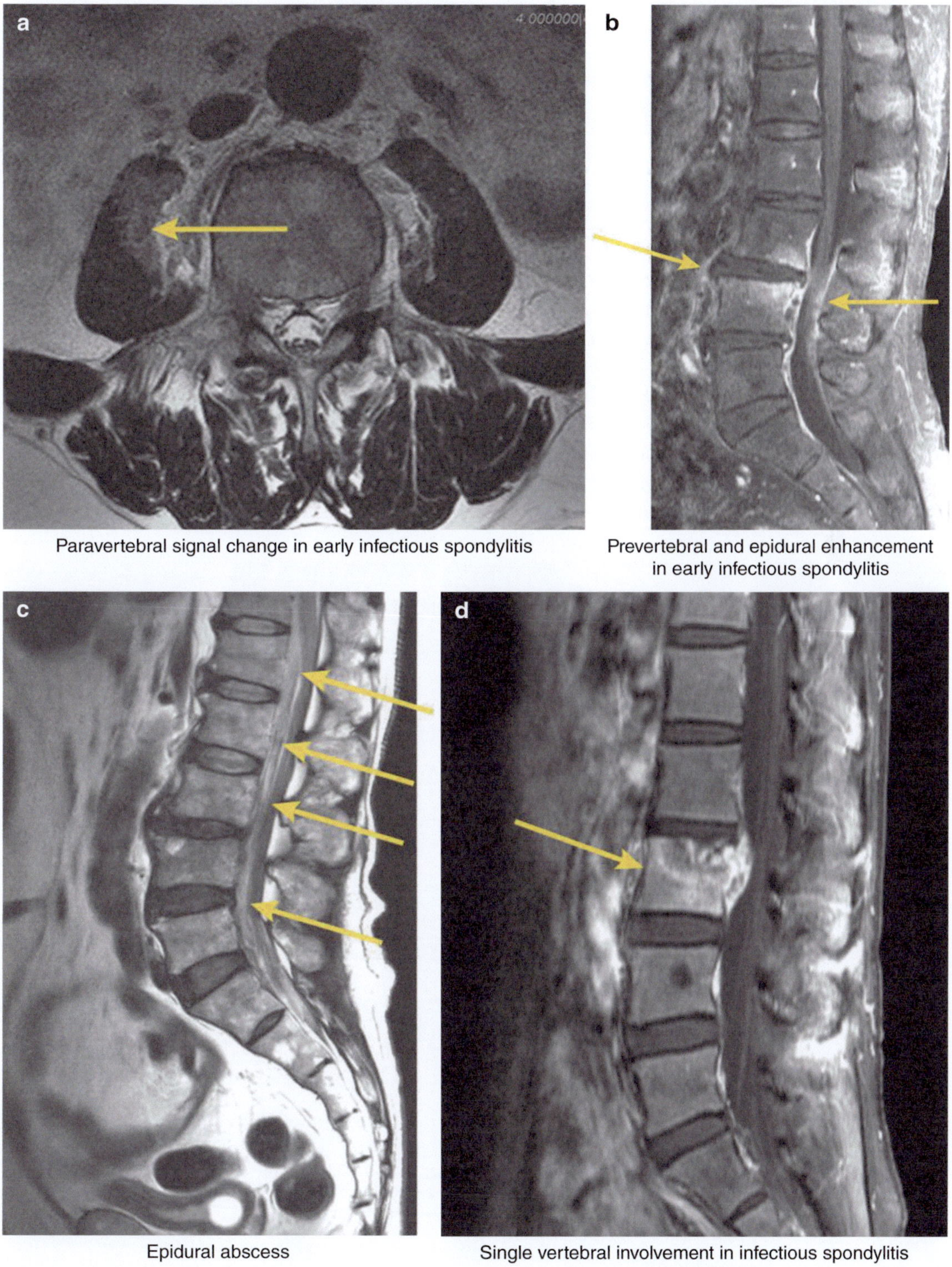

Fig. 18.6 Infectious spondylitis. (**a**) Paravertebral signal change in initial infectious spondylitis. (**b**) Prevertebral and epidural enhancement in initial infectious spondylitis. (**c**) Epidural abscess. (**d**) Single vertebral involvement in infectious spondylitis

18.7 Question 7

Is there a way to distinguish between pre-existing lesions and trauma-induced lesions in trauma patients?

18.7.1 Answer 7 (Fig. 18.7)

It's not easy. In the case of the cervical spine, if a T2-high signal shadow is seen in the cord in patients with a history of trauma, it is a method to distinguish whether this finding is due to trauma or pre-existing compressive myelopathy, such as the pattern of T2-high signal lesions in the cord and the presence or absence of surrounding ligament damage. In the case of spinal cord injury, the range of T2-high signal shadows in the spinal cord is wide up and down, the center of the high signal shadow is located at the disc level where central canal narrowing is present, and the margin of the high signal shadow is often unclear. If T2 hypointense shadow is observed within the high signal shadow, this suggests bleeding, making the possibility of cord contusion more certain and indicating a poor prognosis. Typically, cord injury occurs in hyperextension injury, so if a high signal shadow is observed in the prevertebral space on T2 fat suppression sagittal images and a high signal shadow is observed within the spinal cord, the likelihood of spinal cord injury increases. Compressive myelopathy can show various patterns, so it cannot be ruled out with a specific pattern. However, if the range of the T2-high signal shadow within the cord is narrow, the center is located slightly below the disc level

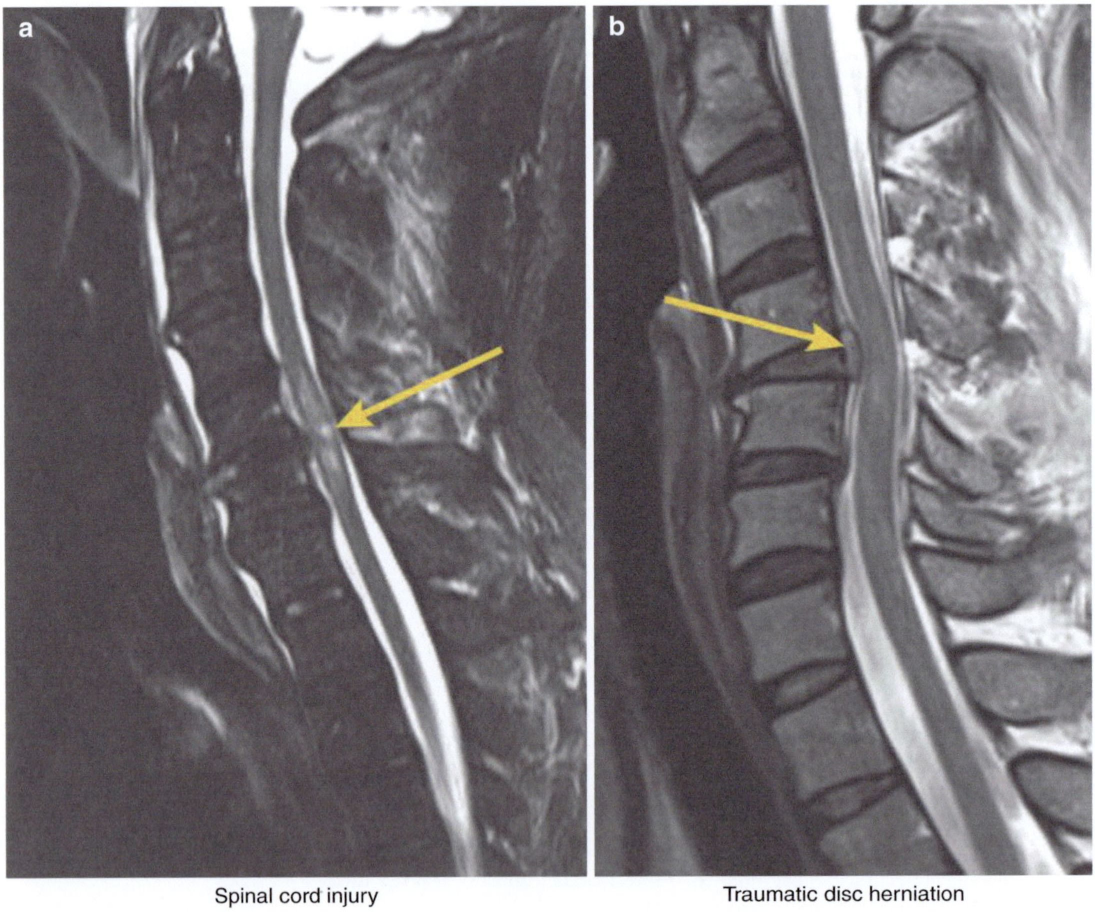

Fig. 18.7 Trauma-related spinal pathology. (**a**) Spinal cord injury. (**b**) Traumatic disc herniation

where canal narrowing is present, and the internal signal intensity is bright and the margin is clear, the possibility of compressive myelopathy is high.

It is not easy to distinguish between traumatic disc herniation and degenerative disc herniation when disc herniation is present. Cases that can be interpreted as traumatic disc herniation are when an injury to the adjacent ligament or bone is accompanied by a T2-high signal shadow observed within the herniated disc. The absence of degeneration in the parent disc and the observation of epidural hematoma are also findings suggesting traumatic disc herniation. If underline disc degeneration is present and osteophytes are observed in adjacent areas or calcification or vacuum is observed within the disc, it can be interpreted as degenerative disc herniation.

18.7.2 Tip 7

Trauma-Related Spinal Pathology

- Spinal Cord Injury
  - The range of the T2-high signal shadow within the spinal cord is wide up and down and the center is located at the disc level where the central canal narrowing is present.
  - The margin of the T2-high signal shadow is unclear.
  - T2 hypointense shadow is observed together within the T2-high signal shadow.
  - High signal shadow is observed in the prevertebral space on T2 fat suppression sagittal images.
- Traumatic disc herniation
  - Injury to adjacent ligament or bone.
  - T2-high signal shadow within the herniated disc.
  - No degeneration of the parent disc.
  - Epidural hematoma.

18.8 Question 8

What should be considered when a high signal shadow is observed in the spinal cord on MR T2 enhanced images?

18.8.1 Answer 8 (Fig. 18.8)

When a high signal shadow is observed in the spinal cord on T2 enhanced images, the possibilities of compressive myelopathy, traumatic cord contusion, and vascular malformation should be ruled out first.

Compressive myelopathy can show very various patterns, so if a T2-high signal shadow is observed in the cord at the level where cord compression is present, the possibility of compressive myelopathy is the highest if there are no findings of cord contusion mentioned earlier. Compressive myelopathy can show all diffuse pattern, fuzzy focal pattern, discrete focal pattern on axial images, and can show signal change over several segments or local high signal shadow just below the disc level on sagittal images. Compressive myelopathy may not enhance, or even if it does, compression it is observed locally only at the level. Occasionally, compressive myelopathy can show a long edema up and down, and in this case, the top and bottom of the edema are characterized by being observed in a fusiform shape.

The possibility of spinal cord injury should be confirmed with the findings mentioned earlier. Also, as time passes after trauma, signal changes can occur within the cord due to Wallerian degeneration, and in this case, signal changes appear along the dorsal column in the upper portion of the traumatic lesion and along the lateral column in the lower portion.

In the case of vascular malformations such as dural or perimedullary arteriovenous fistula (AVF), signal changes are observed in the cord due to congestive myelopathy caused by perimedullary venous hypertension. In this case, prominent flow voids due to perimedullary venous engorgement around the cord are observed, and these flow voids show tortuosity. If such prominent tortuous perimedullary flow voids are observed and T2-high signal shadows are observed in the cord, the possibility of dural or perimedullary AVF is highest.

If compressive, traumatic, vascular etiology is ruled out, tumorous conditions and non-tumorous conditions must be distinguished. The characteristics of a tumorous condition are that the expansion of the cord is severe, there is a T2-low signal shadow part, this part is enhanced, and it is accompanied by syrinx or hemorrhage. If there is a part where enhancement is strong and perimedullary venous engorgement due to intratumoral AV shunt is observed around it, there is a possibility of a hypervascular tumor such as hemangioblastoma. Non-tumorous condition is characterized by less cord expansion in T2 enhanced images, no T2-low signal shadow, and enhancement is observed locally only in some areas compared to the T2-high signal shadow area. Such enhancement is often asymmetrical and is peripheral and patchy.

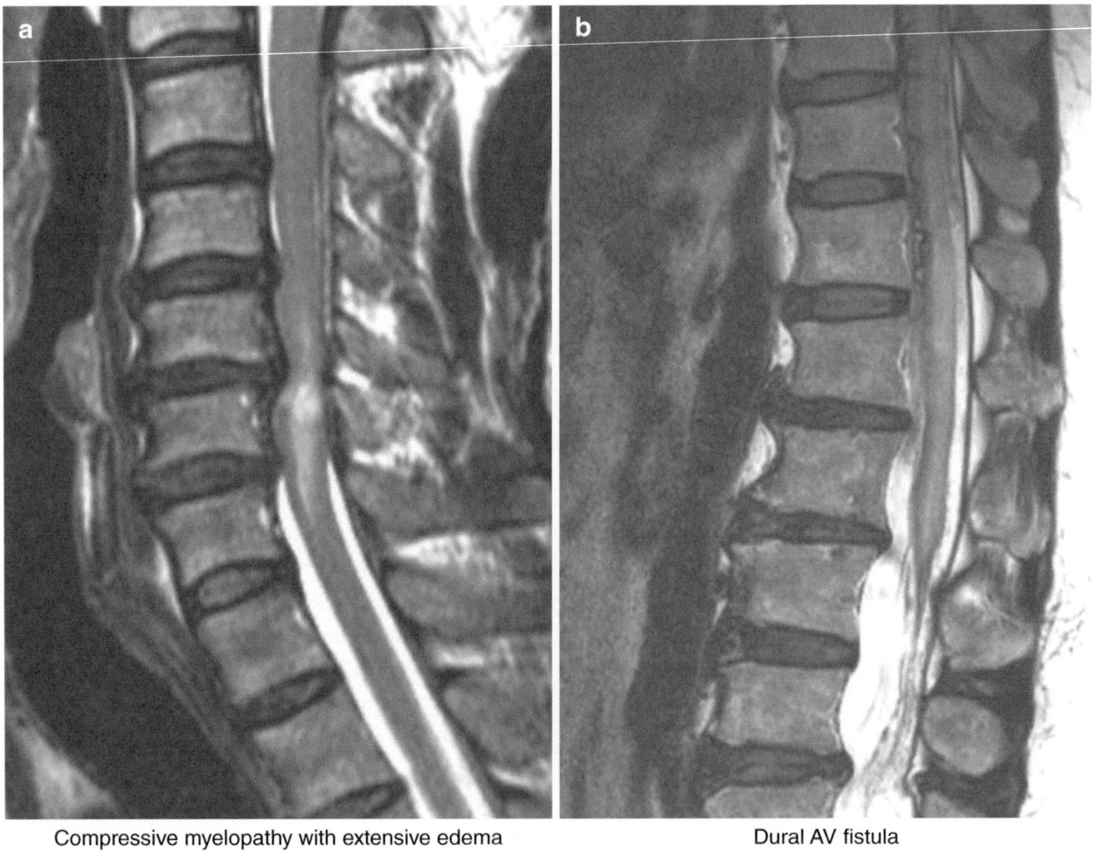

Fig. 18.8 Myelopathy. (**a**) Compressive myelopathy with extensive edema. (**b**) Dural AV fistula. (**c**) Anaplastic astrocytoma. (**d**) Idiopathic acute transverse myelitis

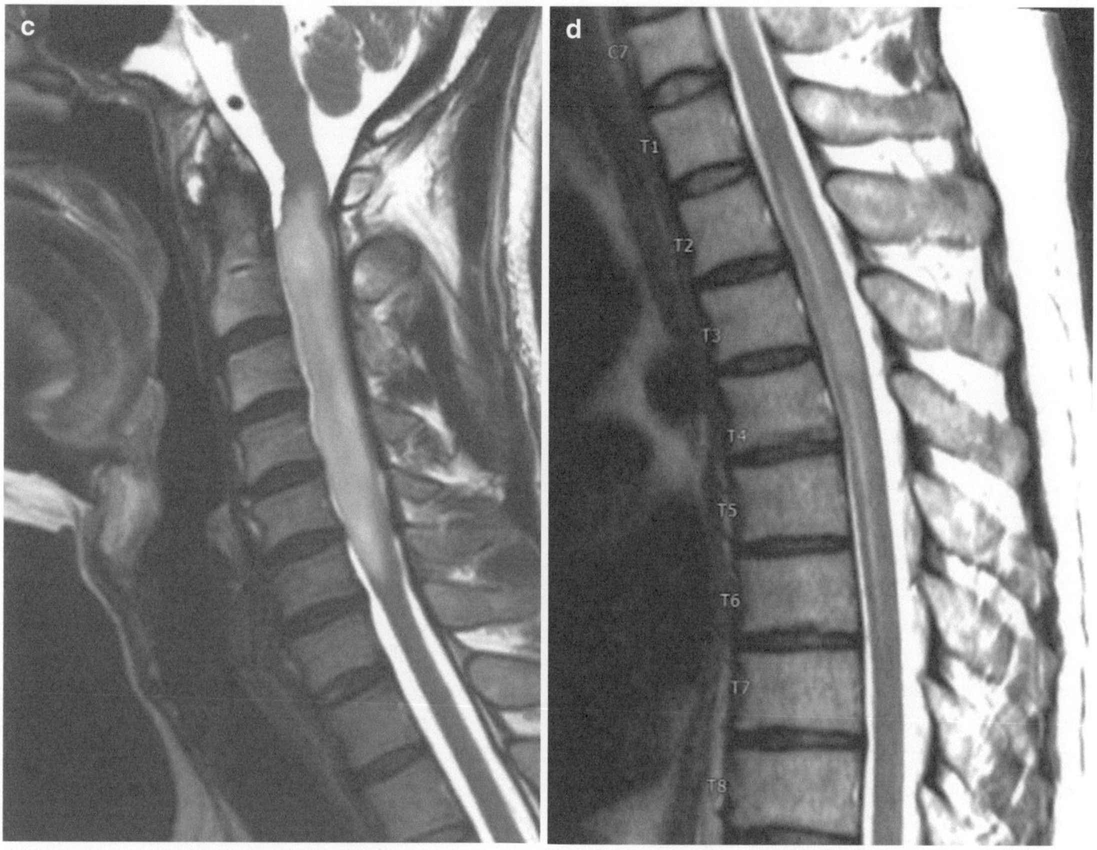

Anaplastic astrocytoma

Idiopathic acute transverse myelitis

Fig. 18.8 (continued)

18.8.2 Tip 8

MR reading tip for myelopathy

- First consider and rule out the possibility of compressive, traumatic, vascular etiology.
- Vascular etiology (dural or perimedullary AVF).
  - Prominent tortuous flow voids due to perimedullary venous engorgement.
- Spinal cord tumor vs non-neoplastic myelopathy.

Spinal cord tumor	Non-neoplastic myelopathy
Severe spinal cord expansion T2-low signal shadow Strong enhancement Syrinx, hemorrhage	Less spinal cord expansion Peripheral, patch enhancement Diffuse or nodular T2-hyperintensity

18.9 Question 9

In T1 enhanced images of the spinal MR, the bone marrow appears mottled. What possibilities should be considered in interpreting this case?

18.9.1 Answer 9 (Fig. 18.9)

If the signal of the bone marrow appears mottled in T1 enhanced images, you should carefully observe the parts that show relatively low signal shadows. If the signal intensity of the low signal shadow part is similar to or shows a high signal shadow compared to the adjacent disc, there is a high possibility of red marrow. If a dot part that is thought to be a fat signal is observed in the center of the low signal intensity part, the possibility of

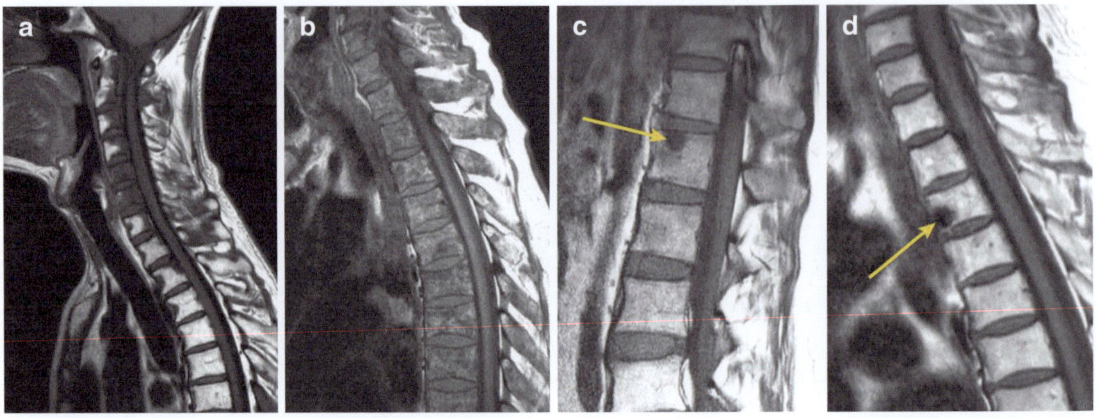

Fig. 18.9 Inhomogeneous bone marrow signal. (**a**) Red marrow reconversion. (**b**) Multiple myeloma. (**c**) Small metastasis. (**d**) Bone island

red marrow increases even more. In cases of chronic anemia or G-CSF treatment, red marrow reconversion can occur, and in this case, red marrow can be observed mottled throughout the spine, each signal intensity is the same as the typical pattern of red marrow, and each shape is geographic or irregular.

Sometimes it can be ambiguous to compare the signal intensity of the T1 low-signal shadow part of the bone marrow with the disc, and in this case, contrast-enhanced images are useful. If only a slight contrast enhancement is observed in the contrast-enhanced image, there is a high possibility of red marrow. If a small nodule that shows a low signal shadow in the T1 enhanced image shows clear contrast enhancement, there is a high possibility of metastasis or multiple myeloma. If many very small T1 low-signal nodules showing a salt and pepper appearance show bright contrast enhancement, the possibility of multiple myeloma is the highest.

It often shows uneven signal intensity adjacent to the endplate of the vertebral body, and care should be taken in differentiation in this case. If a nodular signal change adjacent to the endplate is observed, it is easy to pass as a Schmorl's node, but sometimes small metastases can also appear as nodules adjacent to the endplate, so be careful. In the case of Schmorl's node, breakage or depression of the adjacent cortex is observed and the margin is relatively clear. Since Schmorl's node can also have vascularization inside, it can be difficult to distinguish by the presence or absence of contrast enhancement. In the case of small metastases, the boundary around the nodule is somewhat ambiguous, the signal tends to fade out, and a little contrast enhancement can be observed around the nodule in contrast enhancement, and the boundary is a little uneven. However, there are cases where it is difficult to distinguish even if various findings are combined, and in this case, correlation with PET-CT or short-term follow-up is necessary.

The main causes of unevenness in bone marrow include red marrow hyperplasia or tumor, as well as endplate degenerative changes classified as Modic type. Although it is divided into Modic type 1 (fibrovascular), 2 (fatty), 3 (sclerosis), in reality, many types are often observed mixed. If you see a pattern where several layers overlap centered on the endplate, and disc degeneration is observed, there is a high possibility of Modic type change due to endplate degeneration.

Other causes include hemangioma, focal fatty change, and bone island. Both hemangioma and focal fatty change often show high signal shadows in T1 enhanced images, and hemangioma is round or diffuse in shape. The trabeculation inside is thickened. Focal fatty changes are irregular in shape and are usually connected to the endplate.

Bone islands all show low signal shadows in both T1 and T2 enhanced images. Bone islands can show radiating spicules and do not enhance. Sometimes, the size of the bone island can grow slightly, making it difficult to distinguish from blastic metastasis. Blastic metastasis can enhance in the changed part and being multiple can be a distinguishing point, but often the distinction between the two is difficult and a biopsy may be needed.

18.9.2 Tip 9

Inhomogeneous bone marrow

- Red marrow in vertebral body
  - Signal similar to or higher than the disc in T1 enhanced images
  - Mild enhancement
  - Preservation of internal trabeculation
- Tiny innumerable nodules with definite enhancement
  - Possibility of multiple myeloma
- Small nodule in subchondral bone near endplate
  - Schmorl's node vs small metastasis–check for breakage of the cortex

18.10 Question 10

What order should you look at when interpreting spine MR?

18.10.1 Answer 10 (Fig. 18.10)

First, check the T2 sagittal image. The T2 sagittal image is used to screen the overall spinal lesions. In the T2 sagittal image, the CSF appears bright, so the spinal canal is well observed and whether there is a pathology that compresses the spinal canal is checked. Also, check if there is an abnormal high signal change within the spinal cord. Check both neural foramen and whether there is a pathology that causes nerve root compression. Check the signal intensity of the disc and whether there is degeneration or herniation.

Next, interpret the T2 axial image while matching it with the T2 sagittal image as a cross link. First, carefully observe the back of the disc to check for a herniated disc. Also, check the part where there is central canal narrowing in the T2 sagittal image and if it is due to degenerative change, check the degree of central canal stenosis. Also, check if the high signal shadow suspected in the T2 sagittal image within the spinal cord is also observed in the axial. If the lesion is only visible in the sagittal image, there is a high possibility of an artifact. Check the pathology of the facet joint and paravertebral space. The paravertebral space is not sufficiently covered sagittally, so it should be carefully observed in the axial image.

Third, check the T1 sagittal image. Check the signal intensities while rechecking the lesions confirmed in the T2 sagittal image. Also, carefully check the bone marrow in the T1 sagittal image for any abnormalities. Check for bone marrow edema, fracture, mass, etc. Especially, check the posterior element of fractures or masses that invade the bone marrow are easy to overlook, so we pay more attention to the posterior elements. Also, fractures or edema of the sacral ala can only be scanned on T1 sagittal images, so we check whether the bone marrow signal of the sacral ala appearing on the first and last slice of the T1 sagittal image is normal.

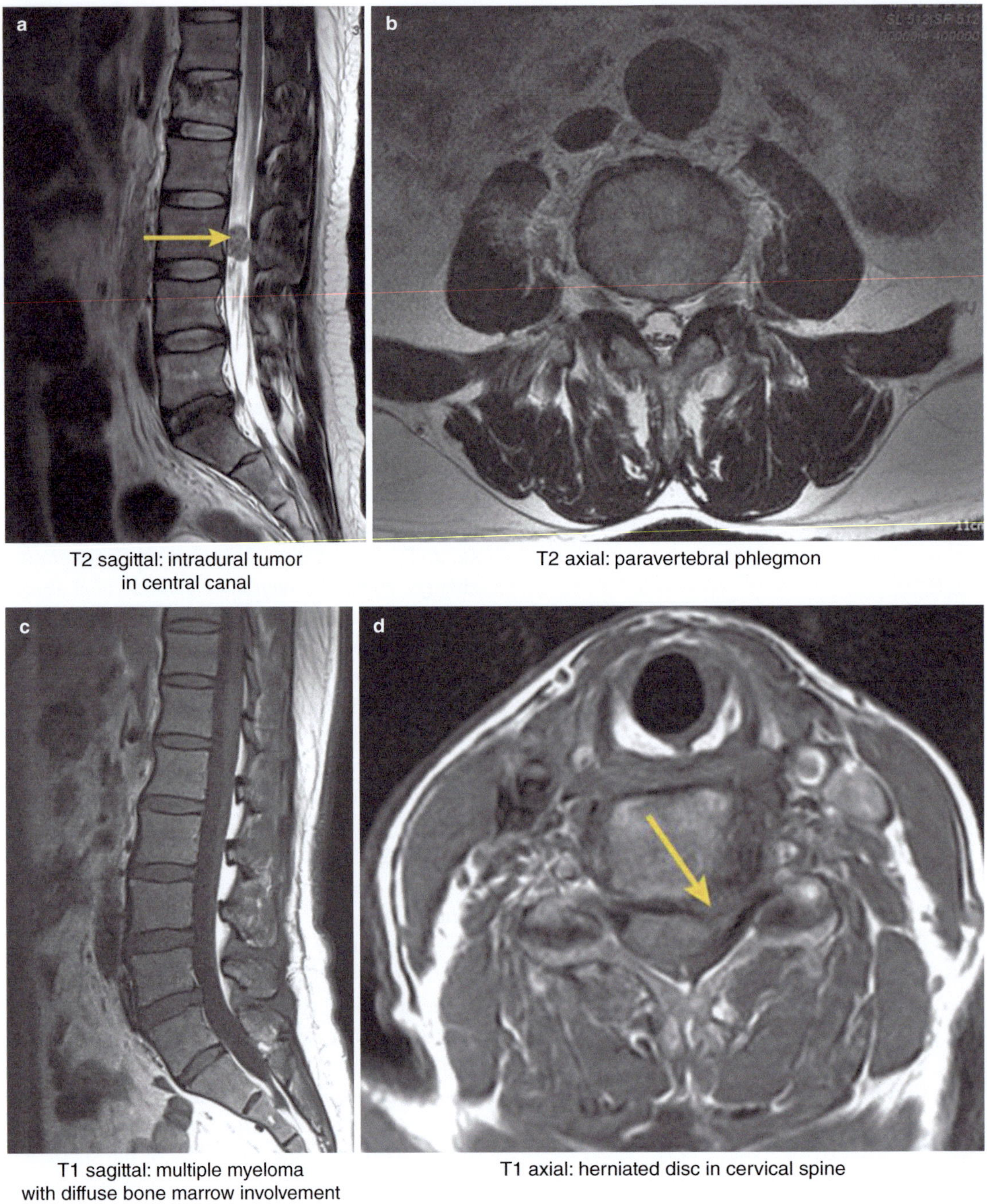

Fig. 18.10 Structures that should be focused on when interpreting spine MR images. (**a**) T2 sagittal: intradural tumor in central canal. (**b**) T2 axial: paravertebral phlegmon. (**c**) T1 sagittal: diffuse bone marrow involvement in multiple myeloma. (**d**) T1 axial: herniated disc in cervical spine

Lastly, we check the T1 axial image. On the T1 axial image, we mainly trace the posterior of the disc to observe if there is disc herniation or osteophytes. Especially in the cervical spine, when there is narrowing in the foramen, the T1 axial image is useful for distinguishing whether this is due to disc herniation or uncovertebral osteophytes. On T1-weighted images, disc herniation shows a signal intensity similar to the parent disc, and osteophytes show a low signal intensity. Also, in the lumbar spine, the nerve root located in the epidural space is well traced because it is surrounded by fat, so we check if there is a nerve root anomaly such as a conjoined nerve root. Also, we check the T1-signal of the lesion observed on the T2 axial image to predict the internal content.

The order described above is the order of interpretation when the lesion is not easily noticeable. Of course, when a lesion is found, you should match the sagittal and axial images, and match the T1- and T2-weighted images. If a lesion is observed while screening sagittally, confirm the lesion axially, and if a lesion is observed axially, the process of checking the sagittal image again is repeated.

18.10.2 Tip 10

Order of interpretation and key structures to focus on in spine MR images

- T2 sagittal → T2 axial → T1 sagittal → T1 axial
  - T2 sagittal: Central canal, spinal cord, nerve root, disc
  - T2 axial: Disc, central canal, paravertebral space
  - T1 sagittal: Bone marrow
  - T1 axial: Posterior margin of disc, nerve root in epidural space

Index

© Panmun Education Co., Ltd. 2025

H. S. Kang, J. W. Lee (eds.), *Spinal Imaging*, https://doi.org/10.1007/978-981-95-1386-4

O

P

Q

R

S

MIX
Papier aus verantwortungsvollen Quellen
Paper from responsible sources
FSC® C105338

If you have any concerns about our products,
you can contact us on
ProductSafety@springernature.com

In case Publisher is established outside the EU,
the EU authorized representative is:
Springer Nature Customer Service Center GmbH
Europaplatz 3, 69115 Heidelberg, Germany

Printed by Libri Plureos GmbH
in Hamburg, Germany